Health Consultants

UNIT 1: A Healthy Foundation

Kristen D. Fink, M.A.
Executive Director, Community of Caring
Arlington, Virginia

Betty M. Hubbard, Ed.D., C.H.E.S.
Professor of Health Education
Department of Health Sciences
University of Central Arkansas
Conway, Arkansas

UNIT 2: Physical Activity and Nutrition

Roberta L. Duyff, R.D., C.F.C.S.
Food and Nutrition Education Consultant
St. Louis, Missouri

Tinker D. Murray, Ph.D.
Professor and Coordinator of Exercise and Sports
    Science Program
Southwest Texas State University
San Marcos, Texas

Don Rainey, M.S.
Instructor, Coordinator of Physical Fitness
    and Wellness Program
Southwest Texas State University
San Marcos, Texas

UNIT 3: Mental and Emotional Health

Lee C. Ancona, Ph.D.
Health Educator
Lamar High School
Arlington, Texas

Betty M. Hubbard, Ed.D., C.H.E.S.
Professor of Health Education
Department of Health Sciences
University of Central Arkansas
Conway, Arkansas

Peter T. Whelley
Adjunct Faculty
University System of New Hampshire
Moultonsborough, New Hampshire

Gordon D. Wrobel, Ph.D.
Consultant, National Association of School
    Psychologists
Bethesda, Maryland

UNIT 4: Promoting Safe and Healthy Relationships

Cheryl Page, C.H.E.S.
Health Education Specialist
Salem Keizer Public Schools
Salem, Oregon

Jeanne Title
Coordinator, Prevention Education
Napa County Office of Education and
    Napa Valley Unified School District
Napa, California

UNIT 5: Personal Care and Body Systems

Patrick M. Forese, M.S.
Allied Health Educator
Slippery Rock University
Grove City High School
Grove City, Pennsylvania

UNIT 6: Growth and Development

Stephanie S. Allen, M.S., R.N.
Senior Lecturer, Baylor University
Louise Herrington School of Nursing
Dallas, Texas

Marilyn Hightower, M.S.N.
Lecturer, Baylor University
Louise Herrington School of Nursing
Dallas, Texas

Alice B. Pappas, Ph.D., R.N.
Associate Dean/Associate Professor
Baylor University
Louise Herrington School of Nursing
Dallas, Texas

Health Consultants (continued)

UNIT 7: Tobacco, Alcohol, and Other Drugs

Nancy S. Maylath, M.P.H., H.S.D.
Director, Student Wellness Office
Purdue University
West Lafayette, Indiana

Jeanne Title
Coordinator, Prevention Education
Napa County Office of Education and
    Napa Valley Unified School District
Napa, California

UNIT 8: Diseases and Disorders

Beverly J. Bradley, Ph.D., R.N., C.H.E.S
Assistant Clinical Professor
University of California, San Diego
San Diego, California

Michael T. Brady, M.D.
Professor and Vice-Chair
Department of Pediatrics
Children's Hospital, Columbus
The Ohio State University
Columbus, Ohio

UNIT 9: Injury Prevention and Environmental Health

David A. Sleet, Ph.D.
Associate Director for Science
Division of Unintentional Injury Prevention
Centers for Disease Control and Prevention
    (CDC)
Atlanta, Georgia

Teacher Reviewers

Pamela R. Connolly
Curriculum Coordinator for Health and
    Physical Education
Diocese of Pittsburgh
North Catholic High School
Pittsburgh, Pennsylvania

Jill English, Ph.D., C.H.E.S.
Assistant Professor
California State University, Fullerton
Fullerton, California

Debra C. Harris, Ph.D.
Department Chair, Health and Physical
    Education
West Linn High School
West Linn, Oregon

Pamela Hoalt, Ph.D.
Professor of Health Education
Malone College
Canton, Ohio

Michael Rulon
Health/Physical Education Teacher
Johnson Junior High School
Adjunct Faculty, Laramie County
    Community College
Cheyenne, Wyoming

Linda B. Salzman
Health Education Consultant and Trainer
Wilmington, North Carolina

Joan Stear
Health and Dance Educator
West Clermont Institute of Performing Arts
Glen Este High School
Cincinnati, Ohio

Contents

UNIT 3   Mental and Emotional Health

UNIT 5 Personal Care and Body Systems

UNIT 6 Growth and Development

Health Skills Activity

Hands-On Health ACTIVITY

Real-Life Application

Exploring Issues

Chapter 1

Living a Healthy Life

How Much Do You Know About Health and Healthy Behaviors?

Health information—and misinformation—is everywhere. Which of these statements do you think is a fact? A myth? Record your opinion for each.

1. Teens need more sleep than adults do.

2. Being an effective communicator can improve your overall health.

3. The health decisions you make as a teen have little impact on your health as an adult.

4. Two 10-minute walks provide nearly the same health benefits as a continuous 20-minute walk.

5. Water is a nutrient.

6. Setting goals can only help you achieve long-term accomplishments, such as establishing a career.

7. Acne flare-ups are a result of eating chocolate and greasy foods.

8. Tanning beds are safe because they use UVA light, which doesn't cause burns.

9. All stress is negative and should be avoided.

10. The relationships you have with family, friends, and peers do not affect your physical health.

HEALTH Online

For instant feedback on your health status, go to Chapter 1 Health Inventory at **health.glencoe.com**.

Quick Write

Using Visuals. Each day you make decisions that affect your health. What you choose to eat, your level of physical activity, how you manage stress, and the types of relationships you have all influence your overall feeling of well-being. Make a list of five decisions you've made this week that have had a positive effect on your health.

Lesson 1

Your Health and Wellness

VOCABULARY

health
wellness
prevention
health education
Healthy People 2010
health literacy

YOU'LL LEARN TO

- Relate the nation's health goals and objectives in *Healthy People 2010* to individual, family, and community health.

- Develop criteria for evaluating health information.

- Discuss the importance of health literacy for achieving and maintaining good health.

QUICK START On a sheet of paper, complete the following statement:
When you have good health, you . . .

▼ **Spending time with friends is an important part of health.** *Give an example of how relationships can have a positive impact on health.*

Suppose someone asks whether you are healthy. How would you answer? Would you consider only your physical health? For example, would you think of how often you are sick? Throughout this course, you will see that health is much more than just the absence of disease. A state of well-being comes from a balance between the physical, mental/emotional, and social aspects of your life. In this chapter you will look at ways to achieve and maintain this balance.

The Importance of Good Health

What is your usual response to the question, "How are you?" A true description of your health would require much more than a simple "fine" or "okay." **Health** is *the combination of physical, mental/emotional, and social well-being*. It is not an absolute state. Being healthy doesn't mean that you will never be sick or that you will be guaranteed a position on the basketball team. Instead, being healthy means striving to be the best *you* can be at any given time.

The Health Continuum

Health is dynamic, or subject to constant change. For example, you might be the top performer for your basketball team on Tuesday and sick in bed with the flu on Wednesday. Think of your health at any moment as a point along a *continuum*. This continuum spans the complete spectrum of health from chronic disease and premature death to a high level of health. Along the continuum are many points where your health could be located at any given time. This point changes from day to day and year to year.

Changes along the continuum may occur suddenly, such as when you get injured playing a sport. At this time of your life, it's even common for your emotions to shift suddenly from moment to moment. Knowing that these emotional shifts are normal can help you maintain a healthful balance as you move along the continuum.

Changes may also be so gradual that you're not even aware that you're moving from one side of the continuum to the other. Take a look at **Figure 1.1.** Where do you fit on the health continuum right now? Where would you like to be in a month? A year?

A person with a balanced life is said to have a high degree of **wellness**, *an overall state of well-being, or total health*. It comes from a way of living each day that includes making decisions and practicing behaviors that are based on sound health knowledge and healthful attitudes. Achieving wellness requires an ongoing, lifelong commitment to physical, mental/emotional, and social health.

When you feel your best, you will perform at your best. *How might maintaining a high level of wellness help you reach your goals?*

FIGURE **1.1**

THE HEALTH CONTINUUM

The continuum shows that your health can be measured on a sliding scale, with many degrees of health and wellness. Name three behaviors that would help you move toward the right side of the continuum.

Premature Death	Loss of Health and Wellness		Improved Health and Wellness	High Level of Health

Chronic disorders — Lack of energy, inattention, minor aches and pains — Free from aches and pains — Moderate level of energy — Optimal level of energy, feeling of well-being

People on this side of the continuum usually do not take responsibility for maintaining their own health.	Many people function below the wellness midpoint.	People on this side of the continuum usually exhibit a high degree of responsibility, discipline, and positive direction in life. They accept responsibility for maintaining their own health.

Promoting Your Health

The decisions you make each day have an impact on your health. What you choose to wear, eat, and do can have personal health consequences that you may or may not have considered. For example, not wearing the proper safety gear when participating in a physical activity increases the chances of serious injury in the event of an accident. Eating high-calorie snacks can result in unhealthful weight gain. Making responsible decisions about health and developing health-promoting habits is crucial to achieving and maintaining wellness.

Lifestyle Factors

Experts have identified habits that affect people's overall health, happiness, and *longevity*—or how long they live. These habits, or *lifestyle factors,* are personal behaviors related to the way a person lives. They help determine his or her level of health. Certain lifestyle factors are linked to specific diseases—for example, smoking and lung cancer. Other lifestyle factors promote good health. These include:

▶ getting 8 to 10 hours of sleep each night.

▶ starting each day with a healthy breakfast.

▶ eating a variety of nutritious foods each day.

▶ being physically active for at least 20 minutes a day, three or more days a week.

▶ maintaining a healthy weight.

▶ avoiding tobacco, alcohol, and other drugs.

▶ abstaining from sexual activity before marriage.

▶ managing stress.

▶ maintaining positive relationships.

▶ practicing safe behaviors to prevent injuries.

Fitting these health-promoting lifestyle factors into your life will help ensure a high level of wellness.

Wellness and Prevention

A key to your wellness is **prevention**—*practicing health and safety habits to remain free of disease and injury.* Wearing safety belts, applying sunscreen, and avoiding unsafe areas are just a few examples of preventive measures. What other actions could you take to prevent illness and injury?

The Importance of Health Education

Health is critical to quality of life. Learning how to become and stay healthy should be a top priority. That's why **health education**—*the providing of accurate health information to help people make healthy choices*—is important. The goal of health education is to give people the tools they need to help them live long, energetic, and productive lives.

The Nation's Health Goals

Health education affects more than just students. *Healthy People 2010* is *a nationwide health promotion and disease prevention plan designed to serve as a guide for improving the health of all people in the United States.* The plan, which is revised every 10 years, aims to promote health and prevent illness, disability, and early death.

GOALS OF *HEALTHY PEOPLE 2010*

Healthy People 2010 has established two main goals for the future: increase quality and years of healthy life for all Americans and remove health differences that result from factors such as gender, race, education, disability, and location. To reach these goals, individuals, families, and communities must work together.

A nation's health depends on the health of the individuals in that nation. Studies have shown, for example, that as people become more educated, the general health of a population improves. Therefore, to benefit the health of the larger community, it is up to each individual to be the best he or she can be. Achieving wellness empowers each individual to improve the community in which he or she lives. This, of course, can be extended to global health issues. As more individuals take charge of their own wellness, the more global health will improve. Individuals, families, and communities each have a role to play:

▶ **Individuals** can take an active role in their own health. You can learn to make informed decisions, master skills that enable you to apply your decisions, access reliable health care information and services, and promote the health of others. The information in this book will help you put many of these strategies into action.

▶ **Families** can shape the attitudes and beliefs that result in healthful behaviors. Parents and guardians play an important role in meeting the nation's health goals when they teach their children the values and skills necessary to maintain good health.

HEALTHY PEOPLE 2010

Understanding and Improving Health

Healthy People 2010 **is a plan designed to promote the health of all Americans.** *What are the nation's health goals as stated in* **Healthy People 2010?**

Learn more about promoting health by using study tools such as eFlashcards, concentration games, and online quizzes at **health.glencoe.com**.

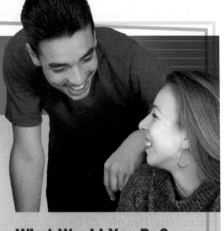

Health Skills Activity

Goal Setting: Health for All

For class James must set a health goal and explain how reaching his goal will help him, his family, and his community. He has asked his sister to help him.

"Becky, how could a person's health affect anyone else?"

"I can think of lots of ways," Becky says.

"Like what?" James asks.

"Cigarette smoking," Becky replies. "If someone in the family smokes, others in the family are exposed. The community is affected, too. Tobacco use means more illness and more health care needs."

"Yeah," James agrees, "and more fires and litter."

"Do you understand the assignment better now?" Becky asks.

James nods. He wonders what goal to set.

What Would You Do?

Put yourself in James's shoes. Choose a goal that will enhance your health and the health of others. Apply the goal-setting steps to help you reach your goal.

1. Identify a specific goal and write it down.
2. List the steps you will take to reach your goal.
3. Identify potential problems and ways to get help and support from others.
4. Set up checkpoints to evaluate your progress.
5. Reward yourself once you have achieved your goal.

▶ **Communities** can offer behavior-changing classes such as tobacco-cessation programs and provide health services. They can also take steps to ensure a safe environment.

The best chances for success occur when individuals, families, and communities work together. For example, a health care professional can provide information to his or her patients and encourage them to practice healthy behaviors. Individuals then have the personal responsibility to put that information into practice.

Becoming Health Literate

Health literacy refers to *a person's capacity to learn about and understand basic health information and services and use these resources to promote his or her health and wellnes*s. This text will give you the information and tools you need to become health literate.

A health-literate individual needs to be

▶ **a critical thinker and problem solver**—a person who can evaluate health information before making a decision and who knows how to make responsible, healthy choices.

▶ **a responsible, productive citizen**—someone who acts in a way that promotes the health of the community and who chooses safe, healthful, and legal behaviors that are consistent with family guidelines and that show respect for the individual and others.

▶ **a self-directed learner**—a person who has developed evaluation criteria for health information. These criteria include whether the information is reliable, accurate, and current. Such information is available through various media, through technology such as the Internet, and from health care professionals.

▶ **an effective communicator**—someone who is able to express his or her health knowledge in a variety of ways.

Helping others make healthy choices is part of being a responsible, productive citizen. *List three ways to help others make healthy decisions.*

 Lesson 1 *Review*

Reviewing Facts and Vocabulary

1. Write a paragraph using the terms *health, wellness,* and *health education.*
2. Relate the nation's health goals and objectives to individual, family, and community health: What can an individual do to address the goals of *Healthy People 2010?*
3. What three criteria can help you evaluate health information?

Thinking Critically

4. **Analyzing.** How can promoting healthy behaviors such as avoiding tobacco help prevent disease?
5. **Evaluating.** Explain how being health literate helps you achieve and maintain good health.

Applying Health Skills

Practicing Healthful Behaviors. Review the health-promoting lifestyle factors discussed in this lesson. For one week, keep track of how many of them you participate in. Then identify three healthy behaviors that you took part in each day. Also identify one or two factors that you could improve.

TECHNOLOGY *OPTION*

SPREADSHEETS You can use spreadsheet software to make a chart for tracking your performance of healthy lifestyle factors. See **health.glencoe.com** for tips on how to use a spreadsheet.

Promoting a Healthy Lifestyle

VOCABULARY
heredity
environment
peers
culture
media

YOU'LL LEARN TO

- Describe the importance of taking responsibility for establishing and implementing health maintenance for individuals of all ages.

- Explain how influences such as heredity, environment, culture, media, and technology have impacted the health status of individuals, families, communities, and the world.

- Analyze the health messages delivered through media and technology.

➡️ **QUICK START**   List three of your favorite activities or hobbies. Then briefly describe the positive effect each has on your health.

🅐 **Participating in fun activities with family members enhances your health.**

How does staying up late affect you in the morning? How do you feel after engaging in physical activity? The actions you take regarding one aspect of your health have an effect on the other aspects as well.

Your Health Triangle

The three elements of health—physical, mental/emotional, and social—are interconnected, like the sides of a triangle. When one side receives too much or too little attention, the whole triangle can become lopsided and unbalanced. To be truly healthy, you need to keep all three sides of your health triangle in balance.

Physical Health

Your physical health has to do with how well your body functions. When you are in good physical health, you have enough energy to perform the activities of daily life and to cope with everyday challenges and stresses. You are also able to resist diseases and protect yourself from injury.

Being physically healthy involves getting adequate sleep and rest, eating nutritious meals, drinking enough water, and being physically active on a regular basis. It also includes practicing good hygiene and getting regular medical and dental checkups and treatments when you need them. Good physical health also involves paying attention to what you put into your body. It means avoiding harmful substances, such as tobacco, alcohol, and other drugs.

Mental/Emotional Health

Your feelings about yourself, how well you meet the demands of daily life, and your ability to process information are all important parts of your mental/emotional health. People with good mental/emotional health enjoy challenges, like learning new things, and see mistakes as opportunities to grow and change. They also accept responsibility for their actions and stand up for their beliefs and values.

People with good mental/emotional health are in touch with their feelings and can express them in appropriate ways. They can usually deal with the frustrations of life without being overwhelmed by them. They avoid dwelling on negative thoughts. Instead, they consider their situation and then use positive thoughts and actions to move forward.

Social Health

Your social health involves the way you get along with others. It includes your ability to make and keep friends and to work and play in cooperative ways, seeking and lending support when necessary. It involves communicating well and showing respect and care for yourself and others.

The health triangle is made up of three elements—physical, mental/emotional, and social health. *How might something affecting the physical side of your health triangle—an injury, for example—affect the other two sides?*

Keeping a Balance

Each side of your health triangle is equally important to your health. You might think of the three areas of health as the legs of a tripod on which a camera is mounted. If one leg is shorter than the other two, the tripod will tilt or fall. It's much the same with your health. An unbalanced health triangle is likely to cause you problems at some point. When you work to keep your physical, mental/emotional, and social health in balance, you are much more likely to function at your highest level.

People from the same family often share many of the same physical traits. *What physical similarities do the people in this family share? What are some health factors that can be inherited?*

Influences on Your Health

I magine that the story of your health were made into a movie. The movie would portray your health from your birth until today. The movie might also focus on the following questions:

▶ What situations and people affected your health at each stage of your life?

▶ How have influences on your health changed through the years?

▶ How do early influences still affect you today?

There are several important influences on your health. They include heredity; environment; media and technology; and, most importantly, your values, attitude, and behavior.

hotlink

heredity For more information on heredity, see Chapter 19, page 498.

Heredity

Your **heredity** refers to *all the traits that were biologically passed on to you from your parents.* You probably are familiar with heredity in terms of your physical traits such as eye color, hair color, and height. Heredity also influences your general level of health. Inheriting specific genes may put you at risk for certain illnesses, such as diabetes, requiring you to take steps to reduce your risk or manage the illness. Other genes may strengthen your resistance to disease. Beyond your physical health, heredity can also influence personality and basic intellectual abilities and talents.

Environment

Your **environment** is *the sum of your surroundings*, including your family, your neighborhood, your school, your job, and your life experiences. Environment includes all the places you go in a given day and the physical conditions in which you live. It also includes all the people in your life, and your culture.

hot link

environment For more information on environmental influences on health, see Chapter 29, page 764.

PHYSICAL ENVIRONMENT

Your physical environment influences every aspect of your health. A person who lives in a safe environment is likely to enjoy good physical and mental/emotional health. In contrast, someone who lives in an area with a high crime rate may experience stress or feel concern for personal safety.

Environmental factors such as air pollution also affect health. Pollen, dust, or smog in the air can cause allergies. Living with a smoker can increase the risk of respiratory problems.

SOCIAL ENVIRONMENT

Your social environment includes your family and other people with whom you come into contact each day. A supportive social environment made up of family and other adult role models can help a person develop positive values, a commitment to learning, and confidence in future success.

As a teen an important part of your social environment is your peers. **Peers** are *people of the same age who share similar interests*. Your peers include your friends and classmates. Loyal and supportive friends who care about their health can have a positive effect on your own health. Peers who take part in dangerous, unhealthy, and illegal behaviors like using tobacco, alcohol, or other drugs could create pressure for you to be "part of the group." Standing up to peer pressure can be challenging. Choosing friends who care about their health and yours supports a positive peer environment.

Climate is one factor that can influence health. *What other aspects of a person's physical environment can affect his or her health?*

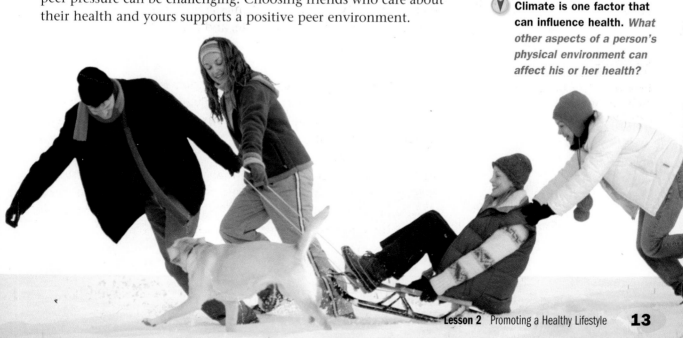

CULTURE

Culture refers to *the collective beliefs, customs, and behaviors of a group*. This group may be an ethnic group, a community, a nation, or a specific part of the world. The language your family speaks, the foods you enjoy, the traditions you have, and the religion you practice are all part of your cultural environment. Your culture gives you a sense of identity. Understanding culture can help you know yourself better and be tolerant of others.

Attitude

The way you view situations—your attitude—greatly affects the choices you make. For example, in order to practice good health habits, you must believe that there is some benefit to you and that problems may result if you don't develop these habits.

Attitude can play a major role in health and wellness. Studies have shown that people who tend to see the positive in situations are more likely to have better health than those who see only the negative. Try to view challenging situations positively and think in realistic terms. Doing so will help you make healthful decisions, reach your goals, and successfully manage your life.

Behavior

Although you have no control over your heredity and only limited control over your environment, you have a great deal of control over your behavior. Suppose your family has a history of heart disease. This doesn't mean that you will "follow in their footsteps." You can lower your risk of developing the disease by practicing healthy habits, such as reducing your intake of high-fat foods and engaging in regular physical activity.

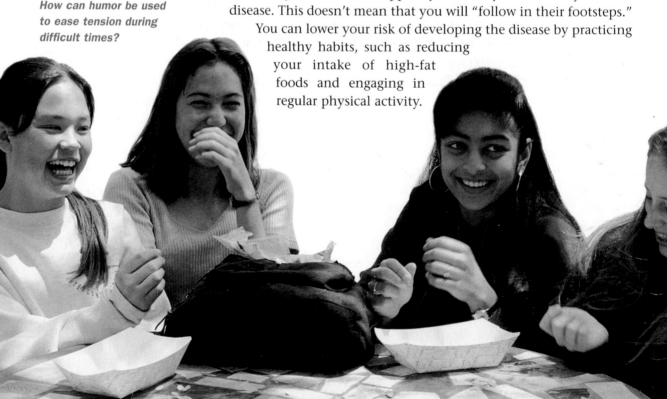

Maintaining a sense of humor can help you handle the difficulties that inevitably occur in life. *How can humor be used to ease tension during difficult times?*

Hands-On Health ACTIVITY

Health Influences

There are many influences on your health each day. In this activity you will record the influences that affect your health for one day.

What You'll Need

- pencil and paper

What You'll Do

1. Divide a sheet of paper into a grid of 12 rows and 3 columns. Label the columns "Activity," "Element of Health" (physical, mental/emotional, social), and "Influence."

2. Throughout the day, record activities that influence your physical, mental/emotional, or social health. Identify the element of health being affected and whether the influence is positive or negative. For example: *Activity:* Worked hard on my science project. *Element:* Mental. *Influence:* Positive because I am learning new information and developing my thinking skills. *Activity:* Watched TV and ate cookies. *Elements:* Physical and mental/emotional. *Influence:* Negative because an ad for cookies made me hungry, and I should be physically active instead of sitting on the couch.

3. Compare your grid with that of a classmate. How are your influences the same, and how are they different? Did you respond to similar influences in different ways? If so, why?

Apply and Conclude

In your private health journal, write a paragraph on what you have learned about health influences. What are the major influences in your life?

Your behavior affects not only your physical health but also your mental/emotional and social health. For example, mastering a new skill can give you a sense of accomplishment and enhance your self-esteem. Learning how to resolve conflicts peacefully can have a positive influence on your relationships with others.

Media

The media is a major influence on health. **Media**, or *the various methods of communicating information*, includes radio, television, film, newspapers, magazines, books, and the Internet. Although the media's main purpose has been to provide information and entertainment, it also plays a powerful role in shaping public opinion.

Advances in information delivery systems, such as the Internet, have put access to information from thousands of sources at your fingertips. Unfortunately, not all sources are reliable or accurate.

To learn more about advances in medical technology, click on Interactive Projects at **health.glencoe.com**.

For example, some advertisers may make exaggerated claims to try to persuade you to buy a product. For reliable information, stick to publications from professional health organizations, such as the American Medical Association, the American Heart Association, and the Centers for Disease Control and Prevention. Generally, Web sites and publications from accredited universities and government agencies are also reliable sources of information.

Technology

Technological advances also influence health. Advances in medical screenings and treatment for diseases such as heart disease, cancer, and AIDS have helped large numbers of people live longer, healthier lives. Other technological advances help keep our air, land, and water clean. However, advances in technology can have a downside. Technology has replaced many of the physical activities that once were part of daily life. People drive or ride instead of walk. They may watch TV, play video games, or work on the computer instead of being physically active. Recognizing the impact of these influences can help you live a more active, healthy life.

 Lesson 2 *Review*

Reviewing Facts and Vocabulary

1. Describe the importance of taking responsibility for health maintenance by keeping the three areas of health in balance.

2. Define the terms *culture* and *media*, and explain how each influences health.

3. Explain how technology has impacted health.

Thinking Critically

4. **Applying.** Select the side of your health triangle that you think is most affected by personal behavior. Explain your choice.

5. **Analyzing.** If you were looking for facts about weight lifting, how might you analyze the health messages delivered through a Web site for a company that sells weight equipment versus information provided by the American Academy of Pediatrics (AAP)?

Applying Health Skills

Analyzing Influences. The United States has many cultures within its population. Investigate which cultures are represented in or near your community. Select one and prepare a presentation on traditions and other factors that might influence the health of people growing up in that particular culture.

PRESENTATION SOFTWARE Presentation software can help you emphasize important points about traditions and culture. Find help in using presentation software at **health.glencoe.com**.

Your Behavior and Reducing Health Risks

VOCABULARY

risk behaviors
cumulative risks
abstinence

YOU'LL LEARN TO

- Describe ways to promote health and reduce risks.

- Associate risk-taking with consequences.

- Analyze the importance of abstinence from risk behaviors, including sexual activity before marriage.

- Communicate the importance of practicing abstinence.

⟹ **QUICK START**   Draw and label a health triangle on a sheet of paper. For each side of the triangle, identify two decisions you have made during the past few days that could affect your health. Place a " + " by those decisions that were healthful and a " − " by those that could have been or were harmful.

P art of becoming an adult is learning how to make responsible decisions. You may already be responsible for buying your own clothes, making your own breakfast or lunch, and managing your schedule. As you move toward adulthood, you become increasingly responsible for decisions regarding your health. It's important to remember that the choices you make during adolescence can have an effect on your health for the rest of your life.

Understanding Health Risks

T he first step in becoming responsible for your health is to increase your awareness of risk behaviors in your life. **Risk behaviors** are *actions that can potentially threaten your health or the health of others*. A second step is to examine your current behaviors and make any necessary changes.

Wearing protective gear is one way to reduce health risks. *What are other ways to reduce health risks when engaging in physical activity?*

Recognizing Risk Behaviors

The Centers for Disease Control and Prevention (CDC) and other public health agencies routinely survey teens nationwide to monitor their risk behaviors. In the most recent youth risk behavior survey, questionnaires on personal risk factors were gathered from teens in grades 9 through 12 in 33 states. The six categories of personal health risk factors and some of the results are shown in **Figure 1.2.**

When you analyze this data, you'll see that there is encouraging news. Most teens are *not* drinking alcohol or using tobacco. Over two thirds of teens wear safety belts when riding in cars. Where do you fit in? Are you making responsible decisions about your own health and well-being? Throughout this course, you will learn strategies for minimizing many types of risks.

▲ Regular physical activity reduces health risks.

FIGURE 1.2

TEEN RISK BEHAVIORS

The majority of teens are avoiding many risk behaviors or are taking preventive measures to improve their health.

The Youth Risk Behaviors Survey (YRBS) gathers data on the following:

- Behaviors that contribute to unintentional and intentional injuries
- Tobacco use
- Alcohol and other drug use
- Sexual behaviors that contribute to unplanned pregnancy and sexually transmitted infections (STIs) (including HIV infection)
- Unhealthy dietary behaviors
- Physical inactivity

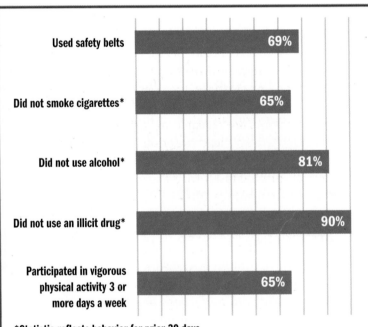

Used safety belts — 69%

Did not smoke cigarettes* — 65%

Did not use alcohol* — 81%

Did not use an illicit drug* — 90%

Participated in vigorous physical activity 3 or more days a week — 65%

*Statistic reflects behavior for prior 30 days.

Source: Based on data from the Centers for Disease Control and Prevention (CDC) and the National Household Survey on Drug Abuse (NHSDA)

Real-Life Application

Analyzing Risk Behaviors

Review Figure 1.2 on page 18. Your teacher will provide you with additional information on youth risk behaviors or instruct you on how to access this information.

Choose one category of personal health risk factors:

- Behaviors that may contribute to intentional and unintentional injuries
- Tobacco use

- Alcohol and other drug use
- Sexual behaviors that contribute to unplanned pregnancy, STIs, and HIV

- Unhealthy dietary behaviors
- Physical inactivity

ACTIVITY

Using the statistics in Figure 1.2 and the additional information you obtained, create a convincing poem, poster, song lyric, or cartoon advocating for risk-reducing behavior among your peers. Share your advocacy message with other students in your class or school.

Cumulative Risks and Consequences

The consequences of risk behaviors may add up over time. These **cumulative risks** are *related risks that increase in effect with each added risk*. Smoking one cigarette, for example, is not likely to result in death. Neither is eating one high-fat meal or getting one sunburn. If these behaviors are repeated over time, however, the negative effects accumulate and lead to serious health consequences.

Cumulative risks may also result from combinations of risk factors. For example, driving faster than the posted speed limit is a risk factor that can have deadly results. Another is not wearing a safety belt when you drive or ride in a car. Driving in bad weather is a third risk factor. The combination of these three factors greatly magnifies the potential for harm to yourself and to others. The more risk behaviors you participate in, the more likely you are to experience negative consequences at some point. Cumulative risks can and do occur in all areas of health and safety.

Did You Know ?

Scientists have discovered that the brain undergoes structural changes during the teen years. Some of those changes may mean that it's natural for teens to want to take on new challenges. *Healthy* challenges include running for class president, trying out for a play, and introducing yourself to a new student.

Abstaining from Risk Behaviors

The only way to avoid the consequences of some of the most serious risk behaviors is to practice abstinence. **Abstinence** is *avoiding harmful behaviors,* including the use of tobacco, alcohol, and other drugs and sexual activity before marriage. Choosing to abstain from high-risk behaviors is one of the most important health decisions you can make as a teen.

Abstaining from Tobacco, Alcohol, and Other Drugs

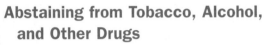

When you abstain from using tobacco, alcohol, and other drugs, you avoid many negative consequences. Using these substances harms all aspects of your health. The physical and psychological effects are well documented—these substances can cause addiction and can seriously harm the body. They can even cause death. Substance use often isolates a person from family and friends, a negative effect on social health. There are legal consequences as well—it is illegal for people under 21 to purchase, possess, or consume alcohol. People under 18 cannot purchase tobacco, and many states restrict purchasing to people over 21. The purchase and use of other drugs are illegal for all people, no matter what their age.

How you behave affects not only yourself but others around you. *What positive effects on others might result from your participation in a campaign that promotes abstinence from substance use?*

Abstaining from Sexual Activity

Abstinence from sexual activity is the preferred choice of behavior for unmarried persons of high-school age. Why? Abstinence from sexual activity protects teens against many negative consequences. Even teens who have been sexually active in the past can choose abstinence. Teens who abstain from sexual activity

▶ never have to worry about unplanned pregnancy.

▶ will not be faced with the difficult decisions associated with unplanned pregnancy, such as being a single parent.

▶ will not have to take on the many responsibilities of caring for a child.

▶ don't have to worry about sexually transmitted infections (including HIV infection).

▶ are free of the emotional problems that usually accompany sexual activity, such as guilt, regret, and rejection.

▶ are making a choice that is always legal.

With the worry of having a sexual relationship eliminated, you are free to establish nonsexual closeness with members of the opposite gender. Through these relationships you can develop genuine feelings of love, trust, and friendship. When you choose to abstain from sexual activity, you can focus on the real priorities of your life: setting and achieving your goals and following your dreams.

Responsible teens abstain from high-risk behaviors. Choosing abstinence will benefit your lifelong health.

 Avoiding high-risk behaviors and choosing friends who do so is one of the best ways to achieve and maintain wellness.

Lesson 3 *Review*

Reviewing Facts and Vocabulary

1. How are risk behaviors associated with consequences?

2. What are *cumulative risks*? Use this term in a complete sentence.

3. Analyze the importance of abstinence from sexual activity before marriage.

Thinking Critically

4. **Analyzing.** Why is it important to learn about risk behaviors in the teen years?

5. **Synthesizing.** How can you communicate the importance of practicing abstinence to other teens?

Applying Health Skills

Accessing Information. Choose one of the health-risk behaviors from Figure 1.2 that is of personal concern to you. Research how student trends in this behavior have changed over the last five years. Present your data in a line graph.

SPREADSHEETS You can use spreadsheet software to make your graph. Click on **health.glencoe.com** to access information on how to use a spreadsheet to represent data graphically.

Teens in the Media

Every day, you make decisions about the media—you choose what television shows to watch, what music to listen to, and what books and magazines to read. These choices can have a significant influence on your overall health.

Think about the TV shows you watch, the music you listen to, and the magazines and books you read. To get an idea of how teens are portrayed in the different forms of media, answer these questions:

Are the teens eating nutritious foods and engaging in regular physical activity?

Do the teens have a positive outlook on life?

Do the teens have healthful family relationships?

Do the teens avoid violence and try to resolve conflicts peacefully?

Do the teens avoid tobacco, alcohol, and other drugs?

Do the teens practice abstinence from sexual activity?

ACTIVITY

Begin a daily journal of your interaction with various forms of media. Record in your journal the names of the programs you watch, the titles of songs you listen to, the titles of books and magazines you read, and the names of Web sites you visit. Ask yourself whether or not the teens depicted in a particular form of media are modeling healthful behaviors and making responsible choices, and write answers to the questions above. Keep the journal for a week.

On the basis of the data in your journal, would you say that there are plenty of healthful images of teens in the media, or do you believe that there is a lack of images of teens making healthful choices and leading healthy lives? Write a paper discussing your view.

EXPRESS YOUR VIEWS

Write a paragraph on how watching TV shows, reading books and magazines, listening to music, or visiting Web sites that promote a healthy lifestyle might positively influence your own health.

CROSS-CURRICULUM CONNECTIONS

Write a Play. Dreaming about the future and setting goals to succeed are part of living a healthy life. Take a few minutes to imagine what lies ahead for you. Write a one-person play about how your life will be if you choose a particular path. Then look at your present reality. Consider what steps you need to take to fulfill your dream. What obstacles or risks might you face? Who will support you on this path?

Write an Analysis. Many technological advances have had a positive impact on health. For example, the development of a medical test known as the computerized tomography (CT) scan has made it possible for certain diseases to be diagnosed earlier and more accurately than before. Use online and print resources to research a technological advance such as the CT scan, and write a short analytical essay on your findings.

Calculate the Amount. Figure 1.2 on page 18 indicates that, according to the Youth Risk Behaviors Survey, in a given 30-day period 65 percent of high-school students did not smoke. Town Center High School has 420 seniors. How many of the seniors at this high school smoked within a given 30-day period?

Present Research Findings. Getting an adequate amount of sleep each night is essential for optimum health and wellness, especially for teens. During sleep, the body passes through several distinct stages, each characterized by specific types of brain activity. Conduct research to find out more about the different stages of sleep. Write up your findings in the form of a report and present it to the class.

Health Educator

Do you have an interest in improving the health of young people? Do you enjoy working with individuals and groups? If so, it might be worth your time to look into health education as a career.

To be a public school health teacher, you must be credentialed. This would include having a four-year college degree and completing an approved teacher-training program. To find out more about this and other health careers, click on Career Corner at **health.glencoe.com**.

Chapter 1 *Review*

> **EXPLORING HEALTH TERMS** *Answer the following questions on a sheet of paper.*

Lesson 1 *Match each definition with the correct term.*

health	health literacy
Healthy People 2010	health education
wellness	prevention

1. The combination of physical, mental/emotional, and social well-being.

2. An overall state of well-being, or total health.

3. The providing of accurate health information to help people make healthy choices.

4. A nationwide health promotion and disease prevention plan designed to serve as a guide for improving the health of all people in the United States.

5. A person's capacity to learn about and understand basic health information and services and use these resources to promote his or her health and wellness.

6. Practicing health and safety habits to remain free of disease and injury.

Lesson 2 *Replace the underlined words with the correct term.*

heredity	media	peers
culture	environment	

7. One part of your <u>culture</u> is where you live.

8. Radio and television are examples of <u>environment</u>.

9. Your <u>heredity</u> influences such things as your language and what you eat.

10. <u>Media</u> is the sum of an individual's traits that were biologically passed along by both parents.

11. People of the same age who share similar interests are your <u>culture</u>.

Lesson 3 *Identify each statement as True or False. If false, replace the underlined term with the correct term.*

risk behaviors	cumulative risks
abstinence	

12. Avoiding harmful behaviors, including sexual activity before marriage and the use of tobacco, alcohol, and other drugs, is known as <u>risk behaviors</u>.

13. <u>Abstinence</u> can potentially threaten your health or the health of others.

14. <u>Cumulative risks</u> are related risks that increase in effect with each added risk.

> **RECALLING THE FACTS** *Use complete sentences to answer the following questions.*

Lesson 1

1. What is the purpose of *Healthy People 2010*?

2. List five lifestyle factors that promote good health.

3. What can communities do to address the goals of *Healthy People 2010*?

Lesson 2

4. Which aspect of health reflects your ability to enjoy challenges and handle frustrations?

5. Identify six categories of influences on health.

6. Over which influences on health do you have the most control?

Lesson 3

7. What is the first step toward becoming responsible for your health?

8. Describe the two ways that cumulative risks occur.

9. List three benefits of abstinence from sexual activity before marriage.

THINKING CRITICALLY

1. **Analyzing.** Review the health continuum shown on page 5. What behaviors would contribute to the loss of health and wellness? What behaviors would move a person toward a high level of health? *(LESSON 1)*

2. **Synthesizing.** John is a good student, has lots of friends, and spends much of his free time practicing the guitar with his band. He eats a lot of fast-food burgers and is 10 pounds overweight. Draw his health triangle. *(LESSON 2)*

3. **Summarizing.** Explain why abstinence from risk behaviors is the most responsible behavior for teens, and provide an example of its application. *(LESSON 3)*

HEALTH SKILLS APPLICATION

1. **Advocacy.** Write a letter to parents informing them of the nation's health goals and the role of *Healthy People 2010.* Highlight things that they can do individually and as a family to impact the health of all people in the United States. *(LESSON 1)*

2. **Analyzing Influences.** Consider how each of the influences on health affects your own wellness. On a sheet of paper, make two columns—one titled *Positive* and the other titled *Negative.* Identify the positive and negative aspects of each influence and record them in the appropriate column. *(LESSON 2)*

3. **Goal Setting.** What would be possible consequences of using an illegal drug? Provide an example of how a goal would be negatively affected by these consequences. *(LESSON 3)*

BEYOND *the* Classroom

Parent Involvement

Analyzing Influences. With a parent, analyze the influence of laws, policies, and practices on a health-related issue. Topics may include regulations for smoking in public buildings, policies and practices for fire and safety in your school, and traffic laws. Write a brief report that summarizes your findings.

The Boulevard
IS NOW SMOKE-FREE
For the convenience of smokers, designated smoking areas are located outside mall entrances.

School and Community

Restaurant Inspection. Talk with a health inspector about food-handling requirements and other health codes for restaurant workers. Find out whether you or a small group of students could observe the inspection of a restaurant. Share what you have learned with your class.

Building Health Skills and Character

Do You Practice Effective Health Skills?

Respond by writing *yes*, *no*, or *sometimes* for each item. Write *yes* only for items that you practice regularly or are sure about.

1. I know how to access reliable health information and services.

2. I care about the well-being of others and encourage them to make healthy choices.

3. I am aware of what influences my actions and decisions.

4. I communicate my thoughts and feelings clearly.

5. I am comfortable saying no to friends and peers who want to engage in risky or unhealthy activities.

6. I use problem-solving skills to resolve conflicts in a peaceful, respectful manner.

7. I engage in regular physical activity and eat nutritious foods.

8. I am aware of sources of stress in my life and know how to reduce or manage them.

9. When making decisions, I consider how the consequences might affect my health and the health of others.

10. I set personal health goals.

For instant feedback on your health status, go to Chapter 2 Health Inventory at **health.glencoe.com**.

Quick*Write*

Using Visuals. List skills that you think would help teens lead healthy lives. What skills are the teens in this photo demonstrating? Which skills do you practice on a regular basis to maintain or improve your health?

Lesson 1

Building Health Skills

VOCABULARY

health skills
interpersonal
communication
refusal skills
conflict resolution
stress management
advocacy

YOU'LL LEARN TO

- Demonstrate communication skills in building and maintaining healthy relationships.

- Develop refusal strategies and conflict resolution skills.

- Apply self-management strategies.

- Analyze influences on behavior.

- Develop criteria for evaluating health information.

→ **QUICK START** On a sheet of paper, list the skills and qualities necessary for effective communication. Then, explain how having strong communication skills can impact your health in positive ways.

FIGURE 2.1

THE HEALTH SKILLS

Developing and practicing these health skills will provide a lifetime of benefits.

Interpersonal Communication
- Communication Skills
- Refusal Skills
- Conflict Resolution

Self Management
- Practicing Healthful Behaviors
- Stress Management

Analyzing Influences

Accessing Information

Decision Making/Goal Setting

Advocacy

The choices you make and the actions you take—including the foods you eat, the friends you choose, and the activities you participate in—can affect your health. Taking responsibility for your health begins with a commitment to take charge of your actions and behaviors in a way that reduces risks and promotes wellness. The first step is to develop *health skills*. **Health skills**, or life skills, are *specific tools and strategies that help you maintain, protect, and improve all aspects of your health.* **Figure 2.1** presents a basic overview of the health skills.

Interpersonal Skills

One of the traits of a health-literate individual is having effective communication skills. Effective communication involves not only making yourself heard but also being a good listener. **Interpersonal communication** is *the exchange of thoughts, feelings, and beliefs between two or more people.*

Strategies for effective **communication** include:

▶ **Clearly say what you mean.** Use *"I" messages* to state your position, for example, "I feel frustrated when our plans change." This helps you avoid placing blame on others.

▶ **Pay attention to *how* you say something.** Use a respectful tone. Make sure your facial expressions and gestures reflect your verbal message.

▶ **Be a good listener.** Avoid interrupting the speaker, and show that you are listening by nodding or asking appropriate questions.

h✺t link

communication For more information on communication skills, see Chapter 10, page 254.

Health Skills Activity

Communication: The Ball's in Your Court

When Mark arrives late at the basketball court, his friend Phillipe throws the ball at him, shouting, "You're a half hour late!"

"Well, excuse me, Mr. Punctual," Mark laughs.

"You're never on time. It's like you assume I have nothing better to do than wait around for you," Phillipe says.

"Sorry, bud, but some things came up," Mark answers.

"Yeah? Well, I'm outta here." Phillipe throws up his hands and turns to walk away.

"Wait, let me explain," Mark says calmly.

Phillipe hesitates, wondering how to respond.

What Would You Do?
How can Mark and Phillipe use effective communication skills to continue their discussion more effectively? Write an ending to this scenario, using the guidelines below.

1. Use "I" messages.
2. Speak calmly and clearly, using a respectful tone.
3. Listen carefully, and ask appropriate questions.
4. Show appropriate body language.

FIGURE 2.2

REFUSAL STRATEGIES

Sometimes you must reinforce your decision to say no.

SAY NO IN A FIRM VOICE.
Do this calmly and clearly. Use expressions such as "I'd rather not."

EXPLAIN WHY.
State your feelings. Tell the other person that the suggested activity or behavior goes against your values or beliefs.

SUGGEST ALTERNATIVES.
Propose a safe, healthful activity to do instead.

USE APPROPRIATE BODY LANGUAGE.
Make it clear that you don't intend to back down from your position. Look directly into the other person's eyes.

LEAVE IF NECESSARY.
If the other person continues to pressure you, or simply won't take no for an answer, just walk away.

CHARACTER CHECK

Respect. When you apply refusal skills to avoid risky situations, you demonstrate respect for yourself and your values. **How can using refusal skills help you uphold your values and the values of your family?**

Refusal Skills

Think about how you handle situations in which you are asked to do something that you know is harmful or wrong. In such circumstances, you need to use refusal skills. **Refusal skills** are *communication strategies that can help you say no when you are urged to take part in behaviors that are unsafe or unhealthful, or that go against your values.* Practicing these strategies, including the ones shown in **Figure 2.2,** will help you resist risky behaviors.

Conflict Resolution Skills

In addition to practicing effective refusal skills, it is important to develop strategies for dealing with conflicts or disagreements. **Conflict resolution** is *the process of ending a conflict through cooperation and problem solving.* The key to conflict resolution is respecting the other person's rights as well as your own. Willingness to compromise will also help achieve a resolution that satisfies everyone. Follow these steps when dealing with a conflict:

▶ Take time to calm down and think through the situation.

▶ When discussing the conflict, speak calmly and listen attentively, asking questions when appropriate.

▶ Use a polite tone and try to brainstorm solutions where no one loses respect. Work to resolve the conflict peacefully.

Self-Management Skills

When you practice self management, you take responsibility for your health and act in specific ways that promote your wellness. Two self-management skills, practicing healthful behaviors and managing stress, help provide a foundation of good health.

Practicing Healthful Behaviors

Choices you make today will affect your health in the future. Healthful behaviors are more than just actions that can protect you from illness or injury. These behaviors support every aspect of your health. Eating nutritious foods and getting regular medical and dental checkups as well as avoiding the use of tobacco, alcohol, and other drugs, are all behaviors that help you maintain and strengthen your overall health. Practicing healthful behaviors also involves expressing your feelings in healthful ways, building your self-esteem, and maintaining healthy relationships.

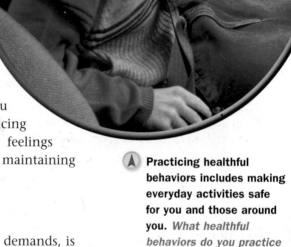

Practicing healthful behaviors includes making everyday activities safe for you and those around you. *What healthful behaviors do you practice on a regular basis?*

Managing Stress

Stress, the body's and mind's reactions to everyday demands, is a natural part of life. Being late to class, balancing many activities, and winning an award can all cause stress. Learning **stress management**, or *ways to deal with or overcome the negative effects of stress,* will become increasingly important as you assume more responsibility for your health and take on additional roles as an adult. Some strategies for managing stress include engaging in physical activity, listening to soothing music, managing time effectively, taking a warm bath, and laughing.

Analyzing Influences

How do you determine what health choices are right for you? Many factors influence your health. *Internal influences,* which include your knowledge, values, likes, dislikes, and desires, are based on your experiences and your perspective on life. You have a great deal of control over your internal influences. *External influences,* which come from outside sources, include your family, your friends and peers, your environment, your culture, laws, and the media. As you become aware of these influences, you will be better able to make healthful choices about everything from your personal behavior to which health products you buy.

Talking to a health professional can help you obtain accurate, reliable information. *Where else can you find valid health information?*

Accessing Information

Learning how to find and recognize trustworthy information will help you be better prepared to make healthful choices. When evaluating health information, check the validity of the source. Keep in mind that reliable sources of health information include:

▶ parents, guardians, and other trusted adults.

▶ library resources, such as encyclopedias and nonfiction books on science, medicine, nutrition, and fitness.

▶ reliable Internet sites, such as those posted by government and educational institutions.

▶ newspaper and magazine articles by health professionals or experts.

▶ government agencies, health care providers, and health organizations.

Advocacy

Advocacy is *taking action to influence others to address a health-related concern or to support a health-related belief.* This skill enables you to positively influence the health of those around you. In this responsible role, you can help others become informed and publicly support health causes that concern and interest you. Encouraging family, friends, peers, and community members to practice healthful behaviors is one way to practice health advocacy.

▶ Lesson 1 *Review*

Reviewing Facts and Vocabulary

1. Define the term *interpersonal communication*, and identify the role of "I" messages.

2. List five refusal strategies.

3. What is *stress management*? Identify three ways to reduce the effects of stress.

Thinking Critically

4. **Analyzing.** What are the advantages of peacefully resolving conflicts?

5. **Applying.** What are two ways you could show support for a health cause or organization?

Applying Health Skills

Stress Management. List all the healthful strategies you used this past week to relieve stress. Which ones helped the most?

TECHNOLOGY *OPTION*

SPREADSHEETS You can keep track of events and organize your thoughts by using a spreadsheet. For help in using spreadsheet software, go to **health.glencoe.com**.

Making Responsible Decisions and Setting Goals

VOCABULARY

decision-making skills
values
goal
short-term goal
long-term goal
action plan

YOU'LL LEARN TO

- Identify decision-making skills that promote individual, family, and community health.

- Summarize the advantages of seeking advice and feedback regarding decision-making skills.

- Identify the processes involved in choosing and achieving goals.

QUICK START What goals have you set for yourself in the past year? What steps did you take to reach your goals?

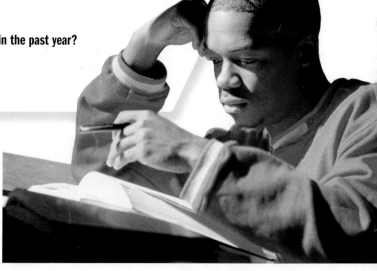

When you make decisions or set goals, you are exercising power over how healthy, happy, and productive you can be. Making responsible decisions and setting meaningful goals are important skills that can have a great impact on your life.

This teen made the decision to study for his exam instead of going out with friends. *What responsible decisions have you made in the past week?*

The Decision-Making Process

Decision-making skills are *steps that enable you to make a healthful decision.* The steps are designed to help you make decisions that protect your rights and health while respecting the rights and health of others. The six basic steps for making a decision are described in **Figure 2.3** on page 34. Often, you will find it helpful to seek advice from those with more experience, such as parents and guardians. Doing so can provide valuable feedback and strengthen family bonds and values.

FIGURE 2.3

STEPS OF THE DECISION-MAKING PROCESS

Step 1: STATE THE SITUATION
Examine the situation and ask yourself: What decisions need to be made? Consider all the facts and who else is involved.

Step 2: LIST THE OPTIONS
What are the possible choices you could make? Remember that sometimes it is appropriate not to take action. Share your options with parents or guardians, siblings, teachers, or friends. Ask for their advice.

Step 3: WEIGH THE POSSIBLE OUTCOMES
Weigh the consequence of each option. Use the word *HELP* to guide your choice.
- **H** *(Healthful)* What health risks, if any, will this option present?
- **E** *(Ethical)* Does this choice reflect what you and your family believe is right?
- **L** *(Legal)* Does this option violate any local, state, or federal laws?
- **P** *(Parent Approval)* Would your parents or guardians approve of this choice?

Step 4: CONSIDER VALUES
Values are *the ideas, beliefs, and attitudes about what is important that help guide the way you live.* A responsible decision will reflect your values.

Step 5: MAKE A DECISION AND ACT ON IT
Use everything you know at this point to make a responsible decision. You can feel good that you have carefully prepared and thought about the situation and your options.

Step 6: EVALUATE THE DECISION
After you have made the decision and taken action, reflect on what happened. What was the outcome? How did your decision affect your health and the health of those around you? What did you learn? Would you take the same action again? If not, how would your choice differ?

Setting Personal Health Goals

Consider your plans for the future. What do you want to do with your life? Do your plans include further education and a family? What kind of career are you interested in pursuing? Setting goals can help you shape your life in positive ways by focusing your energy on behaviors that you want to develop or change. A **goal** is *something you aim for that takes planning and work.* Goal setting is also an effective way to build self-confidence, increase your self-esteem, and improve your overall health.

Types of Goals

Every goal involves planning. When you set a goal and plan strategies to reach it, you will need to consider how much time it will take to accomplish the goal. A **short-term goal**, such as finishing a project by Friday or cleaning your room before dinner, is *a goal that you can reach in a short period of time.* A **long-term goal** is *a goal that you plan to reach over an extended period of time.* Examples include improving your grades for the semester or making the cross country team next season. A long-term goal may take months or even years to accomplish. Often, short-term goals are steps in a plan to achieve a long-term goal. What kinds of short-term goals might help a person become a physician or a computer technician?

Health Minute
Setting Goals

Some guidelines to remember:

► Make sure that your goals are your own, not someone else's.

► Set a goal because it will help you grow, not because you want to outdo someone.

► If you do not achieve your goal, use what you've learned to set a new goal.

Hands-On Health ACTIVITY

Setting Your Personal Health Goal

In this activity, you will set a personal health goal and work to achieve it.

What You'll Need

• notebook   • pencil

What You'll Do

For the next week, use your notebook as a personal health goal journal. Record your efforts to reach your goal. At the end of the week, write a reflective summary of what you learned in the process.

1. **Set a goal.** Do you want to get along better with family members? Eat more nutritiously? Be more active? Set a realistic health goal, and write it down. Explain why you have chosen this goal and what changes you hope to accomplish.

2. **List steps to meet the goal.** Examine a variety of options to achieve the goal you have set. List the steps you will take to reach your goal.

3. **Identify sources of help.** List the names of people who can help and support you as you work toward your goal.

4. **Evaluate your progress, and adjust plans if necessary.** If there have been obstacles, give yourself more time, and work to overcome them. If you are moving ahead of schedule, you may want to set a more challenging goal.

Apply and Conclude

After a week, examine your progress. Has your plan been effective? How can it be strengthened? Extend your one-week plan to four weeks. Make it a habit to continue to set and work toward new health goals.

Achieving Your Goals

To establish and reach your goals, create an **action plan**, or *a multistep strategy to identify and achieve your goals*. Follow these steps:

► **Set a specific, realistic goal, and write it down.** State your goal as something positive. This will help motivate you.

► **List the steps you will take to reach your goal.** Look for ways to break your goal into smaller, short-term goals.

► **Identify sources of help and support.** Such sources might include friends, family members, peers, teachers, or neighbors.

► **Set a reasonable time frame for reaching your goal.** After deciding on a reasonable time, put it in writing.

► **Evaluate your progress by establishing checkpoints.** Periodically check how you are progressing, and make any necessary adjustments that will help you reach your goal.

► **Reward yourself for achieving your goal.** Enjoy the personal satisfaction reaching a goal brings. You might celebrate your achievement with your family or friends.

Lesson 2 *Review*

Reviewing Facts and Vocabulary

1. What are the six steps of the decision-making process?

2. Summarize the advantages of seeking advice regarding decision-making skills.

3. Explain the difference between short-term and long-term goals, and provide an example of each.

Thinking Critically

4. **Applying.** Identify a major health-related decision that teens might have to make. How can teens access information and use decision-making skills to make an informed choice?

5. **Synthesizing.** Explain and defend this statement: *Decision making and goal setting are interrelated.*

Applying Health Skills

Decision Making. Cari's friends want her to skip school to go to the beach with them. Apply the six steps of decision making to Cari's situation, and help her make a responsible choice.

WORD PROCESSING Use word-processing software to present your application of the decision-making steps. See **health.glencoe.com** for tips on using word-processing programs.

Building Character

YOU'LL LEARN TO

- Discuss the importance of good character for self, others, and community.
- Apply communication skills and practice behaviors that demonstrate consideration and respect for self, family, and others.
- Identify ways to demonstrate good character.

QUICK START On a sheet of paper, complete this sentence: *I am taking responsibility when I* . . . Then, write a paragraph explaining your statement.

A s you have learned, it is important to consider and act on your most important beliefs and values when making a decision. Values shape your priorities, and they help you distinguish right from wrong. The values that help you make healthful, well-informed decisions are also traits of good character. **Character** can be defined as *those distinctive qualities that describe how a person thinks, feels, and behaves.*

What Is Good Character?

G ood character is an outward expression of inner values. A person with good character demonstrates *core ethical values,* such as responsibility, honesty, integrity, and respect. These values are held in high regard across all cultures and age groups. Core ethical values are the highest of all human values, and they guide you toward healthy, responsible choices. When your behavior reflects such standards, you can feel confident that you are demonstrating the traits of a person with good character.

Character helps shape behavior. *What values might prompt the teen in the photo to return the found wallet?*

FIGURE 2.4

TRAITS OF GOOD CHARACTER

A person of good character demonstrates these traits in his or her actions and behaviors.

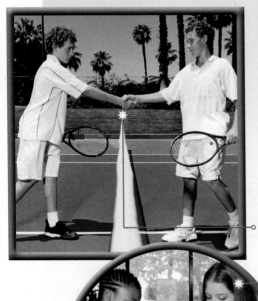

Trustworthiness: If you are trustworthy, you are honest, loyal, and reliable—you do what you say you'll do. You have the courage to do the right thing, and you don't deceive, cheat, or steal.

Respect: Showing respect means being considerate of others and tolerant of differences. It also means using good manners. You make decisions that show you respect your health and the health of others. You treat people and property with care.

Responsibility: Being responsible means using self-control—you think before you act and consider the consequences. You are accountable for your choices and decisions—you don't blame others for your actions. Responsible people try to do their best, and they persevere even when things don't go as planned.

Fairness: If you are fair, you play by the rules, take turns, and share. You are open-minded, and you listen to others. You don't take advantage of others, and you don't assign blame to others.

Caring: A caring person is kind and compassionate. When you care about others, you express gratitude, you are forgiving, and you help people in need.

Citizenship: If you advocate for a safe and healthy school and community, you are demonstrating good citizenship. A good citizen obeys laws and rules and respects authority. Being a good neighbor and cooperating with others are also parts of good citizenship.

Character and Health

Because your character plays a significant role in your decisions, actions, and behavior, it impacts all aspects of your health. Developing good character enhances each side of your health triangle. For example, if you view yourself with respect and value your physical health, you are more likely to take care of your body by eating nutritious foods and keeping physically active. When you act with responsibility and fairness, both your mental/emotional and social health will improve. When you feel good about yourself, your relationships with others are strengthened.

Traits of Good Character

There are several different traits that contribute to good character. **Figure 2.4** identifies six primary traits of good character. Developing and strengthening these traits will assist you in becoming the best person you can be.

HEALTH *Online*

Learn more about putting good character into action by clicking on Web Links at **health.glencoe.com.**

Developing Your Character

Character and core ethical values are learned when you're young and developed throughout your life. To take a more active role in your character development:

► Stand up for your beliefs.

► Learn from people who demonstrate good character traits. Ask family members for tips on strengthening values.

► Join volunteer groups in your school or community. Form friendships with people who exhibit core ethical values.

Real-Life Application

Character in Action

A person with good character can inspire people to make a difference in the world. The teen showcased here began a pen-pal program that links young people suffering from life-threatening illness with other teens around the country.

Character Traits: Compassion, caring, and courage.

Mission: Create a support network among teens with life-threatening diseases.

Taking Action: Contact hospitals and other organizations to establish a network.

ACTIVITY

Choose an organization with volunteer opportunities. Research information on the organization's mission and programs. Which character traits do members of the organization display? Why are these traits necessary to meet the organization's goals? Write a paragraph summarizing your findings.

Should Service Learning Be Required?

Since volunteering is a valuable experience, do you think schools should require service learning?

Viewpoint 1: Chad D., age 16

My experience of volunteering at a senior center through a school service learning program was very positive and taught me a lot of things that can't be learned in a classroom. I wouldn't have known about this opportunity if my school didn't require it. I think it's a great idea to require service learning in schools; it'll open people's eyes to volunteer and career opportunities.

Viewpoint 2: Lisa H., age 15

Isn't the whole point of volunteering that it's done by choice? I'm afraid that forcing it on students may turn them away from the idea. Some teens already have jobs, family commitments, or roles in their faith community that help them demonstrate good character. Service learning should be an *option* in the curriculum. That way, students can make their own decisions about how, when, and where they want to give back to the community.

What do you think? Do you agree with Chad that service learning offers benefits not available in the classroom? What do you think of Lisa's argument that mandatory service learning is a contradiction in terms? Present your views in a one-page essay.

▼ **Teens can be important role models for younger students.**

Positive Role Models

Having positive role models is important in developing and strengthening good character traits. A **role model** is *someone whose success or behavior serves as an example for others.* Many people look to their families for role models. Parents, grandparents, and siblings are often the people who best support your goals and promote your health. They can inspire and encourage basic values such as working hard, staying focused, planning ahead, being honest, and engaging in safe and healthful behaviors. Other role models may include teachers, coaches, religious leaders, and volunteers.

Think about the character traits that your role models demonstrate. Do you show the same traits in your daily actions? When your behaviors reflect good character, you may inspire others to act in kind, responsible ways, too. In return, you will experience increased feelings of self-worth, satisfaction, and a sense of purpose.

Demonstrating Character

By demonstrating good character, you practice behaviors that have a positive effect on both yourself and others at home, at school, and in your community.

▶ **Make a difference at home.** You demonstrate trustworthiness and reliability at home when you carry out your responsibilities. By showing respect and caring in daily actions, you will also strengthen your family relationships.

▶ **Make a difference at school.** At this stage in life, you are probably beginning to evaluate the rules that others have set for you. By observing school rules, you show respect for teachers and fellow students.

▶ **Make a difference in your community.** Good citizenship means obeying laws, respecting the needs of others, and being tolerant of differences. Take advantage of the opportunity you have to model good character and be a positive influence on those around you.

▶ Lesson 3 *Review*

Reviewing Facts and Vocabulary

1. What is *character*? How is good character related to values?
2. Name the six primary traits of good character.
3. List three ways of demonstrating good character in your home, your school, and your community.

Thinking Critically

4. **Synthesizing.** Why do you think that caring, responsibility, and respect are values that exist across cultures?
5. **Applying.** In what ways can you use communication skills to demonstrate consideration and respect for self, family, and others?

Applying Health Skills

Advocacy. Prepare a message about an important health cause or organization. The message should be appropriate for a specific audience, such as children, teens, parents, or individuals with a disability.

TECHNOLOGY *OPTION*

PRESENTATION SOFTWARE You can use presentation software to include images in your advocacy message. Find help in using presentation software at **health.glencoe.com.**

Health Advocacy in the Media

Advocacy organizations are usually nonprofit companies that raise awareness about and raise money for different social, political, or health causes. A high-profile media personality can benefit the cause of an advocacy organization by bringing attention to the cause. In this activity, you will examine how good citizenship and media attention can have a positive impact on various public health issues.

Name of organization and its purpose

Media Campaigns

Type of media: charity golf tournament	Type of media: TV game show	Type of media:	Type of media:
Purpose: to raise funds for research	**Purpose:** to raise money and raise public awareness	**Purpose:**	**Purpose:**
Celebrity involvement: [Name of celebrity] sponsors the event and encourages media to attend.	**Celebrity involvement:** [Name of celebrity] enters game show as a contestant to win money for the cause.	**Celebrity involvement:**	**Celebrity involvement:**

ACTIVITY

Identify a high-profile media personality who is involved in a health advocacy organization or cause. Research the purpose of the organization and the role the celebrity plays in advocating for its cause. Review the media attention the organization gets and by what means. Organize the information you collect into a chart like the one above.

EXPRESS YOUR VIEWS

Write a proposal that suggests how you can help bring local attention to the cause of the health advocacy organization you have researched. Include strategies on how to use local media to help raise awareness or to help raise money for the issue or cause.

CROSS-CURRICULUM CONNECTIONS

Campaign for Character. Demonstrating good character can promote your health and bring you personal satisfaction. Create a poster for younger students that stresses the importance of developing good character. Present and explain the six primary traits of good character, and encourage your audience to take an active role in strengthening these traits. To back up your message, you might include anecdotes from your own experiences as well as examples of people you admire.

Write a Report. Louis Pasteur, Clara Barton, and Jonas Salk are all individuals who have made significant contributions to community health. Choose one of these historical figures or another individual who has striven to improve the health of others. Research that person's life and accomplishments, focusing on his or her contributions to the field of health. What qualities and actions helped this individual achieve his or her goals?

Add Up Your Goal. Laurie has set a long-term goal to make the swim team next year. To help her reach that goal, she has decided she will swim three days a week for the next thirty weeks. For each session, she plans to swim five laps. How many laps will Laurie swim by the end of the thirty weeks?

Research a Topic. Managing stress is an important aspect of developing good health skills. In recent years, the old adage "laughter is the best medicine" has been proven by scientists and medical researchers to be more fact than myth. Research laughter, how it affects the body, and particularly, how it affects brain chemistry. Write a brief report explaining how laughter works and why laughter might be an important part of developing your personal health skills.

Family Counselor

Do you have a keen understanding of how values direct behavior within a family? Are you able to deal with people from varied backgrounds? If so, a career as a family counselor might be for you. These professionals work with entire families or with individual family members to solve problems and improve relationships.

To enter this profession, you'll need a four-year college degree and a master's degree in counseling. Find out more about this and other health careers by clicking on Career Corner at **health.glencoe.com**.

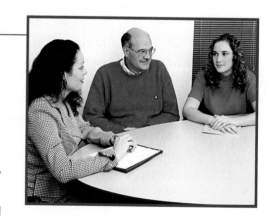

Chapter 2 *Review*

➤ EXPLORING HEALTH TERMS *Answer the following questions on a sheet of paper.*

Lesson 1 *Replace the underlined words with the correct term.*

conflict resolution	advocacy
refusal skills	stress management
interpersonal communication	
health skills	

1. "I" messages are a form of <u>refusal skills</u>.

2. <u>Advocacy</u> is a process to help you resolve conflict through cooperation and problem solving.

3. People use <u>conflict resolution</u> to manage the body's reactions to everyday demands.

4. <u>Stress management</u> is a responsible role in which you influence others' health behaviors.

Lesson 2 *Match each definition with the correct term.*

action plan	goal
decision-making skills	values
long-term goal	short-term goal

5. Something you aim for that takes planning and work.

6. A goal that you can plan to reach over an extended period of time.

7. A multistep strategy for identifying and achieving your goals.

8. The ideas, beliefs, and attitudes about what is important that help guide the way you live.

Lesson 3 *Fill in the blanks with the correct term.*

character	role model

A person with high standards usually exhibits good (_9_). This person often makes a positive (_10_).

➤ RECALLING THE FACTS *Use complete sentences to answer the following questions.*

Lesson 1

1. List the strategies for effective communication.

2. What are refusal skills?

3. What steps should you follow to resolve a conflict?

4. Why are self-management skills important? Give an example of two of these skills.

Lesson 2

5. What are decision-making skills?

6. Define the term *value*.

7. Explain how the word *HELP* can assist you in weighing the possible consequences of a decision and making the right choice.

8. What are the six steps of a goal-setting action plan?

Lesson 3

9. Describe what it means to demonstrate the character trait of trustworthiness.

10. How does character impact your health?

11. How can you take an active role in your character development?

12. What are some benefits of being a positive role model?

➤ THINKING CRITICALLY

1. **Synthesizing.** Gwen tries her best to fit in with a group that she recognizes takes unnecessary risks. She follows along anyway and usually suffers the consequences of her decisions. What skill does Gwen need to develop? Explain how this skill could improve her overall health. *(LESSON 1)*

2. **Analyzing.** Why is recognizing consequences important when using the decision-making process? How do values enter into the decision-making process? *(LESSON 2)*

3. **Evaluating.** Identify a trait of good character that you possess, and list ways that you demonstrate that trait. *(LESSON 3)*

➤ HEALTH SKILLS APPLICATION

1. **Communication Skills.** List examples of body language that you or others use when communicating. Pick two examples, and explain how they reinforce verbal messages. *(LESSON 1)*

2. **Decision Making.** Imagine that you are trying to improve your grades to make the basketball team. Which activity would you attend if they occurred at the same time—an extra basketball practice or a study session? Use the decision-making steps to help you make your choice. *(LESSON 2)*

3. **Analyzing Influences.** Do all individuals who are famous because of their achievements make positive role models? Why or why not? *(LESSON 3)*

BEYOND the Classroom

Parent Involvement

Advocacy. Learn more about a nonprofit organization in your community. With your parents, find out how your family could become involved. By volunteering your time, you can help the organization achieve its mission, get firsthand knowledge of how it operates, and help individuals with special needs in your community.

School and Community

Conduct an Interview. In certain professions—teaching and law, for example—effective communication is especially critical. Interview an individual from one of these professions, and learn about the guidelines he or she uses to ensure good communication.

Chapter 3

Being a Health-Literate Consumer

What's Your Health Status?

Read each statement below and respond by writing *yes* or *no* for each item.

1. As a consumer of health care products and services, I understand that choices are influenced by a variety of factors.

2. I know my rights as a consumer.

3. I have regular medical and dental checkups.

4. I am knowledgeable about where to go for specific health concerns.

5. I read directions and warnings carefully before using any health care product.

6. I evaluate advertisements and confirm any health claims before purchasing a product.

7. I pay attention to the effectiveness of the health care products that I use and the medical treatments that I receive.

8. I know where and how to get help with a consumer problem.

9. I know about public health agencies and their functions.

10. I am aware of specific public health agencies in my community.

HEALTH Online

For instant feedback on your health status, go to Chapter 3 Health Inventory at **health.glencoe.com**.

Quick*Write*

Using Visuals. What is one way to make sure that you are purchasing the product that best meets your needs? Read the label. Make a list of the different types of information you have seen on product labels. How have you used this information to decide what to purchase?

Making Consumer Choices

VOCABULARY

**health consumer
media
advertising
comparison shopping
warranty
online shopping**

YOU'LL LEARN TO

- Identify the factors that influence consumer decisions about health care products and services.

- Analyze the health messages delivered through advertising in the media.

- Demonstrate ways to utilize criteria to evaluate health products for appropriateness.

⟶ QUICK START List five influences on your choice of health care products or services. Circle the two that most often affect your decisions.

▲ Part of being a wise consumer involves making informed purchasing decisions about health- and fitness-related products.

Many health care products and services are available to the consumer. Supermarket and drug store shelves are lined with dozens of well-known brands of personal care products. Phone books list hundreds of different types of health care professionals, clinics, and other health services. What information do you need before you make a decision regarding health care products and services?

Being an Informed Health Consumer

In the years to come, you will become more responsible for decisions regarding your health. Although most decisions about health services are still in the hands of your parents or guardians, you are probably already making choices about such products as shampoo, skin cleansers, or deodorant. Learning about available health products and services and understanding how to judge their effectiveness and reliability will help you become an informed health consumer. A **health consumer** is *anyone who purchases or uses health products or services.*

Influences on Your Decisions

Many factors influence your decision to buy specific products and services. Internal factors, such as habit and personal taste, can play a role, as can such external factors as the opinions of family members and friends, and cost. One important external factor that influences purchasing decisions is the **media**, or *the various methods of communicating information*. Television, radio, newspapers, magazines, and the Internet are all forms of media.

Media and Advertising

Many health products and services are promoted through advertising. **Advertising** is *a written or spoken media message designed to interest consumers in purchasing a product or service*. Advertisements provide information that can help you make purchasing decisions. Remember, however, that the primary purpose of advertising is to get your attention so that you will want to buy the product featured in the ad. **Figure 3.1** lists some of the techniques that advertisers use to convey a certain message to the consumer and persuade him or her to buy a product. These hidden messages are often designed to appeal to the emotions of potential buyers.

FIGURE 3.1

HIDDEN MESSAGES IN ADVERTISING

Advertisers use several techniques to persuade consumers to purchase their products.

Technique	Example	Hidden Message
Bandwagon	Group of people using a product or service	Everyone is using it—you should too.
Rich and famous	Product displayed in expensive home	It will make you feel rich and famous.
Free gifts	Redeemable coupons for merchandise	It's too good a deal to pass up.
Great outdoors	Scenes of nature	If it's associated with nature, it must be healthy.
Good times	People smiling and laughing	The product will add fun to your life.
Testimonial	People for whom a product has worked	It worked for them, so it will work for you, too.

Comparing Choices

Advertising is one source of information about products and services. However, keep in mind that this information may be misleading, since advertising is designed to inform and persuade you to purchase a product. As a consumer, how do you make wise purchasing decisions? One way is to comparison shop. **Comparison shopping** is *a method of judging the benefits of different products by comparing several factors, such as quality, features, and cost.* Here are some criteria to consider as you evaluate products and services.

Accessing product information before you go to the store makes comparison shopping easier. *Where can you find information on the safety and effectiveness of protective equipment?*

▶ **Cost.** Decide on a price range for your purchase. Then compare prices of the same brand or similar brands at different stores.

▶ **Features.** Decide which product features are important to you. This will allow you to avoid paying for features that you don't need and will help ensure that you purchase products with features that you find especially useful or desirable.

▶ **Quality.** Well-made products offer superior performance. An inexpensive product is no bargain if it falls apart or doesn't work.

▶ **Warranty.** Before you purchase a product, especially one that is costly, ask about the warranty. A **warranty** is *a company's or a store's written agreement to repair a product or refund your money should the product not function properly.* Always read a warranty in its entirety—including the fine print—and make sure that you understand its terms. Some warranties cover only certain aspects of a product or its use.

▶ **Safety.** Safety considerations should be foremost in your mind when choosing sports, recreation, or home-safety products.

- The **Underwriters Laboratory (UL)** is a product-safety testing and certification organization. The UL logo on electrical appliances, fire extinguishers, and other products indicates that the product has passed strict safety standards.

- **Snell,** a nonprofit foundation, and the **American National Standards Institute (ANSI)** monitor safety standards for helmets and other protective equipment. Look for their logos on any equipment you are thinking of buying.

▶ **Recommendations.** Talk to people who have used the product that you are considering purchasing. Parents or other trusted adults are good sources of information. Independent testing organizations such as the Consumers Union rate products.

Real-Life Application

Reading Product Labels

You can use the information on a product label to make an informed decision about whether to purchase the product. Study the label below, and then complete the activity for practice in evaluating products.

SPF 35 **SUNBUSTER LOTION**

ACTIVE INGREDIENTS: Avobenzone, Octocrylene, Octyl Salicylate, Oxybenzone

PRODUCT'S INTENDED USE: Provides protection against both UVA and UVB rays to help prevent sunburn, premature aging, and skin cancer.

PRECAUTIONS: Discontinue use if signs of irritation or rash appear. Avoid contact with eyes.

DIRECTIONS FOR USE: Apply liberally to all exposed areas before sun exposure. Waterproof for up to 80 minutes of swimming. Reapply after swimming, excessive perspiration, or vigorous activity.

MANUFACTURER'S CONTACT INFORMATION: Call **800-555-1234** Weekdays 9 a.m. to 9 p.m. Eastern Time.

- If two different brands have the same ingredients, which would be the wiser purchase?
- Why should a consumer read this section carefully?
- How can ignoring this section pose a risk to one's health?
- Why might a consumer need this information?

ACTIVITY

Bring in the container or label of a personal care product that you use. Draw the label on a large sheet of construction paper. Using the above sample as a guide, draw arrows and label the different types of information. Use online Internet or library resources to find out more about the product. Write this additional information on the back of the paper. Tell the class about your product. Discuss whether you will continue using this product, and explain why or why not.

PRODUCT LABELS

One way to compare two similar products is to read their labels. Important information on product labels includes the product's name and intended use, directions for use, precautions and warnings, manufacturer's information, and the amount in the container. On most labels you'll also find the ingredients listed by weight in descending order. The label will also identify the active ingredients— the ones that make the product effective. This means that when you are comparing two acne medications, for example, you can compare labels to determine which contains more of the active ingredient.

Your Rights as a Consumer

As a consumer you have certain rights, both before and after you purchase a product or service. **Figure 3.2** summarizes these rights. Usually, consumer rights are recognized and respected. Most stores and service providers strive to keep their customers satisfied. Sometimes, however, consumers need help resolving a complaint. You will learn more about how to handle consumer problems in Lesson 3.

Today's Consumer Choices

Consumers today have more choices than ever before when it comes to product selection and ways to shop. **Online shopping** involves *using the Internet to buy products and services.* Below are some points to consider when shopping online.

▶ **Price.** Online sources sometimes offer lower prices. However, some of these savings may be lost by the added cost of shipping.

▶ **Convenience.** Items are delivered directly to the home. For many people this convenience outweighs the potential problem of repackaging and mailing items that may need to be returned.

FIGURE 3.2

YOUR CONSUMER RIGHTS

- **The right to safety.** You have the right to purchase products and services that will not harm you or others.
- **The right to choose.** You have the right to select from many products at competitive prices.
- **The right to be informed.** You have the right to truthful information about products and services.
- **The right to be heard.** You have the right to join in the making of laws that govern buying and selling.
- **The right to have problems corrected.** You have the right to seek compensation when you have been treated unfairly.
- **The right to consumer education.** You have the right to learn the skills necessary to help you make wise choices.

▶ **Product information.** Online descriptions provide only limited information about a product, and you can only view a picture of an item—you can't actually examine it or try it on before you buy.

If you decide to purchase products online, there are some safeguards you should consider. First, get permission from your parents or guardians. Next, make sure that the site is secure. This means that information such as credit card numbers will not be accessible to others. Check the organization's return policy, and make sure that you understand it completely. Finally, write down any confirmation numbers or other information related to your purchase. You will need these numbers if a problem arises.

Ⓨ **Be sure to get your parents' or guardians' permission before ordering merchandise online.** *What else should you consider before placing an online order?*

 Lesson 1 *Review*

Reviewing Facts and Vocabulary

1. Why might some health messages delivered through advertising in the media be misleading?

2. What is a *warranty*? Why it is important to read a warranty in its entirety?

3. List three safeguards you should consider when shopping online.

Thinking Critically

4. **Synthesizing.** Demonstrate ways to utilize criteria to evaluate health products for appropriateness: What factors would you consider when deciding which of two bicycle helmets to buy? List the factors in order of importance.

5. **Analyzing.** Explain the advantages and disadvantages of seeking information about a product from someone who uses the product.

Applying Health Skills

Analyzing Influences. Recall a purchase you have made recently. List all the factors that influenced your decision. Include any advertising you have seen for the product, recommendations of family and friends, safety considerations (if any), and incentives such as coupons or sales. Review your list, circle the most influential factor, and explain why that factor was most important in your purchasing decision.

SPREADSHEETS Making a list is easy when you use a spreadsheet. See **health.glencoe.com** for help in using spreadsheet software.

Choosing Community Health Services

VOCABULARY

health care system
primary care physician
specialist
preventive care
health insurance
medical history

YOU'LL LEARN TO

- Identify situations requiring professional health services, such as primary and preventive care, for people of all ages.

- Identify, describe, and assess available health-related services in the community that relate to disease prevention and health promotion.

- Compare and analyze the cost, availability, and accessibility of health services for people of all ages.

QUICK START Identify three situations for which you might require professional health services, as well as the type of health care professional that would provide that service.

▲ Most schools require that a student get a physical exam before participating in a sports program.

Being a health-literate consumer means more than just being informed about products. It also involves understanding your options in health care services.

Types of Health Services

You have probably received immunizations and had your ears and eyes checked during health screenings. The health care professionals you have seen are part of a **health care system**, which includes *all the medical care available to a nation's people, the way they receive care, and the method of payment.* Health care can be divided into general care and specialized care. General care includes **primary care physicians**, or *medical doctors who provide physical checkups and general care,* as well as school nurses and dentists. Specialized care includes **specialists**, or *medical doctors trained to handle particular kinds of patients or medical conditions.* **Figure 3.3** lists a variety of health care specialists.

FIGURE 3.3

SOME HEALTH CARE SPECIALISTS

Specialist	Specializes In
Allergist	allergies
Dermatologist	skin diseases
Gynecologist	care of female reproductive system
Neurologist	nervous system problems
Oncologist	cancer
Ophthalmologist	care of eyes
Orthodontist	adjustments of teeth to improve bite and jaw alignment
Orthopedist	skeletal deformities or injuries
Pediatrician	primary care for children
Psychiatrist	mental health
Urologist	urinary tract problems

An orthopedist is a specialist who treats injuries of the skeletal system. *Describe the difference between a primary care physician and a specialist.*

Whenever you've seen a doctor for a checkup or a dentist for an oral exam, you've used preventive care. **Preventive care** involves *actions that prevent the onset of disease or injury.* Many teens have had preventive care in the form of vision and hearing screenings, sports physicals, and testing for scoliosis (a spinal disorder).

Facilities for Health Care Services

Communities may have more than one type of health care facility. The services provided by these facilities may be offered as inpatient care or outpatient care. *Inpatient care* requires the patient to stay at the facility overnight and is provided for patients with a serious injury or illness. *Outpatient care* allows the patient to be treated and then return home. Health care facilities include:

▶ **Private practices.** Physicians in private practice work for themselves. Most of their patients are seen at an office on an outpatient basis, although the physicians are usually associated with a hospital in case inpatient care is required.

▶ **Clinics.** Physicians may provide outpatient care in a community clinic rather than an office.

Health Skills Activity

Decision Making: Getting a Sports Physical

Dan and two of his friends have just signed up for cross-country.

"Hey, Dan," Brent says. "Mike and I are getting together to practice before the tryouts. Want to join us?"

"I'd like to," Dan answers, "but I haven't had my sports physical yet."

Mike says, "You don't need that to practice with Brent and me."

Dan replies, "I'll feel better about running if I have my physical first."

"Look, Dan," Brent says, "There's only a few days left before tryouts. You'd better get in some practice time, or you might not make the team."

Dan wonders what he should do.

What Would You Do?

Apply the steps to help Dan make a health-enhancing decision.

1. State the situation.
2. List the options.
3. Weigh the possible outcomes.
4. Consider values.
5. Make a decision and act.
6. Evaluate the decision.

▶ **Group practices.** Doctors in a group practice share office space, equipment, and support staff. Otherwise, they function in the same manner as those in private practice.

▶ **Hospitals.** Hospitals generally offer both inpatient and out-patient care. Some physicians work at the hospital. Those in private or group practice are there only when needed.

▶ **Emergency rooms.** Located within most hospitals, emergency rooms provide care for potentially life-threatening illnesses or injuries.

▶ **Urgent care centers.** These centers, staffed by primary care physicians, usually handle emergencies that are not life threatening. Patients may go to these centers if their primary care physician is unavailable or if they don't have one.

How People Pay for Health Services

Health care can be a major expense. Many families have some form of **health insurance**, *a plan in which private companies or government programs pay for part or all of a person's medical costs.* To maintain membership in such a plan, the insured person pays a periodic *premium,* or fee, for coverage. In conventional insurance plans, the insured person pays for doctor visits and other forms of treatment out of pocket. An *out-of-pocket expense* is one that the patient must pay for. The patient is then reimbursed by the insurance company for a fixed portion, often 80 percent of the cost of the visit. Hospital care is covered in much the same way. In most insurance plans, members must also pay a *deductible*. This is an amount a member must pay in out-of-pocket expenses before the plan will start reimbursing for health care services.

Managed Care

Some insurance plans are called *managed care plans*. These plans emphasize preventive care and offer reduced physician charges for their members in an attempt to control costs. There are several types of managed care plans:

▶ **Health Maintenance Organizations (HMOs).** Members of an HMO pay a monthly premium but receive most or all medical services with few or no out-of-pocket expenses. Some HMOs require a small co-payment for an office visit. Usually HMO members can see only those physicians who have signed an agreement with the HMO.

▶ **Preferred Provider Organizations (PPOs).** Medical providers connected with PPOs agree to charge the organization less than their regular fee for member usage. Members pay a monthly premium to use providers in the plan but can choose a provider outside the plan. Using outside providers, however, results in higher out-of-pocket expenses.

▶ **Point of Service (POS) plans.** Members of this type of plan can choose providers inside or outside the plan. Choosing an outside provider often results in higher premiums and higher out-of-pocket expenses.

How do people get health insurance?

There are several ways for people to obtain health insurance. Many people who work are insured through their employers. Often employees can choose from several plans to find the one that best meets their needs. Self-employed people often purchase their own insurance. People who cannot afford insurance may be covered by Medicaid, the federal government's medical insurance program.

Most managed care plans offer preventive health services to their members. *Why is preventive care important?*

Most health care providers request a medical history from their first-time patients.

Trends in Health Care

To help reduce expenses and improve the quality of care, the health community continually updates the types of care offered and the procedures used to implement care. Current trends include the following:

▶ **Birthing centers** are homelike settings that involve family members in the delivery of a baby. Birthing centers are usually less expensive than hospitals. However, they are appropriate only for women with low-risk pregnancies.

▶ **Drug treatment centers** specialize in treating people with drug and alcohol problems, usually outside of a hospital setting.

▶ **Continuing care and assisted living facilities** provide short- and long-term care for people who need help with daily tasks but who do not require professional medical care. Many older adults benefit from this kind of care.

▶ **Hospices** provide care for people who are terminally ill. Hospice workers are experts at managing pain and providing emotional support for the patient and his or her family.

▶ **Telemedicine** is the practice of medicine over distance through the use of telecommunications equipment. A medical specialist located hundreds of miles away can be brought into an examination room through a live interactive electronic system.

You and Your Health Care

A good doctor-patient relationship is critical to quality health care. This relationship requires open communication and a sense of trust. A health care professional can treat you and make recommendations for your health, but you need to take an active role in your medical care. Your relationship with your health care provider is a partnership—each of you must apply skills to effectively maintain your health. A good place to start is with an awareness of your own **medical history**, *complete and comprehensive information about your immunizations and any health problems you have had to date*. Most doctors' offices will ask you to fill out a medical history during your first visit. This form usually requires you to provide information about your own health habits, as well as the health of close family members. Ask your parents to help you obtain this information. The information in your medical history gives a health care provider an idea of your overall level of wellness.

Patient Skills

These tips can help you make the most out of your next medical appointment:

▶ Before you go, write down your reasons for seeing the doctor.

▶ While you are at the office, ask questions about any diagnoses, medications, or procedures that you do not understand or are unsure about.

▶ Inform the staff of any allergies you have or any medications you are taking. If a prescription is needed, this information can help the physician determine the right medication for you.

MEDICINE USE

If the physician prescribes a medicine for you, ask the pharmacist any questions you have about the medication. If the doctor recommends an over-the-counter medication, compare products by reading labels and make sure that you understand what symptoms each medicine is intended to treat.

A pharmacist is a reliable source of information about both prescription and over-the-counter medications. *What types of questions might you ask a pharmacist?*

Lesson 2 *Review*

Reviewing Facts and Vocabulary

1. Distinguish between *primary care physicians* and medical *specialists.*
2. Identify situations requiring primary and preventive care.
3. List three actions that can help you make the most of your next medical appointment.

Thinking Critically

4. **Analyzing.** Compare and analyze the cost, availability, and accessibility of health services for people who don't have health insurance.
5. **Applying.** The incidence of type 2 diabetes is increasing in teens in the United States. Some of the factors that lead to this disease are being overweight and inactive. How might information in a teen's medical history aid a health care professional in diagnosing this disease?

Applying Health Skills

Accessing Information. Use your local telephone book and other sources to identify available health-related services in your community that relate to disease prevention and health promotion. Make a table that describes and assesses each of these services.

SPREADSHEETS You can create a table by using spreadsheet software. For help in using spreadsheet software, see **health.glencoe.com.**

Managing Consumer Problems

VOCABULARY
fraud
health fraud
malpractice
consumer advocates

YOU'LL LEARN TO
- Identify potential problems with health care products and services.
- Understand how to resolve problems related to health care products and services.
- Explore methods for addressing critical health issues that result from fraud.

→ **QUICK START** Suppose that you purchased a new hair dryer that broke the first time you used it. Explain how you would deal with the problem.

Most health care products and services you purchase will live up to their claims. However, some products and services may be faulty, useless, or even potentially harmful. Thus, it's important to learn how to handle consumer problems.

Always keep your sales receipt. Some stores require receipts as part of their return policy, and many manufacturers require receipts to validate a product's warranty.

Problems with Products

Sometimes products are defective. Find out about a seller's return policy before purchasing a product. Many items can be returned to the store from which they were purchased. Others may need to be sent back to the manufacturer. Information in the product warranty will help you determine which course of action to follow. Before you attempt to return a product, reread the instructions to make sure that you are using the product correctly. If the product is truly defective, you must then decide whether you want a replacement or your money back. Put your reasons for returning the item in a letter, and keep a copy for future reference. Return the item in its original packaging. If you are mailing the item, be sure to get a shipping receipt to prove that you sent it.

Health Fraud

Fraud is *deliberate deceit or trickery.* Some individuals and businesses employ fraud to sell defective products or ineffective services. These people often go out of business as soon as consumer complaints expose them. **Health fraud**, also known as quackery, is the *sale of worthless products or services that claim to prevent diseases or cure other health problems.*

Fraudulent Products

Several types of products are particularly susceptible to health fraud:

▶ **Weight-loss products.** Ads for some diet pills, fad diets, and exercise equipment claim that a person can lose weight virtually overnight. Weight loss is effectively achieved only through healthful eating habits and regular physical activity.

▶ **Beauty and anti-aging products.** Many tooth whiteners, hair enhancers, and wrinkle creams may work temporarily, but none offer permanent results. Products that aren't approved by the Food and Drug Administration (FDA) may harm you.

Fraudulent Treatments

Another type of health fraud is clinics that specialize in "miracle" cures for ailments such as arthritis or that feature a remarkable and unusual treatment, such as consuming substances extracted from peach pits to cure cancer. These methods are ineffective and may even be dangerous. Of course, not all clinics offering specialized treatments are fraudulent. Check with a health care professional before seeking treatment at such a clinic.

OTHER PROBLEMS WITH HEALTH SERVICES

Some people experience problems with their regular health care providers. Sometimes these problems can be solved by changing health care professionals. Other concerns are more complicated. Health care professionals can sometimes be negligent or guilty of **malpractice**—*failure by a health professional to meet accepted standards.* To make sure that you are getting the best medical treatment possible, always get a second opinion from another health care professional for any major health concern, such as those involving surgery or other extensive treatment. If you have a serious problem with a health care professional, you may be able to get help from a regulatory organization such as the American Medical Association or from a state licensing board.

Having an open, trusting relationship with your health care provider can help resolve many concerns about a diagnosis or treatment. *Why should you get a second opinion for any serious health concern?*

Real-Life Application

Writing a Letter of Complaint

A carefully written letter of complaint can help secure fair treatment for yourself if a product or service does not meet your expectations. Study the letter and answer the questions. Then compose your own letter of complaint.

```
Name of Company
Street Address
City, State, ZIP code

Dear (contact person):

On (date), I (bought, had repaired)
a (name of product) at (location).
Unfortunately, your product has not
performed well. (state the problem).

To resolve the problem, I would appreciate
(state what you want—money back, exchange,
repair). Enclosed are copies (do not send
originals) of my records (include receipts
and other documents).

I look forward to your reply and a reso-
lution to the problem and will wait until
(set a time limit) before seeking help
from a consumer protection agency or the
Better Business Bureau. Please contact me
at (phone number and address).

Sincerely,

Your name (signed)
```

Why is it important to provide this information early in the letter?

Why do you need to be specific here? Why should you not send the original documents?

Why might mentioning a consumer protection agency or the Better Business Bureau make the company more likely to act on your letter?

Source: Federal Consumer Information Center, U.S. General Services Administration.

ACTIVITY

With a partner, identify a health care product with which you might not be or have not been satisfied. Develop a three-part complaint letter about the product, using the sample above as a guide. Read your completed letter to the class. Have your classmates evaluate the letter, and adjust it on the basis of their feedback.

Help for Consumer Problems

If you try to resolve a problem with a product and are dissatisfied with the result, seek help from one of these groups:

▶ **Business organizations** such as the Better Business Bureau (BBB) deal with complaints against local merchants. The core services of the BBB include dispute resolution and truth-in-advertising complaints.

▶ **Consumer advocates** are *people or groups whose sole purpose is to take on regional, national, and even international consumer issues.* Some groups, like the Consumers Union, test products, inform the public, and play a role in protecting consumers when problems arise. Others work to expose fraud and teach consumers about their rights and responsibilities.

▶ **Local, state, and federal government agencies** ensure that consumers' rights are protected. The federal government, for example, has established a number of specialized agencies that deal with health-related products and services. The Federal Trade Commission works to prevent false or deceptive advertising. The Food and Drug Administration ensures that medicines are safe, effective, and properly labeled. The Consumer Product Safety Commission protects consumers against harmful products and can recall dangerous ones. Small claims courts are state courts that handle legal disputes involving amounts of money below a certain limit. The consumer and the merchant present their case to a judge, who then makes a decision.

HEALTH Online

Go to **health.glencoe.com** to learn more about the U.S. Consumer Product Safety Commission.

Lesson 3 *Review*

Reviewing Facts and Vocabulary

1. Define the term *fraud.*
2. Under what circumstances might you want to seek a second medical opinion?
3. When might a person file suit in small claims court?

Thinking Critically

4. **Analyzing.** Why is health fraud considered one of the worst types of fraud?
5. **Evaluating.** List several criteria you would use to distinguish between an effective complaint against a health care product that didn't fulfill its claim and an ineffective complaint.

Applying Health Skills

Communication Skills. Imagine that your aunt sent away for a wrinkle cream that was "guaranteed to make you look ten years younger in only three weeks." After using the product for a month, she finds that not only does she not look younger, but her skin is red and irritated. Write a dialogue in which you explain to your aunt the likelihood that she is a victim of health fraud and explore methods for addressing this critical health issue.

TECHNOLOGY *OPTION*

WORD PROCESSING Use word-processing software to write and edit your dialogue. For help in using word-processing software, see **health.glencoe.com**.

Understanding Public Health Services

VOCABULARY
public health
epidemiology

YOU'LL LEARN TO
- Analyze the impact of the availability of health services in the community and the world.
- Explain the benefits of positive relationships among community health professionals in promoting a healthy community.

> **QUICK START** On a sheet of paper, list a few public health agencies with which you are familiar. What service does each provide to the public?

▲ Non-profit organizations like the American Red Cross promote community health in various ways.

Thanks to advances in **public health**, *a community-wide effort to monitor and promote the welfare of the population,* Americans are living longer, healthier lives.

Public Health Agencies

Public health issues are addressed at the local, national, and global level.

Health at the Local Level

State, county, and city health departments focus on disease prevention. Their functions include overseeing standards for water and sewage systems, waste disposal, and the sanitation of restaurants. A local health inspector, for example, may close a restaurant for failing a routine inspection. Nonprofit agencies have local chapters that are devoted to particular health concerns. The March of Dimes, for example, works to reduce birth defects.

Health at the National Level

Several agencies also work at the national level to protect health.

▶ **The National Cancer Institute (NCI)** is the federal government's principal agency for **cancer** research.

▶ **The Environmental Protection Agency (EPA)** is responsible for protecting the country's air, water, and land.

▶ The U.S. Department of Labor's **Occupational Safety and Health Administration (OSHA)** works to prevent injuries and safeguard the health of workers across the country.

▶ **The United States Department of Agriculture (USDA)** leads the federal antihunger effort with food stamp, school lunch, and school breakfast programs. One agency of the USDA, the **Food Safety and Inspection Service (FSIS),** is responsible for the safety of meat, poultry, and egg products.

▶ **The Department of Health and Human Services (DHHS)** oversees more than 300 health-related programs. These programs are administered by 13 agencies, which include the following:

• **The Centers for Medicare and Medicaid Services (CMS)** administer federal insurance programs, which help provide health care to low-income and elderly Americans.

• **The Food and Drug Administration (FDA)** ensures the safety of food, drugs, and cosmetics.

• **The National Institutes of Health (NIH)** conduct medical research and provide funding for medical research carried out at other institutions.

• **The Substance Abuse and Mental Health Services Administration (SAMHSA)** provides programs that aid substance abusers and people with mental/emotional disorders.

• **The Centers for Disease Control and Prevention (CDC)** conduct research and collect data that help control the spread of diseases. Part of the CDC's job involves **epidemiology,** or *the scientific study of patterns of disease in a population.*

• **The Federal Trade Commission (FTC)** was established to enforce antitrust and consumer protection laws. The FTC works to promote fair competition in the nation's markets and to ensure that consumers are given the right to make informed choices.

hot link

cancer To learn more about cancer, see Chapter 26, page 681.

OSHA inspectors work to prevent injuries and protect the health of workers in the United States. *How might periodic inspections of a workplace help ensure workers' safety?*

Raising Awareness of Public Health Programs

In this activity your group will create a public service announcement (PSA) to highlight the mission of a public health agency or program.

What You'll Need

- paper and pen
- telephone directory (one per group)
- Internet access (optional)

What You'll Do

1. In your group, examine the list of agencies in the "Government" section of the phone directory. Agencies will often list specific offices that indicate what they do, such as "Lead Poisoning Program" or "Food Safety."

2. Find out the mission and history of one agency or office. What health problems does this agency seek to address? What services does it provide? If possible, research this information online.

3. Write a PSA script that promotes the agency or office. Make sure that you convey how this agency promotes public health. Target the message to high-school students.

4. Arrange with your teacher and school administrators to present your PSA to your school.

Apply and Conclude

As a class, brainstorm a list of other ways of highlighting the contributions of public-health agencies or programs. Then write a paragraph describing the importance of raising people's awareness of these organizations and programs.

Public Health on a Global Scale

Some countries don't have the medical technologies or services that are available in the United States and other developed nations. War, drought, floods, or other crises can lead to starvation, unsanitary living conditions, and uncontrolled disease. Government agencies and private organizations from around the world extend aid to developing countries in times of crisis. One key organization is the World Health Organization (WHO). An agency of the United Nations with a membership of nearly 200 countries and territories, WHO has programs to eradicate diseases such as polio and cholera and to address pollution. Another organization, the International Committee of the Red Cross, provides emergency aid to victims of armed conflict, disease outbreaks, and natural disasters.

FIGURE 3.4

ADVOCATING FOR PUBLIC HEALTH

There are many ways that teens can advocate for public health.
Here are just a few:

- Follow all health and safety laws and ordinances; for example, keep your immunizations up to date.
- Set an example by practicing healthful behaviors, such as always wearing a helmet when biking or skating.
- Avoid actions that could endanger the health or safety of others, such as reckless driving.
- Get involved in events that promote public health. Participating in events such as community walks or 10K runs for charity improves your own health as well as the health of others.
- Find out which community groups deal with public health issues. Identify their goals and support them.
- Inform the proper authorities if you notice a condition or activity that threatens public health.

Advocacy—Taking Action for Public Health

Individuals can play a critical role in promoting public health. **Figure 3.4** lists some of the ways you can help promote public health in your own community.

Lesson 4 *Review*

Reviewing Facts and Vocabulary

1. Define the term *public health*.
2. Identify the public health agency that provides insurance programs for low-income and older Americans.
3. List two organizations that work to maintain world health.

Thinking Critically

4. **Applying.** Why might restaurant inspections be handled by government agencies rather than the restaurants themselves?
5. **Analyzing.** Analyze the impact of the availability of health services in the community and the world.

Applying Health Skills

Accessing Information. Research public-health agencies in your community. Make a four-column chart in which you list the name of each agency, describe what each one does, tell whether each is a government or private agency, and describe opportunities for volunteering to advocate for public health. Share this information with your class.

SPREADSHEETS Making a table is easy when you use a spreadsheet. Find help in using spreadsheets at **health.glencoe.com**.

Today's "Health Beat"

Many newspapers have a health beat or a health section. What kinds of health topics do newspapers cover? How does your local newspaper compare with newspapers in other locations? In this activity, you will examine the health coverage in various newspapers and consider the impact that increased coverage of health topics may have on a community or state or on the nation as a whole.

- **Name of newspaper:**
- **Date:**
- **Title of health article:**
- **Type of article:** (preventive health, nutrition, fitness, disease outbreaks, federal or state legislative health issues, and so on)
- **Length of article:**
- **Intended audience:** (youths, older adults, males/females, registered voters, legislators or government officials, African Americans, Hispanic Americans, other minority groups, and so on)
- **Brief summary:**

ACTIVITY

Choose a specific newspaper, and look through it for health articles or the health section. Examine articles in two different editions of the newspaper you've selected, recording information about each article in a chart like the one above. Compare the information you have collected with others. In a class discussion, consider the following questions: How does the health coverage in the newspaper you examined compare with that in other papers? Do the papers cover the same kinds of topics? Do they devote similar amounts of space to health topics?

EXPRESS YOUR VIEWS

Use the questions as a starting point for a one-page opinion paper: Why do you think media coverage of health topics has increased in recent years? What impact might increased coverage of health topics have on your community or state or on the nation as a whole?

CROSS-CURRICULUM CONNECTIONS

Publish a Newspaper. As a class, create a newspaper that includes news stories and feature articles on health products and services as well as editorials on consumer health concerns that are relevant to teens. Your teacher will organize the class into teams and assign each team a news beat. Create a final product, and obtain permission to distribute your publication to the entire school.

Give an Oral Report. Consumer and health advocacy groups safeguard citizens from unreliable or hazardous products and services. Select and research an independent testing source such as the Consumers Union, a government agency such as the Federal Trade Commission, or a consumer activist such as Ralph Nader. Determine what led to the development of the organization or what motivated the individual to become a consumer activist. Give a short oral report to your class.

Calculate the Better Value. You are trying to decide which brand of energy drink to buy. One ounce equals 0.029574 liters. Zippy is $1.50 for 32 ounces; Get-Going is $1.35 for a liter. Assuming that both products have the same ingredients in the same proportions, which is the better deal?

Conduct Research. Chlorofluorocarbons (CFCs) were once used as aerosol propellants in health care products such as deodorant. In the 1970s it was determined that CFCs were significantly depleting the ozone layer, and their use has been progressively banned throughout the world. Research the history of the use of CFCs and the legislation enacted to eliminate the use of these and other ozone-depleting substances.

CAREER Corner

Public Health Specialist

Are you interested in a career in health education and wellness? Do you have a real concern for the welfare of your community? If so, then a career as a public health specialist might be a good choice for you.

To enter this profession, you need a bachelor's degree with a specialization in a biological, medical, or physical science; food science or technology; chemistry; nutrition; engineering; epidemiology; or another related scientific field. For more information on this and other health careers, click on Career Corner at **health.glencoe.com**.

➤ EXPLORING HEALTH TERMS *Answer the following questions on a sheet of paper.*

Lesson 1 *Match each definition with the correct term.*

advertising   media
comparison shopping   online shopping
health consumer   warranty

1. Anyone who purchases or uses health products or services.
2. Using the Internet to buy products and services.
3. A method of judging the benefits of different products by comparing several similar factors for each one.
4. The various methods of communicating information.

Lesson 2 *Fill in the blanks with the correct term.*

health care system   preventive care
health insurance   primary care physician
medical history   specialist

5. The _____ includes all the medical care available to a nation's people, the way they receive care, and the method of payment.
6. Actions that prevent the onset of disease or injury are known as _____ .
7. _____ is a plan in which private companies or government programs pay for part or all of a person's medical costs.
8. Complete and comprehensive information about your immunizations and any health problems you have had to date is your _____ .

Lesson 3 *Replace the underlined words with the correct term.*

consumer advocate   health fraud
fraud   malpractice

9. Deliberate deceit or trickery is <u>malpractice</u>.
10. When a health care professional fails to meet accepted medical standards, he or she is guilty of <u>consumer advocacy</u>.
11. A person or group whose sole purpose is to take on regional, national, and even international consumer issues is a <u>health fraud</u>.

Lesson 4 *Answer each question with the correct term.*

epidemiology   public health

12. What is a community-wide effort to monitor and promote the welfare of the population?
13. What is the scientific study of patterns of disease in a population?

➤ RECALLING THE FACTS *Use complete sentences to answer the following questions.*

Lesson 1

1. List two internal factors that can influence your buying decisions.
2. List three techniques advertisers use to persuade consumers to buy their products.
3. How are ingredients listed on a product label?

Lesson 2

4. Describe the health care that is provided by emergency rooms and urgent care centers.
5. What is a deductible?
6. Why do health care professionals have new patients fill out a medical history?

Lesson 3

7. List the steps to follow before you try to return a product.
8. What should you do if you have an unresolved problem with a health care provider?
9. Which government office can recall a dangerous product from the marketplace?

Lesson 4

10. What is the focus of state, county, and city health departments?
11. Identify the federal government's principal agency for cancer research.
12. List three ways you can advocate for public health.

➤ THINKING CRITICALLY

1. **Synthesizing.** Think of a health-related product or service that you recently purchased. What factors influenced your decision to buy the product or service? Distinguish between the internal and external factors. *(LESSON 1)*

2. **Evaluating.** What advantages over a private practice would a group practice provide a physician who is just starting out? *(LESSON 2)*

3. **Applying.** Jerome bought an exercise machine that promised to produce "rock-hard abs" in only three weeks. He used the machine according to the instructions, but after a month he was dissatisfied with the results. What conclusion might he draw from this experience? *(LESSON 3)*

4. **Analyzing.** What benefits are gained from positive relationships among community health professionals in promoting a healthy community? Explain your answer. *(LESSON 4)*

➤ HEALTH SKILLS APPLICATION

1. **Accessing Information.** Investigate a type of health-related product, such as a piece of sports equipment or a sports drink. Choose three products in that category and compare costs, quality, and any other appropriate factors. After you have done your research, decide which item you would purchase and explain why. *(LESSON 1)*

2. **Practicing Healthful Behaviors.** Identify those actions you presently take that could be considered preventive care. What additional actions could you take to protect yourself from disease? *(LESSON 2)*

3. **Advocacy.** Create an awareness campaign to help educate older adults in your community about the problem of health fraud. You may wish to create a poster, newsletter, or videotape to present your health message. *(LESSON 3)*

4. **Accessing Information.** Interview the manager of a local restaurant. Find out what state and local health laws the restaurant must follow. Share the information with your class. *(LESSON 4)*

✦ *BEYOND* the Classroom

Parent Involvement

Interpersonal Communication. Sit down with your parents, and discuss their choice in health insurance plans. Talk about the plan's coverage, costs of premiums, choices in physicians, and any out-of-pocket expenses your parents might incur. If your parents have no insurance, discuss with them what you have found out about health insurance plans in class.

School and Community

Community Health Services. Research a health service for people of all ages that is available in your community. Identify its purpose, funding, and programs. Find out what volunteer opportunities, if any, are available at the organization. Summarize your findings in a one-page report that you present to the class.

Chapter 4

Physical Activity for Life

What's Your Health Status?

Read each statement below and respond by writing *yes, no,* or *sometimes* for each item. Write *yes* only for items that you practice regularly.

1. I participate in some form of physical activity every day.

2. Whenever possible, I walk rather than drive or get a ride.

3. My level of physical activity helps me maintain a healthy weight range.

4. I enjoy a wide variety of physical activities and sports.

5. I participate in aerobic activities such as cycling, swimming, or in-line skating.

6. I follow a nutritious diet; avoid harmful substances such as tobacco, alcohol, and other drugs; and get adequate rest.

7. I do at least 20 minutes of nonstop vigorous exercise a minimum of three times a week.

8. When I buy athletic equipment, safety is a primary consideration.

9. I take proper precautions to minimize the risk of injury while engaging in physical activities.

10. I know and follow safety rules for the activities in which I participate.

HEALTH Online

For instant feedback on your health status, go to Chapter 4 Health Inventory at **health.glencoe.com**.

Quick *Write*

Using Visuals. You know that being active is important to your physical health, but do you realize how it affects your mental/emotional and social health? Give two examples of how the physical activity pictured here helps these teens keep their health triangles in balance.

Physical Activity and Your Health

VOCABULARY

physical activity
physical fitness
sedentary
   lifestyle
osteoporosis
metabolism

YOU'LL LEARN TO

• Understand the importance of regular physical activity for enhancing and maintaining personal health throughout the life span.

• Examine the effects of regular physical activity on body systems.

• Analyze the relationship between regular physical activity and disease prevention.

• Discover ways to incorporate physical activity into daily life.

QUICK START On a sheet of paper, make a list of the physical activities in which you participate on a regular basis. Then add to your list three others you would like to try. Briefly describe why each of these activities appeals to you.

What kinds of physical activities do you enjoy? Do you like to play basketball? Maybe you prefer skiing, riding mountain bikes, or playing volleyball. Whatever your preference, regular physical activity enhances your health.

Tasks such as vacuuming, raking leaves, or washing the car can help you fit more physical activity into your life. *What physical activities do you include in your daily routine?*

What Is Physical Activity?

Physical activity is *any form of movement that causes your body to use energy.* It may be purposeful, such as when you exercise or play sports. It may also occur as part of your regular routine—for example, when you wash the car or take the dog for a walk. Many forms of physical activity can improve your level of **physical fitness**, *the ability to carry out daily tasks easily and have enough reserve energy to respond to unexpected demands.* Maintaining a high level of physical fitness gives you a sense of total well-being and is an important lifelong health goal.

What Are the Benefits of Physical Activity?

Physical activity provides health benefits that last a lifetime. It helps strengthen not only the physical but also the mental/emotional and social sides of your health triangle.

Benefits to Physical Health

Physical activity makes your body stronger, increases your energy, and improves your posture. It can reduce chronic fatigue and stiffness and can improve motor responses. It strengthens your muscles and bones and helps reduce the risk of many serious diseases.

Regular physical activity also contributes to the functioning of many body systems, including the following:

▶ **Cardiovascular System.** Regular physical activity strengthens the heart muscle, allowing it to pump blood more efficiently.

▶ **Respiratory System.** When you engage in regular physical activity, your respiratory system begins to work more efficiently—you can breathe larger amounts of air, and the muscles used in respiration don't tire as quickly. This helps you perform such activities as running farther without getting out of breath.

▶ **Nervous System.** By helping you respond more quickly to stimuli, physical activity can improve your reaction time. This is especially helpful when driving or cycling.

hot link

cardiovascular and respiratory systems To learn more about the cardiovascular and respiratory systems, see Chapter 16, page 414.
nervous system For more information on the nervous system, see Chapter 15, page 399.

Benefits to Mental/Emotional Health

Being physically active has many positive effects on your mental/emotional health. It can help reduce stress. Doing some stretching exercises before bed, for example, can help you relax tense muscles and sleep better after a difficult day at school. Physical activity also allows you to manage anger or frustration in a healthy way. By stimulating the release of certain chemicals that affect the brain, physical activity can improve your

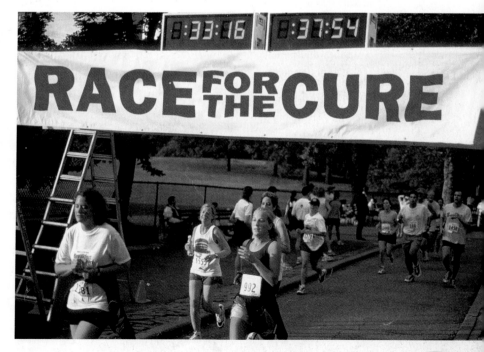

Participating in a community event such as the one shown here is a good way to be physically active, to help others, and to engage in positive social interaction.

mood and decrease your risk of depression. Other ways that physical activity benefits your mental/emotional health include

▶ helping you look and feel better, which can increase your self-confidence.

▶ contributing to a positive self-concept by giving you a sense of pride and accomplishment in taking care of yourself.

▶ reducing mental fatigue by bringing more oxygen to the brain. This improves your concentration, allowing you to think more clearly and work more productively.

▶ giving you a "can-do" spirit when faced with new challenges.

Hands-On Health ACTIVITY

Promote the Benefits of Physical Activity

In this **activity** you will think of ways that different **activities** benefit all three parts of the health **triangle**. Then you'll choose an activity **and create** a plan to try it out.

What You'll Need

- paper **and** pencil
- **markers** or colored pencils

What You'll Do

1. Make a four-column chart on a sheet of paper. Label the columns "Activity," "Physical," "Mental/Emotional," and "Social."

2. Work in a group of three. Take turns identifying and recording a physical activity that you enjoy. Then work together to think of a physical, mental/emotional, and social benefit of each activity listed. Record these in the appropriate columns.

3. Choose one of the activities on your chart. Using markers or colored pencils, create an ad that illustrates the physical, mental/emotional, and social benefits of that activity. Present your finished ad to the class.

Apply and Conclude

Based on class presentations, choose an activity that you're interested in but have never tried. Write a plan to try the activity to see if you like it.

Benefits to Social Health

Are you a member of a recreational or school team? Do you swim laps at a neighborhood pool? Do you like hiking or exploring trails in your community? If so, you have probably met—and possibly formed friendships with—others who share your interests. Participating in a fitness regimen with friends can be fun and may motivate you to stick with your fitness program; in turn, you can help motivate your friends. Physical activity can also benefit social health by

▶ building self-confidence, which helps you cope better in social situations, such as when you meet new people.

▶ giving you the opportunity to interact and cooperate with others.

▶ helping you manage stress, which can enhance your relationships with others.

Risks of Physical Inactivity

According to the Centers for Disease Control and Prevention (CDC), some teens do not make physical activity a part of their lives. The CDC's findings, compiled in its *CDC Fact Book 2000/2001*, include these troubling facts about the level of physical activity among U.S. high school students.

▶ More than one in three teens (35 percent) do *not* participate regularly in vigorous physical activity (that is, for at least 20 minutes three times a week).

▶ Regular participation in vigorous physical activity declines significantly during the teen years, from 73 percent of ninth graders to 61 percent of twelfth graders.

▶ Only 29 percent of teens attend a daily physical education class—a serious decline from 42 percent in 1991.

Clearly, many teens have a **sedentary lifestyle**, or *a way of life that involves little physical activity.* They may spend much of their time watching TV, playing video games, or working on the computer rather than being physically active. The negative effects of a sedentary lifestyle may include

▶ unhealthful weight gain, which is linked to several potentially life-threatening conditions, including cardiovascular disease, type 2 diabetes, and cancer. Cardiovascular disease is the leading cause of death among Americans. **Diabetes** is a serious disorder that prevents the body from converting food into energy.

CHARACTER CHECK

Responsibility. When you participate in regular physical activity, you take responsibility for your health. By taking care of yourself, you are saying that you are worth investing in. Be positive about the benefits these activities bring you, and don't forget to compliment yourself: "I like how I feel, and I like how I look!" **Write three other positive statements that reflect the benefits you receive from regular physical activity.**

hotlink

diabetes For more information on reducing your risk of developing diabetes, see Chapter 26, page 691.

▶ an increased risk of **osteoporosis**, *a condition characterized by a decrease in bone density, producing porous and fragile bones.* Porous and fragile bones fracture more easily than healthy bones.

▶ a reduced ability to manage stress.

▶ decreased opportunities to meet and form friendships with active people who value and live a healthy lifestyle.

You can lower your risk of these and many other health problems by including more physical activity in your daily life. For example, when you go shopping, walk to the store or, if you have to drive, park farther away from the entrance. **Figure 4.1** suggests other healthful alternatives to sedentary activities.

FIGURE 4.1

APPROACHES TO EVERYDAY ACTIVITIES

Instead of . . .	Try . . .
• Taking an elevator or escalator	• Taking the stairs
• Playing video or computer games	• Playing soccer, basketball, or tennis
• Getting a ride to a friend's house	• Walking, skating, or riding your bike there
• Using a shopping cart	• Carrying groceries to the car
• Watching TV or taking a nap	• Gardening or mowing the lawn
• Taking the car through a car wash	• Washing the car yourself

Physical Activity and Weight Control

The CDC reports that more than one-half of American adults and 14 percent of teens are overweight. This situation can be traced to a sedentary lifestyle and overeating. To stay within a weight range that is healthy for you, it's important to develop good eating habits and be physically active on a regular basis.

Understanding how the food you eat gets converted into energy can help you maintain a healthy weight. **Metabolism** is *the process by which your body gets energy from food.* Food's energy value is measured in units of heat called calories. Your body needs a sufficient number of calories each day to function properly. Additional calories must be burned through physical activity or they will be stored in the body as fat. When you are physically active, your metabolic rate rises and your body burns more calories than when it is at rest. The number of calories burned depends in part on the nature of the activity. When you stop being active, your metabolic rate slowly returns to normal. For several hours afterward, however, you continue to burn more calories than you did before you began the activity.

Hiking is a physical activity that you can enjoy throughout your life. *Name two safety considerations to keep in mind while hiking.*

Fitting Physical Activity into Your Life

Health professionals recommend that teens incorporate 60 minutes of moderate physical activity into their daily lives. This may sound difficult, but it doesn't have to be. Any activities that get you moving count toward your daily total. For example, walk or bike to school instead of getting a ride. Suggest to your family that you go for a hike or a swim on the weekend. Organize a basketball game with friends. Be sure to include some activities that you can participate in throughout your life. Hiking, swimming, golfing, biking, racquetball, tennis, and bowling are just a few examples of lifelong activities.

 Lesson 1 *Review*

Reviewing Facts and Vocabulary

1. What is the difference between *physical activity* and *physical fitness*?
2. Examine and briefly describe the effects of regular physical activity on three body systems.
3. Analyze the relationship between regular physical activity and disease prevention.

Thinking Critically

4. **Analyzing.** Explain why watching television and walking affect metabolism differently.
5. **Synthesizing.** Why does it take longer to get the maximum health benefit from a leisurely walk than from swimming laps?

Applying Health Skills

Advocacy. Design a pamphlet with eye-catching headlines and graphics to educate younger students about the importance of physical activity. Your pamphlet should encourage and guide them to determine and then participate in the types of physical activity best suited to their interests and abilities.

WORD PROCESSING Word processing can give your pamphlet a professional look. See **health.glencoe.com** for tips on how to get the most from your word-processing program.

Fitness and You

VOCABULARY

**cardiorespiratory
  endurance
muscular strength
muscular endurance
flexibility
body composition
exercise
aerobic exercise
anaerobic exercise**

YOU'LL LEARN TO

- Identify and describe the five areas of health-related fitness.

- Examine the relationship among body composition, diet, and fitness.

- Understand how to improve each of the five areas of health-related fitness.

- Examine the effects of fitness on body systems.

→) **QUICK
START**   What does it mean to be physically fit? Write "Physical Fitness" at
the top of a sheet of paper. Then write all the ways you can think of to describe a
person's level of physical fitness.

Do you have trouble running a mile even though you work out three times a week? Does your best friend excel at track but have a hard time doing push-ups? As you can see from these examples, every person's level of physical fitness is different.

Elements of Fitness

To have total fitness, you need to take into account the five areas of health-related fitness. These are the areas that affect your overall health and well-being.

**These teens are improving
their fitness levels.** *Explain
how this activity improves
cardiorespiratory
endurance.*

▶ **Cardiorespiratory endurance**—*the ability of the heart, lungs, and blood vessels to utilize and send fuel and oxygen to the body's tissues during long periods of moderate-to-vigorous activity.*

▶ **Muscular strength**—*the amount of force a muscle can exert.*

▶ **Muscular endurance**—*the ability of the muscles to perform physical tasks over a period of time without becoming fatigued.*

▶ **Flexibility**—*the ability to move a body part through a full range of motion.*

▶ **Body composition**—*the ratio of body fat to lean body tissue, including muscle, bone, water, and connective tissue such as ligaments, cartilage, and tendons.*

Various activities and tests can help you evaluate each area of fitness. When you know your strengths and weaknesses, you can take steps to improve your physical fitness through exercise. **Exercise** is *purposeful physical activity that is planned, structured, and repetitive and that improves or maintains personal fitness.*

Measuring Cardiorespiratory Endurance

Cardiovascular disease is the leading cause of death in the United States. Keeping your cardiovascular system healthy is the most effective way of reducing your risk of developing this life-threatening disease. Cardiovascular health depends on maintaining good cardiorespiratory endurance. Can you run a mile without stopping or hike for most of the day without getting tired? If so, you have good cardiorespiratory endurance.

CARDIORESPIRATORY ENDURANCE—STEP TEST

The three-minute step test can be used to measure your cardiorespiratory endurance. This test enables you to determine the rate at which your heart beats following a period of physical activity.

1. Use a sturdy bench about 12 inches high. Fully extending each leg as you step, step up with your right foot and then with your left. Then step down with your right foot first.

2. Repeat at the rate of 24 steps per minute for three minutes.

3. Take your pulse. To do this, find a pulse point on your wrist using the first two fingers of your other hand. *Do not use the thumb, which has its own pulse.* If you have trouble finding the pulse in your wrist, try finding the pulse point in your neck just below your jaw. Count the number of beats you feel for one minute.

4. Find your pulse rate on the chart to evaluate your cardiorespiratory endurance.

Measuring Muscular Strength and Endurance

You need muscular strength for activities that involve lifting, pushing, or jumping and muscular endurance to perform such activities repeatedly. Having good muscular strength and endurance gives you the necessary power to carry out your daily tasks without becoming fatigued. People with good muscular strength and endurance often have better posture and fewer back problems.

V **As you do the step test, your heart rate increases.** *Explain why physical activity causes your heart to beat faster.*

STEP TEST SCORING CHART	
Beats/ Minute	Rating
85–95	Excellent
96–105	Good
106–125	Fair
126 or more	Needs Improvement

Curl-ups measure abdominal strength. *How might abdominal strength improve your posture?*

CURL-UPS HEALTHY RANGE SCORING CHART

Age	Male	Female
13	21 or more	18 or more
14+	24 or more	18 or more

The arm hang is used to measure upper body strength and endurance. *What are the benefits of having good upper body strength and endurance?*

ARM HANG HEALTHY RANGE SCORING CHART

Age	Male (Time in Seconds)	Female (Time in Seconds)
12	7–14	7–14
13–15	12–20	7–14

ABDOMINAL MUSCLE STRENGTH AND ENDURANCE—CURL-UPS

The body has different muscle groups, so there are different ways to measure muscular strength and endurance. Curl-ups often are used to measure abdominal strength.

1. Lie on your back with your knees bent at about a 45-degree angle and your feet slightly apart. Position your arms at your sides.

2. With your heels flat on the floor, curl your shoulders slowly off the ground, moving your arms forward toward your feet as you rise.

3. Slowly return to the original position. Do one curl-up every three seconds; continue until you can't do any more at the specified pace.

4. Find your score on the chart to rate your abdominal strength.

UPPER BODY STRENGTH AND ENDURANCE—ARM HANG

The arm hang is one test that is used to measure upper body strength and endurance. For this test, work with two other people.

1. Grasp the horizontal bar with your palms facing away from you.

2. Raise your body so that your chin is above the bar and your elbows are flexed to hold your chest near the bar. One person should act as a spotter to make sure that you are not swinging as you hang from the bar.

3. Hold the position described in Step 2 for as long as possible. The third person will time you with a stopwatch and will stop the watch if your chin touches the bar, your head tilts backward, or your chin falls below the bar.

4. Compare your score with those in the chart to rate your upper body strength and endurance.

Measuring Flexibility

When sitting on the floor with your legs outstretched, can you reach forward and touch your toes? If so, you have good flexibility. Being flexible can increase your athletic performance, help you feel more comfortable, and reduce the risk of muscle strains and other injuries. It can also help prevent lower back problems. Some track and field events, gymnastics, ballet and other forms of dance, figure skating, and the martial arts require a great deal of flexibility.

BODY FLEXIBILITY—SIT-AND-REACH

You can use the back saver sit-and-reach test, developed by the Cooper Institute of Aerobics Research in Dallas, Texas, to assess the flexibility of your lower back and the backs of your thighs. Before taking the test, do some light stretching to warm up your muscles.

1. Tape a yardstick on top of a 12-inch-high box so that it protrudes 9 inches toward you. The "zero" end should be nearest you. Put the back of the box against a wall.

2. Sit on the floor. Remove your shoes, and fully extend one leg so that the sole of your foot is flat against the side of the box beneath the yardstick. Bend your other knee so that your foot is flat on the floor two to three inches from the side of the extended leg.

3. Place the palm of one hand over the back of the other hand. Extend your arms over the yardstick, reaching forward as far as you can.

4. Repeat Step 3 four times. On the fourth try, hold the position for at least one second and notice where your fingertips are on the yardstick. Record your score to the nearest inch.

5. Switch the position of your legs and repeat the test.

6. Find your scores on the chart to determine your flexibility.

SIT-AND-REACH HEALTHY RANGE SCORING CHART	
Gender	Number of Inches
Male	8
Female	10 (ages 13–14) 12 (ages 15+)

Measuring Body Composition

Being physically active and eating a balanced diet can improve the way you look. These healthful practices can also help you avoid the health problems associated with being overweight. To look and feel your best, it is helpful to have some idea of your body composition—that is, how much of your body is composed of fat and how much is composed of everything else. In general, males with 25 percent or more body fat and females with 30 percent or more body fat are at risk of developing cardiovascular problems. Carrying too much weight also places added stress on the skeletal system. To maintain a healthy body composition, eat a nutritious, balanced diet and participate in regular physical activity.

The "pinch test" is a common method of determining body composition. It is conducted with a tool called a *skinfold caliper*, a gauge that measures the thickness of the fat beneath a fold of skin. The tester measures folds of skin on three to seven different parts of the body, usually including the back of a shoulder, the back of an arm, the abdomen, hip, and thigh. The average of the measurements is then calculated to estimate the total proportion of body fat.

Improving Your Fitness

You can choose from many different physical activities and exercises to improve your fitness level, but most fall into one of two categories: aerobic exercise or anaerobic exercise. **Aerobic exercise** is *any activity that uses large muscle groups, is rhythmic in nature, and can be maintained continuously for at least 10 minutes three times a day or for 20 to 30 minutes at one time.* Examples of aerobic exercise include running, cycling, swimming, and dancing.

The pinch test is often used to determine how much of a person's body is composed of fat.

Real-Life Application

Targeting Cardiovascular Fitness

Use these steps to find your target heart range—the ideal range for your heart rate during aerobic activity. Then do the activity to help you apply this information.

Maximum target heart rate. Exercising above this rate can result in injury.

Target heart range. To safely build cardiorespiratory endurance, keep your heart rate within this range. Take your pulse for 6 seconds and multiply this number by 10 to determine the number of beats per minute.

Minimum target heart rate. Exercising below this rate will not build cardiorespiratory endurance.

ACTIVITY

Prepare a written plan describing how you will apply this information. Include your target heart range (with your calculations), two aerobic activities, how you will check your heart rate while you are doing each activity, and how you will keep your heart rate within the target range.

Finding Your Target Heart Range

1. Sit quietly for five minutes, and then take your pulse. This is your resting heart rate. Suppose that it is 66 beats per minute.
2. Subtract your age from 220 to find your maximum heart rate. For example, if you are 16, your maximum heart rate will be 204.
3. Subtract your resting heart rate from your maximum heart rate. (Example: 204 − 66 = 138)
4. Multiply the number you arrived at in Step 3 by 60 percent and again by 85 percent. Round to the nearest whole numbers. (Example: 138 × 0.60 = 83; 138 × 0.85 = 117)
5. Add your resting heart rate to the numbers you arrived at in Step 4. (Example: 83 + 66 = 149; 117 + 66 = 183) The resulting totals represent your target heart range (between 149 and 183).

Anaerobic exercise involves *intense short bursts of activity in which the muscles work so hard that they produce energy without using oxygen.* Running a 100-meter dash and lifting weights are examples of anaerobic exercises.

Improving Cardiorespiratory Endurance

When you do aerobic exercises, your heart rate increases and your heart sends more oxygen to your muscles to use as energy. Over time, this strengthens the heart muscle, allowing it to pump blood more efficiently. Aerobic exercise also affects your respiratory system by increasing the lungs' capacity to hold air. **Caution:** Don't force yourself to continue an aerobic activity if you become exhausted. Before beginning a fitness program that includes aerobic activities, consult a health care professional. This is especially important if you have asthma or another respiratory disorder. It is also recommended for people with heart disease.

Improving Muscular Strength and Endurance

Anaerobic exercises improve muscular strength and endurance. The more work the muscles do, the stronger they become. Sprinting is an example of an anaerobic activity. Resistance or strength training, which builds muscles by requiring them to move in opposition to a force, is also a form of anaerobic exercise. Free weights, exercise machines, or your own body weight can provide resistance. In addition to building and strengthening muscle, resistance exercises help the body keep blood sugar levels normal and help maintain healthy **cholesterol** levels.

As indicated in **Figure 4.2,** there are three types of resistance training exercise. Exercises such as these tone muscles, improve muscular strength, and increase muscular endurance.

Improving Flexibility

When you have good flexibility, you can easily bend, turn, and stretch your body. You can improve your flexibility through regular

h⊙t link

cholesterol See Chapter 5, page 118 for information on cholesterol.

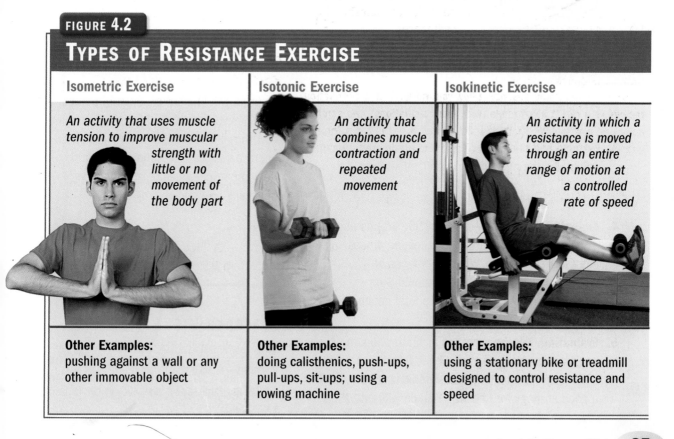

FIGURE 4.2

TYPES OF RESISTANCE EXERCISE

Isometric Exercise	Isotonic Exercise	Isokinetic Exercise
An activity that uses muscle tension to improve muscular strength with little or no movement of the body part	An activity that combines muscle contraction and repeated movement	An activity in which a resistance is moved through an entire range of motion at a controlled rate of speed
Other Examples: pushing against a wall or any other immovable object	**Other Examples:** doing calisthenics, push-ups, pull-ups, sit-ups; using a rowing machine	**Other Examples:** using a stationary bike or treadmill designed to control resistance and speed

Regular, gentle stretching of muscles and joints helps increase flexibility. *What exercises do you include in your routine to increase your flexibility?*

stretching exercises. Just be sure to move slowly and gently. For example, to stretch the muscles of your upper body, stand with your arms extended behind your back, hands clasped; raise your arms until you feel tightness in your shoulders and chest; and hold for 20 seconds.

Improving and Maintaining Bone Strength

The decisions you make concerning physical activity and nutrition can affect the health of your skeletal system now and later in life. You probably already know that calcium—found in dairy products and certain green vegetables—is essential for building strong bones. Resistance training and weight-bearing aerobic activities—those that force you to work against gravity, such as walking and stair climbing—can also help increase bone mass, strengthening your skeletal system.

It's very important to build strong bones during your teen years because this time period is your last opportunity to significantly increase bone mass. During a person's late twenties and early thirties, bone mass and density begin to decline. This can lead to osteoporosis.

 Lesson 2 *Review*

Reviewing Facts and Vocabulary

1. Identify and describe the five areas of health-related fitness.

2. Examine and briefly describe the relationship among body composition, diet, and fitness.

3. Examine and briefly describe the effects of resistance training on the muscular and skeletal systems.

Thinking Critically

4. **Analyzing.** Sam has been doing 50 curl-ups each day. Explain what area of health-related fitness this exercise benefits. What other types of physical activities or exercises should Sam add to his routine to improve his total health-related fitness?

5. **Evaluating.** Keesha, who has asthma, wants to begin an exercise program. She is thinking of signing up for a high-impact aerobic class. Is this a good strategy for Keesha? Explain your answer.

Applying Health Skills

Practicing Healthful Behaviors. Help family members determine their target heart ranges. Then make a list of aerobic activities you could do together. Determine how you all could use this information to improve your cardiorespiratory endurance. Remember: get a health screening before beginning an exercise program.

SPREADSHEETS Using spreadsheet software, design a table that lists target heart ranges for people of various ages and with different resting heart rates. See **health.glencoe.com** for information on how to use a spreadsheet.

Planning a Personal Activity Program

VOCABULARY

overload
progression
specificity
warm-up
workout
F.I.T.T.
cool-down
resting heart rate

YOU'LL LEARN TO

- Set realistic fitness goals.

- Synthesize information and apply critical-thinking, decision-making, and problem-solving skills to develop a personal physical activity program.

- Identify the basic principles of a physical activity program.

QUICK START   List the physical activities in which you have participated during the past week. Classify each activity as *aerobic, anaerobic,* or *other*, and explain your choice.

Knowing the many health benefits of physical activity may inspire you to begin a personal activity program—but having a reason or goal for being physically active is even more inspiring. Setting fitness goals can help you get started by providing you with a plan of action.

Setting Physical Activity Goals

How can you be sure to include physical activity in your daily routine? The first step is to set realistic fitness goals. Then you can develop a plan to meet your goals. To meet the USDA recommendations, teens should get 60 minutes of physical activity every day. This may include all sorts of activities, from participating in physical education classes and playing sports to doing household tasks such as mowing the lawn and cleaning your room.

▲ Participating in a school sports program may inspire you to set fitness goals and begin a physical activity program.

Your school or community may offer programs that provide a variety of fun and healthful physical activities.

Getting Started

Figure 4.3 provides suggestions about how to divide your time when doing various types of physical activity.

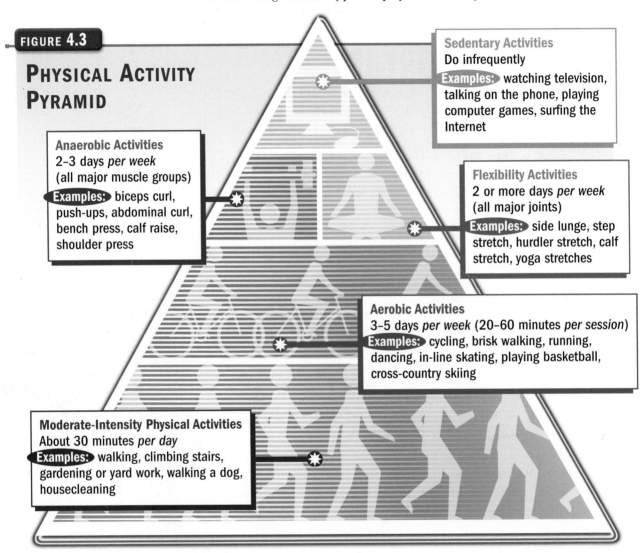

FIGURE 4.3

PHYSICAL ACTIVITY PYRAMID

Sedentary Activities
Do infrequently
Examples: watching television, talking on the phone, playing computer games, surfing the Internet

Anaerobic Activities
2–3 days *per week* (all major muscle groups)
Examples: biceps curl, push-ups, abdominal curl, bench press, calf raise, shoulder press

Flexibility Activities
2 or more days *per week* (all major joints)
Examples: side lunge, step stretch, hurdler stretch, calf stretch, yoga stretches

Aerobic Activities
3–5 days *per week* (20–60 minutes *per session*)
Examples: cycling, brisk walking, running, dancing, in-line skating, playing basketball, cross-country skiing

Moderate-Intensity Physical Activities
About 30 minutes *per day*
Examples: walking, climbing stairs, gardening or yard work, walking a dog, housecleaning

Choosing Activities

Including different types of physical activities in your fitness program can help make it more enjoyable. As your fitness level increases and your interests change, you can alter your program. Other factors that may affect your activity choices include:

▶ **Cost.** Some activities require specialized—and possibly expensive—equipment. Think about what you can afford, and keep in mind that you may discover after a time that an activity just doesn't suit you.

- ▶ **Where you live.** For convenience you'll want to choose activities that you can do locally, without spending a lot of time traveling. Think about the features of your local area. Is the land flat or hilly? What type of climate do you live in? To what activities does the region best lend itself?

- ▶ **Your level of health.** Some health conditions have risks that need to be considered when planning physical activities. For example, some types of physical activity can aggravate **asthma,** a disease of the respiratory system.

- ▶ **Time and place.** Build your program into your daily routine. Do not schedule jogging at 6:00 a.m. if you are not a morning person. Design your schedule to help you achieve your goals.

- ▶ **Personal safety.** Think about your **personal safety** as you develop a fitness program. If you plan to run long distances, avoid going through unsafe areas or running after dark.

- ▶ **Comprehensive planning.** Select activities that address all five areas of health-related fitness.

hot link

asthma To learn more about asthma, see Chapter 26, page 690.

personal safety For more information on issues related to personal safety, see Chapter 13, page 330.

Health Skills Activity

Goal Setting: Starting a Physical Activity Program

William wants to start a physical activity program, but he's not sure where to begin. He really wants to improve his cardiorespiratory and muscle endurance, and he knows that his flexibility and muscle strength need work, too. He's also thinking about signing up for soccer; tryouts are in three months. What can William do to improve his fitness level and make the soccer team?

What Would You Do?
Apply the five goal-setting steps to William's situation.

1. Identify a specific goal and write it down.
2. List the steps you will take to reach your goal.
3. Identify potential problems and ways to get help and support from others.
4. Set up checkpoints to evaluate your progress.
5. Reward yourself once you have achieved your goal.

Cross Training

Engaging in a variety of physical activities to strengthen different muscle groups is known as cross training. Jumping rope, swimming, jogging, and cycling are good cross-training activities for athletes.

Basics of a Physical Activity Program

Because it focuses on *your* goals and interests, your fitness program is unique. However, all effective fitness programs are based on these three principles:

▶ **Overload**, *working the body harder than it is normally worked*, builds muscular strength and contributes to overall fitness. It is achieved by increasing repetitions or by doing more sets (groups of 6 to 12 repetitions) of an exercise.

▶ **Progression** is *the gradual increase in overload necessary to achieve higher levels of fitness*. As an activity becomes easier to do, increase the number of repetitions or sets or increase the amount of time spent doing the activity.

▶ **Specificity** indicates that *particular exercises and activities improve particular areas of health-related fitness*. For example, resistance training builds muscular strength and endurance, while aerobic activity improves cardiorespiratory endurance.

To gain the most benefit from an exercise program, you'll want to include three basic stages for each activity. These are the *warm-up*, the *workout*, and the *cool-down*. Include each stage in every session even when you're in a hurry.

The Warm-Up

The **warm-up**, *an activity that prepares the muscles for work*, is the first stage in any physical activity routine. Begin the warm-up by taking a brisk walk to raise your body temperature. Then, slowly stretch large muscles to increase their elasticity and reduce the risk of injury. After stretching individual muscles, perform the physical activity slowly for about five minutes. For example, if you are running, jog slowly for about five minutes and then increase your pace to a run. Warming up allows your pulse rate to increase gradually. A sudden increase in pulse rate places unnecessary strain on the heart and blood vessels.

The Workout

The part of an exercise program when the activity is performed at its highest peak is called the **workout**. To be effective, the activity needs to follow the *F.I.T.T.* formula—*frequency, intensity, time/duration,* and *type of activity*—outlined in **Figure 4.4.**

FREQUENCY

You should schedule workouts three to four times each week, with only one or two days between sessions. The frequency of your workouts depends partly on your fitness goals and the type of activity you do—as well as on your schedule and possibly even the weather. Exercising more than three times each week for six months should help *get* you physically fit. To *maintain* your fitness level, continue your program at least three times each week.

INTENSITY

Working your muscles and cardiorespiratory system at an intensity that allows you to reach overload will help you improve your fitness level. Begin slowly to build endurance. Doing too much too soon is harmful and can cause chronically sore muscles.

When weight training, start with a light weight and build to heavier weights. For aerobics, work toward your target heart range. If you are out of shape, it may take about six months before you can work out for 20 to 30 minutes within your target heart range.

TIME/DURATION

Slowly build up the amount of time you spend doing aerobic exercises. The goal in aerobics is to work within your target heart range for 20 to 30 minutes. When weight training, do the exercises slowly, taking at least two seconds to lower a weight. Rest for one or two minutes between sets. Also, vary the exercises to strengthen your muscles in the full range of motion.

TYPE

To get the maximum health benefits from your workout routine, devote 75–80 percent of your workout time to aerobic activity and 20–25 percent to anaerobic activity. Choose activities that you enjoy, or you may find it difficult to complete your workouts.

The Cool-Down

Ending a workout abruptly can cause your muscles to tighten and may make you feel dizzy. To avoid these effects, you need to cool down after a workout. The **cool-down** is *an activity that prepares the muscles to return to a resting state.*

FIGURE 4.4

THE *F.I.T.T.* FORMULA

Include each of these elements in your workout.

F requency
how often you do the activity each week

I ntensity
how hard you work at the activity per session

T ime/duration
how much time you devote to a session

T ype
which activities you select

 The warm-up is an important part of any physical activity routine. *Explain how stretching prepares muscles for exercise and prevents injuries.*

Begin the cool-down by slowing down the activity. Continue the activity at this slower pace for about five minutes, then stretch for five minutes.

Monitoring Your Progress

To monitor your progress, keep a fitness journal. In your journal, list your goals and note the frequency, intensity, duration, and type of each activity in which you participate. At the end of 12 weeks, and every 6 weeks after that, compare the figures to evaluate your progress.

Resting Heart Rate

Your **resting heart rate** is *the number of times your heart beats in one minute when you are not active.* Your resting heart rate can also be used to evaluate your progress. A person of average fitness has a resting heart rate of about 72 to 84 beats per minute. Just four weeks of a fitness program can decrease that rate by 5 to 10 beats per minute. A resting heart rate below 72 indicates a good fitness level.

 Lesson 3 *Review*

Reviewing Facts and Vocabulary

1. How can using the Physical Activity Pyramid help you meet your fitness goals?

2. Identify and define the three principles upon which all effective fitness programs are based.

3. What do the letters in the *F.I.T.T.* formula stand for?

Thinking Critically

4. **Analyzing.** How is your resting heart rate an indication of your level of fitness?

5. **Synthesizing.** Maria is a runner. Describe how she could include the three stages of an effective exercise program in her fitness routine.

Applying Health Skills

Goal Setting. Use the goal-setting steps to develop a personal fitness program. Synthesize information from this lesson and apply critical-thinking and decision-making skills to determine what activities to include and how you will incorporate them into a formal plan. Think of obstacles that could prevent you from following your plan, and apply problem-solving skills to figure out how to overcome these obstacles.

TECHNOLOGY *OPTION*

SPREADSHEETS Use spreadsheet software to design a table that can help you organize your physical activity schedule and track your progress. See **health.glencoe.com** for information on how to use a spreadsheet.

Training and Safety for Physical Activities

VOCABULARY

training program
hydration
anabolic steroids
health screening

YOU'LL LEARN TO

- Recognize health-promoting strategies that can enhance a training program.

- Understand the importance of preventive health screenings before beginning a physical activity program.

- Identify safety concerns related to various physical activities.

QUICK START Divide a sheet of paper into two columns. In the first column, list five physical activities you enjoy doing. In the second column, list any special equipment, including safety gear, needed for each activity.

A physical education teacher or coach can help you establish your goals for a training program.

Beginning a new physical activity can be exciting. It also requires some preparation to make sure that you stay safe and get the most out of the activity.

Training and Peak Performance

The first step in becoming fit is to take good care of your body. Eat nutritious foods and drink plenty of fluids, especially water. Getting adequate rest is also essential. To keep your body in top form, it is also important that you avoid harmful substances such as tobacco, alcohol, and other drugs.

The next step in improving fitness often involves beginning a training program for your chosen activity. A **training program** is *a program of formalized physical preparation for involvement in a sport or another physical activity*. Consult your physical education teacher, coach, or another trusted adult to help you set your training goals.

Drinking water is important before, during, and after vigorous physical activity. *Explain why hydration is so important during any physical activity.*

h⬤t link

anabolic steroids For more information on the harmful effects of anabolic steroids, see Chapter 23, page 601.

Nutrition and Hydration

What you eat and drink is an important part of any training program. Food provides the energy necessary for peak performance. You will learn more about nutrition and healthy food choices in Chapter 5. Equally important is hydration, especially when you are engaged in vigorous physical activity. **Hydration** is *taking in fluids so that the body functions properly*. When you are adequately hydrated, you are more alert and focused, your reaction time is faster because your muscles respond more quickly and are less likely to cramp, and your endurance is greater. To stay hydrated, drink plenty of water before, during, and after vigorous physical activity.

Adequate Rest

Sleep, which helps your body rest and reenergize, is also essential for any training program. Getting too little sleep can disrupt the nervous system, causing slowed reaction time, lack of concentration (increasing the possibility of errors and accidents), forgetfulness, irritability, and even depression. On average, teens need 8 to 10 hours of sleep every night to function at their best.

Avoiding Harmful Substances

Avoiding harmful substances such as tobacco, alcohol, anabolic steroids, and other drugs is another part of maintaining an athletic training program.

ANABOLIC STEROIDS

Anabolic steroids are *synthetic substances that are similar to the male hormone testosterone*. Because these substances cause the body to make muscle tissue, some athletes take them to increase muscle mass and enhance performance. However, anabolic steroids have very harmful effects, including increased risk of cancer and heart disease; sterility, or the inability to produce children; skin problems such as acne and hair loss; unusual weight gain or loss; sexual underdevelopment and dysfunction; and violent, suicidal, or depressive tendencies.

It is illegal to use anabolic steroids without a prescription, and those who test positive for steroid use are disqualified from competitions. Thus, abstinence is the best choice when it comes to the use of steroids.

NUTRITIONAL SUPPLEMENTS

Nutritional supplements are nonfood substances that contain one or more nutrients that the body needs, such as vitamins or minerals. The best way to get nutrients is from food, but sometimes a multiple vitamin and mineral supplement may be appropriate.

Should Random Drug Testing of Athletes Be Performed?

A number of high schools in the United States have adopted a policy of random drug testing of student athletes even if there is no indication that the athletes are using drugs. What's your position on the subject of random drug testing of school athletes? Here are two points of view.

Viewpoint 1: Maya D., age 17

Random drug testing of school athletes is unfair and an invasion of privacy, especially if there's no evidence that the person has been using drugs. Students who want to participate in school sports shouldn't have to give up their privacy just to be on an athletic team. Besides, why should athletes be singled out—isn't that discrimination?

Viewpoint 2: Graham H., age 16

I understand Maya's argument, but I think that schools have a right to know whether students are using drugs. They aren't out to catch us doing something wrong. They're concerned about our health and the environment in which we live and learn. People may not like the rules, but schools must follow the policy. We don't want our school to be represented by athletes who use drugs and get away with it. That's dangerous *and* embarrassing.

ACTIVITIES

1. **Take the pro or con position, and expand upon it. Use online or print resources to back up your views. Be sure to investigate each supporting point raised in an argument.**

2. **Some school districts are advocating drug testing of all students who want to be involved in any extra-curricular activities. What might be the pros and cons of such an approach?**

A health care provider can advise you about whether you need this type of supplement. It's important to take the recommended dosage of any supplement. High doses, or *megadoses*, of a nutritional supplement can be harmful.

Safety First!

Safety should be a major concern when you participate in sports and other physical activities. You can reduce your risk of injury by

▶ visiting a health care professional for a health screening before beginning a new activity. A **health screening** is *a search or*

What Are Herbal Supplements?

Herbal supplements are chemical substances derived from plants that may be sold as dietary supplements. Little research has been conducted on their effects or safety, and not much is known about how they work. Nutritionists recommend eating a variety of fruits, vegetables, and whole grains to get the plant chemicals your body needs.

check for diseases or disorders that an individual would otherwise not have knowledge of or seek help for. This screening helps ensure that you do not have a health condition that could make the activity dangerous for you and that you're fit enough to begin the activity you've chosen.

▶ using the proper safety equipment for your chosen activity.

▶ being alert to the surrounding environment, including other players and spectators.

▶ playing at your skill level and knowing your physical limits.

▶ warming up before and cooling down after every activity.

▶ staying within areas that have been designated for physical activities, such as skateboarding parks and bicycle paths.

▶ obeying all rules and restrictions—for example, those that restrict swimming to certain areas or that prohibit skateboarding on sidewalks.

▶ practicing good sportsmanship.

If you should become injured or ill during physical activity, tell a physical education teacher, coach, or another adult immediately.

Personal Safety

You can reduce risks to your personal safety by selecting the right time and place for your activity. This is especially true if you work out alone. If you run or jog, choose a well-used park during daylight hours, when other people are there. If you can't avoid nighttime physical activity, wear reflective clothing so that others can see you. Wearing a whistle that you can blow to attract attention if you are in danger is also a good idea. Also, be aware of the effects of weather: bicycling or running—and even walking—can be a health risk when it's wet and slippery outside.

To avoid sports injuries, choose the proper athletic gear. *Match each piece of equipment with an appropriate sport or other physical activity.*

Using Proper Equipment

Before you begin any new physical activity, learn to use the equipment involved. Check the equipment to make sure that it fits and is in good condition. Always wear the safety gear recommended for that particular activity. Many sports have strict requirements for protective equipment. These tips may also help.

▶ Wear a helmet when bicycling, skateboarding, or skating. Also, when skateboarding or skating, wear knee and elbow pads, gloves, and wrist guards.

▶ Avoid riding at night, if possible. If you must, make sure your bike has reflective tape, a rear reflector, and a headlight. Skateboards and skates also should be outlined with reflective tape. When participating in any outdoor activity at night, wear light-colored clothing with reflective patches on the front and back so that drivers and pedestrians can see you more easily.

▶ Males participating in contact sports—such as football and hockey—should wear athletic supporters or cups to protect the groin area. Females should wear sports bras to prevent stretching of the ligaments that support the breasts.

Proper footwear and clothing also are important. Athletic shoes should be comfortable and should have a cushioned heel, good arch support, and ample toe room. Laced shoes are best for proper control of your foot in the shoe. Wear socks to cushion your feet and keep them dry. In general, choose comfortable, nonrestrictive clothing. When it's warm outside, dress lightly. In cool weather, wear several loose-fitting layers that you can easily remove as you warm up.

Whatever activity you choose, it's essential to use the proper safety equipment. *What safety equipment are the teens pictured here using?*

 Lesson 4 *Review*

Reviewing Facts and Vocabulary

1. Define the term *hydration*.

2. What are *anabolic steroids*? Name three ways they can harm health.

3. Why is it important to get a preventive health screening before beginning a physical activity program?

Thinking Critically

4. **Evaluating.** How can practicing good sportsmanship help you stay safe when participating in a sport?

5. **Analyzing.** Enrique wants to play on the school football team in the fall. To prepare, he plans to participate in a training program in the spring and summer. List five things Enrique should do before and during his training program.

Applying Health Skills

Accessing Information. Working with a classmate, search the Web for three schools that have adopted the policy of random drug testing of school athletes. Compare your school's policy with theirs, noting both similarities and differences.

TECHNOLOGY *OPTION*

WEB SITES   Use the information you find to develop a Web page explaining your school's approach to random drug testing of school athletes. See **health.glencoe.com** for help in planning and building a Web site.

Physical Activity Injuries

VOCABULARY

overexertion
heat cramps
heatstroke
frostbite
hypothermia
muscle cramp
strain
sprain

YOU'LL LEARN TO

- Identify weather-related risks associated with various physical activities.
- Analyze strategies for preventing and responding to accidental injuries related to physical activity.
- Identify physical activity injuries requiring professional health services for people of all ages.

QUICK START List activities you do only during specific seasons of the year. Next to each activity, describe how you prepare for the weather conditions of that season.

These teens are taking specific precautions to prevent sports injuries.
What safety precautions did you take in your most recent outdoor activity?

With any activity that involves movement, there is always a risk of accident or injury. The risk of injury during physical activity increases when a person is not in good physical condition or has not sufficiently warmed up or cooled down. Attempting physical activities that are beyond your level of ability also increases the risk of injury.

Weather-Related Risks

Taking your physical activity routine outdoors can be a great change of pace, but some weather-related health problems need to be taken into consideration. These problems can be avoided by not participating in outdoor physical activity when temperatures are extremely high or extremely low. Factors such as wind, humidity, and air pollution can increase your risk of injury or illness. Be aware of wind chill factors, ultraviolet (UV) indexes, and air quality alerts. You also should pay attention to weather warnings. Stay inside if there is a threat of tornadoes, thunderstorms, flash floods, or blizzards.

Hot-Weather Health Risks

Two concerns during hot weather are dehydration, or excessive loss of water from the body, and poor air quality. Smog can damage the lungs, so avoid outdoor physical activities during smog alerts. To avoid dehydration, drink plenty of water before, during, and after physical activity.

Many hot-weather health problems are related to **overexertion**, or *overworking the body*. For example, heat exhaustion—an overheating of the body that results in cold, clammy skin and symptoms of shock—is caused by overexertion in a hot, humid atmosphere. Other symptoms include dizziness, headache, shortness of breath, and nausea. Heat exhaustion may be preceded or accompanied by **heat cramps**, *muscle spasms that result from a loss of large amounts of salt and water through perspiration*. If you experience any of these symptoms, move to a cool place and lie down with your feet elevated. Take small sips of water as you start to recover. If symptoms are severe, or if vomiting occurs, get medical help immediately.

Continuing to exercise with the symptoms of heat exhaustion and dehydration can lead to **heatstroke**, *a condition in which the body loses the ability to rid itself of excessive heat through perspiration*. This causes hyperthermia, a sudden increase in body temperature, which can be life-threatening. A person suffering from heatstroke may have difficulty breathing and may collapse suddenly. If heatstroke occurs, immediately call for medical help. Then move the person to a cool place, and sponge him or her with cold water until help arrives.

Cold-Weather Health Risks

When participating in cold-weather activities, dress in three layers to keep warm. The first layer should pull moisture and perspiration away from your body. Many synthetic fabrics have been specifically developed to help keep the skin dry. The middle layer should provide insulation. Wool or synthetic fleece fabrics can help keep you warm even if they get wet. A coated nylon windshell as the top layer will help keep warmth in and water and wind out. A hat is also a must—70 percent of the body's heat is lost through the head. Removing layers as you warm up or adding them as the temperature drops can help you adjust to changes in the weather.

When you begin any cold-weather activity, start slowly and be sure to warm up your muscles. Staying hydrated is as important in

Staying hydrated is essential when working out in hot or cold weather. *What other steps can this player take to protect himself from health problems associated with working out in hot weather?*

Did You Know ?

Altitude sickness is a risk in some mountain sports. It usually occurs at altitudes of 7,000 feet or higher, where there are lower levels of oxygen. Symptoms include severe headache, nausea, and weakness. The best ways of preventing altitude sickness are to give yourself time to adjust to activity at high altitudes, to drink plenty of water, and to avoid alcohol and caffeine.

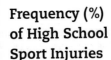
Helmets, goggles, and gloves are proper equipment when snowboarding.

cold weather as it is in hot weather. Two specific health risks from cold weather are particularly important to keep in mind: frostbite and hypothermia.

▶ **Frostbite** is *a condition that results when body tissues become frozen*, and it requires professional medical treatment. You can avoid frostbite by dressing warmly and covering all exposed skin—especially the ears, face, feet, and fingers, where frostbite most often occurs. An early warning sign of frostbite, called frostnip, is a whitening of the skin of the toes, fingers, nose, or ears. If this happens or if you notice a lack of feeling in any exposed area, get indoors right away and warm the area with warm water.

Real-Life Application

Being Safe While Physically Active

Sports and recreational activities are the second most frequent cause of injury for teens. Many such injuries can be prevented by being cautious and by wearing proper equipment. Examine the graph, and choose a sport or recreational activity in which you or your friends participate. Using reliable online and print resources, research your sport to find injury statistics. For example, what injuries are most common for this sport? How many teens are injured each year in this sport? How many of these injuries are treated in emergency rooms? What protective equipment and precautions can reduce injury in this sport?

Frequency (%) of High School Sport Injuries

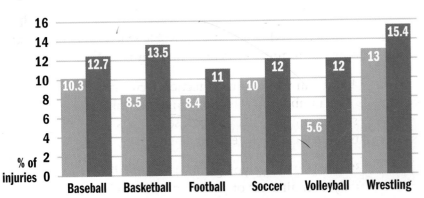

Major Moderate

Source: Based on data from the National Athletic Trainers' Association

ACTIVITY

Using the activity you have researched, create a poster that explains how teens can get injured while participating in the activity and presents ways of staying safe. Make your poster colorful and attention-getting to appeal to a teen audience. Be sure to give it a catchy title.

▶ **Hypothermia** is *a condition in which body temperature becomes dangerously low*. It is usually associated with cold weather, but it also can result from lengthy exposure to wind or rain or from submersion in cold water. When hypothermia occurs, the body loses the ability to warm itself. As body temperature drops, the brain cannot function and body systems begin to shut down. A person with this condition may become disoriented and lose motor control. Because hypothermia can lead to death, it requires immediate medical attention.

When participating in cold-weather activities, pay attention to your body. Shivering is a sign that your body is losing heat. If you begin to feel cold or to shiver, go to a warm, dry place; wrap yourself in a blanket; and drink warm liquids to slowly raise your body temperature.

Protecting Yourself from Sun and Wind

Prolonged exposure to sun and wind is another weather-related risk of outdoor physical activity. Windburn occurs when skin is exposed to freezing wind, causing it to become red, tight, and sore to the touch. Reduce the risk of windburn by wearing protective clothing and using lip balm. The sun's UV rays cause *sunburn*, a burning of the outer layers of the skin. Mild sunburn makes your skin red and slightly sore. Severe sunburn causes blistering of the skin, swelling, and pain. In addition to increasing the risk of sunburn, repeated or prolonged exposure to the sun speeds the skin's aging process and increases your risk of developing **skin cancer.** The most dangerous hours for UV exposure are from 10:00 a.m. to 4:00 p.m. To protect yourself against sunburn:

▶ Cover as much of the body with clothing as possible when outdoors and wear broad-brimmed hats on sunny days.

▶ Use sunscreen and lip balm with a sun protection factor (SPF) of *at least* 15. The SPF number indicates the sunscreen's ability to screen out the sun's harmful UV rays. Because UV rays penetrate clouds, you need to wear sunscreen on cloudy days, too.

▶ Apply sunscreen 30 minutes before you go outside, spreading it liberally and evenly over all areas of your skin that will be exposed. Reapply it at least every two hours.

UV rays can also damage your eyes. A *cataract*, a cloudy covering over the lens of the eye, is caused in part by sun exposure. Wear a visor or a hat with a brim, and use sunglasses, even during the winter months. Because sunlight is reflected off snow, those participating in winter sports need to wear goggles to protect their eyes from both UV exposure and glare.

▼ **Apply sunscreen frequently when you participate in outdoor activities.** *Why is it important to use sunscreen in both hot and cold weather?*

hot link

skin cancer For more information about skin cancer, see Chapter 26, page 683.

Ligaments are strong bands of tissue that connect the bones to one another at a moveable joint. Sprains result if these bands are stretched or torn.

Minor Injuries

Have you ever had sore muscles after a physical activity or experienced the pain of a twisted ankle? Muscles are often sore 24 to 48 hours after a strenuous workout. Warming up, cooling down, and stretching can prevent or reduce muscle soreness. Other minor injuries that affect the skeletal or muscular systems include muscle cramps, strains, and sprains. A **muscle cramp** is *a spasm or sudden tightening of a muscle*. It happens when a muscle is tired, overworked, or dehydrated. Drinking cool water may ease muscle cramping. A **strain** is *a condition resulting from damaging a muscle or tendon*. A **sprain** is *an injury to the ligament surrounding a joint*. Symptoms of a sprain include pain, swelling, and difficulty moving. Severe sprains require medical treatment. Warming up can help prevent muscle strains and sprains.

Treatment for Minor Injuries

Minor injuries such as muscle cramps, strains, and some sprains are easily treated. Muscle cramps can be relieved through light massage. Minor strains and sprains can be treated using the *R.I.C.E.* procedure described in **Figure 4.5.**

Major Injuries

Pain—especially extreme pain—may signal that you have a major injury. If you experience extreme pain, numbness, or disorientation or hear a "cracking" sound during a fall, get appropriate medical treatment immediately.

Many minor sports injuries can be treated by following the *R.I.C.E.* procedure. *Which part of the R.I.C.E. procedure is pictured here?*

FIGURE 4.5

THE *R.I.C.E.* PROCEDURE

Rest Avoid using the affected muscle or joint. This may mean not using the affected area for several days.

Ice Ice helps reduce pain and swelling. Place ice cubes in a plastic bag, and wrap the bag in a towel. Hold the towel-wrapped bag on the affected area for 20 minutes. Remove the bag for 20 minutes, and then reapply the bag for another 20 minutes. Repeat this process every three waking hours over the course of 72 hours.

Compression Light pressure through the use of an elastic bandage can help reduce swelling. The bandage should not be so tight that it cuts off the blood supply to the area, and it should be loosened at night.

Elevation Raising the affected limb above the level of the heart helps reduce pain and swelling, especially at night.

Major injuries include:

▶ **Fractures and Dislocations.** Fractures are any break in a bone. A fracture causes swelling and often extreme pain, and it usually requires immobilization to heal properly. Dislocations result when a bone is forced from its normal position at a joint. A dislocation sometimes causes a "popping" sound when it occurs. A physician must put the bone back into place and immobilize the joint so that the tissue can heal.

▶ **Tendonitis.** This is a condition in which the tendons, bands of fiber that connect muscles to bones, are stretched or torn from overuse. Treatment includes rest, medication, and physical therapy.

▶ **Concussions.** Concussions result from blows to the head and can cause swelling of the brain, resulting in unconsciousness or even death. Concussions can lead to serious neurological problems. If you receive any blow to the head and experience headache, dizziness, or loss of memory or consciousness, see a health care professional immediately.

This teen's safety gear helps protect him from serious injury. *What type of serious injury might the face mask prevent?*

Lesson 5 *Review*

Reviewing Facts and Vocabulary

1. What is *hypothermia*? With which types of weather is this condition often associated?
2. Analyze and describe strategies for preventing muscle soreness after a workout.
3. Identify which injuries described in this lesson require the attention of professional health services.

Thinking Critically

4. **Evaluating.** Explain why muscle cramps might be more dangerous for a swimmer than for a jogger.
5. **Analyzing.** On a hot day, a runner begins to have trouble breathing and also becomes pale, dizzy, and nauseous. From what condition is this runner likely to be suffering? How might the condition have been prevented? Analyze and describe strategies for responding to this condition.

Applying Health Skills

Communication Skills. Imagine that your friend has suffered a minor sprain to her ankle while in-line skating. Analyze and describe how she could use the *R.I.C.E.* procedure to respond to this accidental injury.

TECHNOLOGY *OPTION*

WORD PROCESSING Use a word-processing program to create your own chart outlining the *R.I.C.E.* procedure. See **health.glencoe.com** for tips on how to get the most from your word-processing program.

Eye ON THE Media

Truth in Fitness Advertising?

TV infomercials for fitness products usually feature in-shape spokespeople with "rock-hard abs" or bulging biceps. Are these typical results from using the advertised product? In this activity you will explore advertising techniques and evaluate the effectiveness of a fitness product.

Before

ACTIVITY

Watch a TV infomercial for a particular fitness product, and answer the following questions.

1. What product is being advertised? What are the claims being made in the infomercial? Note any key statements describing the product's advantages.

2. What specific information does the advertiser provide about using the product? For instance, how often must a person use the product in order to get the desired results?

3. Who is the spokesperson? Does this person lend any credibility to the advertiser's claims?

Compare your notes with those of your classmates. Discuss the claims made in these infomercials in light of what you have learned in your text about improving various aspects of health-related fitness.

EXPRESS YOUR VIEWS

Write a paragraph expressing your overall impressions of the infomercial you watched. How much of what is being advertised is based on accurate statements? Explain whether you think the product might provide any fitness benefits, and compare that with the advertiser's claims. If you thought that the product claims were exaggerated, include suggestions on how the advertiser could present a more realistic advertisement about the product's capabilities.

CROSS-CURRICULUM CONNECTIONS

Compose an Essay. "Ripping through the water while swimming laps" or "straining and puffing while on a daily jog" are examples of phrases that illustrate the sensory details of physical activity. Capture the sights, sounds, feel, taste, and smell of your favorite physical activity in a brief descriptive essay. Focus on using adjectives, adverbs, and action verbs. Use metaphors to create an even more vivid picture.

Create a Visual Aid. One of the earliest examples of organized exercise is the Olympic Games in 776 B.C.E. At these first Games, the Greeks hosted just one event—the *stade,* a 180-meter distance race. Research a historical aspect of physical exercise and design a visual aid, like a poster, to present your findings to the class.

Compute the Calories. A foot-pound (ft-lb) is the amount of energy required to lift a 1-pound object one foot. Kilocalories are units of heat that measure food energy as well as the energy used by the body. Kilocalories can be converted to foot-pounds as follows: 1 kcal = 3088.025 ft-lb. Walking up one flight of stairs is equal to lifting yourself 10 feet. How many calories would a 180-pound man use walking up one flight of stairs?

Conduct Research. There are three different types of muscles in the human body: skeletal, smooth, and cardiac. Skeletal muscles are used for voluntary motion and are the ones we think of when playing sports or lifting weights. Cardiac and smooth muscles produce the involuntary activities of the body, controlling movement in the heart (cardiac), arterial, and digestive systems. Research the different muscle tissue types, and discuss what kind of exercise is best for each.

CAREER Corner

Sports Medicine

Would you like to work with athletes and others who lead physically active lives? If so, you may enjoy a career in sports medicine. Physicians specializing in sports medicine treat injuries related to sports and other physical activities.

To enter this profession, you will need to complete a four-year college program, four years of medical school, and from one to seven years of residency training. Learn more about this and other related health careers by clicking on Career Corner at **health.glencoe.com**.

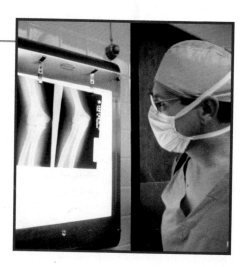

Chapter 4 Review

> **EXPLORING HEALTH TERMS** *Answer the following questions on a sheet of paper.*

Lesson 1 *Replace the underlined words with the correct term.*

physical activity   osteoporosis
physical fitness   sedentary lifestyle
metabolism

1. <u>Osteoporosis</u> refers to the process by which your body gets energy from food.

2. Watching television and taking naps are characteristic of a <u>physical activity</u>.

3. <u>Physical fitness</u> is a condition characterized by a decrease in bone density, producing porous and fragile bones.

Lesson 2 *Fill in the blanks with the correct term.*

body composition   muscular strength
exercise   aerobic exercise
flexibility   anaerobic exercise
muscular endurance
cardiorespiratory endurance

Purposeful physical activity that is planned, structured, and repetitive and that improves or maintains fitness is (_4_). (_5_) is any rhythmic activity that uses large muscle groups and can be maintained continuously for 20 to 30 minutes at one time. (_6_) involves short bursts of activity in which the muscles work so hard that they produce energy without using oxygen.

Lesson 3 *Replace the underlined words with the correct term.*

overload   workout
progression   cool-down
specificity   F.I.T.T.
warm-up   resting heart rate

7. The part of an exercise program when the activity is performed at its highest peak is called the <u>overload</u>.

8. A <u>workout</u> is an activity that prepares the muscles for work.

9. An activity that prepares the muscles to return to a resting state is a <u>progression</u>.

Lesson 4 *Match each definition with the correct term.*

health screening   hydration
training program   anabolic steroids

10. A program of formalized physical preparation for involvement in a sport or another physical activity.

11. Taking in fluids so that the body functions properly.

12. A search or check for diseases or disorders that an individual would otherwise not have knowledge of or seek help for.

Lesson 5 *Identify each statement as True or False. If false, replace the underlined term with the correct term.*

overexertion   hypothermia
heatstroke   muscle cramp
heat cramps   strain
frostbite   sprain

13. Many hot-weather health problems, such as heat exhaustion and heat cramps, are related to <u>hypothermia</u>.

14. <u>Frostbite</u> is a condition that results when body tissues become frozen.

15. A <u>muscle cramp</u> is an injury to the ligament surrounding a joint.

> **RECALLING THE FACTS** *Use complete sentences to answer the following questions.*

Lesson 1

1. Examine and briefly describe the effects of regular physical activity on the nervous system.

2. Analyze the relationship between regular physical activity and disease prevention: How can engaging in regular physical activity now and in adulthood reduce your risks of cardiovascular disease, type 2 diabetes, and cancer?

3. What are three ways to incorporate physical activity into your daily life?

Lesson 2

4. What is muscular strength, and how is it measured?
5. Examine and briefly describe how aerobic exercise benefits the cardiovascular and respiratory systems.
6. What are the three types of resistance training exercises?

Lesson 3

7. In the context of physical activity, what is meant by the term *progression*?
8. What three elements should be part of every physical activity session?
9. How can the *F.I.T.T.* formula help you meet your fitness goals?

Lesson 4

10. Why are proper nutrition and adequate rest important factors in a physical activity training program?
11. Why is starting a fitness program a situation that requires a preventive health screening?
12. List three ways to stay safe when exercising alone outdoors.

Lesson 5

13. What are two advantages to dressing in layers when outside in cold weather?
14. Analyze and describe a strategy for responding to minor strains and sprains.
15. What symptoms signal a major injury that requires treatment by professional health services?

▶ THINKING CRITICALLY

1. **Analyzing.** Why do you think many teens lead a sedentary lifestyle? *(LESSON 1)*
2. **Evaluating.** Samantha does not enjoy participating in formal group exercise programs such as those at a health club. What physical activities might she include in her daily life to obtain the benefits of both aerobic exercise and anaerobic exercise? *(LESSON 2)*
3. **Synthesizing.** Develop a physical activity program that includes all areas shown in the Physical Activity Pyramid in Figure 4.3. *(LESSON 3)*
4. **Explaining.** Why is it important to be alert to the surrounding environment when playing a sport? Give two specific examples. *(LESSON 4)*
5. **Applying.** Brianna is an enthusiastic but inexperienced skier. She accepts an invitation to go skiing even though it is 10°F below zero. What strategies would you give her for preventing illness and injury while participating in this activity? *(LESSON 5)*

▶ HEALTH SKILLS APPLICATION

1. **Practicing Healthful Behaviors.** Identify three sedentary activities from your daily life and suggest a physical activity you could do in place of each. *(LESSON 1)*
2. **Goal Setting.** Identify two areas of your health-related fitness that need improvement. Use the goal-setting steps to develop a plan for improving these areas. *(LESSON 2)*
3. **Advocacy.** Prepare a short presentation in which you encourage teens to develop their own fitness programs based on the principles of overload, progression, and specificity. *(LESSON 3)*
4. **Refusal Skills.** With a classmate, role-play a scenario in which you refuse a friend's offer of an herbal supplement that claims to enhance athletic performance. *(LESSON 4)*
5. **Accessing Information.** Locate three sources in your community from whom you can request information about sports injuries. Summarize the information you receive from each source, and share your findings with the class. *(LESSON 5)*

Chapter 5

Nutrition and Your Health

What Do You Know About Healthful Eating?

Read the statements below and respond by writing *Myth* or *Fact* for each item. You may want to jot down reasons for each of your choices.

1. Meat should make up the largest part of my daily food intake.

2. The foods I eat now can affect my health later in life.

3. It's *what* I eat that really counts, not how much I eat.

4. To help maintain a healthy weight, I must balance the energy in the foods I eat with the energy I use in physical activity.

5. The calories in a doughnut are more likely to be converted to fat in my body than the calories in a piece of fruit.

6. The Food Guide Pyramid provides a good guideline for my daily food intake.

7. Eating a healthy breakfast each day can help me perform better in school.

8. The best way for me to get the nutrients I need is to take a daily vitamin and mineral supplement.

HEALTH Online

For instant feedback on your health status, go to Chapter 5 Health Inventory at **health.glencoe.com**.

Quick *Write*

Using Visuals. Food and social activities often go together. Describe how friends and family members influence your eating habits and food choices.

Nutrition During the Teen Years

VOCABULARY

nutrition
calories
nutrients
hunger
appetite

YOU'LL LEARN TO

- Explain the relationship between nutrition, quality of life, and disease.

- Evaluate various influences on food choices.

- Explain the immediate and long-term benefits of nutrition on body systems.

QUICK START On a sheet of paper, list six of the foods you eat most often for meals or snacks. Then describe why you eat each of these foods. Do you base your choice on their health benefits? Their taste or appearance? Their convenience?

▲ Choosing fresh fruit as a snack is a good way to supply your body with the nutrients it needs.
What's your favorite healthful snack?

Picture yourself biting into a crisp, juicy apple or a slice of cheese pizza with zesty tomato sauce. Do these foods appeal to you? What other foods do you like? Enjoying a wide variety of healthful foods is an important part of good **nutrition—** *the process by which the body takes in and uses food.* Because not all foods offer the same benefits, making healthful food choices is important to your overall level of health.

The Importance of Good Nutrition

Good nutrition enhances your quality of life and helps prevent disease. It provides you with the calories and nutrients your body needs for maximum energy and wellness. **Calories**, or more correctly, kilocalories, are the *units of heat that measure the energy used by the body and the energy that foods supply to the body.* This energy fuels everything you do, from exercising and playing sports to doing your homework and talking with friends. **Nutrients** are the *substances in food that your body needs to grow, to repair itself, and to supply you with energy.* Making healthy food choices will provide your body with the nutrients it needs to help you look your best and perform at your peak.

What Influences Your Food Choices?

Have you ever wondered why you choose the foods you do? Taste, of course, plays an important part in your choice of foods. You probably won't eat a food—even if you know it's healthful—if you don't like its taste. To gain insight into your eating habits, it's important to understand the difference between your physical *need* for food and your psychological *desire* for food—between hunger and appetite. Distinguishing between the two can help you make more healthful food choices.

Hunger and Appetite

Hunger, an unlearned, inborn response, is *a natural physical drive that protects you from starvation.* When your stomach is empty, its walls contract, stimulating nerve endings. The nerves signal your brain that your body needs food. When you eat, the walls of the stomach are stretched and the nerve endings are no longer stimulated. You have satisfied your physical need for food.

The physical need for food isn't the only reason people eat. Have you ever eaten something "just to be sociable" or in response to a familiar sensation—for example, the aroma of freshly baked bread? In such cases you are eating in response to appetite rather than to hunger. **Appetite** is *a desire, rather than a need, to eat.* Whether you are responding to hunger or to appetite when you eat, many factors influence your food choices and eating habits, including your emotions and a number of factors in your environment.

Food and Emotions

Food is sometimes used to meet emotional needs. For example, do you tend to eat more—or less—when you feel stressed, frustrated, or depressed? Do you sometimes snack just because you're bored? Do you reward yourself with a food treat when you've achieved a goal? Using food to relieve tension or boredom or to reward yourself can result in overeating and unhealthful weight gain. On the other hand, if you lose interest in eating whenever you're upset, you may miss getting enough of the nutrients your body needs. Recognizing when emotions are guiding your food choices can help you break such patterns and improve your eating habits.

Food and Your Environment

A number of environmental factors influence food choices:

▶ **Family, friends, and peers.** Many of your eating habits were shaped as you were growing up, when adults planned your meals. Now you may prefer certain foods because you've grown up eating them. Friends and peers can influence you to try new foods.

Should Soft Drinks and Snacks Be Taxed to Fund Health Education Programs?

Some health advocates have recommended that soft drinks and high-calorie snacks be taxed. They believe that these foods are partly to blame for the recent rise in obesity rates. Each item would be taxed one to two cents, and the money would fund programs that promote healthful eating and physical activity. Read what two teens have to say about this issue:

Viewpoint 1: Zack H., age 16

I'd pay an extra penny or two for snacks if the money was being used for a good cause. Cigarettes and alcohol are taxed—why not soft drinks and high-calorie snacks? Every year, obesity causes almost as many deaths as tobacco. Health advocates have shown that antitobacco messages can change behavior. I think nutrition campaigns could do the same thing.

Viewpoint 2: Songhee L., age 16

How can you compare soft drinks and snacks to tobacco and alcohol? People have to eat. There are no good or bad foods, just unhealthful eating patterns. The answer to obesity is making the right food choices. A sedentary lifestyle also contributes to overweight and obesity. Why not tax video games and computer software? Also, why stop at soft drinks and snack foods? Why not tax cheese, butter, and salad dressing?

ACTIVITIES

1. **Do you think campaigns or formal programs on nutrition would influence people to make healthful eating choices? Why or why not?**

2. **Should the government be responsible for individual eating choices? Explain.**

▶ **Cultural and ethnic background.** Your food choices may reflect your cultural heritage or ethnic background. For example, corn, beans, and tortillas might be common foods in many Mexican-American households.

▶ **Convenience and cost.** Convenience and cost of foods may be top priorities for some people. For example, busy families may rely on foods that can be prepared quickly, such as microwavable meals.

▶ **Advertising.** Advertisers spend millions of dollars each year to influence your decisions about food. Part of making informed food choices involves carefully analyzing the health messages delivered through food advertisements. Then you, rather than advertisers, will control your food choices.

Nutrition Throughout the Life Span

Good nutrition is essential for health throughout life but particularly during adolescence—one of the fastest periods of growth you'll experience. Healthful eating provides you with the nutrients you need for growth and development, gives you energy for sports and other activities, enables you to stay mentally alert, and helps you feel good and look your best. A healthful and balanced eating plan also helps prevent unhealthful weight gain, obesity, and type 2 diabetes—conditions that have become more common among children and teens in recent years. Making healthful food choices now also lowers your risk of developing many life-threatening conditions as you get older. These conditions include heart disease and stroke, certain cancers, and osteoporosis.

 Eating nutritious meals as a family can contribute to the health of all family members.

 Lesson 1 *Review*

Reviewing Facts and Vocabulary

1. Briefly explain the relationship between nutrition, quality of life, and disease.
2. Define the term *appetite*.
3. Name three influences—other than family—on people's food choices.

Thinking Critically

4. **Evaluating.** Give examples of how your family has influenced your food choices.
5. **Applying.** How does what you eat now affect your health, both now and as you grow older?

Applying Health Skills

Analyzing Influences. Look through magazines and find five food advertisements that contain specific health claims. Analyze the health message that each advertisement delivers about its product. How might it influence your food choice? Present your findings in the form of a table.

TECHNOLOGY | *O P T I O N*

SPREADSHEETS Spreadsheet software can be used to create your table. For help in using spreadsheet software, go to **health.glencoe.com**.

Nutrients

VOCABULARY

carbohydrates
fiber
proteins
lipid
vitamins
minerals

YOU'LL LEARN TO

- Describe the functions of the six basic nutrients in maintaining health.

- Demonstrate knowledge of nutrients in a variety of foods.

- Analyze the relationship between good nutrition and disease prevention.

QUICK START What's your idea of a healthful meal? On a sheet of paper, describe a nutritious meal that you would enjoy. Then make a list of the health benefits that you think you would get from this meal.

Each of these foods is rich in one or more nutrients. *Which of these foods do you eat regularly?*

To survive, the human body needs the nutrients found in food. These nutrients are classified into six groups: carbohydrates, proteins, fats, vitamins, minerals, and water. Each plays a unique part in maintaining the normal growth and functioning of your body. Together, they are essential to your overall health and wellness.

Carbohydrates

Do you like potatoes, pasta, and bread? These foods are rich in carbohydrates. **Carbohydrates** are *the starches and sugars present in foods*. Made up of carbon, oxygen, and hydrogen, carbohydrates are the body's preferred source of energy, providing four calories per gram. Your body uses energy from carbohydrates to perform every task, including sitting and reading the words on this page. Depending on their chemical makeup, carbohydrates are classified as either simple or complex. Most nutritionists recommend that 55 to 60 percent of your daily calories come from carbohydrates, mainly complex carbohydrates.

Simple and Complex Carbohydrates

Simple carbohydrates are *sugars,* such as fructose and lactose (found in fruit and milk, respectively). You're probably most familiar with sucrose. It occurs naturally in many plants, such as sugarcane and sugar beets, and is refined to make table sugar. Sugars are added to many manufactured food products.

Complex carbohydrates, or *starches,* are found in whole grains, seeds, nuts, legumes (dried peas and beans), and tubers (root vegetables such as potatoes). The body must break down complex carbohydrates into simple carbohydrates before it can use them for energy.

The Role of Carbohydrates

Your body converts all carbohydrates to glucose, a simple sugar that is the body's main source of energy. Glucose that your body does not use right away is stored in the liver and muscles as a starch-like substance called glycogen (GLI-coh-jen). When more energy is needed, your body converts the glycogen back to glucose. However, it's possible to take in more carbohydrates than your body can use right away or can store as glycogen. When this happens, your body converts and stores the excess carbohydrates as body fat. You can avoid consuming excess carbohydrates by learning to make informed food choices and maintaining healthful eating habits.

Fiber

Fiber is *an indigestible complex carbohydrate* that is found in the tough, stringy parts of vegetables, fruits, and whole grains. Although it can't be digested and used as energy, fiber helps move waste through the digestive system and thereby helps prevent intestinal problems such as constipation. Eating enough fiber throughout your life may reduce your risk of heart disease. Some types of fiber have also been shown to help control diabetes by reducing blood glucose levels.

To stay healthy, eat 20 to 35 grams of fiber each day. Fruits and vegetables with edible skins and whole-grain products such as bran cereals, oatmeal, and brown rice are excellent sources of fiber.

Health Minute

Getting More Fiber into Your Diet

To get 20-35 grams of fiber daily:

► Start your day with a whole-grain breakfast cereal, such as oatmeal.

► Choose whole fruit instead of fruit juice.

► Make sure you eat at least five servings of fruits and vegetables each day.

► Select high-fiber snacks (popcorn, raw vegetables, nuts, and fruit with edible skins).

► Eat legumes at least two or three times a week.

► Substitute whole-grain ingredients (whole-wheat flour, bran) for low-fiber ingredients (white flour) in recipes whenever possible.

Each of these foods is a rich source of carbohydrates.

Proteins

A vital part of every cell in your body, **proteins** are *nutrients that help build and maintain body cells and tissues.* Proteins are made of long chains of substances called amino acids. Your body can manufacture all but 9 of the 20 different amino acids that make up proteins. The 9 that your body can't make are called *essential amino acids*—you must get them from the foods you eat.

Complete and Incomplete Proteins

The proteins in food are classified into two groups, *complete proteins* and *incomplete proteins.*

▶ **Complete proteins** contain adequate amounts of all nine essential amino acids. Animal products—such as fish, meat, poultry, eggs, milk, cheese, and yogurt—and many soybean products are good sources of complete proteins.

▶ **Incomplete proteins** lack one or more of the essential amino acids. Sources include beans, peas, nuts, and whole grains. Consuming a combination of incomplete proteins, for example, rice and beans or peanut butter and bread, is equivalent to consuming a complete protein. You don't have to combine the incomplete proteins in one meal to get this benefit, you just need to eat them both over the course of the day.

The Role of Proteins

Proteins have many functions. During major growth periods, such as infancy, childhood, adolescence, and pregnancy, the body builds new cells and tissues from the amino acids in proteins. Throughout your life your body replaces damaged or worn-out cells by making new ones from protein. The body also uses protein to make enzymes, hormones, and antibodies. Enzymes are substances that control the rate of chemical reactions in your cells. Hormones regulate the activities of different cells, and antibodies help identify and destroy disease-causing organisms. Proteins also supply the body with energy, although they are not the body's main energy source. Like carbohydrates, proteins provide four calories per gram and excess protein is converted to body fat.

▼ **Each of these foods is a good source of protein.** *Which of these foods contain complete proteins? Which contain incomplete proteins?*

Fats

Some fat in the diet is necessary for good health. Fats are a type of **lipid** (LIHP-uhd), *a fatty substance that does not dissolve in water.* Fats provide more than twice the energy of carbohydrates or proteins—nine calories per gram.

The building blocks of fats are called fatty acids, molecules made mostly of long chains of carbon atoms, with pairs of hydrogen atoms and single oxygen atoms attached. Fatty acids that the body needs, but cannot produce, are called *essential fatty acids.* Depending on their chemical composition, fatty acids are classified as either saturated or unsaturated. Most fats are a mixture of these two types.

Saturated and Unsaturated Fatty Acids

A *saturated fatty acid* holds all the hydrogen atoms it can. Fats high in saturated fatty acids are usually solid at room temperature. Animal fats and tropical oils—such as palm oil, palm kernel oil, and coconut oil—have a high proportion of saturated fatty acids. Fats in beef, pork, egg yolks, and dairy foods are higher in saturated fatty acids than are the fats in chicken and fish. A high intake of saturated fats is associated with an increased risk of heart disease.

Most vegetable fats—including olive, canola, soybean, corn, and cottonseed oils—contain a high proportion of unsaturated fatty acids. An *unsaturated fatty acid* has at least one unsaturated bond—a place where hydrogen can be added to the molecule. Unsaturated fats are usually liquids (oils) at room temperature. In contrast to saturated fats, unsaturated fats have been associated with a reduced risk of heart disease.

The Role of Fats

Besides providing a concentrated form of energy, fats are essential for other important health functions. They transport vitamins A, D, E, and K in your blood and serve as sources of *linoleic* (lih-noh-LAY-ihk) *acid,* an essential fatty acid that is needed for growth and healthy skin. Fats also add flavor and texture to food, and, because they take longer to digest than carbohydrates or proteins, they help satisfy hunger longer than other nutrients do. Foods that are high in fats also tend to be high in calories, and consuming excess amounts of fat increases your risk of unhealthful weight gain and obesity. Therefore, most nutritionists recommend eating only moderate amounts of fat—no more that 20 to 30 percent of your total daily calorie intake.

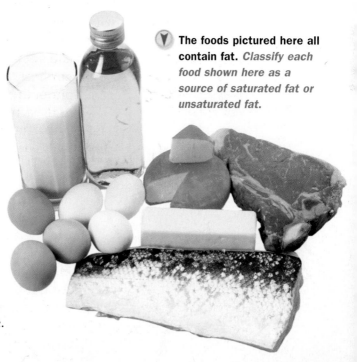

The foods pictured here all contain fat. *Classify each food shown here as a source of saturated fat or unsaturated fat.*

Hands-On Health ACTIVITY

Reducing Your Intake of Fats

Consuming too much fat can increase the risk of heart disease and unhealthful weight gain. Most teen boys need no more than 84 grams of fat each day. Most teen girls need no more than 66 grams each day. Analyzing the amount of fat in fast foods and snacks can help you see how to reduce your consumption of fats.

What You'll Need

- paper and pencil

What You'll Do

1. List every fast-food and snack item you eat and the portion size of each over the next three days. Next to each item, record how many grams of fat were in that portion. You can find fat grams in snacks by reading the label on packaged food products or by using a computerized dietary analysis program. Fast-food restaurants can provide a list of nutritional information about their products.

2. Determine the total number of fat grams you consumed over the three-day period. Then divide by three to find your daily average. What did you discover? Were there any surprises?

3. Using your dietary analysis as a guide, set a goal to reduce your fat intake for the next three days. Write a detailed plan describing the steps you will take to reach your goal.

Apply and Conclude

Follow your plan for three days. As a class, share which low-fat substitutions you tried and enjoyed.

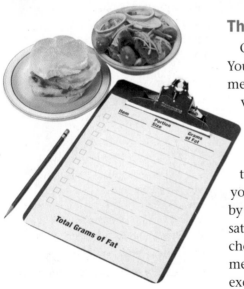

The Role of Cholesterol

Cholesterol is a waxy lipidlike substance that circulates in blood. Your body uses the small amount it manufactures to make cell membranes and nerve tissue and to produce many hormones, vitamin D, and bile, which helps digest fats. Excess blood cholesterol is deposited in arteries, including the arteries of the heart. This increases the risk of heart disease.

High cholesterol may be hereditary, and cholesterol levels tend to rise as people age. Although heredity and age are out of your control, you can significantly reduce your risk of heart disease by eating a diet low in saturated fats and cholesterol. A high intake of saturated fats is linked to increased cholesterol production. Dietary cholesterol is found only in animal products such as egg yolks, meats (especially organ meats), and high-fat milk products. Losing excess weight can also lower cholesterol levels.

Vitamins

Vitamins are *compounds that help regulate many vital body processes, including the digestion, absorption, and metabolism of other nutrients.* Vitamins are classified as either water- or fat-soluble.

Water-soluble vitamins, listed in **Figure 5.1,** dissolve in water and pass easily into the blood during digestion. The body doesn't store these vitamins, so you need to replenish them regularly through the foods you eat. Fat-soluble vitamins are absorbed, stored, and transported in fat. Your body stores these vitamins in your fatty tissue, liver, and kidneys. Excess buildup of these vitamins in your body can be toxic. **Figure 5.2** on page 120 provides more information about fat-soluble vitamins.

FIGURE 5.1

WATER-SOLUBLE VITAMINS

Vitamin/Amount Needed Each Day	Role in Body	Food Source
C (ascorbic acid) Teen female: 60 mg Teen male: 60 mg	protects against infection, helps form connective tissue, helps heal wounds, maintains elasticity and strength of blood vessels, promotes healthy teeth and gums	citrus fruits, cantaloupe, tomatoes, cabbage, broccoli, potatoes, peppers
B_1 (thiamine) Teen female: 1.1 mg Teen male: 1.5 mg	converts glucose into energy or fat, contributes to good appetite	whole-grain or enriched cereals, liver, yeast, nuts, legumes, wheat germ
B_2 (riboflavin) Teen female: 1.3 mg Teen male: 1.8 mg	essential for producing energy from carbohydrates, fats, and proteins; helps keep skin healthy	milk, cheese, spinach, eggs, beef liver
Niacin Teen female: 15 mg Teen male: 20 mg	important for maintenance of all body tissues; helps in energy production; needed by body to utilize carbohydrates, to synthesize body fat, and for cell respiration	milk, eggs, poultry, beef, legumes, peanut butter, whole grains, enriched and fortified grain products
B_6 Teen female: 1.5 mg Teen male: 2.0 mg	essential for amino acid and carbohydrate metabolism, helps turn the amino acid *tryptophan* into serotonin (a messenger to the brain) and niacin	wheat bran and wheat germ, liver, meat, whole grains, fish, vegetables
Folic acid Teen female: 180 mcg Teen male: 200 mcg	necessary for production of genetic material and normal red blood cells, reduces risk of birth defects	nuts and other legumes, orange juice, green vegetables, folic acid-enriched breads and rolls, liver
B_{12} Teen female: 2.0 mcg Teen male: 2.0 mcg	necessary for production of red blood cells and for normal growth	animal products such as meat, fish, poultry, eggs, milk, and other dairy foods; some fortified foods

FIGURE 5.2

FAT-SOLUBLE VITAMINS

Vitamin/Amount Needed Each Day	Role in Body	Food Source
A Teen female: 800 mcg Teen male: 1,000 mcg	helps maintain skin tissue, strengthens tooth enamel, promotes use of calcium and phosphorous in bone formation, promotes cell growth, keeps eyes moist, helps eyes adjust to darkness, may aid in cancer prevention	milk and other dairy products, green vegetables, carrots, deep-orange fruits, liver
D Teen female: 5 mcg Teen male: 5 mcg	promotes absorption and use of calcium and phosphorous, essential for normal bone and tooth development	fortified milk, eggs, fortified breakfast cereals, sardines, salmon, beef, margarine; produced in skin exposed to sun's ultraviolet rays
E Teen female: 8 mg Teen male: 10 mg	may help in oxygen transport, may slow the effects of aging, may protect against destruction of red blood cells	present in vegetable oils, apples, peaches, nectarines, legumes, nuts, seeds, wheat germ
K Teen female: 55 mcg Teen male: 65 mcg	essential for blood clotting, assists in regulating blood calcium level	spinach, broccoli, eggs, liver, cabbage, tomatoes

▼ You get many of the minerals your body needs from these types of foods.

Minerals

Minerals are *substances that the body cannot manufacture but that are needed for forming healthy bones and teeth and for regulating many vital body processes.* Several key minerals are described in **Figure 5.3.**

Water

Water is vital to every body function. It transports other nutrients to and carries wastes from your cells. Water also lubricates your joints and mucous membranes. It enables you to swallow and digest foods, absorb other nutrients, and eliminate wastes. Through perspiration, water helps maintain normal body temperature. It's important to drink at least 8 cups of water a day to maintain health. Plain water, milk, and juice are the best sources of this nutrient. Beverages containing caffeine, such as tea, coffee, and some soft drinks, are not good choices—they cause you to lose some water through increased urination. Certain foods, such as fruits and vegetables, also contain some water.

FIGURE 5.3

SOME IMPORTANT MINERALS

Mineral/Amount Needed Each Day	Role in Body	Food Source
Calcium Teen female: 1,300 mg Teen male: 1,300 mg	building material of bones and teeth (skeleton contains about 99% of body calcium), regulation of body functions (heart muscle contraction, blood clotting)	dairy products; leafy vegetables; canned fish with soft, edible bones; tofu processed with calcium sulfate
Phosphorous Teen female: 1,250 mg Teen male: 1,250 mg	combines with calcium to give rigidity to bones and teeth, essential in cell metabolism, helps maintain proper acid-base balance of blood	milk and most other dairy foods, peas, beans, liver, meat, fish, poultry, eggs, broccoli, whole grains
Magnesium Teen female: 360 mg Teen male: 410 mg	enzyme activator related to carbohydrate metabolism, aids in bone growth and muscle contraction	whole grains, milk, dark green leafy vegetables, legumes, nuts
Iron Teen female: 15 mg Teen male: 12 mg	part of the red blood cells' oxygen and carbon dioxide transport system, important for use of energy in cells and for resistance to infection	meat, shellfish, poultry, legumes, peanuts, dried fruits, egg yolks, liver, fortified breakfast cereal, enriched rice

Lesson 2 *Review*

Reviewing Facts and Vocabulary

1. Compare the energy provided to the body by carbohydrates, proteins, and fats.

2. Analyze the relationship between good nutrition and disease prevention: How can reducing your saturated fat intake help lower the risk of heart disease?

3. What are *vitamins*?

Thinking Critically

4. **Analyzing.** Your friend Steve wants to cut down on his intake of saturated fats and cholesterol. What advice would you give him?

5. **Synthesizing.** What are the benefits of eating a variety of fruits and vegetables?

Applying Health Skills

Goal Setting. Copy your school's weekly lunch menus, and examine each day's options. Using what you've learned about nutrients in this lesson, list the most healthful food choices available each day. Then set a goal to eat healthful school lunches for the next week. Use the goal-setting steps to help you create a plan.

SPREADSHEETS   Use spreadsheet software to keep track of the meals you create from each day's school menu. Find help in using spreadsheet software at **health.glencoe.com**.

Guidelines for Healthful Eating

VOCABULARY
Dietary Guidelines for Americans
Food Guide Pyramid

YOU'LL LEARN TO

• Evaluate the concepts of balance, variety, and moderation, using the Food Guide Pyramid and national dietary guidelines.

• Examine the effects of healthful eating behaviors on body systems.

• Select healthful meals and snacks as part of a balanced diet.

QUICK START Make a word web of healthful eating habits. Write "Healthful Eating" in the middle of a sheet of paper. Then, around the edges of the paper, add phrases such as "Eat five fruits and vegetables a day"—one phrase for each of the major food groups. Connect these to the center phrase with lines.

Choosing nutritious foods from the thousands of products available can be a challenge. *What are some factors to consider when shopping for food?*

No single food provides all the nutrients your body needs. That's why it is so important to eat a balanced variety of nutrient-rich foods each day. There are tools to help you select the most nutritious foods in the appropriate amounts.

Dietary Guidelines for Americans

The U.S. Department of Agriculture (USDA) and the Department of Health and Human Services (DHHS) have published a booklet titled *Nutrition and Your Health: Dietary Guidelines for Americans*. The **Dietary Guidelines for Americans** is *a set of recommendations for healthful eating and active living.*

The recommendations in the *Dietary Guidelines* are grouped into three broad areas known as the ABCs of good health. Following the ABCs will help you stay fit and will ensure variety, balance, and moderation in your food choices. It can also help lower your risk of developing chronic diseases, such as those of the cardiovascular system.

A: Aim for Fitness

The "A" in the ABCs of good health deals with fitness goals. In addition to healthful eating, regular physical activity is important to staying well. To improve or maintain fitness, follow these guidelines.

▶ **Aim for a healthy weight.** Maintaining a healthy weight helps you look and feel good. A health care professional can help you determine a healthy weight for your height and age and the best way to achieve or maintain that weight.

▶ **Be physically active each day.** Daily physical activity benefits your overall health and can improve fitness. To maintain fitness, try to include at least 60 minutes of moderate physical activity in your daily routine.

B: Build a Healthy Base

The "B" in the ABCs relates to building a healthful eating plan. The "base" of this food plan is the **Food Guide Pyramid**, *a guide for making healthful daily food choices.* The following guidelines can help you build a healthy base.

▶ **Make your food choices carefully.** Eat the recommended number of daily servings from each of the five major food groups in the Food Guide Pyramid.

▶ **Choose a variety of grain products, especially whole grains.** Most of your daily food choices should be grain products. Whole-grain products are rich in complex carbohydrates and fiber, as well as some vitamins and minerals. Examples of whole-grain products include whole-wheat bread, oatmeal, and brown rice.

▶ **Choose a variety of fruits and vegetables daily.** Fruits and vegetables are rich in vitamins and minerals; some are high in fiber. Eating a variety of these foods will keep you healthy and may help protect you from many chronic diseases.

▶ **Keep food safe to eat.** You can reduce your risk of illness by cooking foods thoroughly, handling food with clean utensils, refrigerating perishable foods, and washing your hands before and after you handle foods. These steps make it less likely that food will cause sickness from harmful organisms and other contaminants.

Choosing a variety of fruits and vegetables each day is an important part of building a healthy base. *What fruits and vegetables would you choose as an afternoon snack?*

The Food Guide Pyramid

The Food Guide Pyramid, shown in **Figure 5.4,** is a useful tool for making healthful food choices each day. Notice that grain products are at the base of the pyramid—this means that most of your daily servings should come from the grain group. By eating the recommended number of daily servings from each food group, you'll achieve a balanced eating plan. The tip of the pyramid (Fats, Oils, and Sweets) is not a food group; these products should be consumed sparingly.

Keep in mind that meals often include foods from more than one group. What groups are represented in a meal of spaghetti with meat sauce?

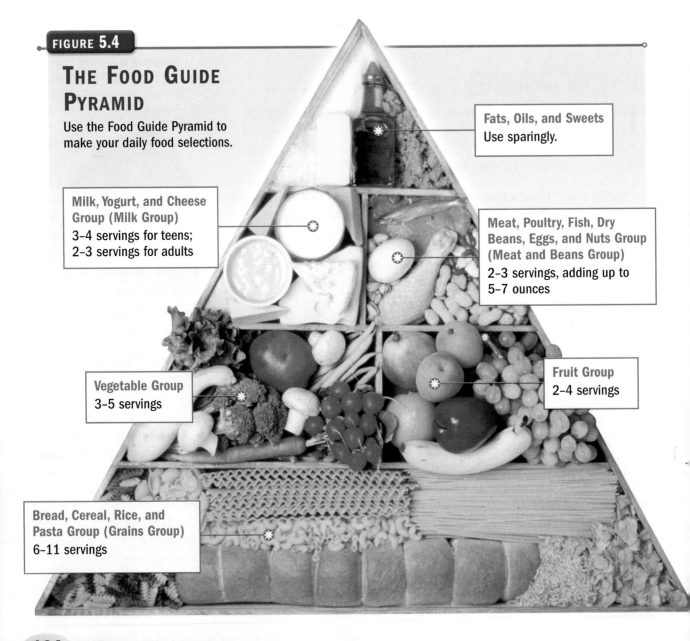

FIGURE 5.4

THE FOOD GUIDE PYRAMID

Use the Food Guide Pyramid to make your daily food selections.

Fats, Oils, and Sweets
Use sparingly.

Milk, Yogurt, and Cheese Group (Milk Group)
3–4 servings for teens; 2–3 servings for adults

Meat, Poultry, Fish, Dry Beans, Eggs, and Nuts Group (Meat and Beans Group)
2–3 servings, adding up to 5–7 ounces

Vegetable Group
3–5 servings

Fruit Group
2–4 servings

Bread, Cereal, Rice, and Pasta Group (Grains Group)
6–11 servings

FIGURE 5.5

SERVING SIZES

Grains Group	Vegetable Group	Fruit Group	Milk Group	Meat and Beans Group
• 1 slice bread • 1 tortilla • ½ small bagel • 1 cup dry cereal • ½ cup cooked cereal, rice, or pasta	• 1 cup raw leafy vegetables • ½ cup cooked or raw vegetables • ¾ cup vegetable juice	• 1 medium apple, orange, pear, or banana • ½ cup chopped, cooked, or canned fruit • ¾ cup fruit juice	• 1 cup milk or yogurt • 1.5 oz. natural cheese, such as Swiss • 2 oz. processed cheese	• 2–3 oz. cooked lean meat, fish, or poultry **Equivalents of 1 oz. of meat:** • ½ cup cooked dry beans/tofu • 1 egg • 2 tbsp. peanut butter • ⅓ cup nuts

Understanding Serving Sizes

The Food Guide Pyramid's recommended number of daily servings may seem like a lot of food to eat in one day. However, understanding what constitutes a serving will help you see how much food is actually being recommended. **Figure 5.5** lists sample serving sizes for each food group. Understanding serving sizes will help you practice portion control. A portion is how much of a food you eat in one meal. Visualizing some common objects can help you estimate serving sizes and control portions. For example, a medium apple is about the size of a tennis ball. One serving of meat is about the size of a regular computer mouse. A piece of meat twice this size equals two servings. To balance your daily food choices, try to eat enough servings from all five major food groups.

C: Choose Sensibly

The "C" in the ABCs of good health involves making sensible food choices, including

▶ choosing a diet that is low in saturated fat and cholesterol and moderate in total fat.

▶ choosing beverages and foods to moderate your intake of sugars.

▶ choosing and preparing foods with less salt.

CHARACTER CHECK

Citizenship. Citizenship means doing what you can to improve your community. For example, there may be people in your community who go hungry. **Find out how to organize an effort to collect nonperishable food items for a local food bank or homeless shelter. How could this benefit the whole community?**

Health Minute

These strategies
can help you make
healthful food choices.

**To limit dietary fat and
cholesterol:**

▶ Aim to get most of your
calories from whole grains,
vegetables, and fruits.

▶ Read labels on prepared
foods to determine how much
total fat, saturated fat, and
cholesterol a serving of the
food contains.

▶ Calculate the percentage
of fat in one serving: Divide
calories from fat by total
calories.

▶ Try to choose foods that
have 3 grams or less of fat
per serving. These foods are
considered low in fat.

Moderation in Fats

While some dietary fats are necessary for good health, most Americans eat too many fats. The *Dietary Guidelines* recommends that no more than 30 percent of daily calories come from fats, yet most Americans consume a diet that averages a significantly higher percentage. Eating less fat, especially saturated fat, lowers your risk of cardiovascular disease. You don't have to completely eliminate your favorite high-fat foods to limit your intake to no more than 30 percent of calories from fat. If you eat high-fat foods at one meal, eat foods that are lower in fats at other meals.

Moderation in Sugar

You might think that you don't eat much added sugar, but sugars are hidden everywhere, including in prepared foods. You can moderate your sugar intake by

▶ learning to identify added sugars by their names on food packages. Corn syrup, honey, and molasses are all types of sugar, as are ingredients ending with -*ose*, such as sucrose and maltose.

▶ balancing foods that have added sugars with foods that have less added sugars.

▶ limiting your intake of foods that have added sugars but few other nutrients. For example, choose 100 percent fruit juice or water instead of regular soda.

▶ choosing fresh fruits or canned fruits packed in water or juice.

Moderation in Salt

Sodium is an essential mineral. It helps transport nutrients into your cells and helps move wastes out. It also helps maintain normal blood pressure and nerve function. However, most Americans consume far too much salt, much of it from processed foods. Consuming less salt can reduce your chances of developing high blood pressure and may also benefit your skeletal system by decreasing the loss of calcium from bone. Try these tips to moderate your salt intake.

▶ Read the Nutrition Facts panel on food labels to find out how much sodium a serving contains.

▶ Season foods with herbs and spices instead of with salt.

▶ When eating at restaurants, ask for foods that are prepared without salt or salty flavorings or with reduced amounts of them.

▶ Taste foods before you salt them, and then go easy with the salt shaker.

▶ Choose fruits and vegetables often. They contain very little salt unless it is added in processing.

Smart Snacking

Eating several small snacks each day can help growing teens get the nutrients they need. You can choose snacks that promote good health without adding too much fat or too many calories.

Nutrition Facts
Serving Size 1 cookie (17g)
Servings Per Container about 27

Amount Per Serving

Calories 90	Calories from Fat 45

	% Daily Value*
Total Fat 5g	**8%**
Saturated Fat 2.5g	**13%**
Cholesterol 5mg	**2%**
Sodium 80mg	**3%**
Total Carbohydrate 11g	**4%**
Dietary Fiber 0g	0%
Sugars 6g	
Protein 1g	

Vitamin A	0% •	Vitamin C	0%
Calcium	0% •	Iron	2%

* Percent Daily Values are based on a 2,000 calorie diet. Your daily values may be higher or lower depending on your calorie needs:

Calories from Fat
Look at this section of the Nutrition Facts panel to find out how much fat is in the snack you are choosing.

Total Fat
This gives you an overview of the fat in the snack. The amount of fat is listed in grams. Remember that fats provide 9 calories per gram, so even small amounts of fats can add a lot of calories.

Saturated Fat
This tells how much of the fat in the snack is saturated. Remember, limiting saturated fats can help reduce the risk of heart disease.

Total Carbohydrate
Under this heading you'll find information about sugars. These, too, are listed in grams. Carbohydrates provide 4 calories per gram.

ACTIVITY

In small groups, examine the snack labels that your group or teacher has brought to class. Use the above callouts to help you identify snacks that are low in fat and sugar. In a paragraph, explain other ways the information on labels can help you choose nutritious snacks.

Healthful Eating Patterns

Whether you eat three meals a day or even more "mini-meals," *variety, moderation,* and *balance* are the foundation of a healthful eating plan. Many people, including teens, find making healthful food choices particularly challenging when having breakfast, snacking, and eating out. Keep in mind that nutrition guidelines apply to all of your daily food choices, not to just a single meal or food. Any food that supplies calories and nutrients can be part of a healthful eating plan. You don't have to deprive yourself of your favorite foods. With a little planning, you can fit them into your diet.

Many types of foods can be part of a healthy breakfast. *Name three nontraditional breakfast foods that you might like to try.*

The Importance of Breakfast

You've probably heard the saying, "Breakfast is the most important meal of the day." While you sleep, your body uses energy for functions such as breathing and keeping your heart beating. By the time you wake up, your body needs a fresh supply of energy. Studies show that eating a nutritious breakfast improves mental and physical performance and reduces fatigue later in the day. If you eat breakfast, you tend to perform better in school, get better grades, and miss fewer days of school. Eating breakfast may also help you maintain a healthy weight. Skipping this meal may cause you to overeat later in the day.

Breakfast foods don't have to be "traditional," such as cereal or eggs. Try eating pizza, peanut butter on toast, or a stuffed tomato. To get enough vitamin C, add citrus juice, fruit, or tomato juice to your meal. Breakfast is also a good time to eat a high-fiber cereal and get one calcium-rich serving of milk, cheese, or yogurt.

Nutritious Snacks

A healthful eating plan can include sensible snacks. When you think about snacks, you might think of potato chips, soft drinks, and candy bars. These foods contain a lot of calories but very few nutrients. They may also be high in fat, added sugars, or salt. More healthful snacks include whole-grain products, fruits, and vegetables. Food companies have also started offering healthier snack choices, such as potato chips that are baked instead of fried. **Figure 5.6** lists some healthful snack items.

FIGURE 5.6

SENSIBLE SNACKS

Food	Food Group	Total Calories per Serving	Calories from Fat
Air-popped popcorn, 3 cups (plain)	Grains	23	0
Apple, 1 medium	Fruit	80	0
Bagel, ½ (small, 2 oz.)	Grains	83	10
Bread stick, 1	Grains	42	6
Frozen juice bar, 4 oz.	Fruit	75	0
Skim milk, 1 cup	Milk	90	0
Sugar-free gelatin (½ cup) with ½ cup sliced banana	Fruit	76	0
Graham cracker squares, 3	Grains	80	15
Pretzel sticks, 50 small	Grains	60	9
Fat-free, sugar-free yogurt, 6 oz.	Milk	86	0

Eating Out, Eating Right

Part of healthful eating is making sensible food choices when you eat out. It might help to use the Food Guide Pyramid when ordering restaurant food. Also, be aware that many menu items may be fried or topped with mayonnaise, butter, or high-fat sauces. For less fat, order foods that are grilled, baked, or broiled, and ask that high-fat sauces not be used at all or be served on the side. Many fast-food restaurants list the calorie counts and other nutrition information for the foods they serve. You can ask to see this list before placing your order.

When eating out, don't forget to think about portion control. The portion sizes of most restaurant meals are much larger than the serving sizes in the Food Guide Pyramid. You may want to eat only part of a portion and take the rest home to enjoy later. As an alternative, offset the larger meal with a smaller meal later.

 When eating out, don't hesitate to ask how a particular dish is cooked or what ingredients it contains. *Name two other ways to make healthy food choices when eating out.*

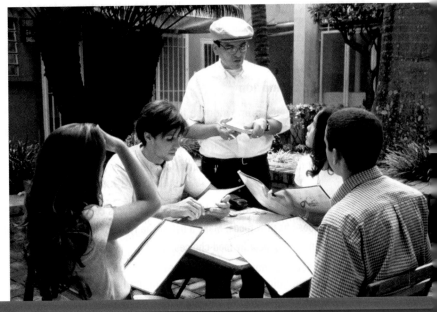

Lesson 3 *Review*

Reviewing Facts and Vocabulary

1. Define the *Dietary Guidelines for Americans.*
2. What is the purpose of the Food Guide Pyramid?
3. Examine the effects of healthful eating behaviors on body systems: How can decreasing salt intake benefit the cardiovascular and skeletal systems?

Thinking Critically

4. **Analyzing.** Why might a person eat fewer servings than recommended by the Food Guide Pyramid and still gain an unhealthful amount of weight?
5. **Evaluating.** For lunch Josh had a cheeseburger, fries, and a nondiet soft drink. What could he choose for his afternoon snack and dinner to balance out his high-fat, high-sugar, high-salt meal?

Applying Health Skills

Advocacy. Work with a partner to create a poster that encourages teens to adopt healthful eating habits. Use pictures cut from magazines, computer graphics, or your own drawings to illustrate your poster.

TECHNOLOGY *OPTION*

WEB SITES   Use information and drawings from your poster to create a Web page encouraging teens to develop healthful eating habits. See **health.glencoe.com** for help with planning and building your own Web site.

Analyzing Food Ads

Being overweight is associated with many serious health problems, including type 2 diabetes. Ads for fast food and high-calorie snacks may influence young people to consume foods that contribute to unhealthful weight gain. In this activity you will learn to recognize the different techniques food advertisers use to appeal to children and teens.

Language	Color	Music	Types of Characters	Editing Methods

ACTIVITY

One way to critique a TV ad is to consider its style. An ad's style includes its use of language, color, and music; types of characters featured; and methods of film editing. Ads for breakfast cereals, for example, often feature cartoon characters to draw in children. Fast-food ads may have a fast-paced editing style, such as that seen in music videos, to appeal to teens.

Critique a TV ad for a food product that is targeted to children or teens. Use a chart like the one above to describe each element of the ad. Then write an essay indicating how the style of the ad is attempting to draw in its target audience. Explain why the advertised food should not be targeted to children or teens. Include information on why the food is a poor nutritional choice for a healthful eating plan.

EXPRESS YOUR VIEWS

Should fast-food and convenience-food manufacturers be required to put warning labels on their products that describe the health risks of consuming a particular food? Hold a class debate on this issue.

CROSS-CURRICULUM CONNECTIONS

Write a Story. Compose a short story about a family enjoying a traditional feast featuring their native cuisine. You may wish to focus on your own cultural or ethnic background, or choose one that you are interested in. Research that culture's cuisine and dining customs to incorporate into your story, and be sure to use vivid, descriptive language to set the scene.

Give an Oral Report. Early settlers in America had to modify their diets based on the foods available in the area where they settled. Your teacher will divide you into groups and assign you a particular U.S. region to study. Research what groups settled in that area and how they adapted their diets to incorporate the foods available in that region. Create a visual aid, and present an oral report to the class.

Calculate the Calories. The USDA's *Dietary Guidelines for Americans* recommends that no more than 30 percent of daily calories come from fat. Mike is a teen whose recommended daily calorie intake is 2,800 calories. Keeping in mind that a gram of fat yields 9 calories, if the total fat content of Mike's breakfast and lunch totals 38.6 grams, how many more calories from fat can he eat that day and still remain within the recommended limits?

Conduct Research. The French chemist Louis-Camille Maillard noticed that certain chemical compounds appeared in foods during the cooking process that were not present in the raw food. This phenomenon is now called the Maillard Reaction. List some common foods, such as bread, meats, and vegetables, and research the compounds produced in the Maillard Reaction when they are cooked.

Dietetic Technician

Do you enjoy planning meals and cooking? Do you like interacting with others? If so, you may enjoy a career as a dietetic technician. This career allows you to assist dietitians in the planning of healthful meals.

To enter this field, you must first complete a two-year associate's degree program. You'll also need to complete an accredited dietetic technician program and pass a national exam. To maintain certification, you'll need to stay up-to-date on nutrition trends. Find out more about this and other health careers by clicking on Career Corner at **health.glencoe.com**.

Chapter 5 *Review*

► EXPLORING HEALTH TERMS *Answer the following questions on a sheet of paper.*

Lesson 1 *Fill in the blanks with the correct term.*

hunger   **nutrition**   **calories**
nutrients   **appetite**

The process by which the body takes in and uses food is (**_1_**). (**_2_**) are the units of heat that measure the energy used by the body and the energy that foods supply to the body. The substances in food that your body needs to function properly are (**_3_**).

Lesson 2 *Match each definition with the correct term.*

vitamins   **lipid**   **carbohydrates**
proteins   **fiber**   **minerals**

4. The starches and sugars present in foods.

5. An indigestible complex carbohydrate.

6. Nutrients that help build and maintain body cells and tissues.

7. A fatty substance that does not dissolve in water.

Lesson 3 *Fill in the blanks with the correct term.*

Food Guide Pyramid
Dietary Guidelines for Americans

8. The _____ is a set of recommendations for healthful eating and active living prepared by the USDA and DHHS.

9. The _____ is a guide for making healthful daily food choices.

Lesson 4 *Match each definition with the correct term.*

food allergy   **pasteurization**
food additives   **cross-contamination**
foodborne illness   **food intolerance**

10. Substances intentionally added to food to produce a desired effect.

11. Another name for food poisoning.

12. The spreading of bacteria or other pathogens from one food to another.

► RECALLING THE FACTS *Use complete sentences to answer the following questions.*

Lesson 1

1. How does hunger differ from appetite?

2. Give an example of how friends and peers can influence food choices.

3. Why is good nutrition especially important during the teen years?

Lesson 2

4. What is the relationship between glucose and glycogen?

5. How does water benefit the body?

6. List three minerals that are important for health.

Lesson 3

7. What are the ABCs of good health?

8. Most of the foods you eat each day should come from which three parts of the Food Guide Pyramid?

9. How many servings should you eat each day from the Milk Group? From the Meat and Beans Group?

Lesson 4

10. What does the Percent Daily Value column of a food label tell you?

11. What are some symptoms of a food allergy?

12. How can you keep picnic foods safe to eat?

▶ THINKING CRITICALLY

1. **Synthesizing.** Use specific examples to explain how strong emotions such as anger and fear might affect your eating habits. *(LESSON 1)*

2. **Evaluating.** Explain why it's important to know whether a fat is saturated or unsaturated. *(LESSON 2)*

3. **Applying.** What would you say to someone who always skips breakfast because he or she isn't hungry in the morning? *(LESSON 3)*

4. **Analyzing.** Several hours after eating dinner, you begin to feel nauseous and feverish and you have some abdominal cramps. What type of problem might these symptoms suggest? *(LESSON 4)*

▶ HEALTH SKILLS APPLICATION

1. **Advocacy.** Watch 30 minutes of television and keep a record of the food commercials shown. Analyze the health messages delivered through these food ads. Then write a script for an advertisement that encourages viewers to try a particular healthful food. *(LESSON 1)*

2. **Goal Setting.** Develop a table that summarizes what you have learned about the nutrients your body needs. Include in your table the name of each type of nutrient, why your body needs the nutrient, and what foods you can eat to make sure you include enough of the nutrient in your eating plan. Then set a goal to improve your intake of one or more of these nutrients. Use the goal-setting steps to reach your goal. *(LESSON 2)*

3. **Accessing Information.** Use reliable online resources to do more in-depth research on the relationship between nutrition and heart disease. How can good nutrition prevent this disease and improve quality of life? Summarize your findings in a one-page report. *(LESSON 3)*

4. **Practicing Healthful Behaviors.** Analyze how healthful practices might reduce the risk of foodborne illness, a communicable disease. Then develop a plan that features safe cooking strategies to reduce the spread of foodborne pathogens. *(LESSON 4)*

 BEYOND *the* Classroom

Parent Involvement

Accessing Information. Work with your family to make a list of the prepared and fast foods you most enjoy eating. Then look through cookbooks to find recipes for similar treats that contain less fat, sugar, and salt. Make a recipe booklet of these healthful alternatives, and set a goal to try one new recipe each week.

School and Community

Meals on Wheels. Many communities have organizations such as Meals on Wheels or other groups that provide nutritious meals to older adults or physically challenged individuals who are unable to prepare meals for themselves. Find out whether your community has such an organization and how you and your classmates can become involved.

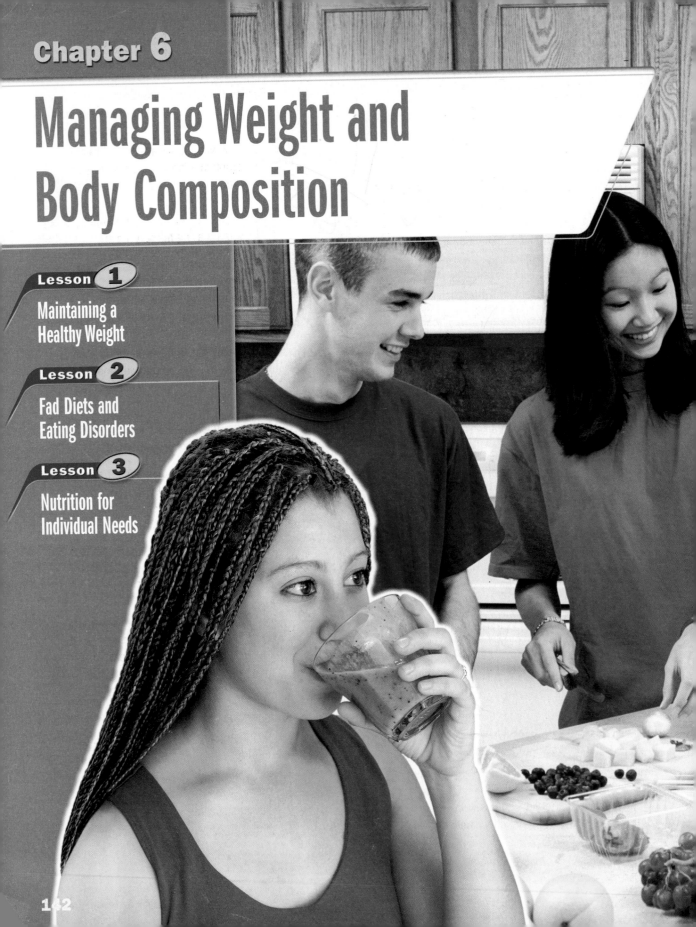

Managing Weight and Body Composition

Kevin's Story

Kevin has always had a weight problem. When he was younger, it didn't seem to matter much that he was a little bigger than the other boys. In fact, the extra weight came in handy when playing his favorite sport—football.

Now Kevin is 15, and things seem very different to him. He's worried about how he looks and feels. "Being overweight is supposed to be a girl's problem," says Kevin. "It's embarrassing that I have to worry about my weight."

Kevin finds it difficult to make healthy food choices. He often eats at fast-food restaurants and snacks on candy bars and potato chips. He also doesn't get much physical activity.

In the past Kevin has tried quick fixes to lose weight. "One time I went on a fad diet, but that didn't really work," says Kevin. "I lost weight at first, but then I started feeling really run down, so I went back to my old way of eating. Before I knew it, I had regained all the weight I lost, plus a few extra pounds."

Kevin knows he has to change his lifestyle in order to lose weight, but he doesn't know what steps to take.

HEALTH Online

For instant feedback on your health status, go to Chapter 6 Health Inventory at **health.glencoe.com**.

Quick*Write*

Using Visuals. Maintaining a healthy weight involves being physically active and making healthful food choices. Write a brief paragraph describing the healthful food choices these teens are making.

Maintaining a Healthy Weight

VOCABULARY

body image
body mass index (BMI)
overweight
obesity
underweight
nutrient-dense foods

YOU'LL LEARN TO

- Examine the relationship among body composition, diet, and fitness.
- Analyze the relationship between maintaining a healthy weight and disease prevention.
- Describe healthful ways to manage weight.

→ **QUICK START**   On a sheet of paper, list three feelings a person might have about his or her body's appearance. Then write down three factors that might influence these feelings.

 Media images can have an impact on a person's body image. *How might messages sent by media images negatively affect body image?*

When you look in the mirror, how do you feel about what you see? Are you happy with the way you look, or do you wish some things were different? *The way you see your body* is called your **body image**. Body image is affected by several factors, including media images and the attitudes of family and friends.

For many people body image is tied to perception of weight. Your own healthy weight probably won't be the same as the weight of a fashion model, a bodybuilder, or your best friend. However, you can use some general guidelines to assess your weight and keep it within a healthy range.

The Weight-Calorie Connection

To understand how to manage your weight effectively, it's important to understand calories. As you've learned, calories are units used to measure energy—both the energy in food and the energy your body uses for life processes and physical activities. Maintaining a healthy weight, even while you're growing, is a matter of energy balance: the calories you consume must equal the calories your body burns.

Calories: Their Source

Some foods have more calories than others. The specific number of calories depends on portion size as well as the amounts of carbohydrates, proteins, and fats in the food. Both carbohydrates and proteins supply four calories per gram. Fats supply more than twice that number—nine calories per gram. For this reason, even small amounts of fat in a food greatly increase its calorie content. The way a food is prepared or cooked also affects the calorie count.

The Energy Equation

Tipping the balance of the energy equation will result in weight loss or gain. If you take in fewer calories than you burn, you lose weight. If you take in more calories than you burn, you gain weight.

One pound of body fat equals about 3,500 calories. Eating 500 fewer calories per day than you need to maintain your weight will result in the loss of one pound of body fat after one week (500 calories per day × 7 days = 3,500 calories). Burning an additional 500 calories per day through physical activity would result in a similar weight loss.

Determining Your Appropriate Weight Range

Your appropriate weight is influenced by several factors, including gender, age, height, body frame, growth rate, metabolic rate, and activity level. As a teen you are still growing, so you need more calories than an adult does. Tall and large-framed people need more calories than short and small-framed people. Because an active person burns more calories than a sedentary person does, he or she can consume more calories without gaining weight than a sedentary person can.

Body Mass Index

One way to evaluate whether your weight is within a healthy range is to determine body mass index. **Body mass index (BMI)** is *a ratio that allows you to assess your body size in relation to your height and weight.* Because BMI for children and teens takes age and gender into account, different charts are used for males and females. **Figure 6.1** on page 146 explains how to determine your BMI. A different chart is used for adults.

As you calculate your BMI, keep in mind that many different ratios of height to weight can be healthy. Teens grow at different rates and in different ways. There is no single size, shape, or growth pattern that's normal for everyone.

Height and gender are two factors that need to be considered when evaluating a person's weight.

FIGURE 6.1

DETERMINING BMI

Use this formula to find your BMI:

$$BMI = \text{weight (in pounds)} \times 703/[\text{height (in inches)}]^2$$

Here's how to find the BMI for a 16-year-old male who weighs 145 pounds and is 65 inches tall:

$$BMI = 145 \times 703 / 65^2$$
$$BMI = 101{,}935 / 4{,}225$$
$$BMI = 24.12 \text{ or } 24$$

Find this result in the chart. This teen's BMI indicates that he is within an appropriate weight range.

Source: Adapted from CDC information

BMI Chart for Boys

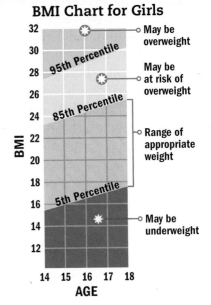

BMI Chart for Girls

If your BMI falls above the 85th percentile or below the 5th percentile, consult a health care professional for further evaluation. However, keep in mind that this does not necessarily mean that you are over- or underweight.

Body Composition

Body composition, or the ratio of body fat to lean body tissue, needs to be taken into account when assessing weight. Diet and fitness affect a person's body composition. For example, a weight-lifting program will increase muscle mass. A high-calorie diet can increase the amount of stored body fat.

Body Weight versus Body Fat

The terms *overweight* and *obesity* are often used interchangeably, but they are not the same. **Overweight** is *a condition in which a person is heavier than the standard weight range for his or her height.* **Obesity** refers specifically to *having an excess amount of body fat.* Being overweight or obese can endanger health. In certain cases being overweight may not pose health risks. Athletes such as bodybuilders or football players may be overweight because of excess muscle tissue rather than excess body fat.

Weight-Related Health Risks

BMI for adults serves as a general guide to evaluate some health risks. Adults with high BMIs are at increased risk of cardiovascular disease; type 2 diabetes; cancer; high blood pressure; and osteoarthritis, a joint disease. Maintaining a healthy weight can help prevent the development of these diseases.

Overweight: A Health Risk

Being overweight is a serious problem in the United States. The latest findings from the CDC indicate that 14 percent of teens are overweight. Excess body fat strains the muscles and the skeletal system. It forces the heart and lungs to work harder and increases the risk of high blood pressure and high blood cholesterol. Being overweight or obese also increases the risk of type 2 diabetes, asthma, and some cancers.

Why are some people overweight? Genetics may play a role, but overweight and obesity usually result from consuming excess calories and from physical inactivity. To maintain a healthy weight and avoid the health risks associated with overweight and obesity, follow the ABCs of good health as described in the *Dietary Guidelines for Americans:*

▶ **Aim for Fitness.** Get 60 minutes of physical activity daily.

▶ **Build a Healthy Base.** Eat the recommended number of daily servings from each of the five major food groups in the **Food Guide Pyramid.**

▶ **Choose Sensibly.** Balance high-fat choices with low-fat foods, and moderate your intake of sugar.

Underweight: A Health Risk

Some teens are very thin while they are growing. Being thin may also be normal because of genetics or a fast metabolism. Other people, however, diet or exercise excessively to stay thin. A person who is too thin has little stored fat to provide the body with an energy reserve and may not be consuming enough calories and nutrients for health and growth. This may lead to fatigue and a decreased ability to fight illness. How do you know whether you are underweight? **Underweight** refers to *a condition in which a person is less than the standard weight range for his or her height.* A health care professional can help you determine whether you are underweight.

hot link

Dietary Guidelines for Americans For more information on the *Dietary Guidelines*, see Chapter 5, page 122.
Food Guide Pyramid See Chapter 5, page 124, to learn more about using the Food Guide Pyramid to make healthy food choices.

▼ **Physical activities such as swimming burn calories and can help you manage your weight.** *What other physical activities can help you manage your weight?*

FIGURE 6.2

THE BEST WEIGHT-LOSS STRATEGY

Eat Fewer Calories

Eat more foods that are high in nutrients and low in calories.

Burn More Calories

Burn more calories through physical activity.

Healthful Ways to Manage Weight

The teen years are a period of rapid growth and change, so some fluctuations in your weight are normal during this time. Following the ABCs of good health will help most teens maintain a healthy weight. However, if you want to begin a formal weight-management plan, these strategies can help:

▶ **Target your appropriate weight.** Speak with a health care professional to determine a weight range that is healthy for you.

▶ **Set realistic goals.** Gaining or losing one-half pound to one pound per week is a safe and realistic goal.

▶ **Personalize your plan.** Think about your food preferences and lifestyle when designing your weight management program.

▶ **Put your goal and plan in writing.** You might also find it helpful to keep a journal of what and when you eat to become more aware of your eating habits.

▶ **Evaluate your progress.** Track your progress by weighing yourself weekly at the same time of day. Remember that time periods when your weight does not change are normal.

Healthy Weight-Loss Strategies

A health care provider is your best source of information about your appropriate weight. If he or she recommends that you lose weight, use the best weight-loss strategy, illustrated in **Figure 6.2.** Here are some other tips for losing weight.

▶ **Eat 1,700 to 1,800 calories daily to meet your body's energy needs.** To reach this goal, eat at least the minimum number of servings from each of the five groups in the Food Guide Pyramid. Eating fewer than 1,400 calories a day may cause you to miss out on essential nutrients.

▶ **Include your favorites in moderation.** Eat smaller portions of your favorite high-calorie foods, and eat them less frequently. Instead of giving up ice cream altogether, for example, have a small scoop once a week.

▶ **Eat a variety of low-calorie, nutrient-dense foods. Nutrient-dense foods** are *foods that are high in nutrients as compared with their calorie content.* Whole-grain products, vegetables, and fruits are examples of low-calorie, nutrient-dense foods.

▶ **Drink plenty of water.** Eight glasses a day will help keep your body functioning at its best.

Exploring Issues

Should Schools Limit the Use of Vending Machines?

In schools across the country, vending machines offer soda, candy, and other snacks. Some schools limit the types of foods offered in vending machines or restrict student access to the machines. Should schools set rules concerning vending machines? Here are two points of view.

Viewpoint 1: Philip S., age 16

Most of the food in vending machines is high in sugar, fat, or salt—definitely not part of a healthful eating plan. I've seen kids eat only the foods from vending machines for lunch. If access to the vending machines were limited, students would have to eat more healthful meals. I think that schools have every right to put limits on access or to change the foods offered.

Viewpoint 2: Katie T., age 15

I don't think schools need to limit the types of snacks in vending machines or restrict students' access to them. It's up to the individual to make responsible decisions about his or her food choices. Besides, eating snacks high in sugar, fat, or salt is okay once in a while.

ACTIVITIES

1. **Are vending machines interfering with students' efforts to eat healthfully? Why or why not?**
2. **Should schools control the contents of vending machines or restrict access to them? Explain your answer.**

Healthy Weight-Gain Strategies

Follow these tips to gain weight healthfully:

▶ **Increase your calorie intake.** Choose foods high in complex carbohydrates, such as breads, pasta, and potatoes. Limit foods high in fat and sugar.

▶ **Eat often and take second helpings.** Choose more than the minimum number of servings from each food group in the Food Guide Pyramid.

▶ **Eat nutritious snacks.** Snack two to three hours before meals to avoid spoiling your appetite.

▶ **Build muscle.** A supervised resistance-training program will help you gain weight by increasing muscle mass.

Health Online

Go to **health.glencoe.com** to learn more about the basics of healthy weight management.

Fruit and vegetable drinks are nutrient-dense snacks that can be part of a healthy weight-management plan.
What are some other examples of nutrient-dense snacks?

Physical Activity and Weight Management

Whether you want to lose, gain, or maintain weight, regular physical activity should be part of your plan. Aerobic exercise burns calories and helps you lose fat. Weight lifting or resistance training will increase muscle mass and produce a firm, lean body shape. Also, since muscle is more efficient than fat at burning calories, having more lean muscle tissue increases the number of calories your body burns, even at rest. Here are some added benefits of regular physical activity:

► It helps relieve the stress that often leads to over- or undereating.

► It promotes a normal appetite response, which helps you gain, lose, or maintain weight.

► It increases self-esteem, which helps keep your plan on track.

Research consistently shows that regular physical activity, combined with healthy eating habits, is the most efficient and healthful way to manage your weight and live a healthy life. Choose activities that you enjoy and that fit your personality. You will soon discover your body's capabilities and begin to look and feel your best.

Lesson 1 *Review*

Reviewing Facts and Vocabulary

1. List three factors that influence what an individual's appropriate weight should be.

2. Explain the difference between the terms *overweight* and *obesity*.

3. Examine and briefly describe the relationship among body composition, diet, and fitness.

Thinking Critically

4. **Analyzing.** How can keeping a food journal help a person manage his or her weight?

5. **Hypothesizing.** Why is it important to eat a variety of low-calorie, nutrient-dense foods if you're trying to lose weight?

Applying Health Skills

Practicing Healthful Behaviors. Vicki wants to be sure that she maintains a healthy weight range as she moves through her teen years. What behaviors can Vicki practice to help her meet this goal? Write a short story that shows how Vicki practices these behaviors.

WORD PROCESSING Word processing can give your short story a professional look. See **health.glencoe.com** for tips on how to get the most out of your word-processing program.

Fad Diets and Eating Disorders

VOCABULARY

fad diets
weight cycling
eating disorder
anorexia nervosa
bulimia nervosa
binge eating
    disorder

YOU'LL LEARN TO

- Describe the risks of fad diets and other dangerous weight-loss strategies.

- Describe the causes, symptoms, and treatment of eating disorders.

- Provide help to someone with an eating disorder.

- Identify the presence of an eating disorder as a situation requiring assistance from professional health services.

QUICK START   Write the term *diet* in the center of a sheet of paper. Around this term, write five to ten words or phrases that come to mind when you hear the word *diet*.

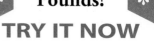
"Miracle patch lets you lose weight without dieting!" "One pill helps you burn fat and lose pounds!" Are you familiar with promises like these? They often appear in print ads and TV commercials. You may hear them on the radio. Such ads promise quick and easy weight loss. What do they actually deliver?

 Fad diets may promise quick and easy weight loss, but any weight lost on these diets is usually regained. *What features does a healthful weight-loss program have?*

Risky Weight-Loss Strategies

A number of weight-loss strategies not only fail to produce long-term results but also can cause serious health problems. Part of being a health-literate consumer involves recognizing the potential health risks associated with some weight-loss plans and products.

Fad Diets

If you see an ad like the one shown here, be wary. Such ads are often for **fad diets**, *weight-loss plans that are popular for only a short time*. These diets often are hard to stick with because they limit food variety. The "grapefruit diet" is an example of a food-limiting fad diet. Some fad diets are costly because they require dieters to buy certain products. Fad diets that severely restrict the foods a dieter eats fail to provide the body with the nutrients it needs for health and growth. Any weight lost on fad diets is usually regained.

> Some weight-loss products contain a substance called *ephedra.* Manufacturers may claim that ephedra can suppress appetite, promote weight loss, and increase energy and physical endurance. However, ephedra can lead to heart attacks, strokes, or even death.
>
> Always read the labels of products before you buy or use them, and never take a product containing ephedra.

Effective weight management involves making healthy lifestyle choices. *What steps can a person take to successfully manage his or her weight?*

Liquid Diets

A person on a liquid diet replaces all of his or her food intake with a special liquid formula. These very-low-calorie diets generally do not meet the body's energy needs. As a result, they often leave the dieter feeling fatigued. Many liquid diets do not provide the body with fiber and needed nutrients. Relying on high-protein, low-carbohydrate liquids as the only source of nutrients can cause serious health problems and even death. Because of the potential dangers associated with liquid diets, the U.S. Food and Drug Administration (FDA) requires these products to carry warning labels and recommends that they be used only under close medical supervision.

Fasting

To fast is to abstain from eating. Although this may seem like a sure way to lose weight, fasting for more than short periods deprives your body of needed nutrients and energy. Without a fresh supply of nutrients each day, your body begins breaking down protein stored in muscle tissue for energy. If the person who is fasting also avoids liquids, he or she may become dehydrated.

Some religious and cultural rituals involve brief periods of fasting. Such fasting is not dangerous for the average person because the fast is of limited duration. However, fasting may not be advisable for those with diabetes or other health conditions. If you are unsure about how cultural or religious fasting may affect a medical condition, consult a health care professional for advice.

Diet Pills

Many diet pills work by suppressing appetite. They may cause drowsiness, anxiety, a racing heart, or other serious side effects. Diet pills may also be addictive. Some cause the body to lose more water than normal, which can lead to dehydration. Diet pills may claim to "burn," "block," or "flush" fat from the body, but a low-risk pill that meets these claims has not yet been developed.

Weight Cycling

Some diet plans or products may seem to help people lose weight quickly, but the weight loss is usually from water, not body fat. Water weight lost is quickly regained. *The repeated pattern of loss and regain of body weight* is called **weight cycling**. Weight cycling is common in people who follow fad diets. Some reports have suggested that weight cycling is harmful, although other studies do not support this finding. In general, slow and steady weight loss is the best strategy for long-lasting results.

Fad Diets Harm Health

In a society obsessed by weight and appearance, the promise of quick weight loss is hard to resist. However, fad diets are not only ineffective in producing long-term weight loss, they're also potentially harmful. In this activity you will create a poster advocating against fad diets.

What You'll Need

- poster board
- markers

What You'll Do

1. As a class, brainstorm potentially harmful effects of fad diets.

2. In groups of two or three, come up with a simple concept that conveys the message that fad diets can harm health. Your concept should be relevant to high school students.

3. Make a poster illustrating your message. Include supporting information about healthful weight-loss strategies in the poster.

4. Ask permission to display your posters at school.

Apply and Conclude

Is your poster persuasive? What advocacy techniques did you use to persuade others? How will your poster have a positive effect on the health of your audience? Why is this an important health issue for teens?

The Risks of Eating Disorders

Sometimes a person's concerns about weight and efforts to lose weight can get out of control. Becoming obsessed with thinness can lead to eating disorders. An **eating disorder** is an *extreme, harmful eating behavior that can cause serious illness or even death*. The exact cause of eating disorders is unknown. They may be brought on by mental or emotional factors such as poor body image, social and family pressures, and perfectionism. Some scientists think that the cause may be partly genetic. Teens with a family history of weight problems, depression, or substance abuse may be more at risk for developing an eating disorder.

About 90 percent of those with eating disorders are female. It's estimated that about one percent of females ages 16 to 18 have this illness. Eating disorders are a serious health problem, and people who suffer from them need professional help.

Anorexia Nervosa

Anorexia nervosa is *a disorder in which the irrational fear of becoming obese results in severe weight loss from self-imposed starvation.* Anorexia nervosa is a psychological disorder with emotional and physical consequences. The disorder relates to an individual's self-concept and coping abilities. Outside pressures, high expectations, a need to be accepted, and a need to achieve are characteristics associated with the development of anorexia. Medical specialists have also found that genetics and other biological factors may play an equally powerful role in the development of this disorder. Hormones and certain brain chemicals have been shown to trigger the illness in some people.

Anorexia develops most often in teenage girls and young women. Symptoms include extremely low caloric intake, an obsession with exercising, emotional problems, an unnatural interest in food, a distorted body image, and denial of an eating problem.

HEALTH CONSEQUENCES OF ANOREXIA NERVOSA

Physical consequences of anorexia are related to malnutrition and starvation. A drastic reduction of body fat may cause females with anorexia to stop menstruating. Other consequences include loss of bone density, low body temperature, low blood pressure, slowed metabolism, and reduction in organ size. People with anorexia may develop serious heart problems, including an irregular heartbeat that can lead to cardiac arrest and sudden death.

Treatment for anorexia nervosa may include a stay at a clinic or hospital where the person can receive nutrients to regain weight and strength. Anorexia nervosa also requires psychological treatment to address the problems that lead to the disorder.

People with anorexia often see themselves as overweight even when they are very thin. *What type of help does an individual with an eating disorder need?*

Bulimia Nervosa

Bulimia nervosa is *a disorder in which some form of purging or clearing of the digestive tract follows cycles of overeating.* A person with bulimia often fasts or follows a strict diet and then *binges*, or quickly consumes large amounts of food. After eating, the person may vomit or take laxatives to purge the food from the body. Following a binge, the person may again try dieting to gain a sense of control and avoid putting on weight. The exact cause of bulimia has not been determined, but societal pressures, self-esteem issues, and family problems may be factors.

HEALTH CONSEQUENCES OF BULIMIA NERVOSA

Repeated binging, purging, and fasting can cause serious health problems or even death. Frequent vomiting and diarrhea can lead to dehydration, kidney damage, and irregular heartbeat. Vomiting also destroys tooth enamel; causes tooth decay; and damages the tissues of the stomach, esophagus, and mouth. Frequent use of laxatives disrupts digestion and absorption and may cause nutrient deficiencies. Laxative abuse can also change the composition of the blood. Treatment of bulimia nervosa usually includes both medication and psychological counseling.

Binge Eating Disorder

People with **binge eating disorder**, *a disorder characterized by compulsive overeating,* consume huge amounts of food at one time but do not try to purge. This disorder may signal the use of food as a coping mechanism for strong emotions or depression. Treatment involves professional psychological counseling and sometimes medication.

Decision Making: Helping a Friend Get Help

Audrey and Rebecca are friends. They are both on the school basketball team. Lately, Audrey has noticed that Rebecca skips lunch and seems to be losing weight.

One day after practice, Rebecca tells Audrey that she is going to jog for at least a mile. Audrey is amazed. "What do you mean? You just ran up and down the court for two full hours."

Rebecca says, "I ate a salad for lunch today. I'm getting fat." Audrey suspects that Rebecca has an eating disorder and wonders how to help her.

What Would You Do?

Apply the decision-making steps to Audrey's problem.
1. State the situation.
2. List the options.
3. Weigh the possible outcomes.
4. Consider values.
5. Make a decision and act.
6. Evaluate the decision.

Psychologists and clinics that specialize in the treatment of eating disorders may offer support groups for people with these disorders. *Why might support groups be helpful to individuals with eating disorders?*

HEALTH CONSEQUENCES OF BINGE EATING DISORDER

Binge eating disorder often results in unhealthful weight gain, which contributes to health problems such as type 2 diabetes, heart disease, and stroke. Gallbladder problems, high blood pressure, high cholesterol, and increased risk of certain types of cancer have also been associated with this disorder.

Help for Eating Disorders

People with eating disorders need professional medical and psychological help. They may also benefit from support groups and clinics. All eating disorders are serious. If you believe a friend might be developing an eating disorder, you may want to discuss the problem with a trusted adult such as a parent, a counselor, or a school nurse. You can also help by encouraging your friend to seek professional help and by being supportive.

Lesson 2 *Review*

Reviewing Facts and Vocabulary

1. Define the term *fad diets*.
2. Describe the causes, symptoms, and treatment of the eating disorder anorexia nervosa.
3. What is *bulimia nervosa*?

Thinking Critically

4. **Evaluating.** Describe the similarities and differences between bulimia nervosa and binge eating disorder.
5. **Analyzing.** Why do people with eating disorders require assistance from professional health services?

Applying Health Skills

Advocacy. Think of ways to inform teens about the dangers of fad diets and other risky weight-loss strategies. With a group of classmates, plan and create a video or public service announcement (PSA) that tells teens about these dangers and gives tips for healthy weight loss.

TECHNOLOGY *OPTION*

WEB SITES Use your video or PSA as part of a Web page you develop on healthy weight management. See **health.glencoe.com** for help in planning and building your own Web site.

Nutrition for Individual Needs

VOCABULARY

electrolytes
rehydration
vegetarian
vegan
dietary supplement
megadose
herbal supplement

YOU'LL LEARN TO

- Understand the specific nutritional needs of different groups.

- Explain the importance of proper nutrition in promoting optimal health for pregnant women, infants, and young children.

- Identify good nutrition as a health-promoting behavior that will enhance and maintain personal health throughout life.

 QUICK START An individual's nutritional needs change throughout his or her life. Brainstorm a list of times in a person's life during which nutritional needs may change. Briefly explain each of your choices.

D oes it seem to you that everyone has a different idea about proper nutrition? Some friends may tell you that eating meat is unhealthy, and others may insist that eating too many carbohydrates is bad for you. What can you believe? In truth, proper nutrition may depend on the individual. A pregnant woman, for example, has different nutritional needs than those of an older adult.

Performance Nutrition

D o you play on a sports team or take aerobics classes? Good nutrition can help you perform your best in any physical activity.

The Training Diet

No single food will help you build muscle or increase speed. The best eating plan for athletes is one that is balanced, moderate, and varied. Your body's need for protein, vitamins, and minerals does not change greatly when training for sports or competition. However, because physical activity burns calories, athletes and other active individuals need to eat more calories from nutrient-dense foods to maintain their weight and energy levels when training.

▲ Eating well-balanced meals and snacks each day is an important part of any training program. *Why is it important for physically active people to have a well-balanced eating plan?*

hot link

heatstroke For more information on the physical effects of heatstroke, see Chapter 4, page 99.

(A) Resistance training helps build muscle mass.

hot link

anabolic steroids For more information about the dangers of anabolic steroids, see Chapter 23, page 601.

HYDRATION

Your body naturally loses fluids through perspiration, breathing, and waste elimination. The amount of fluids lost increases during physical activity, especially in hot weather. These fluids must be replaced to avoid dehydration and **heatstroke.** Becoming dehydrated can lead to an imbalance of **electrolytes,** *minerals that help maintain the body's fluid balance.* The minerals sodium, chloride, and potassium are all electrolytes.

To maintain your body's electrolyte balance, you must take in as much water and electrolytes as you lose through perspiration and body wastes. Drink 16 to 24 ounces of fluids two to three hours before a heavy workout and 6 to 12 ounces of fluids every 15 to 20 minutes during heavy workouts. **Rehydration,** or *restoring lost body fluids,* is important after physical activity and competition. Drink 16 ounces of fluid for every pound of body weight lost through sweat. It's best to drink plain water to replenish fluids lost during exercise.

"Making Weight"

In sports such as wrestling and boxing, participants compete in specific weight classes, so maintaining a certain weight is important. Always compete at a weight that's right for you.

LOSING WEIGHT

Competing in a weight class that is below your healthy weight can be dangerous. Fasting, crash dieting, or trying to sweat off extra weight before weigh-in can cause dehydration and harm your performance and your health. Over time, such practices may also lead to a loss of muscle mass. Athletes who need to lose weight should follow a sensible plan and try to lose only one-half pound to one pound each week.

GAINING WEIGHT

A program that combines balanced nutrition and exercise is the healthful way to gain weight. A supervised resistance-training or weight-lifting program can help build muscle mass. The extra calories you need for gaining weight should come from nutrient-dense foods, not from protein supplements. For best results, a slow, steady weight gain of no more than one to two pounds per week is recommended. Using **anabolic steroids** or other bodybuilding drugs to build muscle mass is not healthy. Many of these drugs have dangerous side effects ranging from acne and breast development in men to heart attacks and liver cancer. Use of these substances is illegal; athletes who test positive for steroids and similar drugs often are disqualified from their sport.

Eating Before Competition

Eating three to four hours before competition allows the stomach to empty yet gives an athlete the necessary energy and keeps him or her free from hunger pangs while competing.

Before competing, choose a meal that's high in carbohydrates and low in fat and protein, both of which stay in the digestive system for a longer period of time. Pasta, rice, vegetables, breads, and fruits are good sources of carbohydrates. Also, remember to drink plenty of water before, during, and after competing.

Vegetarianism

A **vegetarian** is *a person who eats mostly or only plant foods.* Some people are vegetarians for religious or cultural reasons. Others make this choice because of their concern for the environment or for how food animals are raised or slaughtered. Many people become vegetarians for health reasons. By cutting out the saturated fats and cholesterol found in many or all animal products, vegetarians may reduce their risk of cardiovascular disease and some cancers. Also, vegetarians may consume more fruits, vegetables, and whole grains—foods that are linked to a reduced risk of many health problems. **Figure 6.3** describes four vegetarian eating styles.

FIGURE 6.3

VEGETARIAN EATING PLANS

No matter which plan a person follows, a vegetarian eating style still involves choosing nutritious foods.

Plan Name	Foods Included
Lacto-ovo vegetarianism	• Dairy *(lacto)* foods and eggs *(ovo)* in addition to foods from plant sources.
Lacto vegetarianism	• Dairy foods in addition to foods from plant sources.
Ovo vegetarianism	• Eggs and foods from plant sources. Fortified soy milk and soy cheese are often substituted for dairy products.
Vegan	• Foods from plant sources only. Fortified soy milk and soy cheese are often substituted for dairy products.

Meatless Meals

Some people have chosen to become vegetarians. A little planning can ensure that vegetarian meals contain sufficient amounts of nutrients.

Fats, Oils, and Sweets
Use sparingly

Dry Beans, Nuts, Seeds, Eggs, and Meat Substitutes Group
2–3 servings daily

Milk, Yogurt, and Cheese Group
0–3 servings daily*
*Vegetarians who choose not to consume dairy products need to select other calcium-rich foods.

Fruit Group
2–4 servings daily

Vegetable Group
3–5 servings daily

Bread, Cereal, Rice, and Pasta Group
6–11 servings daily

Source: American Dietetic Association

ACTIVITY

Use the Vegetarian Food Pyramid above to plan a full day's menu for a vegetarian. Plan a breakfast, a mid-morning snack, a lunch, a mid-afternoon snack, and an evening meal.

MEETING NUTRIENT NEEDS

Vegetarians need to eat a variety of incomplete proteins in a way that will yield complete protein over the course of a day. They must also make sure they get enough iron, zinc, and B vitamins, nutrients often found in animal products. For vegetarians the key to getting complete proteins and enough vitamins lies in eating adequate amounts of various nutrient-dense foods, including fruits, vegetables, leafy greens, whole grains, nuts, seeds, and legumes, as well as dairy foods or eggs. **Vegans** are *vegetarians who eat only plant foods.*

Because vegans consume no meat or dairy products, they must obtain vitamin D, vitamin B$_{12}$, and calcium from other sources.

Dietary Supplements

Do you take a multivitamin and mineral supplement regularly? These tablets are one type of **dietary supplement**, *a non-food form of one or more nutrients*. Dietary supplements may contain vitamins, minerals, fiber, protein, or herbs. Supplements can be in pill, capsule, powder, or liquid form.

Eating healthful meals and snacks based on the Food Guide Pyramid can provide you with all the nutrients your body needs. However, taking a multivitamin and mineral supplement may sometimes be appropriate. A health care provider may recommend these supplements to people with certain lifestyles or medical conditions. For example, a calcium supplement may be recommended for vegans or for people who are lactose intolerant. Iron tablets might be recommended for someone with iron-deficiency anemia.

Vitamin and mineral supplements may also be recommended for older adults, pregnant or nursing women, people receiving certain medical treatments, and those recovering from illness. If you are in doubt about your own requirements, ask a health care provider.

Risks of Dietary Supplements

Dietary supplements must be used carefully. Taking a **megadose**, or *a very large amount of a dietary supplement*, can be dangerous. Vitamins A, D, E, and K, for example, are stored in body fat and may cause toxicity if taken in large amounts.

An **herbal supplement** is a *chemical substance from plants that may be sold as a dietary supplement*. These substances are often sold as "natural" nutrition aids. However, the safety and nutritional claims of many of these products are not based on conclusive scientific evidence. Currently, manufacturers of herbal products are responsible for product safety and label claims unless the product is known to be dangerous. The Center for Food Safety and Applied Nutrition (CFSAN) of the U.S. FDA alerts consumers to potentially dangerous dietary supplements. Some herbal supplements known to have dangerous side effects include ephedra, lobelia, yohimbe, and chaparral.

Are herbal products safe because they're natural?
Just because something is natural doesn't mean it's harmless. Certain herbs are poisonous. Others may be harmless on their own, but may interact dangerously with prescription or over-the-counter drugs. Consult a health care provider before taking any herbal supplement.

Labeling laws require manufacturers to include information about a supplement's ingredients. *Where would you go to find reliable information about supplements?*

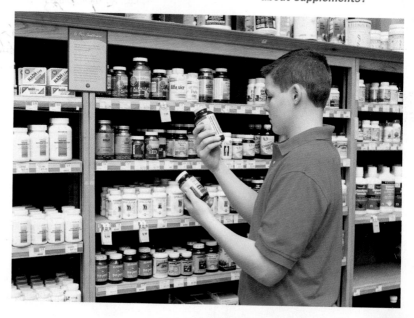

Nutrition Throughout the Life Span

People have different nutritional needs at different stages of life. Many children and most teens, for example, need more calories each day than less active adults. While the nutritional needs of these groups vary slightly, most people can get all the calories and nutrients they need each day by following the recommendations from the *Dietary Guidelines* and the Food Guide Pyramid.

Nutrition During Pregnancy

A developing fetus depends on its mother for all its needs, so it's important for pregnant females to eat healthfully and to avoid harmful substances such as tobacco, alcohol, and other drugs. In addition to eating properly, pregnant females are encouraged to increase their intake of foods rich in the nutrients listed below. A health care provider may also recommend that a pregnant female take a multivitamin and mineral supplement to help meet these nutrient needs.

▶ **Folate.** Getting enough folate, or folic acid, early in pregnancy can prevent spinal defects in the developing fetus. Sources of this B vitamin include fruits, dark green leafy vegetables, and fortified grain products.

▶ **Iron.** Increased blood volume during pregnancy produces an increased demand for this mineral. Found in meat, poultry, fish, dark green leafy vegetables, and enriched grain products, iron helps build and renew hemoglobin, the oxygen-carrying compound in blood cells.

▶ **Calcium.** Calcium helps build the bones and teeth of the developing fetus and replaces any calcium taken from the mother's bones. Calcium is found in most dairy products, dark green leafy vegetables, canned fish with edible bones, and calcium-fortified cereals and juices.

Good nutrition during early childhood is important for the health of the individual throughout his or her life span. *Why is it important to provide a variety of foods to young children?*

Nutrition for Infants and Young Children

Breastfeeding is the best way to feed infants. If breastfeeding isn't possible, fortified formulas provide the nutrients that infants need. As a baby grows through its first year, breast milk or formula is supplemented with a variety of solid foods, usually starting with cereal grains, then vegetables and fruits, and then meat or poultry.

After a child's first birthday, many parents substitute whole milk for formula or breast milk. The fats in whole milk provide essential nutrients for a child's developing nervous system. By this time most children are eating a variety of foods. This variety provides the energy and nutrients needed for growth and encourages the child to enjoy different foods.

Between a child's second and fifth birthdays, parents should gradually replace whole milk with low- or non-fat milk to meet calcium and vitamin D needs while reducing fat intake.

 Proper nutrition and active lifestyles help many of today's older adults remain in good health.

Nutrition and Older Adults

Most older adults can get all the calories and nutrients they need each day by following the recommendations in the *Dietary Guidelines* and the Food Guide Pyramid. Older adults may be advised to follow a special diet if they have a specific health problem.

In certain cases, health care providers might recommend that older adults take a dietary supplement to help meet their nutrient needs. For example, some older adults may take medications that interfere with nutrient absorption.

Lesson 3 *Review*

Reviewing Facts and Vocabulary

1. What type of meal should an athlete eat before competing?
2. Define the term *vegetarian*.
3. Explain what a *megadose* is and why it may be dangerous.

Thinking Critically

4. **Synthesizing.** Explain why proper nutrition is especially important in promoting optimal health for pregnant women, infants, and young children.
5. **Analyzing.** How does good nutrition enhance and maintain personal health throughout life?

Applying Health Skills

Advocacy. Many people think that taking vitamins, minerals, and herbal supplements will improve their health. Develop a pamphlet to educate others about the best ways of getting the nutrients needed for good health. Include information on the safe use of supplements.

PRESENTATION SOFTWARE By using presentation software, you can include art and graphics in a slide show on the importance of good nutrition. Find help in using presentation software at health.glencoe.com.

Body Image in Teen Magazines

Teen magazines often feature images of very thin and fit models. Readers who feel that they don't "measure up" to these models in terms of weight may develop a negative body image. Use the activity below to help you examine messages in teen magazines about weight.

ACTIVITY

Look through a number of teen magazines. What sorts of images of teens do the magazines contain? Are a variety of body types featured? What is the magazine's take on weight management? Do the articles and ads focus on having a moderate, balanced eating plan and increasing physical activity as ways of managing weight healthfully?

As a class, produce a magazine devoted to the topic of healthy weight management for teens. Be sure to include all the elements of a magazine, including feature articles on exercise, nutrition, and body composition; a cover; letters from readers; an advice column; and advertisements. You might also want to include recipes, fictional stories, and a Buyer's Guide/Buyer Beware column.

EXPRESS YOUR VIEWS

Some teen magazines refuse to publish articles and ads on dieting because of the potential these items have for contributing to teens' negative body image. Others continue to feature such articles and ads. As a class, discuss whether magazines should contain information and ads on dieting.

CROSS-CURRICULUM CONNECTIONS

Create a Flyer. Many communities are encouraging their members to eat healthfully and be more physically active. Using a persuasive writing style, create a flyer that gives teens tips on how to develop healthy eating habits and include more physical activity into their lives. Obtain permission from the proper school officials to distribute your flyer to the school community.

Write a Report. Eating disorders have been recorded as early as ancient Greek and Roman times. Research the history of eating disorders in the last three decades. Address theories on the possible causes of eating disorders, and determine why it was not until the 1970s that public awareness of these illnesses increased. Write a report based on your research.

Calculate Calorie Ranges. Nutritionists recommend that 55 to 60 percent of daily calories come from complex carbohydrates. What is the range of calories that should come from complex carbohydrates for a teen who consumes 2,200 calories per day? What is the range for a teen who consumes 2,800 calories per day?

Investigate the Topic. Reducing calorie intake can slow down a person's metabolism, a process that is similar to what happens in people who are suffering from starvation. Research this biological process and explain why the body responds to decreased caloric intake in this way. Present your findings in a brief report.

Registered Dietitian

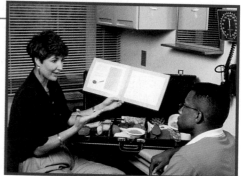

Are you interested in the special nutritional needs of athletes, older adults, or pregnant women? Would you like to inspire others to make healthful food choices? If you answered yes to these questions, you may enjoy a career as a registered dietitian.

Registered dietitians use a variety of skills in their jobs. They must be critical thinkers to analyze an individual's eating habits. They must base their nutritional advice on sound science. Good communication skills are necessary to help people understand how to make food choices. Registered dietitians must show sensitivity to people's needs, cultures, and lifestyles. Find out more about becoming a registered dietitian or working in a related field by clicking on Career Corner at **health.glencoe.com**.

Chapter 6 *Review*

► EXPLORING HEALTH TERMS *Answer the following questions on a sheet of paper.*

Lesson 1 *Replace the underlined words with the correct term.*

Body Mass Index (BMI)	**underweight**
overweight	**obesity**
nutrient-dense foods	**body image**

1. The way you see your body is your <u>BMI</u>.
2. The ratio of weight to height used to assess body size is <u>body image</u>.
3. Fruits and vegetables are <u>nutrient-poor foods</u>.
4. <u>Obesity</u> refers to weighing less than the standard weight range for a certain height.

Lesson 2 *Identify each statement as True or False. If false, replace the underlined term with the correct term.*

bulimia nervosa	**eating disorder**
fad diets	**anorexia nervosa**
weight cycling	**binge eating disorder**

5. The repeated pattern of loss and regain of body weight is <u>bulimia nervosa</u>.
6. An extreme, harmful eating behavior that can cause serious illness or even death is an <u>eating disorder</u>.
7. <u>Anorexia nervosa</u> is a condition in which the irrational fear of becoming obese results in severe weight loss from self-imposed starvation.
8. Compulsive overeating is called <u>weight cycling</u>.

Lesson 3 *Match each definition with the correct term.*

dietary supplement	**rehydration**
electrolytes	**vegan**
herbal supplement	**vegetarian**
megadose	

9. Restoring lost body fluids.
10. A person who eats only plant foods.
11. A nonfood form of one or more nutrients.
12. A chemical substance from plants that may be sold as a dietary supplement.

► RECALLING THE FACTS *Use complete sentences to answer the following questions.*

Lesson 1

1. Explain the relationship between energy balance and a healthy weight.
2. Analyze the relationship between maintaining a healthy weight and disease prevention. Name three diseases that can be prevented by maintaining a healthy weight.
3. List three weight-management strategies.
4. How does regular physical activity help promote a healthy weight?

Lesson 2

5. What are some risks of long-term fasting?
6. Name three risks associated with diet pills.
7. Describe the causes, symptoms, and treatment of the eating disorder bulimia nervosa.
8. Describe the causes, symptoms, and treatment of binge eating disorder.

Lesson 3

9. Explain how dehydration and electrolyte imbalance are related.
10. How can a vegetarian diet benefit health?
11. Why might taking an herbal supplement be risky?
12. Why might a pregnant woman need to take a dietary supplement?

▶ THINKING CRITICALLY

1. **Synthesizing.** Why might a person who is on a weight-loss plan become undernourished? How can this condition be avoided? *(LESSON 1)*

2. **Analyzing.** Find two diet plans featured in magazines. Use what you know about good nutrition and the Food Guide Pyramid to identify the strengths and weaknesses of each plan. *(LESSON 2)*

3. **Applying.** Apply what you have learned about nutrition and vegetarian eating by using the Food Guide Pyramid to plan a sample one-day vegan menu. *(LESSON 3)*

▶ HEALTH SKILLS APPLICATION

1. **Analyzing Influences.** Many factors, including media messages, influence body image. Identify the three factors that you think have the greatest effect on a teen's body image. Explain what role you think each factor plays in determining body image and whether the effect is positive or negative. *(LESSON 1)*

2. **Communicating.** Your friend Amy confides that she maintains her weight by alternating periods of fasting with eating large amounts of food. After eating, she vomits to rid her body of the food. Amy says that this practice is not harmful and helps her control her weight. Write a script describing what you would say to Amy. With a partner, role-play your scenario for the class. *(LESSON 2)*

3. **Accessing Information.** Use reliable online and print resources to find information on at least three dietary supplements known to have harmful side effects. Make a two-column chart that lists in the first column the health claims the supplement manufacturers use to promote their products and, in the second column, the potential side effects of using or abusing the product. Ask permission to post your findings in the weight-training room at your school. *(LESSON 3)*

BEYOND
the Classroom

Parent Involvement

Goal Setting. Sometimes it's easier to set and achieve goals if you work with others. With family members, draw up a plan for achieving a specific nutritional health goal. Your goal may be to lose weight, eat more fruits and vegetables, or anything else that applies to your own needs. Use the goal-setting steps to help you reach your goal.

School and Community

Overeaters Anonymous. Overeaters Anonymous (OA) is a group that offers support to those who are trying to overcome eating problems. Contact a branch of this organization in your community. Find out what services OA provides and how "sponsors" are used to help support people in recovery. Share your findings in a brief report.

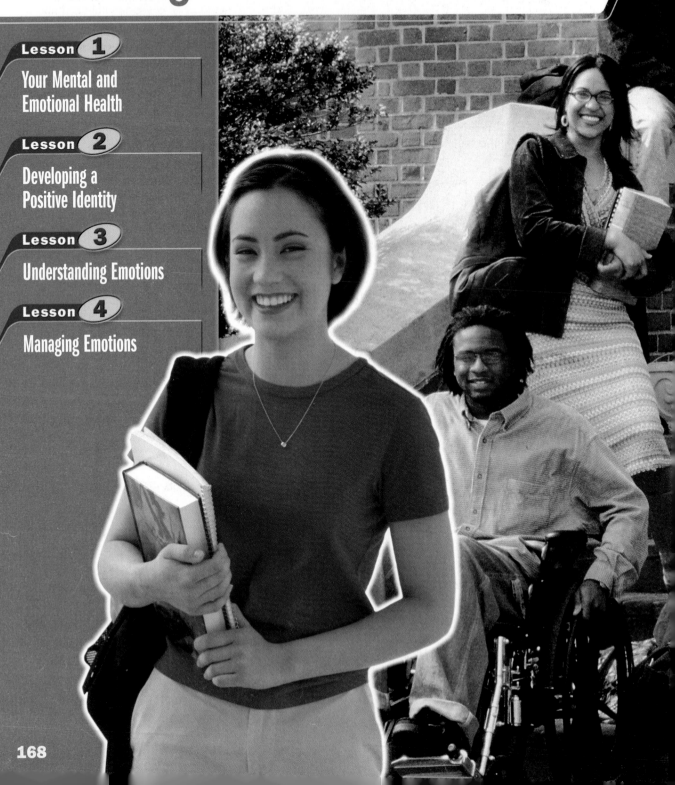

Chapter 7

Achieving Good Mental Health

Lesson 1
Your Mental and Emotional Health

Lesson 2
Developing a Positive Identity

Lesson 3
Understanding Emotions

Lesson 4
Managing Emotions

What's Your Health Status?

Read each statement below and respond by writing *yes*, *no*, or *sometimes* for each item. Write *yes* only for items that you practice regularly.

1. I take responsibility for and consider the consequences of my personal behavior.

2. I express emotions in positive ways.

3. I recognize my personal strengths and weaknesses.

4. I accept and learn from constructive criticism.

5. I have values that benefit me and the people around me in healthful ways.

6. I accept new challenges and face problems rather than avoid them.

7. I think that I am important to other people.

8. I resist negative peer pressure.

9. I am proud of who I am.

10. I have a generally positive outlook on life.

HEALTH Online

For instant feedback on your health status, go to Chapter 7 Health Inventory at **health.glencoe.com**.

Quick *Write*

Using Visuals. Being mentally and emotionally healthy means building a healthy identity and learning to express your emotions in appropriate ways. How do family and friends influence your mental and emotional health?

Your Mental and Emotional Health

VOCABULARY

**mental/emotional
health
hierarchy of needs
self-actualization
personality
modeling**

YOU'LL LEARN TO

- Identify the characteristics of good mental and emotional health.

- Explain the importance of meeting needs in healthful ways.

- Analyze the importance and benefits of abstinence as it relates to emotional health.

- Analyze the relationship between mental health promotion and disease prevention.

→ *QUICK START*   Fold a sheet of paper in half. On one half, write as many characteristics as you can think of that describe a person with good mental health. Circle those characteristics that apply to you. Then select a characteristic that you would like to develop. On the other half of your paper, write what you can do to strengthen that characteristic.

Ⓐ **A person with good mental/emotional health has positive self-esteem.** *What are some of the positive feelings you have about yourself?*

How do you see yourself? Would you describe yourself as serious, friendly, confident, or shy? Do you think you have a positive outlook? Are you generally a happy person? Do you look forward to facing life's challenges? Your responses to these questions reflect aspects of your mental/emotional health.

The Characteristics of Good Mental/Emotional Health

Mental/emotional health is the *ability to accept yourself and others, adapt to and manage emotions, and deal with the demands and challenges you meet in life.* Someone who is mentally and emotionally healthy can usually handle a wide variety of feelings and situations. He or she can make wise choices that demonstrate both strong values and responsible behavior.

People with good mental/emotional health demonstrate the following characteristics:

▶ **Positive Self-Esteem.** Your feelings of confidence and self-esteem are directly related to your general level of wellness. A person with positive self-esteem is better able to accept challenges and take failure in stride.

▶ **Sense of Belonging.** Having emotional attachment to family members, friends, teachers, and other people around you provides comfort and assurance. It promotes stability and makes you feel a part of your community.

▶ **Sense of Purpose.** Recognizing your own value and importance enables you to set and achieve goals and engage in activities that are personally rewarding, such as working hard in school, participating in sports, or doing community service.

▶ **Positive Outlook.** Seeing the bright side and having hope about life reduces stress and increases your energy level. It also increases the possibility of success.

▶ **Autonomy.** Having the confidence to make responsible and safe decisions promotes self-assurance and a sense of independence.

How would you assess your own mental/emotional health? How many of the attributes of good mental/emotional health listed in **Figure 7.1** apply to you?

FIGURE 7.1

SIGNS OF GOOD MENTAL/ EMOTIONAL HEALTH

In general, teens with good mental/emotional health

* are realistic about their strengths and weaknesses.
* are responsible for their personal behavior.
* avoid high-risk behaviors, such as using tobacco, alcohol, or other drugs.
* are open-minded, flexible, and able to see several sides of an issue.
* are fun-loving and able to relax alone or with others.
* respect both their own needs and the needs of others.
* respect each person's value as a human being—including their own.
* invest time and energy in developing nurturing relationships.
* express their emotions in ways that do not hurt themselves or others.
* put their talents and abilities to good use.
* view change as a challenge and an opportunity.

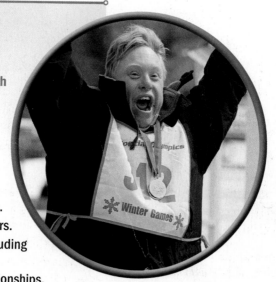

A Pyramid of Needs

Many theories have been developed to explain human development and mental health by examining behavior. One important theory was created by Abraham Maslow, a pioneer in psychology. Maslow organized human needs in the form of a pyramid, as shown in **Figure 7.2**. This **hierarchy of needs** is *a ranked list of those needs essential to human growth and development, presented in ascending order, starting with basic needs and building toward the need for reaching your highest potential.*

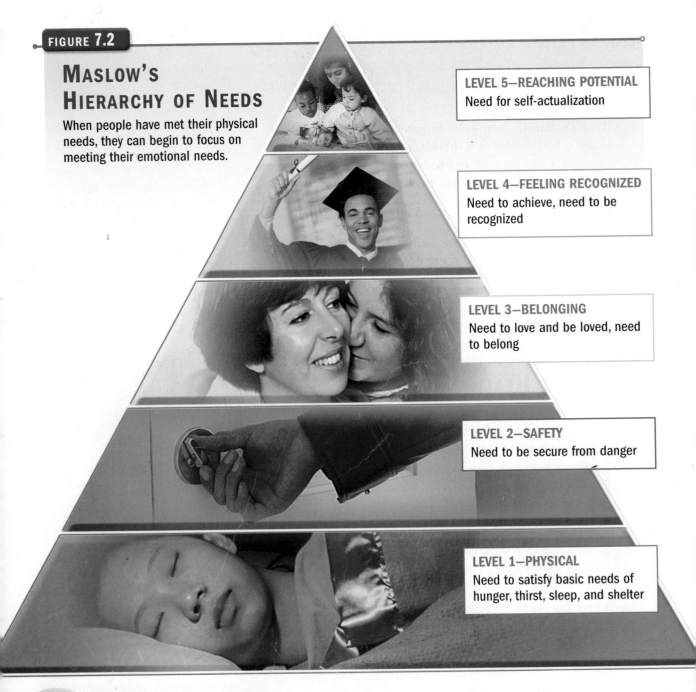

FIGURE **7.2**

MASLOW'S HIERARCHY OF NEEDS

When people have met their physical needs, they can begin to focus on meeting their emotional needs.

LEVEL 5—REACHING POTENTIAL
Need for self-actualization

LEVEL 4—FEELING RECOGNIZED
Need to achieve, need to be recognized

LEVEL 3—BELONGING
Need to love and be loved, need to belong

LEVEL 2—SAFETY
Need to be secure from danger

LEVEL 1—PHYSICAL
Need to satisfy basic needs of hunger, thirst, sleep, and shelter

Physical Needs

Survival needs such as food, water, sleep, and shelter from the elements are among the needs at the bottom of the pyramid. People who are denied these basic needs become physically weak and may develop illnesses. Many people in our society take for granted that basic physical needs are easily met. However, there are many people for whom food, clean water, and shelter are not easily obtained. For example, people who are homeless may face many difficulties meeting their basic physical needs.

Need for Safety

Satisfying the need for safety includes more than just safeguarding yourself against physical harm. In fact, the safety needs that are essential to your personality can also be psychological in nature. You need the safety of familiar places and people that help you feel secure, such as your home, your family, or trusted friends.

Need to Be Loved and to Belong

Everyone needs to give love and to know that he or she is loved in return. Babies who are denied emotional attention may be stunted mentally. They may fail to thrive, and they may even develop behavioral problems later.

Humans are social beings. We need to interact with other people and to know that we are valued members of a group that enhances our physical, mental, or social health. Most people generally want to belong to a community, such as a family, a circle of friends, or a social group such as a school club or a sports team. Feeling a sense of belonging can increase your confidence and strengthen your mental/emotional health.

Need to Be Valued and Recognized

Most of us feel a need to be appreciated, to be personally valued by family, friends, and peers. One way you might meet this need is by participating in productive activities, such as studying hard for exams, playing an instrument or sport, volunteering at a hospital, or writing short stories. By being able to do something well, you gain respect and a feeling of self-worth.

Compassion is a trait that you can express when you understand the needs of others. People who are compassionate are not just aware of other's distress; they have a desire to ease suffering. Homelessness is a growing problem in all communities, both urban and rural. How can you show compassion for people who are unable to meet their basic need for shelter?

Participating in team sports can give teens a sense of belonging. *What other positive actions can teens take to fulfill this need?*

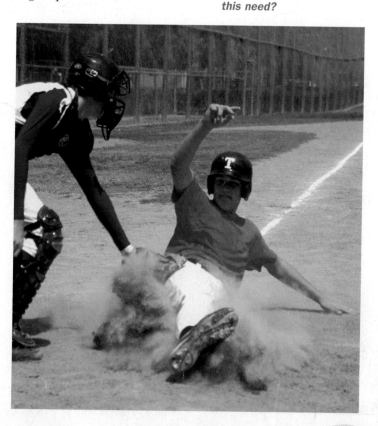

Need to Reach Your Potential

At the top of the pyramid is the need to reach your full potential as a person. This quest for **self-actualization**—*the striving to become the best you can be*—includes having goals that motivate and inspire you. Self-actualization means having the courage to make changes in your life in order to reach your goals and grow as a person. During your teen years, you begin to recognize your potential and set goals for your future. You see more clearly what your talents are, what your dreams are, and who it is you want to become. Self-actualization is a lifelong process. Part of the process is learning the self-discipline you need to reach your goals.

Meeting Your Needs

The ways you choose to meet your needs affect your mental/emotional health. For example, meeting the need for affection by building and maintaining respectful, loving relationships with people you care about will strengthen your mental/emotional health. However, sometimes people choose risky ways to fulfill their needs. Some teens may decide to join a gang to feel a sense of belonging or engage in sexual activity in an attempt to feel loved. Such decisions carry dangerous consequences. Gang membership can lead to physical harm and trouble with the law. Sexual activity can result in unplanned pregnancy, sexually transmitted diseases, and the loss of self-respect and the respect of others. Practicing **abstinence** and finding healthful ways to meet emotional needs are critical in developing and maintaining good mental health.

hot link

abstinence For more information about the benefits of abstinence, see Chapter 12, page 318.

Practicing abstinence and meeting needs in healthy ways will strengthen your mental/emotional health. *What other decisions can you make to promote your health?*

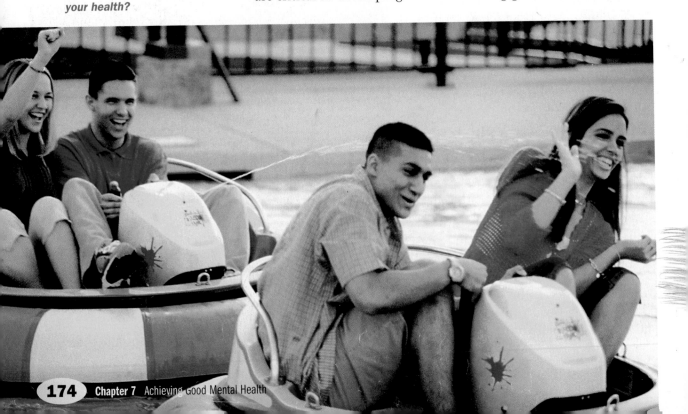

Understanding Your Personality

Your **personality** is *a complex set of characteristics that makes you unique.* It's what makes you different from everyone else and determines how you will react in certain situations. Personality is an important factor in how you choose to meet your needs. Thus, it plays a major role in your overall mental health.

Influences on Your Personality

Personality includes an individual's emotional makeup, attitudes, thoughts, and behaviors. It is composed of tendencies that you were born with and characteristics that you have developed in response to life situations and experiences. The two main influences on your personality are heredity and environment.

PERSONALITY AND HEREDITY

Just as you inherit physical traits such as hair and eye color, you inherit some personality traits from your biological parents and ancestors. Heredity plays a role in determining a person's basic intellectual abilities and temperament, or emotional tendencies. There is also evidence that heredity may influence behaviors such as risk-taking and talents such as athletic or artistic abilities. This doesn't mean that you have no control over how smart you become or what you do. Your inherited brain chemistry is only one of the many factors contributing to your personality and behavior.

PERSONALITY AND ENVIRONMENT

Your environment includes everything that surrounds you in your day-to-day life. This means your family, friends, peers, home, neighborhood, school, and every other person, place, object, event, or activity in your life. All of these influences can have an impact on your developing personality.

Among the people in your environment are some who serve as role models for your behavior. Most people naturally engage in **modeling**, or *observing and learning from the behaviors of those around you*, sometimes without even thinking about it. If the behavior of your role model is healthful, the effect on your developing personality will also be healthful. The values you learn from your role models help shape the person you are and the way you live your life.

Many influences can help shape personality traits, such as a sense of self-discipline and the desire to excel. *Who are the role models in your life who have helped shape your personality?*

Should Learning Styles Be Taken Into Account in the Classroom?

Academic performance affects many teens' view of themselves. Being a good student is one way teens can meet the need to be valued and recognized. Because students learn and demonstrate their knowledge in different ways, some teachers use different testing methods. For instance, teachers may test students according to the way each one learns best—through seeing, through hearing, or through doing. Do you think teachers should use multiple methods to accommodate different learning styles? Here are two points of view.

Viewpoint 1: Melissa J., age 15

I'm proud of my grades. I study every night and always work extra hard before exams. It's not fair to apply different standards just because some students can't handle a written test. Why should I have to write an essay while someone else in class has fun drawing a picture or building a diorama? How can the teacher possibly grade these different projects fairly? It's like comparing apples and oranges. Students should be given real tests, not whatever makes them feel good. That's not the way the real world works after graduation. Those students just need to work harder.

Viewpoint 2: Gary D., age 16

I do study hard for tests, but even when I know the content, I still do lousy on multiple-choice tests. If that's the only way I can demonstrate my knowledge, I end up looking stupid. Students have different strengths and weaknesses—and so do people in the real world. Look at athletes or dancers. They demonstrate their knowledge and talent by performing, not by taking a written test. I'm not saying you should get rid of all pencil-and-paper tests or forget about writing papers. I just think teachers should offer students a variety of approaches to accommodate different ways of learning. It's only fair.

ACTIVITIES

1. **Research one of the different learning styles mentioned above, including visual (seeing), auditory (hearing), and tactile/kinesthetic (touching, doing). Describe the style and how students in that category learn best.**

2. **Write a paragraph explaining which viewpoint you favor and why. Be sure to link your discussion to the issue of school performance and self-esteem.**

Personality and Behavior

The one aspect of your personality over which you have the most control is your behavior. How you make decisions, what decisions you make, whether you recognize the consequences of those decisions, and what actions you take can make a great difference in the quality of your life and in your levels of physical and mental/emotional health.

Promoting Mental/Emotional Health

Knowing the factors that affect your mental/emotional health will help you choose behaviors that promote health. Being mentally and emotionally healthy can improve your physical health and help prevent some diseases. For example, meeting needs in healthful ways by abstaining from risk behaviors such as gang involvement and sexual activity will protect you from physical harm. People who are able to cope with their emotions and deal with the stress in their lives are also less susceptible to illnesses such as colds and other upper-respiratory infections. Engaging in behaviors that promote mental/emotional health may help prevent disease, and it will strengthen all three sides of your health triangle.

Showing respect and caring are outward signs of positive aspects of your personality. *In what positive ways do you demonstrate your personality through your daily behaviors?*

 Lesson 1 *Review*

Reviewing Facts and Vocabulary

1. Define the term *mental/emotional health*. Identify three characteristics of a mentally and emotionally healthy person.

2. List the needs included in Maslow's hierarchy of needs.

3. How does heredity influence personality?

Thinking Critically

4. **Evaluating.** Analyze the importance and benefits of abstinence as it relates to emotional health.

5. **Synthesizing.** Analyze the relationship between mental health promotion and disease prevention.

Applying Health Skills

Practicing Healthful Behaviors. The need to belong and to be loved is a basic human need. What are some healthy choices that provide positive ways for meeting this need? What are the consequences of meeting this need in negative ways? Make a two-column table to organize your thoughts.

WORD PROCESSING Sometimes it's easier to organize and display your thoughts if you use a word-processing program. See **health.glencoe.com** for tips on how to use a word processor to create a table.

Developing a Positive Identity

VOCABULARY

personal identity
developmental assets
constructive criticism

YOU'LL LEARN TO

- Recognize developmental assets.

- Explore strategies for developing a healthy identity.

- Relate how self-esteem and a positive outlook benefit your mental/emotional health.

QUICK START On a sheet of paper, list your talents and abilities. What are your special qualities? What other traits make you the person you are?

Your personal identity is made up of many different pieces. *What are some aspects of your identity that make you unique?*

If you were to write an essay describing who you are, you might begin by giving your name and age. Then you might identify your various roles, such as a son or daughter, brother or sister, student, club member, or athlete. You might also describe your talents, interests, hobbies, and accomplishments. All these elements help define the person you are. They contribute to your **personal identity**, *your sense of yourself as a unique individual.*

Your Personal Identity

During the teen years, you begin to develop a stronger sense of who you are. You learn about yourself through your interactions and relationships with other people. The knowledge you gain from your experiences will help you see yourself more clearly. Developing your personal identity is like putting a jigsaw puzzle together. The pieces of this puzzle include

▶ your interests.

▶ your likes and dislikes.

▶ your talents and abilities.

▶ your values and beliefs.

▶ your goals.

Your Developmental Assets

As you mature, it is important to recognize the developmental assets that will help you build a healthy, positive identity. **Developmental assets** are the *building blocks of development that help young people grow up as healthy, caring, and responsible individuals.* These assets, listed in **Figure 7.3,** can help you achieve wellness as you mature into a dependable, conscientious adult. Remember that developmental assets can be found in many aspects of your life and that you can always work to strengthen these assets.

FIGURE 7.3

DEVELOPMENTAL ASSETS

The Search Institute, a nonprofit organization, compiled this list of 40 assets that can help young people make healthful decisions on the road to adulthood.

Support—family support, positive family communication, relationships with other adults, caring neighborhood, caring school climate, parental involvement in schooling

Empowerment—being valued by adults in the community; serving a purpose by having a role in the community; feeling safe at home, at school, and in the neighborhood

Boundaries and Expectations—family boundaries (clear rules and consequences), school boundaries, neighborhood boundaries, adult role models, positive peer influences, high expectations

Constructive Use of Time—creative activities, youth programs, time at home, sports

Commitment to Learning—being motivated to achieve, being involved at school, doing homework, reading for pleasure

Positive Values—compassion, equality and social justice, integrity, honesty, responsibility, self-control

Social Competencies—planning and decision making, interpersonal communication, having knowledge and tolerance of different cultures, resistance skills, peaceful conflict resolution skills

Positive Identity—personal power, self-esteem, sense of purpose, positive view of personal future

Real-Life Application

Identify and Strengthen Your Developmental Assets

Developmental assets increase the likelihood that a person will behave in ways that will enhance his or her health. Use the chart and questions to help you analyze the influences in your life and strengthen your developmental assets.

External Assets

- **Support**
- **Empowerment**
- **Boundaries and Expectations**
- **Constructive Use of Time**

External developmental assets are the positive experiences that support and empower you as you grow up. They include the standards set by parents or guardians, the expectations and encouragement of teachers, and the laws and rules established by the community.

Internal Assets

- **Commitment to Learning**
- **Positive Values**
- **Social Competencies**
- **Positive Identity**

Internal developmental assets are the personal strengths, commitments, and values that you use to guide the decisions you make. For example, if you respect yourself, you will not harm your health by using tobacco, alcohol, or other drugs.

ACTIVITIES

1. Identify the external developmental assets in each of the following areas, and describe at least one way that each asset provides a positive influence in your life: family relationships, peer relationships, the school environment, the community environment.

2. Identify your internal developmental assets, and explain why these are personal strengths. Consider the following: accomplishments, strengths, and values.

3. Write a summary about the assets in your life. Reflect on the positive influences these assets have on the decisions you make. Use the following sentence beginnings in your summary:

   I learned that . . . I am proud that . . . I was surprised that . . . I would like to improve . . .

Working Toward a Healthy Identity

Once you recognize your developmental assets as important influences on your personal identity, you can take active steps to strengthen these assets and build a healthy identity. This process requires both self-acceptance and self-improvement.

Recognize Your Strengths and Weaknesses

An essential step in developing a healthy identity is viewing your strengths and weaknesses in honest, realistic ways. Accept and take pride in your strengths and accomplishments. Whether you are a caring family member, a trustworthy friend, an honor student, a good basketball player, or a talented singer, you should feel proud of the positive aspects of your identity.

At the same time, assess your weaknesses without being overly self-critical, and set goals for improvement. For example, if you tend to put things off, or procrastinate, try to develop new work habits that will lessen the pressure of having to do everything at the last minute. You may be able to use one of your strengths to help you address a weakness. For example, your strength might be that you are a fast learner and will quickly learn new work habits. Using your strengths and addressing your weaknesses helps you develop competence and effectiveness.

Demonstrate Positive Values

Your values, or your beliefs and ideas about what is important in your life, guide your actions and influence the decisions you make. You can demonstrate your values in many ways. For instance, you show honesty and integrity when you don't cheat on tests. When you comfort a sad friend, you demonstrate caring and compassion. Making sure that your behavior reflects your personal values and standards will reinforce your positive identity.

Develop a Purpose in Your Life

Think of having a sense of purpose as a framework for your mental health as you grow toward adulthood and work to build a healthy identity. Having a sense of purpose means establishing goals and working to achieve them. Some of the goals you establish will be short-term, such as studying for and passing an exam. Others will be long-term, such as making plans for higher education and acquiring job skills.

Form Meaningful Relationships

Relationships provide one means of developing a sense of purpose in your life. Family and friends enable you to express yourself and share your experiences, beliefs, and feelings. Positive relationships with family, friends, teachers, and coaches also give you a support system that will help you build confidence and develop a sense of security and belonging.

The relationship between this coach and her team is part of a caring school climate. *Explain how having this asset can help teens build a healthy identity.*

People with high self-esteem:

▶ take responsibility for their behavior.

▶ generally have a positive outlook on life.

▶ like and accept who they are overall.

▶ try to learn from their successes as well as from their mistakes.

▶ build and maintain healthy relationships.

To improve self-esteem:

▶ think of appropriate ways to share your positive attributes.

▶ engage in behaviors that will promote your health.

Contribute to the Community

Your community is an extended support system for you and your family; it provides services and resources to meet many of your needs. Giving back to the community is part of being a good citizen, and it helps you feel a sense of accomplishment. For example, you might help out a neighbor or participate in a community clean-up campaign. Apply your strengths to improving others' quality of life, and strengthen your sense of belonging in the process.

Avoid Unhealthful Risk Behaviors

Risk-taking is a normal part of growing up—it helps define and develop identity. Healthful risk-taking has a positive effect on development. Engaging in sports, artistic or creative activities, public speaking, travel, and making friends all involve some risk. Such risks challenge you to develop skills and mature in new ways.

Unhealthful risk-taking, such as using tobacco, alcohol, or other drugs; reckless driving; and gang affiliation, can be dangerous. Refuse to participate in such behavior. Keep in mind the aspects of your identity, such as your values, that you are trying to uphold.

Self-Esteem and Positive Outlook

When you have a healthy identity, you will experience increased self-esteem and a higher level of mental/emotional health. Self-esteem comes from the understanding that you are a unique and valuable human being. How you feel mentally and physically and how you take care of yourself are all affected by what you think of yourself. Teens with high self-esteem are in a strong position to meet the challenges of adult life.

Along with self-esteem, having a positive outlook is also directly related to your general level of wellness. Studies have shown that people with a positive outlook live longer and are healthier, both mentally and physically. Remind yourself that no matter what happens, there is always hope. Then, when something goes wrong, make a plan to address the problem. Try to see challenges as opportunities for growing and learning.

▶ **Teens find many ways to contribute to their community, including building houses for the homeless.** *How does helping others contribute to a positive identity?*

Realistic Patterns of Thinking

In order to increase your self-esteem and develop a positive outlook on life, it is essential to see events realistically. Some people fall into a pattern of seeing events as worse than they actually are. For example, a teen who has just failed an exam may think that he or she is stupid and will always fail. By looking at the situation realistically, the teen will realize that he or she was simply unprepared for that day's work and will resolve to study harder next time.

Sometimes, to help yourself see events more realistically, you might seek **constructive criticism**, or *nonhostile comments that point out problems and encourage improvement.* Constructive criticism can help you view a situation more objectively, without the emotional influences that can alter your perception and thinking.

ANALYZING YOUR SELF-TALK

Listen to your self-talk. Replace negative messages with constructive criticism. If you make a mistake, tell yourself that all people make mistakes; learn from yours and move on. Also, don't be afraid of telling yourself "Good job!" when you've done something that deserves praise. Such positive self-talk will benefit your self-esteem, your general outlook on life, and your mental/emotional health.

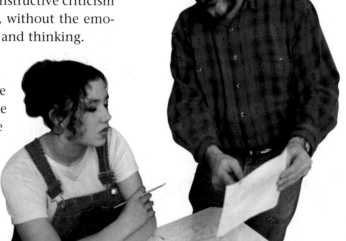

This teen uses constructive criticism from the teacher to improve her skills and thus raise her self-esteem. *Why is self-esteem important to mental and emotional health?*

 Lesson 2 *Review*

Reviewing Facts and Vocabulary

1. Define *personal identity*. List five elements that contribute to one's personal identity.
2. Name three of the positive values listed as developmental assets.
3. List three strategies for building a positive identity.

Thinking Critically

4. **Synthesizing.** Why do you think developmental assets increase the likelihood that a person will not engage in risk behaviors?
5. **Analyzing.** Describe how positive identity and high self-esteem help you with goal setting, developing relationships, and contributing to your community.

Applying Health Skills

Goal Setting. Evaluate aspects of your identity. Is there an area you would like to improve? Make a specific goal to strengthen one aspect of your identity. Using the steps of goal setting, write down plans and strategies to help you achieve your goal.

TECHNOLOGY *OPTION*

SPREADSHEETS Using a spreadsheet can help you organize a list. To learn more about how to use a spreadsheet, see **health.glencoe.com**.

Understanding Emotions

YOU'LL LEARN TO

• Analyze how emotions influence your overall health.

• Appraise the significance of changes occurring during adolescence.

• Explore ways to demonstrate empathy toward others.

• Demonstrate communication skills in building and maintaining healthy relationships.

QUICK START In one minute, list as many emotions as you can. Then compare your list with those of your classmates. Which emotions are most common? Why might some emotions, such as empathy, be on fewer lists?

Actors portray strong emotions by using body language and changes in their voices. *What emotions are these actors trying to express?*

A rt imitates life. This familiar phrase is particularly true in regard to drama. Acting requires the performer to express a character's emotions both verbally and physically. How might an actor express joy or sorrow as part of a play?

Understanding Your Emotions

E **motions** are *signals that tell your mind and body how to react.* Sometimes referred to as feelings, emotions are your responses to certain thoughts and events. To communicate emotions, you use combinations of words or other sounds, facial expressions, and body language. Emotions affect all sides of your health triangle.

▶ Joy can prompt the release of brain chemicals that cause you to experience warmth and a sense of well-being. Feeling this way promotes mental/emotional health and positively influences your relationships and thus your social health.

▶ Fear can trigger physical changes, including increased perspiration, a rise in heart rate, and a tightening of muscles. This "fight-or-flight" response enables you to defend yourself or flee the scene.

► Strong emotions like anger can cause both physical and mental responses, such as a rise in heart rate and feelings of distress. Inappropriate responses, such as lashing out, can be harmful to you or to people around you.

Identifying Your Emotions

Sometimes you know exactly what you are feeling and why. At other times, you may experience emotions that seem to have no apparent cause. Moreover, the many changes brought on by hormones during puberty can affect your emotions. A **hormone** is *a chemical secreted by your glands that regulates the activities of different body cells*. Hormones may cause you to swing quickly between extreme emotions such as elation and depression. Mixed emotions, such as when you feel both jealous of and happy for a friend, also can be challenging. Accurately identifying what you are feeling is an important first step toward knowing how to respond in a healthy way.

Happiness

Think of other words that might describe how you feel when you are happy. You might say you are pleased or that you feel good or carefree. Happiness can be described as being satisfied or feeling positive. When you are happy, you usually feel energetic, creative, and sociable.

Sadness

Sadness is a normal, healthy reaction to difficult events. Causes of sadness can range from being disappointed or rejected to experiencing the loss of a loved one. Feelings of sadness may be mild and fleeting, or they may be deep and long-lasting. When you are sad, you may feel easily discouraged and have less energy.

Love

Love involves strong affection, deep concern, and respect. It includes supporting the growth and individual needs of another person and respecting that person's boundaries and values. Love can be expressed through words or actions, such as good deeds. It comes in many forms, such as caring about family and friends, loyalty to siblings, and a deep sense of being connected to your community and country.

Sadness may bring feelings of hurt, isolation, or helplessness. *How can you comfort a friend who is feeling down?*

Empathy

Empathy is *the ability to imagine and understand how someone else feels*. When you feel empathy, you feel connected to another person's emotions. An empathetic person listens attentively and communicates understanding when people express their feelings. Demonstrating empathy can help strengthen your emotional bonds and enhance your relationships.

Fear

When you are startled by someone or something, you probably feel some degree of fear. Feelings of fear can increase your alertness and help you escape from potentially harmful situations. However, fear that results from an imagined threat can prevent people from leading normal lives. For example, an exaggerated fear of being in a crowd can result in a life of solitude. This type of fear is called a **phobia** and requires professional help.

hot link

phobia To learn more about phobias, see Chapter 9, page 225.

Health Skills Activity

Communication: Expressing Your Feelings

Tara feels a knot in her stomach when she sees her friend Suzanne. The last time she agreed to go to a concert with Tara, Suzanne failed to show up. It hurt Tara's feelings that Suzanne didn't care enough about their friendship to show up.

Suzanne says excitedly, "Tara, did you see who's playing this weekend? Let's get there early, okay?"

Tara feels torn between two choices. She could ignore her feelings by keeping them bottled up. Her other option would be to communicate her hurt and disappointment, but that would risk hurting Suzanne's feelings.

What Would You Do?

Use the following communication skills to write a dialogue in which Tara expresses her hurt and disappointment in a way that spares Suzanne's feelings.

1. Use "I" messages.
2. Keep your tone respectful.
3. Provide a clear, organized message that states the problem.
4. Listen to the other person's side without interrupting.

Guilt

Guilt often results from acting against one's values or from failing to act when action might have brought about a better outcome. Although guilt can eat at you, it can also act as your conscience and motivate you to make some positive changes in your behavior. Sometimes, people may feel guilty for things they have no control over. For example, some teens blame themselves when parents divorce even though they are not the cause of the separation. Being able to recognize when you are not responsible for a negative outcome will save you from needless guilt.

Anger

Anger is a common reaction to being emotionally hurt or physically harmed. When anger isn't handled in constructive ways, it can result in violence, bringing physical and emotional harm to you and others. **Hostility**, *the intentional use of unfriendly or offensive behavior*, can be particularly damaging, not only to others but also to the hostile person. People who show chronic hostile behavior are four to seven times more likely to die of heart disease than those who are not prone to hostility. Knowing what causes your anger and how you can respond to it healthfully can help you gain control.

HEALTH *Online*

Explore more about emotions and the role they play in our lives at **health.glencoe.com**.

 Lesson 3 *Review*

Reviewing Facts and Vocabulary

1. How can emotions influence your overall health?
2. Define *empathy*. How can a person demonstrate empathy?
3. How might guilty feelings lead to positive results?

Thinking Critically

4. **Evaluating.** Appraise the significance of changes occurring during adolescence: What effects do changing hormone levels have on emotions?
5. **Synthesizing.** List three situations that may cause a teen to feel anger. Then, explain how each of these situations can be dealt with in healthful ways.

Applying Health Skills

Conflict Resolution. Write a skit in which unpleasant emotions cause a conflict between two friends. Your skit should demonstrate positive communication skills that aid the teens in handling their strong emotions and resolving their differences.

TECHNOLOGY *OPTION*

WORD PROCESSING Word-processing software can help you write and revise your skit. For more information on using word-processing software, click on **health.glencoe.com**.

Managing Emotions

VOCABULARY
defense mechanisms
suppression

YOU'LL LEARN TO

• Evaluate the effects of peers, family, and friends on emotional health.

• Demonstrate strategies for communicating emotions and needs in healthful ways.

→ **QUICK START** There are many ways to communicate emotions to others. List three emotions, and describe how you usually communicate them.

▼ Healthful expression of feelings increases your ability to enjoy life. *What are some positive ways to express emotions?*

Emotions are neither good nor bad. How you deal with your emotions, however, can strongly influence your overall level of health. Learning to recognize emotions and dealing with them in healthful ways are especially important to good mental health.

Dealing with Emotions in Positive Ways

As you were growing up, you learned various ways of expressing your emotions from others, from your environment, and from your experiences. Perhaps your family members talk openly about their feelings and encourage sharing them. Maybe your friends express themselves indirectly with looks or smiles or with behaviors such as laughing or hugging. Perhaps some of your peers don't talk about or express feelings much, and you've learned from their example that emotions are private. Regardless of what you have learned, it is important to evaluate methods of communicating feelings and practice healthful ways of expression.

Negative ways of dealing with feelings do nothing to solve problems. Exaggerating emotions for effect, pretending that feelings are not there at all, or intentionally hurting another person while expressing feelings can worsen the situation and create new problems.

Responding to Your Emotions

You can use some of the following strategies for interpreting and responding to most emotions.

▶ Look below the surface of your emotion. Ask yourself: What am I really reacting to? Does the intensity of my emotion match the situation?

▶ Consider whether or not the situation to which you are reacting will matter tomorrow, next week, or next year.

▶ Don't take action on a strong feeling until you have thoroughly considered the possible consequences of your action.

▶ Use positive feelings to inspire yourself. Relieve negative or upsetting feelings by engaging in physical activities or by talking to a family member or trusted friend.

▶ If a negative feeling doesn't go away, seek help from a parent, another trusted adult, or a health care professional.

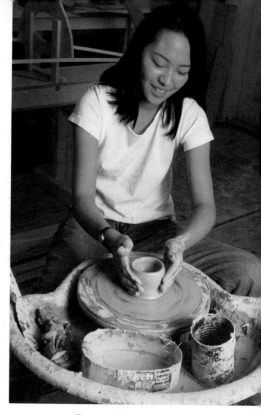

Creating art is a healthful way to handle your emotions. *The next time you feel a strong emotion, try doing something creative.*

Managing Difficult Emotions

You've probably been overwhelmed by strong emotions at one time or another. Intense emotions can affect your attitude and behavior in ways that are upsetting. However, you can learn to manage strong emotions. When you feel your emotions building, recognize the feeling and manage it by taking slow, deep breaths and relaxing. You might also get away from the situation to compose yourself. Sometimes you can control your feelings by analyzing the situations that cause the feelings. Writing in a private journal, playing music, or talking your feelings over with a parent or trusted friend can help you reflect on both your emotions and the situation that led to them.

Defense Mechanisms

Because of the way emotions affect you, you may try to avoid the ones that cause you discomfort by using **defense mechanisms**. These are *mental processes that protect individuals from strong or stressful emotions and situations*. **Figure 7.4** on page 190 lists some of the most common defense mechanisms. Sometimes, these responses occur unconsciously and may help protect you from feeling too much emotional pain. For instance, the use of **suppression**, *holding back or restraining*, can provide a temporary escape from an unpleasant situation. In the long run, however, defense mechanisms may keep you from facing what is really troubling you. That's why it's important to develop strategies for dealing with difficult emotions in healthful ways.

FIGURE 7.4

COMMON DEFENSE MECHANISMS

- **Repression.** Involuntary pushing of unpleasant feelings out of conscious thought.
- **Suppression.** Conscious, intentional pushing of unpleasantness from one's mind.
- **Rationalization.** Making excuses to explain a situation or behavior rather than directly taking responsibility for it.
- **Regression.** Reverting to behaviors more characteristic of an earlier stage of development rather than dealing with the conflict in a mature manner.
- **Denial.** Unconscious lack of acknowledgement of something that is obvious to others.
- **Compensation.** Making up for weaknesses and mistakes through gift-giving, hard work, or extreme efforts.
- **Projection.** Attributing your own feelings or faults to another person or group.
- **Idealization.** Seeing someone else as perfect, ideal, or more worthy than everyone else.

Handling Fear

Fear is an emotion many people work to overcome. Overcoming fear requires a strategy. The first step is to identify your fear. Analyzing the situation that causes the fear often helps. Talking about your fear with someone you trust may also give you a fresh outlook. This person may remind you of other fears you have faced successfully or know of resources that can help you. Some fear is healthy and natural; only when fear is irrational or uncontrollable should you consider it a problem.

Dealing with Guilt

Guilt can be a very destructive emotion. When you feel guilty about something, try to get at the underlying source and address that issue. If you have hurt someone, for example, admit your mistake and make amends. Learn from the experience, and resolve to be more careful and responsible in the future. Discussing the situation with family or friends can also help make you feel better. Keep in mind that some situations may not be in your control. Viewing such circumstances realistically and honestly will help you see that you are not responsible and should not feel guilty for them.

Managing Anger

Anger can be one of the most difficult emotions to handle. The first step in constructively dealing with anger is similar to dealing with guilt—you must try to get at the underlying source and address it. Even if there is nothing you can do about the source of your anger, you can find ways to cope with your feelings. Refer to the Hands-On Health Activity for some general anger-management techniques.

Hands-On Health ACTIVITY

Managing Anger

In this activity you'll identify and develop healthy strategies to handle anger.

What You'll Need

- pencil and paper

What You'll Do

1. Write the following headings on your paper.
   - Do something to relax.
   - Rechannel your energy.
   - Talk to someone you trust.
   - Get some physical activity.

2. Under each heading, list at least two *specific* activities you can try.

3. Compare your list with a partner's. How are your techniques similar or different? What does this tell you about how individuals handle anger?

Apply and Conclude

Working with your partner, create a comic strip that illustrates at least one effective anger management skill.

Lesson 4 Review

Reviewing Facts and Vocabulary

1. List three strategies for interpreting, responding to, and communicating an emotion in healthful ways.
2. What are five common defense mechanisms?
3. Give four examples of anger-management techniques.

Thinking Critically

4. **Analyzing.** Evaluate the effects of various relationships on emotional health: In what ways do peers, family, and friends influence how you express and manage emotions?
5. **Explaining.** Describe the results that may occur when you take time to reflect before responding to a strong emotion.

Applying Health Skills

Communication Skills. Write a one-act play. Focus on someone using the strategies listed at the beginning of this lesson to decide how to react to and express a specific feeling.

WORD PROCESSING   You can use word-processing software to help you draft, revise, and edit your play. See health.glencoe.com for tips on using a word-processing program.

Emotional Health in TV Programs

There are healthy and unhealthy ways of dealing with your emotions. In this activity, you will examine the ways in which emotions are expressed on different television programs and analyze the messages these programs send on the subject of emotional health.

Emotion	How it was expressed	How other characters reacted
Frustration	The character snapped at a younger sibling.	His mother made him apologize and then asked him to discuss what was wrong.

ACTIVITY

Watch a sitcom, drama, reality show, or talk show. Record the ways in which different emotions are expressed throughout the program. Use a chart like the one above to help organize your notes.

Consider the overall message the program sends regarding emotional health. Do the characters demonstrate healthy ways of dealing with difficult emotions? Do they suffer consequences as a result of inappropriate behavior? Are unhealthful ways of expressing emotions corrected? Rate the emotional health of the program, using a scale of 1 to 5, with 5 being the highest and 1 being the lowest.

EXPRESS YOUR VIEWS

Write a one-page review of the program that includes a synopsis of the plot and characters and a description of the consequences of the characters' behaviors. Indicate whether the program provided a positive or negative example of how to express or deal with emotions. Support your viewpoint with specific examples from the program.

CROSS-CURRICULUM CONNECTIONS

Create a Poem. Reaching for the stars means striving to become the best you can be. Working toward this self-actualization is an important aspect of good mental health. Poet Langston Hughes described it this way: "We have tomorrow, bright before us like a flame." Using Hughes's words as a model, choose a symbol that represents you and your quest to fulfill your potential. Write a poem about your self-image and incorporate your symbol.

Research a Biography. Developing a sense of purpose in your life means moving beyond your own needs to contributing to your community. Many successful people, such as Nelson Mandela and Mother Theresa, have chosen paths of self-sacrifice in life. Write a short research report on a well-known figure who has worked to improve the quality of life of others. Determine why helping others was a priority for this person.

Calculate Demographics. According to the U.S. Department of Health and Human Services, the percentage of females reporting significant emotional problems is 22 percent among adolescents aged 14 to 17. Suppose that the study surveyed 3.7 million girls ages 14 to 15 and 3.5 million girls ages 16 to 17. How many girls aged 14 to 17 would have reported significant emotional problems?

Investigate a Body System. Hormones play an important role in influencing mental and emotional health. The endocrine system produces hormones in ductless glands located throughout the body. These hormones transmit chemical signals to which the body responds. Create a chart showing the glands of the endocrine system, their location in the body, the hormones they secrete, and the function of each in the body. Discuss the problems that might arise from imbalances in the system and what conditions can cause them.

 CAREER Corner

School Counselor

Do you have empathy, and do you like helping others? Are you interested in teaching and working with students and their families? If so, a career as a school psychologist or counselor might be for you. These professionals assist students with personal, family, educational, and mental health problems.

To enter this profession, you'll need a four-year college degree and at least a two-year graduate degree. Find more information about this and other health careers by clicking on Career Corner at **health.glencoe.com**.

Chapter 7 Review

> **EXPLORING HEALTH TERMS** *Answer the following questions on a sheet of paper.*

Lesson 1 *Match each definition with the correct term.*

hierarchy of needs   self-actualization
mental/emotional health   modeling
personality

1. The sum of behavioral and emotional tendencies that affect a person's life.
2. A ranked list of those needs essential to human growth and development.
3. Striving to become the best you can be.
4. Observing and learning from the behavior of others.

Lesson 2 *Replace the underlined words with the correct term.*

constructive criticism   personal identity
developmental asset

5. Constructive criticism is made up of elements such as interests, abilities, values, and goals.
6. A personal identity is a building block of development that helps you grow up as a healthy, caring, and responsible individual.
7. Giving thoughtful recommendations on how a friend can improve a skill is an example of developmental asset.

Lesson 3 *Fill in the blanks with the correct term.*

emotion   hormone
empathy   hostility

A(n) **(8)** _____ tells your mind and body how to react. A change in the level of a(n) **(9)** _____ can affect how you react to situations and thus can affect your emotions. Anger sometimes results in **(10)** _____, which can damage a relationship.

Lesson 4 *Identify each statement as True or False. If false, replace the underlined term with the correct term.*

suppression   defense mechanisms

11. People sometimes use defense mechanisms to avoid dealing with an unpleasant emotion.
12. Projection is the intentional pushing of unpleasantness out of one's mind.

> **RECALLING THE FACTS** *Use complete sentences to answer the following questions.*

Lesson 1

1. In general, teens with good mental/emotional health demonstrate what characteristics?
2. Why is it important to meet needs in positive ways?
3. List four environmental influences that can affect the development of someone's personality.

Lesson 2

4. Identify the eight categories of developmental assets.
5. What does it mean to develop a sense of purpose?
6. How can healthful risk-taking have a positive effect on development?
7. How does high self-esteem and a positive outlook affect a person's health?

Lesson 3

8. List seven basic emotions.
9. Why is it harmful to feel hostile often?
10. Identify two causes of guilt.

Lesson 4

11. What are some ways of managing strong emotions?
12. Identify two strategies for dealing with guilt.

► THINKING CRITICALLY

1. **Evaluating.** Identify a positive role model in your life. Explain the qualities and characteristics that make her or him a positive role model. *(LESSON 1)*

2. **Synthesizing.** Identify three of your strengths and three of your weaknesses. Outline ways that you can use your strengths to address your weaknesses. *(LESSON 2)*

3. **Analyzing.** Why is empathy an important characteristic? Explain actions you can take to demonstrate empathy. *(LESSON 3)*

4. **Evaluating.** List three unhealthful responses to a difficult emotion such as guilt or anger. Explain why these responses are unhealthful, and then provide healthier alternatives for dealing with the emotion. *(LESSON 4)*

► HEALTH SKILLS APPLICATION

1. **Analyzing Influences.** Make a list of the factors that you think have the strongest influence on your personality. Identify which of these are hereditary influences and which are environmental influences. *(LESSON 1)*

2. **Communication Skills.** Think of a person in your life who has given you constructive criticism or positive feedback. Write a thank-you letter to this person. Indicate how this feedback has affected your feelings of self-esteem. *(LESSON 2)*

3. **Advocacy.** Create a small booklet that promotes emotional health by explaining positive ways for teens to deal with difficult emotions or mood swings. *(LESSON 3)*

4. **Practicing Healthful Behaviors.** For one week, maintain an "anger log." After each instance of anger, rate the experience from 1 (mildly irritated) to 10 (hostile). Include the trigger for your anger, what you felt like doing at the time, and how you actually handled the emotion. If necessary, determine ways to improve your anger-management skills. *(LESSON 4)*

BEYOND the Classroom

Parent Involvement

Advocacy. Learn more about local charities and shelters in your community. With your parents or guardians, find out what items and experience are needed and what volunteer positions are available. Use this information to make leaflets or posters that inform others of ways they can help individuals meet their needs.

School and Community

Service Learning. Find out whether your school has a service-learning program. If it does, determine what community volunteer opportunities exist. If your school doesn't have such a program, run a Web search for the Corporation for National and Community Service to locate specific opportunities in your community in fields that interest you.

Chapter 8

Managing Stress and Anxiety

Using Visuals. Communicating with friends, family members, and other people you trust can help you handle the stress of the teen years and help you get through the ups and downs of life. What other strategies can help relieve stress?

Zoe's Story

Zoe has always been focused and well organized. She's known since she was a very young girl that she wanted to be a dancer and has done everything she can to ensure that she would achieve this goal.

Lately, however, Zoe feels as though her life is getting out of control. Homework is taking up too much time. Her friends expect her to go out with them when she has dance practice. Her family always seems to have something big planned when she needs to prepare for an exam or finish a project.

These pressures are beginning to take a toll on Zoe's health. She's been having trouble sleeping and gets angry very easily. She often feels overwhelmed, as if she can't cope with the demands of everyday life. Being tired all the time is having a negative effect on her school-work and dancing. Zoe knows that she needs to do something about her problem but isn't sure what steps to take.

What advice would you give Zoe? Write a sentence or two describing what you would say to her. Reread this story and your response when you complete the chapter. Identify how stress might be affecting *your* life and what you do to manage it.

HEALTH Online

For instant feedback on your health status, go to Chapter 8 Health Inventory at **health.glencoe.com**.

Effects of Stress

VOCABULARY

stress
perception
stressor
psychosomatic
  response
chronic stress

YOU'LL LEARN TO

- Examine causes of stress.

- Describe the effects of stress on body systems.

- Analyze how stress can affect physical, mental/emotional, and social health.

- Discuss how substance abuse harms mental and emotional health.

QUICK START List five situations that you think cause teens to feel stressed. Next to each item, write down why you think that particular situation is a source of stress for teens.

A Disagreements with friends can be a source of stress that affects all aspects of your health triangle. *How does your perception change the way an event affects you?*

Everyone experiences stress—it's a natural part of life. **Stress** is *the reaction of the body and mind to everyday challenges and demands.* You might experience stress during your daily routine, such as when you're running late or when you can't find your keys. Taking an important exam, playing in a state championship basketball game, missing the bus, or arguing with a friend can all be sources of stress. No matter what the source, stress can affect your physical, mental/emotional, and social health. Learning how to manage stress is an important part of staying healthy.

Stress in Your Life

How much stress you feel depends in part on your perception of events that cause stress. **Perception** is *the act of becoming aware through the senses.* One way to manage stress is to change how you perceive and react to events that cause it. Imagine, for example, that you and your best friend have just had an argument. You believe that this disagreement has destroyed your friendship. Your friend, on the other hand, sees the argument as a simple disagreement that you will eventually work out. Because of your perception of the event, you are more likely to experience a higher level of stress than your friend.

➤ THINKING CRITICALLY

1. **Summarizing.** Examine the causes and effects of stress. Write a paragraph describing common stressors and effects of stress. *(LESSON 1)*

2. **Synthesizing.** Describe one potentially stressful situation for which planning might reduce your stress. Make an outline of a plan for that situation. *(LESSON 2)*

3. **Analyzing.** Compare the physical symptoms of anxiety with those of depression. What do anxiety and depression have in common? *(LESSON 3)*

4. **Evaluating.** How might learning about people of other cultures or ethnic backgrounds strengthen your resiliency? *(LESSON 4)*

➤ HEALTH SKILLS APPLICATION

1. **Accessing Information.** Using library resources or the Internet, research the relationship between stress and disease. Write a paragraph explaining what you learned. Identify your sources, and explain why you think they are reliable. *(LESSON 1)*

2. **Refusal Skills.** Describe a scenario in which using refusal skills effectively could help you avoid a potentially stressful situation. Then, write three effective refusal statements you could use to avoid the situation. *(LESSON 2)*

3. **Communication Skills.** Suppose you have a friend who is showing symptoms of depression. For example, he or she has withdrawn from activities you used to share and enjoy. How would you talk with your friend? How could you tell whether he or she needed professional help? *(LESSON 3)*

4. **Analyzing Influences.** Consider the protective factors in your life. Which have the strongest influence on your health behaviors? Why do you think this is so? *(LESSON 4)*

⭐ *BEYOND* the Classroom

Parent Involvement

Accessing Information. With a parent, investigate stress-management resources in your community. Your local Yellow Pages may be a good place to start. Make a list of agencies and their services. Discuss which resource your family members would most likely use if daily stress were to become a health concern. Which resource would be most helpful in dealing with a highly stressful event?

School and Community

Stress Management Classes. Contact a wellness center in a hospital in your area. Ask whether there are stress management seminars or classes that you could observe. Attend a session and report to your class on what you have learned.

Chapter 9
Mental and Emotional Problems

Myth or Fact?

What Do You Know About Mental and Emotional Disorders?

Read the statements below and respond by writing *Myth* or *Fact* for each item. You may want to record reasons for each of your choices.

1. People who have mental and emotional disorders are typically violent.

2. Mental and emotional disorders are true medical illnesses like heart disease and diabetes.

3. Most people can "snap out of" their depression if they try hard enough.

4. Depression and other mental or emotional disorders do not affect children or adolescents.

5. People are less likely to seek treatment for mental disorders than for physical disorders.

6. People who talk about suicide should always be taken seriously.

7. Being treated for a mental or an emotional disorder means that an individual has failed in some way or is responsible for the problem.

8. Getting help for a mental problem is difficult and expensive.

HEALTH Online

For instant feedback on your health status, go to Chapter 9 Health Inventory at **health.glencoe.com**.

Quick *Write*

Using Visuals. Taking time to be with supportive people and setting aside time to be alone can help keep your emotions in balance. Sometimes, however, feelings such as anger, loneliness, fear, or sadness can seem overwhelming. How do you manage these strong emotions? When should a person seek help in dealing with intense feelings?

Mental Disorders

VOCABULARY

mental disorder
anxiety disorder
post-traumatic
  stress disorder
mood disorder
conduct disorder

YOU'LL LEARN TO

• Distinguish types of mental disorders.

• Identify situations requiring professional mental health services.

• Identify and describe the types of mental disorders that affect our society.

QUICK START On a sheet of paper, write as many words as you can think of when you hear the term *mental disorder*. Categorize the words as positive or negative. What might this indicate about attitudes regarding mental disorders?

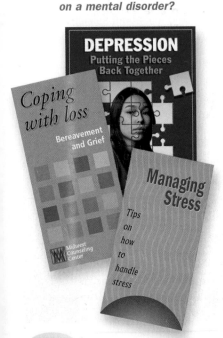

Information about mental disorders is available in most health clinics. *Where else could you find reliable information on a mental disorder?*

Almost everyone experiences periods of sadness, anxiety, and anger. For most people, these feelings are short-lived. For millions of others, however, these feelings persist for weeks, months, and even years. If such feelings begin to interfere with an individual's behavior or daily activities, he or she may be suffering from a mental disorder.

What Are Mental Disorders?

A **mental disorder** is *an illness of the mind that can affect the thoughts, feelings, and behaviors of a person, preventing him or her from leading a happy, healthful, and productive life.* People who suffer from some form of mental disorder are often identified by their inability to cope in healthy ways with life's changes, demands, problems, or traumas. Each year, about 20 percent of the U.S. population—54 million people—are affected by some form of mental disorder. Even though professional help is necessary, fewer than 8 million people with mental disorders actually seek treatment. Of the 20 percent of children and adolescents who suffer from mental health problems, only one-third receive the help they need.

Some people are reluctant to seek treatment for mental/emotional problems because they feel embarrassed or ashamed. Another reason is the stigma associated with mental disorders. A *stigma* is a negative label or a mark of shame. Misconceptions and stereotypes may prevent some people from seeing mental disorders as medical conditions. However, mental disorders require medical attention just as physical illnesses do. In fact, many mental and emotional disturbances involve imbalances in brain chemistry. The sooner a person seeks treatment, the sooner he or she will be on the road to recovery.

Types of Mental Disorders

Mental disorders are classified as either organic or functional. An *organic disorder* is caused by a physical illness or an injury that affects the brain. Brain tumors, infections, chemical imbalances, exposure to drugs and toxins, or injuries resulting in brain damage may lead to organic mental disorders.

A *functional disorder* has a psychological cause and does not involve brain damage. These disorders may result from heredity, stress, emotional conflict, fear, ineffective coping skills, or other conditions. Often, functional disorders are tied to disturbing events in childhood, such as abuse, serious illness, or the traumatic death of a close relative. These disorders may also be tied to recent events, such as divorce, economic hardships, or natural disasters.

Anxiety Disorders

About 4 million Americans suffer from **anxiety disorder**, *a condition in which real or imagined fears are difficult to control.* An anxiety disorder is characterized by chronic fear. People with anxiety disorders often arrange their lives to avoid situations that make them feel anxious or fearful. Anxiety disorders can be classified according to four main types: phobias, obsessive-compulsive disorders, panic disorders, and post-traumatic stress disorders.

PHOBIA

A phobia is a strong and irrational fear of something specific, such as high places or dogs. People with phobias do everything they can to avoid the object of their fear. As a result, a person with a phobia may be unable to live a normal life. For example, people with *agoraphobia* have a fear of open or public places. Their phobia may make them prisoners in their own homes. Some mental health professionals believe that certain phobias are caused by childhood experiences. The fear resulting from these experiences lasts far past the actual threat.

Why are mental disorders a critical health issue?
In the United States, half of the people suffering from mental disorders are untreated, 40 percent of the homeless have some form of mental/emotional problem, and about 20 percent of people in prison have a mental disorder. It is a national concern to get professional mental help for those who need it.

Source: National Alliance for the Mentally Ill

Arachnophobia, a fear of spiders, is a common phobia. People with phobias can seek help from classes, support groups, and mental health professionals.

Post-traumatic stress disorder may occur in the aftermath of a crisis.
What can members of a community do to support one another during crises?

OBSESSIVE-COMPULSIVE DISORDER

A person with obsessive-compulsive disorder is trapped in a pattern of repeated thoughts or behaviors. The term *obsessive* refers to persistent, recurrent, and unwanted thoughts that prevent people from attending to normal daily activities. *Compulsive* refers to repeated, irresistible behaviors. A person with obsessive-compulsive disorder might, for example, feel the urge to wash his or her hands constantly throughout the day.

PANIC DISORDER

A person with a panic disorder has sudden, unexplained feelings of terror. These "panic attacks" are accompanied by symptoms such as trembling, a pounding heart, shortness of breath, or dizziness. Panic disorder is a condition in which fear and anxiety get in the way of a person's ability to function and enjoy life. Panic attacks may occur at any time or place, but most are triggered by a particular object, condition, or situation.

POST-TRAUMATIC STRESS DISORDER

Post-traumatic stress disorder is *a condition that may develop after exposure to a terrifying event that threatened or caused physical harm.* This disorder is common after a personal assault, such as rape; natural or human-made disasters, such as earthquakes or bombings; accidents, such as plane crashes; or military combat. Symptoms may include flashbacks (sudden recall of a terrifying event), nightmares, emotional numbness, sleeplessness, guilt, and problems with concentration. The disorder may arise weeks or months after the event that caused it.

Mood Disorders

A **mood disorder** is an *illness, often with an organic cause, that involves mood extremes that interfere with everyday living.* These extremes are not the highs and lows that everyone experiences, nor are they the mood swings sometimes experienced during adolescence. The emotional swings of mood disorders are extreme in both intensity and duration.

CLINICAL DEPRESSION

Most people who say they are depressed are suffering from a passing case of the blues. For some people, however, depression doesn't go away. Their feelings of sadness, hopelessness, or despair last for more than a few weeks and interfere with daily interests and activities. This type of depression, known as clinical depression, can affect a person's ability to concentrate, sleep, perform at school or work, or handle everyday decisions and challenges. Clinical depression is a chemical imbalance that a person cannot overcome without professional help.

Approximately 19 million Americans are affected by clinical depression each year. Depression often runs in families and can be biologically based, but it can also be caused by life events. Sometimes it may be a symptom of substance abuse or addiction, because alcohol and other drugs can affect brain chemistry.

BIPOLAR DISORDER

This disorder, also known as manic-depressive disorder, is marked by extreme mood changes, energy levels, and behavior. Characteristics of the manic "highs" and depressive "lows" of this disorder are described in **Figure 9.1.** Although adults with bipolar disorder may behave normally between episodes of extreme emotion, teens with the disorder tend to alternate rapidly between the two extremes with few clear periods of wellness between episodes.

Eating Disorders

Psychological pressures, possible genetic factors, and an obsession with body image and thinness can lead to an **eating disorder.** People with eating disorders such as anorexia and bulimia suffer from life-threatening disturbances in eating behavior. Eating disorders are not a failure of will or behavior; they are real, treatable medical illnesses. A person who suffers from an eating disorder can experience a wide range of physical health complications, including serious heart conditions and kidney failure, which may lead to death. It is therefore critical that a person with an eating disorder get help immediately.

HEALTH Online

Learn more about teens and depression by clicking on Health Updates at health.glencoe.com.

hot link

eating disorders For more information about eating disorders, see Chapter 6, page 153.

FIGURE 9.1

MANIA AND DEPRESSION—FLIP SIDES OF MOOD DISORDERS FOR TEENS

Manic Symptoms:

- **Severe changes in mood**—is either excessively happy or silly, or very irritable, angry, agitated, or aggressive
- **Grandiosity**—unrealistically high self-esteem, feeling all-powerful
- **Very high energy level**—including the ability to go with little or no sleep for days without feeling tired
- **Pressured speech**—talks too much, too fast, changes topics too quickly, and does not allow interruption
- **Distractibility**—attention moves constantly from one thing to another
- **Repeated high-risk behavior**—alcohol or drug use, reckless driving, or sexual activity

Depressive Symptoms:

- **Irritability,** persistent sadness, frequent crying
- **Preoccupation with death** or suicide
- **Loss of enjoyment** in favorite activities
- **Frequent physical complaints** such as headaches or stomachaches
- **Low energy level,** fatigue, poor concentration, boredom
- **Dramatic change in eating or sleeping patterns,** such as overeating or oversleeping

Source: American Academy of Child and Adolescent Psychiatry

Conduct Disorders

Children and adolescents who act out their impulses toward others in destructive ways may have a **conduct disorder**, *a pattern of behavior in which the rights of others or basic social rules are violated.* Examples include lying, theft, aggression, violence, truancy, arson, and vandalism. The condition is more common among males than females. Although they may project an image of toughness, people with this disorder usually have low self-esteem. They may also have symptoms of other mental disorders including anxiety, depression, and substance abuse. Without treatment, many teens with this disorder will be unable to adapt to the demands of adulthood and will continue to have problems relating to others, holding a job, and behaving in appropriate ways.

Schizophrenia

Schizophrenia (skit-suh-FREE-nee-uh) is a severe mental disorder in which a person loses contact with reality. Symptoms of schizophrenia include delusions, hallucinations, and thought disorders. Causes of this condition may be a combination of genetic factors and chemical and structural changes in the brain. The disease affects about 1 percent of the population. Schizophrenia affects both men and women and usually first appears between the ages of 15 and 35.

People who suffer from schizophrenia have difficulty understanding the difference between real and imaginary events. This inability leads to unpredictable behavior, difficulty functioning, and lack of good health habits. A common misconception about people who suffer from this disorder is that all of them are violent or have multiple or split personalities. However, schizophrenic people are usually not a threat to others. Professional help and medication are necessary to successfully treat schizophrenia.

Teens with a conduct disorder may act with aggression, but they often have low self-esteem.
How might an untreated conduct disorder affect a teen's future?

Personality Disorders

The term *personality* refers to an individual's unique traits and behavior patterns. People with healthy personalities can cope with the day-to-day challenges of life. However, people afflicted with personality disorders think and behave in ways that make it difficult for them to get along with others. Over the course of their lives, usually beginning in adolescence, they are in constant conflict with others—family, friends, teachers, coworkers, or supervisors. About 10 percent of the population has one of the several types of personality disorder. Counseling, and sometimes medication, are recommended as treatment.

▶ **Antisocial personality disorder.** People with this disorder tend to be irritable, aggressive, impulsive, and violent. In many cases, they are unable to show remorse for their behavior.

▶ **Borderline personality disorder.** People with this disorder frequently experience a series of troubled relationships. They tend to engage in high-risk activities, and many have poor self-esteem. Although they fear abandonment, they frequently lash out violently at the people they need most.

▶ **Passive-aggressive personality disorder.** People with this disorder are often uncooperative. They resent being told what to do, yet they rely on others' direction. Angry over issues of control, they show their anger, but only indirectly. For example, a passive-aggressive person who doesn't want to take part in an activity either may forget to show up or may arrive late and leave early.

As with all mental and emotional problems, it is important to recognize the signs of personality disorders and seek professional help.

Improving Attitudes About Mental Disorders

To help defeat the social stigma of mental disorders:

▶ Use respectful language when referring to a person with a mental disorder.

▶ Emphasize abilities over limitations.

▶ Express disapproval if someone shows disrespect or inconsideration toward people with mental disorders.

▶ Encourage people who have emotional problems to seek help.

 Lesson 1 *Review*

Reviewing Facts and Vocabulary

1. Define the term *mental disorder,* and explain how organic and functional disorders differ.

2. What do clinical depression and bipolar disorder have in common?

3. Compare and contrast the characteristics of schizophrenia and antisocial personality disorder.

Thinking Critically

4. **Synthesizing.** Although scientific evidence shows that mental disorders are medical conditions, the stigma attached to these illnesses persists. Why do you think this is so?

5. **Analyzing.** How do eating disorders differ from the other types of mental disorders?

Applying Health Skills

Advocacy. Teens suffering from mental disorders often feel confused, isolated, scared, or ashamed. Create a Bill of Rights for people with mental disorders; your list should advocate demonstrating empathy. Focus on specific ways for students to be supportive, patient, and understanding.

PRESENTATION SOFTWARE Using presentation software, you can highlight certain points that you want to make. Find help in using presentation software at **health.glencoe.com.**

Suicide Prevention

VOCABULARY

alienation
suicide
cluster suicides

YOU'LL LEARN TO

- Identify the warning signs of suicide.
- Analyze strategies for preventing suicides.
- Develop strategies for coping with depression.
- Develop strategies for coping with feelings in the aftermath of a tragedy.

QUICK START Write down three danger signs you might detect in someone who is thinking about suicide. Then explain why you think these are warning signs of suicide. What do you think family members and friends can do to help a loved one who is exhibiting these signs?

A Recognizing signs of depression and seeking help is critical to suicide prevention.

L ife can be difficult for everyone at times. Challenges, respon- sibilities, and pressures can pile up and seem overwhelming. These feelings can be further complicated by troubling life events, such as the divorce of parents or the death of a friend or family member. For some people, this emotional overload can lead to depression or **alienation**, *feeling isolated and separated from every- one else.* When such painful feelings become unbearable, some peo- ple may try drastic, self-destructive measures to escape their pain. **Suicide**, the most drastic of all measures, is *the act of intentionally taking one's own life.* Suicide is a serious problem, but it is preventable.

Suicide Risk Factors

M ost suicidal thoughts, behaviors, and actions are expressions of extreme distress, not bids for attention. More than 90 percent of the people who kill themselves are suffering from depression or another mental disorder or are abusing alcohol or drugs. Other suicidal risk factors include a history of physical or sexual abuse, a history of previous suicide attempts, or a family history of emotional disorders or suicides.

FIGURE 9.2

TEEN SUICIDE: RECOGNIZING THE WARNING SIGNS

The warning signs of suicide should be taken seriously. The more signs a person exhibits, the more likely he or she is thinking about suicide.

Verbal Signs	Nonverbal or Behavioral Signs
• Direct statements such as these: "I want to die." "I don't want to live anymore." "I wish I were dead." • Indirect statements such as these: "I won't have to put up with this much longer." "I just want to go to sleep and never wake up." "They'll be sorry when I'm gone." "Soon this pain will be over." "I can't take it anymore." "Nothing matters." "I won't be a problem for you much longer." "What's the use?" • Writing poems, song lyrics, or diary entries that deal with death. • Suicide threats or insinuations that are either direct or indirect.	• An unusual obsession with death • Withdrawal from friends • Dramatic changes in personality, hygiene, or appearance • Impulsive, irrational, or bizarre behavior • An overwhelming sense of guilt, shame, or rejection; negative self-evaluation • Significant deterioration in schoolwork or recreational performance • Preoccupation with giving away personal belongings • Substance abuse • Frequent complaints about physical symptoms such as stomachaches, headaches, fatigue • Persistent boredom and indifference • Violent actions, rebellious behavior, or running away • Intolerance for praise or rewards

Sources: National Mental Health Association; American Academy of Child and Adolescent Psychiatry

Preventing Suicide

Although most thoughts about committing suicide are impulsive and temporary, the unfortunate consequence—death or debilitating injury—is permanent. The warning signs of suicide are described in **Figure 9.2.** Your ability to recognize these signs in yourself or others can mean the difference between life and death. When a teen talks about committing suicide—whether it's done in a serious, casual, or even humorous way—*he or she must be taken seriously.* Never bargain with someone who is thinking about suicide. Any discussion or suggestion about suicide requires immediate intervention. Seek adult assistance without delay.

Despite the fact that depression is very treatable, untreated depression is the leading cause of suicide. People who appear to have mental health problems need to be encouraged repeatedly to seek help—especially if they seem suicidal. With adequate help and support, people suffering from depression, extreme stress, or other mental and emotional problems can often find new purpose and happiness.

Health Skills Activity

Decision Making: When a Friend Seems Troubled

When Ian started exhibiting signs of depression, his friend Jordan tried to persuade him to get help. Ian admitted that he was unhappy. However, he told Jordan, "I appreciate your trying to help me, but it's okay; I'm handling my problems by myself."

Jordan knows that Ian is a private person, but Jordan has never seen his friend this "down" before. Jordan wants to tell someone about his concerns, but he is hesitant about betraying a confidence.

What Would You Do?

Apply the six steps of the decision-making model to Jordan's concerns.

1. State the situation.
2. List the options.
3. Weigh the possible outcomes.
4. Consider values.
5. Make a decision and act.
6. Evaluate the decision.

Did You Know ?

You can use *CLUES* to remember how to communicate effectively with a friend who is suffering emotionally.

Connect (Make contact.)

Listen (Take time and pay attention.)

Understand (Let the person know that you empathize with his or her feelings.)

Express Concern (Say that you care, and stay with the person.)

Seek Help (Encourage the person to talk to an adult, and tell an adult yourself.)

Source: University of Minnesota Extension Service

Helping Others

Suicidal people often believe that their death will not matter to anyone. For this reason, it is critical to show concern and empathy for someone who is talking about suicide. All talk of suicide must be taken seriously. Remember, the suicidal person needs professional help—immediately. When you are with someone who appears to be suicidal, show you care by following these steps.

► **Initiate a meaningful conversation.** Showing interest and compassion for a person is an important first step. Listen closely to what that person says; be patient and understanding.

► **Show support and ask questions.** Remind the person that most problems have solutions. Make it clear that you understand that the person wants to end his or her pain, but emphasize that suicide is *not* the answer. Share the fact that most suicide survivors later express gratitude that they did not die.

► **Try to persuade the person to seek help.** Encourage the person to talk with a parent, counselor, therapist, or other trusted adult. Offer to go with the person to get help.

Multiple Suicides

Sometimes within a teen population, **cluster suicides** occur. These are *a series of suicides occurring within a short period of time and involving several people in the same school or community*. Studies have shown that cluster suicides in the United States occur mainly among teens and young adults and may account for as much as 5 percent of all suicides in any given year. Some cluster suicides are the result of pacts or agreements between two or more people to take part in suicide. Others result when individuals commit suicide in response to the suicide of a friend or a suicide that has been sensationalized in the media.

The Centers for Disease Control and Prevention (CDC) has developed guidelines for preventing cluster suicides. Among their recommendations is the evaluation and counseling of close friends and relatives of suicide victims because these people may themselves be at high risk for suicide. The CDC also recommends that the media report on suicide in a way that does not glorify the victim, over-simplify the victim's motivation, or portray the suicide as an understandable response to pressure or emotional pain.

Suicide can affect people beyond the victim's immediate family and friends. *Why might a teen be affected by the suicide of someone who is a stranger?*

Lesson 2 *Review*

Reviewing Facts and Vocabulary

1. Name five warning signs of suicide.
2. List three risk factors of suicide.
3. Describe some of the strategies for suicide prevention.

Thinking Critically

4. **Analyzing.** How might support from family, friends, or mental health professionals help prevent suicides? What strategies might each of those groups offer to help an individual cope with stress, depression, and anxiety?
5. **Synthesizing.** Why is empathy important when talking with a suicidal person?

Applying Health Skills

Accessing Information. Compile a list of local resources for suicide prevention. This list should include mental health professionals, school counselors, hospital emergency rooms, suicide hot lines, and local authorities (including representatives of the police and fire departments).

TECHNOLOGY OPTION

WEB SITES Researching valid Web sites can provide additional information on resources for suicide intervention. See **health.glencoe.com** for more information on using Web sites.

Getting Help

VOCABULARY

psychotherapy
behavior therapy
cognitive therapy
group therapy
biomedical
   therapy

YOU'LL LEARN TO

• Relate the importance of early detection and warning signs that prompt people to seek mental health care.

• Explore the methods for addressing critical mental health issues.

• Identify and describe mental health services.

QUICK START On a sheet of paper, explain why some people may find it difficult to seek help for mental and emotional problems.

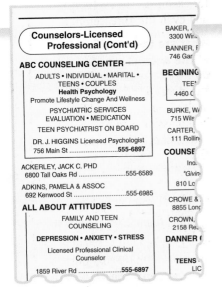

Counselors-Licensed Professional (Cont'd)

ABC COUNSELING CENTER
ADULTS • INDIVIDUAL • MARITAL •
TEENS • COUPLES
Health Psychology
Promote Lifestyle Change And Wellness
PSYCHIATRIC SERVICES
EVALUATION • MEDICATION
TEEN PSYCHIATRIST ON BOARD
DR. J. HIGGINS Licensed Psychologist
756 Main St **555-6897**

ACKERLEY, JACK C. PHD
6800 Tall Oaks Rd 555-6589
ADKINS, PAMELA & ASSOC
692 Kenwood St 555-6985

ALL ABOUT ATTITUDES
FAMILY AND TEEN
COUNSELING
DEPRESSION • ANXIETY • STRESS
Licensed Professional Clinical
Counselor
1859 River Rd **555-6897**

BAKER,
3300 Win
BANNER,
746 Gar

BEGINING
TEE
4460 C

BURKE, W
715 Wils
CARTER,
111 Rollin
COUNSE
Ina.
Givin
810 Lo

CROWE &
8855 Lon
CROWN,
2158 Re
DANNER
TEENS
LIC

Many sources of help are available to people who have mental health concerns. *How would you evaluate sources of help for appropriateness?*

Recognizing the early symptoms of mental and emotional problems is critically important to getting help for them. Knowing some specific symptoms of mental disorders can help a person determine if he or she should seek help.

Knowing When to Get Help

It can be difficult to ask for help in coping with mental or emotional problems. Our thoughts are private, and we tend to hide those that embarrass us or those we can't control. However, we usually need help most when we feel like asking for it least. Seek help if any of the feelings or behaviors listed below persist over a period of days or weeks and begin to interfere with other aspects of daily living.

▶ You feel trapped with no way out, or you worry all the time.

▶ Your feelings affect your sleep, eating habits, school work, job performance, or relationships.

▶ Your family or friends express concern about your behavior.

▶ You are becoming involved with alcohol or other drugs.

▶ You are becoming increasingly aggressive, violent, or reckless.

Signs That Professional Help Is Needed

Some symptoms that are severe enough to require intervention by a mental health professional include: prolonged sadness for no specific reason; frequent outbursts of anger; overwhelming fear, anxiety, or anger at the world; unexplainable change in sleeping or eating habits; and social withdrawal. Of course, if you have any doubt about your mental health, you should always get assistance. Like most forms of sickness, mental disorders may get worse if left untreated.

Real-Life Application

Evaluating Sources of Self-Help

Thousands of self-help materials are available in print, on tapes and CDs, and online. Many people have benefited from self-help resources, but others have wasted time and money and sometimes risked their health. Use these questions to evaluate self-help materials.

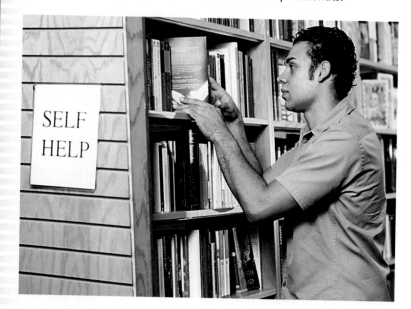

Are you being advised to try medication or some other remedy?
Check first with a health professional. Certain herbs, for example, can be harmful and even life-threatening.

What are the qualifications of the authors?
Do they have university-based training in mental health? Have they published in professional journals? For books, check the reference section for citations from professional journals.

Is the material backed by a nationally known and respected mental health organization?
Look for recommendations from organizations such as the American Psychological Association or the National Institute of Mental Health.

Is a cost involved?
If you are asked online for a credit card number or personal information, use caution and check with a parent or guardian.

ACTIVITY

Choose a self-help book, magazine article, CD, or Web site and evaluate the information using the criteria listed here. Share your findings with the class, and recommend any useful and appropriate sources to the school librarian.

FIGURE 9.3

MENTAL HEALTH PROFESSIONALS

- **Psychiatrist**—a physician who specializes in diagnosing and treating mental disorders and can prescribe medications
- **Neurologist**—a physician who specializes in organic disorders of the brain and nervous system
- **Clinical Psychologist**—a professional who diagnoses and treats emotional and behavioral disorders by means of counseling but cannot prescribe medications
- **Counselor**—a professional who works to help people with personal and educational matters
- **Psychiatric Social Worker**—a professional who provides guidance and treatment for clients with emotional problems, usually in the setting of a mental hospital, mental health clinic, or family service agency
- **School Psychologist**—a professional who specializes in the assessment of learning, emotional, and behavioral problems of schoolchildren

Seeking Help

Most people tend to wait too long before seeking help even though there are many people in their lives who are willing and eager to assist them. Besides parents and guardians, who are usually the most accessible, there are teachers, school psychologists, counselors, coaches, clergy members, and crisis hot lines. According to the Surgeon General, school is the place where children and teens are most likely to receive treatment. **Figure 9.3** provides a list of mental health professionals to whom a person might be referred for help.

STUMBLING BLOCKS TO SEEKING HELP

Some people are afraid to seek help for mental or emotional problems. They see these problems as a sign of weakness, not as a legitimate illness. If you or someone you know is reluctant to seek help, remember these facts.

▶ Asking for help from a mental health professional does not mean that a person is weak. Rather, asking for needed help is a sign of strength. It shows responsibility for one's own wellness.

▶ People who have mental disorders often cannot get better on their own. Serious disorders, clinical depression, compulsions, and addictions are complex and require professional intervention.

▶ Sharing your deepest thoughts with a "stranger" is not painful or embarrassing. In fact, most people are surprised and happy to find that unloading problems is a great relief.

Therapy Methods

A mental health professional may use any of several treatment methods, depending on his or her area of expertise and the needs of the patient. The following are the most commonly used therapy methods.

▶ **Psychotherapy** is *an ongoing dialogue between a patient and a mental health professional.* The dialogue is designed to find the root cause of a problem and devise a solution.

▶ **Behavior therapy** is *a treatment process that focuses on changing unwanted behaviors through rewards and reinforcements.*

▶ **Cognitive therapy** is *a treatment method designed to identify and correct distorted thinking patterns that can lead to feelings and behaviors that may be troublesome, self-defeating, or self-destructive.*

▶ **Group therapy** *involves treating a group of people who have similar problems and who meet regularly with a trained counselor.*

▶ **Biomedical therapy** is *the use of certain medications to treat or reduce the symptoms of a mental disorder.* It is sometimes used alone, but is often combined with other treatment methods, such as those listed above.

Most forms of therapy involve counseling. *What are some short-term and long-term benefits of receiving help for a mental health problem?*

 Lesson 3 *Review*

Reviewing Facts and Vocabulary

1. Identify three signals that may indicate a person needs help with a mental or an emotional problem.
2. Why do some people delay seeking help for mental or emotional problems?
3. Define *group therapy*, and use the term in a sentence.

Thinking Critically

4. **Synthesizing.** Identify at least three personal qualities one would need to fill a position at a mental health clinic.
5. **Analyzing.** What factors might determine from whom you would seek help for a mental problem?

Applying Health Skills

Decision Making. Imagine that you have a friend who is always making negative comments and seems to be withdrawing from his or her normal activities. Use the six steps of decision making to determine what actions to take.

WORD PROCESSING Using a word-processing program can help you better organize your thoughts. See **health.glencoe.com** for information on using word-processing software.

Understanding Death and Grief

VOCABULARY

coping
grief response
mourning

YOU'LL LEARN TO

- Describe the different kinds of emotional loss.

- Identify the stages of the grieving process.

- Discuss the ways in which people cope with emotional loss.

- Examine issues related to death and grieving.

- Analyze the importance of using community mental health services to help cope with grief.

→ *QUICK START* What words come to mind when you imagine dealing with the loss of someone or something of great value? Write the word *grief* at the center of a sheet of paper. Write words you associate with grieving on your paper, and make a word web by drawing lines from those words to the word *grief*.

▲ Flowers and cards are appropriate expressions of sympathy for someone who has suffered a loss. *In what other ways can you show support?*

L oss is a part of life. Although it is always difficult and painful to lose someone you love or care for, learning to cope with grief is an important part of human development. The strong bonds we form with others can help us deal with loss in appropriate ways and accept it as a part of the entire life experience.

Different Kinds of Loss

Y ou have probably experienced losses that resulted in emotional distress. Perhaps you missed a chance to play in a championship game because of an injury or failed to get the grade you needed on an important exam. You may have experienced rejection; the breakup of a relationship; or the loss of a pet, friend, or family member to death. Maybe you have had to move or change schools and have felt the loss of whatever—or whomever—you left behind. A strong emotional attachment can make loss deeply painful.

Expressions of Grief

Coping is *dealing successfully with difficult changes in your life.* When a loss occurs, it's common and natural to experience a **grief response**, *an individual's total response to a major loss.* The way a person responds to loss is unique to the situation and to the individual. If a death is sudden or traumatic, for example, the response is likely to be somewhat different from the response to a death that resulted from a long-term illness. A person's perspective on the lost relationship and his or her ability to remain open to interaction in other relationships might also affect the response to loss.

The Grieving Process

Mental health professionals have recognized a common phenomenon, called the *grieving process*, that occurs during the grief response. The purpose of this process is to reach closure, or acceptance of a loss. There is no correct way of experiencing loss, but the stages of grief reflect a variety of reactions that may occur as people work through the process. The reactions, which were identified in part by the noted Swiss American doctor Elisabeth Kübler-Ross, include the following:

▶ **Denial or Numbness.** In this stage, the person cannot believe the loss has occurred. This part of the process protects the person from being overwhelmed by his or her emotions.

▶ **Emotional Releases.** These reactions come with recognition of the loss and often involve periods of crying, which is important to the healing process.

▶ **Anger.** Feeling powerless and unfairly deprived, the person may lash out at whatever is perceived to be responsible for the loss. Sometimes a general resentment toward life sets in.

▶ **Bargaining.** As the reality of the loss becomes clear, the person may promise to change if only what was lost can be returned, even for a little while.

▶ **Depression.** Beyond the natural feelings of sadness, feelings of isolation, alienation, and hopelessness occur as the person recognizes the extent of the loss.

▶ **Remorse.** The person may become preoccupied with thoughts about what he or she could have done to prevent the loss or make things better.

▶ **Acceptance.** This stage can involve a sense of power, allowing the person to face reality in constructive ways and make significant and meaningful gestures surrounding the idea of loss.

▶ **Hope.** Eventually the person reaches a point when remembering becomes less painful and he or she begins to look ahead to the future.

Health Minute

Breaking Up

The breakup of a relationship can cause a person to experience many of the stages of grief. These feelings are a natural part of the healing process.

Overcoming a breakup:

▶ Allow yourself to feel the pain associated with the breakup. Denying your feelings only prolongs the grief process.

▶ Recognize that self-blame and guilt are defenses against feeling out of control. Remember that you can't control another person's decisions or behaviors.

▶ Be thankful for the good times you've had and the contributions the relationship has made to your life.

▶ Give yourself time to heal. Allow yourself to have new experiences and to make new friends, but avoid comparing new relationships with the one that has ended.

An Encouraging Word

Much of the day-to-day comforting of terminally ill persons is carried out by dedicated volunteers. These volunteers often experience a profound sense of loss when the patient passes away. A word of support in the form of a card will encourage these volunteers to continue their important work.

What You'll Need

- card stock paper
- felt-tip pens in different colors
- computer with clip art software (optional)

What You'll Do

1. On 8½" x 11" notebook paper, compose several versions of a message. Many volunteers report that inspirational messages are helpful.

2. Sketch the artwork you will include in your card. The artwork should emphasize serenity, peace, or hope. You may want to examine clip art options from a computer program for ideas.

3. Decide what "goodies," such as a flower or candy, to include with your card.

4. Create your card, using card stock paper and felt-tip pens or computer clip art.

Apply and Conclude

Send your card to a hospital, hospice, or other facility in which volunteers provide support for terminally ill people. Then compose a reflective essay describing what you have learned about dealing with loss and grieving by empathizing with those who work with terminally ill patients.

Coping with Death

To help cope with death, allow some time to reflect on who you were before the loss and who you will be after grieving. Focus on what you were able to do in the relationship, not what you could or should have done. Remember the wonderful things about the person and the good times you've shared. Another way to reach closure is by seeking support from others or writing a letter to say good-bye.

Did You Know ?

Unresolved grief tends to affect the grieving process at the next occurrence of a loss—causing a person to express some emotions and responses that have been held back. The surfacing of unresolved grief reactions can slow and complicate the healing process.

Helping Others Through the Grieving Process

Support from family and friends is important during **mourning**, or *the act of showing sorrow or grief*. While it is up to the individual to go through the grieving process, he or she doesn't have to do it alone. You can help by showing empathy or just being there to listen. Share your memories and appreciation of the person who is gone. Talking about experiences and memories can help survivors bridge the transition.

Grief Counseling

Seeing a counselor or therapist who specializes in grief can help people through the grieving process. These specialists often can be found through community mental health services, such as hospices.

Memorial services are times for remembering and showing respect.
What are some other ways to remember a loved one?

Coping with Disasters and Crises

Traumatic or sudden events, such as natural disasters, can leave people feeling a range of emotions from numb and helpless to horrified and afraid. Using effective coping mechanisms can ease the process of recovery.

▶ Spend time with other people, and discuss your feelings.

▶ Get back to daily routines as quickly as possible.

▶ Eat nutritious foods, exercise, and get enough rest and sleep.

▶ Do something positive to help your community through the event, such as assisting with cleanup or raising money for aid.

 Lesson 4 *Review*

Reviewing Facts and Vocabulary

1. Name the stages that may be involved in the grieving process.
2. Define the term *grief response*.
3. List three strategies for coping with disasters and crises.

Thinking Critically

4. **Analyzing.** How might coping with a death resulting from a long-term illness differ from coping with a sudden death caused by an accident?
5. **Applying.** Recall a story of personal loss that you saw in a movie or on a TV show or that you read about in a magazine article or book. Write a paragraph that describes the process the grieving character went through to reach closure.

Applying Health Skills

Communication Skills. How could you express support to a friend who is suffering from a tragic loss? Make a list of things you could say to comfort someone in such a situation. Your statements should show consideration, respect, and empathy.

SPREADSHEETS Spreadsheets offer a quick and easy way to organize and edit a list. See health.glencoe.com for tips on using spreadsheets.

Creating Positive Media Influences

In April 2002, President George W. Bush's New Freedom Commission on Mental Health initiated a comprehensive study to assess the mental health care system in the United States. The commission's efforts brought national media attention to the issue of mental health. In this activity, you will help design a media campaign in your community that will promote awareness of mental health issues.

"Our country must make a commitment: Americans with mental illness deserve our understanding, and they deserve excellent care."

ACTIVITY

Based on what you have learned, you and your class will design a positive media campaign that will accomplish the following: encourage people to seek help when faced with mental or emotional problems; convey empathy for people who suffer from mental or emotional problems; and teach the public that people with mental illnesses should be treated fairly.

Your teacher will divide the class into groups to create the following components of your media campaign:

a slogan, a direct mail marketing piece, a billboard, and a print ad for a newspaper or magazine.

EXPRESS YOUR VIEWS

In a class discussion, share your views on the potential impact of media portrayals of mentally ill people. What can television dramas and local news programs do to help educate the public about mental health issues?

CROSS-CURRICULUM CONNECTIONS

Write a Poem. Knowing that they have the love and support of friends and family can help people through the grieving process. Imagine that a friend has suffered the loss of a loved one. Write a poem expressing sympathy, support, and hope to help the friend through the difficult time.

Research Cultural Rituals. Rituals to help people cope with death go back to ancient times. Study various burial traditions and ceremonies from throughout the ages, and share your findings in a short oral presentation to your class. How are these customs similar to or different from the ways Americans confront death today?

Calculate Percentage. Among children and adolescents, the portion of those who suffer from mental health problems is 20 percent. If a third of these individuals receive treatment, what percentage of these children and adolescents do *not* get help for mental disorders?

Research Neurotransmitters. Abnormal levels of neurotransmitters can contribute to mental illness. Research the following neurotransmitters: dopamine, serotonin, glutamate, phenylethylamine, epinephrine, norepinephrine, acetylcholine, oxytocin. Create a chart that shows their relationship to the forms of mental disorders discussed in the chapter.

Psychologist

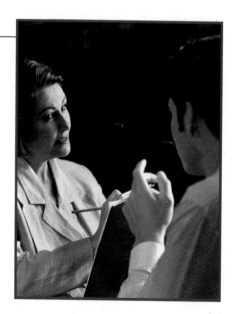

Are you interested in human behavior and the mental processes related to behavior? Do you enjoy talking with people and helping them with their problems? If so, a career as a psychologist might be for you. Psychologists counsel individuals to help them resolve mental and emotional problems.

If you want to be an advocate for children, you might consider specializing in school psychology. A school psychologist specializes in educational assessment, childhood development, behavioral management, individual and group counseling, and consultation.

To become a psychologist, you will need at least a master's degree. A doctoral degree is required for clinical counseling. Find out more about this and other health careers by clicking on Career Corner at **health.glencoe.com**.

Chapter 9 *Review*

➤ **EXPLORING HEALTH TERMS** *Answer the following questions on a sheet of paper.*

Lesson 1 *Match each definition with the correct term.*

anxiety disorder	conduct disorder
eating disorder	mental disorder
post-traumatic stress disorder	mood disorder

1. An illness of the mind that can affect the thoughts, feelings, and behaviors of a person, preventing him or her from leading a happy, healthy, productive life.
2. An illness, often with an organic cause, that relates to emotions and may involve mood extremes that interfere with everyday living.
3. A pattern of behavior in which the rights of others or basic social rules are violated.

Lesson 2 *Fill in the blanks with the correct term.*

suicide	cluster suicide
alienation	

A (_4_) can occur in a community when a local (_5_) is sensationalized in the media. These behaviors often result from feelings of depression and (_6_).

Lesson 3 *Replace the underlined words with the correct term.*

behavior therapy	biomedical therapy
cognitive therapy	group therapy
psychotherapy	

7. <u>Psychotherapy</u> usually involves several people.
8. A psychiatrist may use <u>behavior therapy</u> if medication is needed in the treatment.
9. A distorted thinking pattern requires <u>group therapy</u>.
10. The therapy that uses rewards and reinforcements is called <u>cognitive therapy</u>.
11. <u>Biomedical therapy</u> involves an ongoing dialogue between a patient and a mental health professional.

Lesson 4 *Match each definition with the correct term.*

mourning	grief response
coping	

12. Dealing successfully with difficult changes in your life.
13. An individual's total response to a major loss.
14. The act of showing sorrow or grief.

➤ **RECALLING THE FACTS** *Use complete sentences to answer the following questions.*

Lesson 1

1. What types of events are associated with post-traumatic stress disorder?
2. Name two eating disorders.
3. Describe antisocial personality disorder.

Lesson 2

4. What should you do if you recognize the warning signs of suicide in yourself or others?
5. List three actions a person can take if he or she is with someone who appears to be suicidal.
6. What are the CDC's guidelines for preventing cluster suicides?

Lesson 3

7. Where are teens and children most likely to receive treatment for mental health problems?
8. Name six types of mental health professionals.
9. List three therapy methods for treating mental disorders.

Lesson 4

10. List three examples of loss.
11. What is one means of reaching closure after the death of a loved one?
12. How can you help someone who is mourning?

➤ THINKING CRITICALLY

1. **Summarizing.** If a teen with a conduct disorder does not get treatment, he or she may have trouble adapting to adulthood. Explain this statement using examples from the text or from your own observations. *(LESSON 1)*

2. **Synthesizing.** How might you respond to someone who expresses the desire to take his or her life and asks you to promise not to tell anyone? *(LESSON 2)*

3. **Applying.** A friend tells you that she is uncomfortable seeking help from a mental health professional for a mental disorder. What could you say to her? *(LESSON 3)*

4. **Synthesizing.** What are some skills a grief counselor should exhibit? Where might you access the help of such a counselor? *(LESSON 4)*

➤ HEALTH SKILLS APPLICATION

1. **Analyzing Influences.** Briefly describe some movies or television shows that have portrayed characters with mental disorders. Do you think that these depictions are realistic, accurate, and sensitive? How do you think media representations of mental disorders affect how the public views mental problems? *(LESSON 1)*

2. **Advocacy.** Write a letter to your school newspaper to raise awareness of teen suicide as a serious problem. Include information on what everyone can do to help prevent teen suicide. *(LESSON 2)*

3. **Accessing Information.** Evaluate the availability of mental health professionals in your community. *(LESSON 3)*

4. **Practicing Healthful Behaviors.** Develop a strategy for coping with loss. Think about what would make you feel better if you were grieving a loss. Make a list of actions you could take to cope with the situation and with your feelings. *(LESSON 4)*

BEYOND the Classroom

Parent Involvement

Accessing Information. Learn more about family counseling centers that are available in your community. With your parents, create a pamphlet that highlights the services offered through the centers, the costs of these services, and where financial assistance for counseling can be found. Provide the pamphlet to your school counselor.

School and Community

Crisis Centers. Identify local crisis centers that help teens deal with mental health problems. Contact the centers to determine how a person could become a volunteer either in the centers or on their associated hotlines.

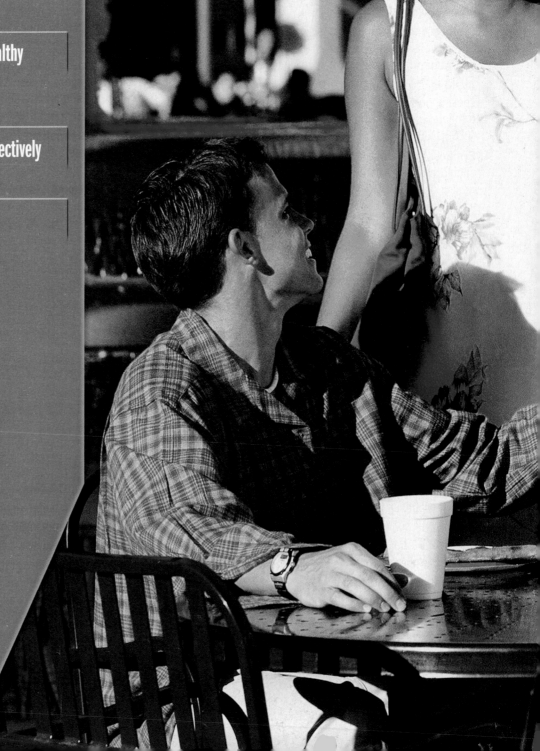

Chapter 10

Skills for Healthy Relationships

Personal Health Inventory

What's Your Health Status?

Read each statement below and respond by writing *yes*, *no*, or *sometimes* for each item. Write *yes* only for items that you practice regularly.

1. I treat others with respect.
2. I am a good team player.
3. I am trustworthy.
4. I resolve differences through compromise.
5. I am willing to work at my relationships.
6. I am a good listener.
7. I communicate well with others.
8. I ask questions when I am uncertain about what is being said.
9. I make eye contact when communicating with others.
10. I am aware of my body language and the messages it sends to others.

HEALTH Online

For instant feedback on your health status, go to Chapter 10 Health Inventory at **health.glencoe.com**.

Quick Write

Using Visuals. Friendships are an important part of our lives. What kinds of skills do you think help friendships remain healthy and strong?

Foundations of Healthy Relationships

VOCABULARY

relationship
friendship
citizenship
role
communication
cooperation
compromise

YOU'LL LEARN TO

- Analyze how relationships with peers, family, and friends affect physical, mental/emotional, and social health.

- Demonstrate strategies for communicating needs, wants, and emotions in healthy ways.

- Identify the qualities and character traits that promote healthy relationships with peers, family, and friends.

➜ **QUICK START** List five characteristics you think are needed for healthy relationships. Rank the characteristics in order of importance, and explain why you ranked each item as you did.

Ⓐ Shared values and mutual respect are essential in healthy relationships.

As you learned in Chapter 7, human beings are social creatures with a need to belong and be loved. We also need to feel safe, secure, valued, and recognized. These needs are met when we form healthy relationships with others. A **relationship** is *a bond or connection you have with other people.*

Healthy Relationships

All of your relationships can have effects on your physical, mental/emotional, and social health. Healthy relationships are based on shared values and interests and mutual respect. You are naturally drawn to those who encourage and support your own best qualities. A healthy relationship is one in which both people benefit and feel comfortable.

Family Relationships

Family relationships, which involve both immediate family (parents or guardians and siblings) and extended family (grandparents, aunts, uncles, and cousins), last your entire life. Healthy family relationships enhance all sides of your health triangle. For example, your parents or guardians provide for your physical health with food, clothing, and shelter. They build your social health by teaching you the values that will guide you throughout your life. The love, care, and encouragement you receive from family members also contribute to your mental/emotional health.

Friendships

A **friendship** is *a significant relationship between two people that is based on caring, trust, and consideration.* Your friends can be of any age, and you can choose them for different reasons. For example, a friend may be someone with whom you share confidences, interests, hobbies, or other friends. Good friends share similar values. They can positively influence your self-concept and behavior and help you resist negative influences. Maintaining a good friendship can sometimes be hard work, but it is well worth the effort.

Community Relationships

Citizenship is *the way you conduct yourself as a member of the community.* Members of a community work together to promote the safety and well-being of the entire community. Citizens may volunteer at hospitals or work to provide food, clothing, or shelter to the homeless. You can demonstrate good citizenship by obeying laws and rules, by being a friendly and helpful neighbor, and by contributing to efforts to improve your school and community.

◀ The roles you play in relationships with family, with friends, and in the community are part of your everyday life. *Name several different relationships and roles that you experience each day.*

h⊙tlink

family relationships For more information on family relationships, see Chapter 11, page 272.

Did You Know ?

Your friends can influence your self-concept greatly. When choosing a friend, ask yourself these questions:
- Does this person have the qualities I admire most?
- Is this someone I can trust with my thoughts and confidences?
- How does this person affect my health triangle?
- What interests and values do we have in common?
- What can I offer in this friendship? What can the other person offer?

Roles with Family and Friends

What roles do you play as you interact with others? A **role** is *a part you play in a relationship.* You may be a daughter or son; a sister or brother; a granddaughter or grandson; a member of the school band or volleyball team; a volunteer at a homeless shelter; an employee; a member of a church, synagogue, or mosque; a best friend; and a girlfriend or boyfriend. You probably play many of these roles—all at the same time!

The role you play in a relationship may be obvious. For example, you know that when you baby-sit a neighbor's child, you are an employee. Sometimes your roles are less clear, and they may change gradually or even suddenly. For example, your relationship with a fellow choir member may change if you begin dating. Such role changes can be confusing and can make it difficult to know how to act.

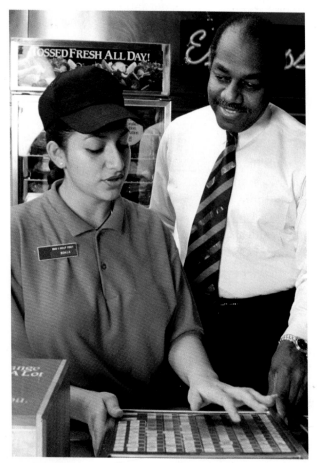

▼ **This teen has a working relationship with her employer.** *What other relationship roles might be part of this teen's life?*

Building Healthy Relationships

For a relationship to succeed, the people involved need certain skills. Three of these skills are communication, cooperation, and compromise—the Three Cs of healthy relationships.

Communication

Communication refers to *your ways of sending and receiving messages.* These messages may be exchanged in words or through gestures, facial expressions, and behaviors. You communicate to let others know your feelings, thoughts, and expectations. Communication also lets you discover the feelings, needs, wants, and knowledge of others. You will learn more about skills for effective communication in the next lesson.

Cooperation

Have you ever helped someone move a heavy object, such as a large piece of furniture? Such activities are almost impossible without **cooperation**, *working together for the good of all.* Working together through cooperation helps build strong relationships. For example, Susan helps prepare dinner each evening because her parents don't get home from work until 6 p.m. Because of her help, Susan's family is able to eat together and enjoy one another's company. Her contribution benefits the entire family.

Compromise

Three friends can't agree on how they'll spend the afternoon: Thomas and Elise want to go biking, but Serena wants to play miniature golf. Have you ever been in a similar situation? If so, you probably used compromise to solve the problem. **Compromise** is *a problem-solving method that involves each participant's giving up something to reach a solution that satisfies everyone*. It can be used to create a win-win situation for everyone involved.

The "give and take" of effective compromise strengthens relationships. By your willingness to give up something in order to reach a solution, you show the other person that you value the relationship. Remember, however, that compromise involves seeking a solution that is acceptable to *all* persons involved. Therefore, it should not lead to a decision that goes against your values or beliefs. In such situations, it's important that you use refusal skills to stand your ground. Learning when—and when *not*—to compromise is a vital relationship skill.

Characteristics of Healthy Relationships

By practicing the Three Cs, you make positive contributions to healthy relationships. In addition, all good relationships—whether with family members, friends, or other members of your community—have certain recognizable characteristics. Some of these characteristics are described below.

▶ **Mutual Respect and Consideration.** In healthy relationships, people show mutual respect even when they disagree. This involves accepting one another's tastes and opinions and being tolerant of different viewpoints. Furthermore, each person shows consideration by being thoughtful about the rights and feelings of others.

▶ **Honesty.** Because of their mutual respect and consideration, participants in a healthy relationship have the confidence to be open and honest about their actions, thoughts, and feelings. Dishonesty can seriously weaken or even destroy a relationship.

▶ **Dependability.** Participants in a healthy relationship are dependable. They are trustworthy and reliable. Each is there for the others when they are needed.

▶ **Commitment.** Healthy relationships require commitment. The participants are willing to work together and make sacrifices that benefit everyone involved. They are loyal to each other, and they are committed to strengthening the relationship.

Isn't compromise really a matter of one person giving in or losing?

If two people can't agree on a compromise between two choices, they should look for a third choice that both can agree on. If there really are only two choices, the compromise might be for one person to "win" this time with the understanding that the next time it will be the other person's turn to "win." If only one person is always giving up something, there is no compromise.

hot link

character For more information about character, see Chapter 2, page 37.

Character and Healthy Relationships

Your **character**—the way you think, feel, and act—has the greatest influence on your relationships with others. Think about the people with whom you enjoy spending time. These people probably have values similar to yours. Your values are the beliefs and ideals that guide the way you live.

You can build a foundation for healthy relationships by demonstrating the six main traits of good character. These traits are described in **Figure 10.1.** Think about ways you can demonstrate each character trait.

FIGURE 10.1

DEMONSTRATING CHARACTER IN RELATIONSHIPS

Trustworthiness	Fairness
You show trustworthiness when you are honest, reliable, and loyal. Trustworthy people don't cheat, steal, or deceive; they have the courage to do what's right. • *Example:* Hector finds a wallet containing $300. He uses the name on the driver's license and the phone book to call the owner so that he can return the wallet.	You show fairness when you play by the rules, take turns, and share. You also don't blame or take advantage of others. A fair person listens to others and is open-minded. • *Example:* Maria shows fairness by telling the referee that the volleyball was on the line and the opposing team won the point.
Respect	**Caring**
You show respect by using good manners, being considerate of others, and being tolerant of differences. You are also respectful when you deal with anger and disagreements in a peaceful way and treat other people and property with care. • *Example:* Sid knows that his dad brought a lot of work home from the office. Sid turns down the volume of his music so he won't disturb his father.	You show that you are caring when you are kind and compassionate. Caring means putting in time and energy to help others. • *Example:* Juanita is entering a store. She holds the door open for a man whose arms are filled with packages.
Responsibility	**Citizenship**
You show that you are responsible when you do what is expected of you and are accountable for your choices. Being responsible also means that you use self-control, think before you act, and always try your best. • *Example:* Sarah's drama rehearsal runs late. She calls her parents to let them know she is going to be late.	You show good citizenship by cooperating and doing your share to improve your school and community. You obey laws and rules and respect authority. Staying informed about issues that affect you and your neighbors, voting when you are of age, and doing your part to protect the environment are other ways to demonstrate good citizenship. • *Example:* Brad sees that someone has left an empty juice bottle on a table in the school cafeteria. He picks up the bottle and puts it in a recycling bin.

Real-Life Application

The Importance of Good Character to Friendships

Discuss how the e-mail below demonstrates good character traits.

Dear Lola,

    I'm sorry I didn't invite you to go with me to the grand opening of the new music store. I didn't think you were interested, so I was surprised when I found out that you were angry about not being invited. I'm not making excuses—I should have thought of you before we left. I don't blame you for feeling hurt and angry.

    I care about our friendship and I hope you'll forgive me. I'll try to be more considerate next time.

Your friend (I hope),

Mieko

Trustworthiness: apologizing, being honest, not making excuses.

Fairness: not blaming Lola.

Caring: saying that she is grateful for the friendship.

Responsibility: realizing that she should have thought before she acted.

ACTIVITY

Write a reply to the e-mail above. Show at least four traits of good character. Next, write a paragraph explaining how the character traits demonstrated in your message can strengthen the friendship.

Lesson 1 Review

Reviewing Facts and Vocabulary

1. Define *relationship*, and evaluate the positive effects of family relationships on your emotional health.
2. What are the Three Cs of healthy relationships?
3. List the six traits of good character.

Thinking Critically

4. **Evaluating.** Identify specific examples of how the roles you play with family and friends differ from those you play in other social groups.
5. **Applying.** Give an example of how you demonstrate consideration, respect, commitment, honesty, and dependability in your relationships with family members.

Applying Health Skills

Advocacy. Design a flip book for children about the six traits of good character. The book should demonstrate the importance of good character and persuade children to develop these traits.

TECHNOLOGY *OPTION*

WORD PROCESSING Make use of clip art, graphics, and fonts in your word-processing software. See **health.glencoe.com** for tips on using your word-processing program.

Communicating Effectively

VOCABULARY

"I" message
active listening
body language
prejudice
tolerance
constructive criticism

YOU'LL LEARN TO

• Classify forms of communication as passive, aggressive, or assertive.

• Demonstrate communication skills needed to build and maintain healthy relationships with family, friends, peers, and others.

• Apply communication skills that demonstrate consideration and respect for oneself, one's family, and others.

QUICK START On a sheet of paper, make a list of eight different ways in which people communicate with one another. Place a check mark beside each communication method you have used in the past two days.

H ow often have you given or received a shrug, a raised eyebrow, or a grin in reply to a comment or question? Although you may not have thought about it at the time, these responses are all forms of communication. Most of the time, you probably talk to let others know about your feelings, wants, and needs. Sometimes you may convey your feelings by writing notes or letters. People also show their feelings through gestures, facial expressions, and behaviors. There are many ways to exchange ideas with others. All of the ways in which you send and receive messages are forms of communication.

Effective Communication

C ommunication is critical to healthy relationships. When you communicate effectively, the messages you send to others are clear. Being an effective communicator also means that you correctly interpret the messages you receive and respond appropriately.

Three basic skills are needed for effective communication: speaking, listening, and body language. Learning to use these skills well takes practice, but the effort is worthwhile because effective communication helps you form and maintain healthy relationships with others. It is a skill from which you will benefit for your entire life.

Writing a note or letter can be an effective way to communicate your feelings.
In what other ways do you communicate with your family, friends, and peers?

Communication Styles

Do you have any friends who always just "go along" with what others decide to do, never saying what they would prefer? Perhaps you know someone who is "pushy," always insisting on getting his or her own way. These examples reflect two of the three styles of communication.

▶ **Passive.** Passive communication involves the inability or unwillingness to express thoughts and feelings. Passive communicators do not stand up for themselves or defend their attitudes or beliefs. They will often do something they'd prefer not to do rather than say how they really feel.

▶ **Aggressive.** Aggressive communicators often try to get their way through bullying and intimidation. They do not consider the rights of others. In disagreements, they attack the other person, not the problem.

▶ **Assertive.** Assertive communication involves expressing thoughts and feelings clearly and directly but without hurting others. Assertive communicators stand up for themselves. They defend their attitudes and beliefs, but they also respect the rights of others. In disagreements, they attack the problem, not the other person.

Assertive communication, which involves effective speaking and listening skills as well as appropriate body language, is an important asset in all healthy relationships.

Speaking Skills

Having good communication skills means that you do not assume that others can read your mind or know your needs and expectations. When you interact with others, you are responsible for making your thoughts and feelings known. For example, you need to say when your feelings have been hurt or when you've been disappointed. You demonstrate good speaking skills when you clearly say what you mean. This is the first step in healthy communication.

Changes in the tone, pitch, or loudness of your voice can affect communication. Kind words spoken in a sarcastic tone, for example, may not be interpreted as kind. Speaking loudly may make you seem bossy or arrogant. Saying "no" too softly can make you sound insincere or uncertain. These examples show that *how* you say something is as important as *what* you say.

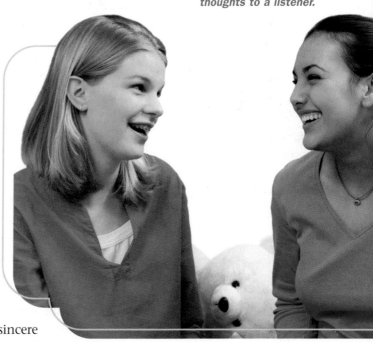

Good communication skills can strengthen a friendship. *List some strategies for effectively communicating your thoughts to a listener.*

FIGURE 10.2

STATING YOUR FEELINGS EFFECTIVELY

Compare the messages and the probable results of these scenes.

 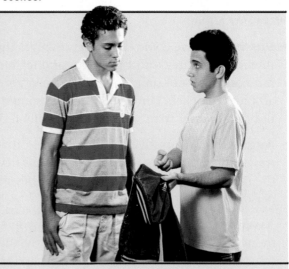

Aggressive Messages	Assertive "I" Messages
(What *not* to say)	**(What to say)**
"You idiot! You took my favorite jacket and got paint all over it! You ruined it, and you'll have to pay for it."	"I'm upset that my favorite jacket was borrowed without my knowledge."
"Why are you always late? It's really annoying."	"I worry about you when you don't show up."
"Why do you always have to get what you want? You never do what I suggest."	"I'll agree to have Mexican food today if I can pick the restaurant the next time we go out."

Did You Know ?

About 45 percent of the average person's communication time is spent listening, and 30 percent is spent speaking.

Reading, on average, occupies about 16 percent of a person's communication time, and writing accounts for only 9 percent of this time.

When you want to deliver messages that have strong emotional content, consider using "I" messages. An **"I" message** is *a statement in which a person describes how he or she feels by using the pronoun "I."* As shown in **Figure 10.2,** using "I" messages can help you communicate your feelings positively, without blame or name-calling. Blaming and name-calling always put people on the defensive because they feel that they are being attacked.

Listening Skills

Speaking is an important communication skill, but listening is equally important. You can make use of **active listening**, *paying close attention to what someone is saying and communicating,* to improve your communication skills. Active listening involves giving your full attention to whatever the speaker is saying without interrupting or making judgments. **Figure 10.3** illustrates some ways of becoming a more active listener.

TECHNIQUES FOR ACTIVE LISTENING

Being a good listener is important to healthy relationships. When you listen to others, you show them that you care about what they have to say and how they feel. Active listeners use several techniques to show others that they are listening. These techniques include:

▶ **Reflective listening.** In reflective listening, you rephrase or summarize what the other person has said. This allows you to be sure you have understood what was intended.

▶ **Clarifying.** Clarifying involves asking the speaker what he or she thinks or how he or she feels about the situation being discussed. It also involves asking questions to help you understand more fully what is being said.

▶ **Encouraging.** You encourage the speaker when you signal that you are interested and involved. You can show your interest by nodding your head or saying "I see," "Uh-huh," or "I understand."

▶ **Empathizing.** When you have **empathy,** you are able to imagine and understand how someone else feels. Empathizing is feeling what the other person feels as you listen. For example, if a friend tells you how disappointed he was when he didn't make the baseball team, you are likely to share his disappointment. Keep in mind that sometimes empathy is not appropriate, such as when what the person is saying goes against your values.

hot link

empathy For more information on empathy, see Chapter 7, page 186.

FIGURE 10.3

TIPS FOR ACTIVE LISTENING

Practicing active listening skills can improve your relationships.

- Make direct eye contact.
- Use body language, such as leaning in toward the speaker, which shows you are listening and giving your full attention.
- Use signals, such as nodding, to show that you are involved and interested.
- Don't interrupt the speaker.
- Put away prejudices, images, or assumptions that you have of the other person so that you can focus on what he or she is saying.

Hands-On Health ACTIVITY

Demonstrating Empathy

One way to be a good friend is to express empathy. Here are some tips:

- Maintain eye contact as you listen.
- Rephrase or summarize what the person has said.
- Avoid judging or offering advice.
- If a loss has been experienced, avoid trying to minimize the sense of loss by stating that it is not that bad.

In this activity you will role-play situations in which friends express empathy for each other.

What You'll Need

- index cards
- pen or pencil

What You'll Do

1. In groups of six, brainstorm three situations that could cause teens to feel sad. Write each one on a separate index card.
2. Your teacher will assign one situation to you and a partner in your group.
3. Practice and then role-play the situation for the class, demonstrating several different ways a friend can show empathy.

Apply and Conclude

Demonstrating empathy during happy moments is just as important as being empathetic during sad times. Make a list of situations in which you might share in a friend's joy or excitement. Explain how showing empathy during these situations can strengthen your friendship.

Nonverbal Communication

Many of the messages you send to others do not involve words. Such messages involve **body language**, *nonverbal communication through gestures, facial expressions, behaviors, and posture.* You use body language when you nod or shake your head to show that you agree or disagree with something that is said. When you hold yourself in a tense posture, you silently communicate that you're feeling nervous or worried.

Nonverbal communication can be subtle, taking place at an unconscious level. For example, if you feel embarrassed or ashamed, you may look at the ground instead of at the person to whom you are speaking. If you are greatly interested in what someone is saying, you may find yourself leaning toward the speaker.

You can help send clearer messages by being aware of your body language. If your words and your body language seem to contradict each other, the person you are speaking to may be confused or unsure of what to believe.

Eliminating Communication Barriers

Have you ever heard the saying, "A chain is only as strong as its weakest link"? The same is true of communication. If one person in a relationship has good communication skills but the other person does not, the entire communication process suffers. Sometimes a person's beliefs or attitudes can make communication difficult. Examples of obstacles to clear communication include:

▶ **Image and identity issues.** Many teens spend at least part of their teen years searching for an **identity**—a sense of who they are and their place in the world. If someone is unsure of his or her values, the uncertainty can complicate the communication process.

ho**t l**i**nk**

identity For more information about the search for identity during the teen years, see Chapter 7, page 178.

Health Skills Activity

Communication: Expressing Disapproval of Bullying

Walking in the school hallway, Marya and Ramone witness Matt intentionally bump into a boy walking the other way. The boy drops his books and papers.

"Hey!" Matt says rudely, "Watch where you're going!"

"Sorry," the boy apologizes, scrambling to pick up his things.

Matt places his foot on one of the boy's papers. "Looking for this?"

Ramone starts to laugh, but Marya frowns. "Matt is just having a little fun," Ramone says.

Marya shakes her head. She wonders how to let Matt know that she disapproves of his bullying.

What Would You Do?

Marya uses body language to communicate to Ramone that she disapproves of Matt's bullying behavior. Now it is important to verbally communicate this message to Matt. Use the following communication skills to role-play a dialog between Marya and Matt that clearly communicates that his behavior is not acceptable.

1. Present a clear, organized statement.
2. Use "I" statements.
3. Show appropriate body language.
4. Listen carefully.
5. Be firm and direct, but avoid being rude or insulting.

Fairness. Fairness is an important quality in any relationship. Whether you are facing an opponent in a student council election or competing with a friend on the tennis court, fairness is a principle that respects the abilities, needs, and contributions of all parties. **Describe three ways that you demonstrate fairness in your relationships.**

Accept constructive feedback positively. This is one way you can learn from others and improve yourself. *Give an example of how a critical statement can be turned into constructive feedback.*

▶ **Unrealistic expectations.** Avoid imposing unrealistic expectations on your listener; this may cause the individual to become frustrated or defensive.

▶ **Lack of trust.** Good communication is built on trust between two people. If you don't trust a person—if you believe that you can't count on him or her to tell you the truth or to keep a confidence—communication is very difficult.

▶ **Prejudice.** Some individuals have a **prejudice** or *an unfair opinion or judgment of a particular group of people.* Prejudice prevents a person from having an open mind and listening to new information. To avoid developing prejudices, you can demonstrate **tolerance**, or *the ability to accept others' differences and allow them to be who they are without your expressing disapproval.* Being tolerant helps you understand the differences among people and recognize the value of diversity.

▶ **Gender stereotyping.** Gender stereotyping is a type of prejudice that involves having an exaggerated or oversimplified belief about people of a certain gender. Assuming that all males like sports and that all females enjoy cooking are examples of gender stereotyping. Such assumptions make it difficult to communicate effectively.

Constructive Feedback

No one, not even your best friend or your teacher, is perfect. It's only realistic to be disappointed in a relationship occasionally. Imagine that you are meeting a friend to see a movie. Your friend is late, causing you to miss the beginning of the show. How would you react in this situation? Some people might resort to name-calling or placing blame. However, when someone lets you down, you may find that giving the person feedback in a more positive manner helps him or her *and* your relationship. The feedback you provide should take the form of **constructive criticism**, *non-hostile comments that point out problems for the purpose of helping a person improve.*

Constructive criticism is intended to bring about positive changes. Consequently, it should not be given in an aggressive way. Verbally attacking the other person will only make things worse. It is very important to begin your discussion by using an "I" message to explain how you feel. Point out what the person is doing or has done, and suggest a better way to do it. For example, you might deal with your friend's lateness by saying in a neutral voice, "I really don't like missing the opening scene of a movie. Let's get here early next time, okay?"

Acknowledgements and Compliments

 Acknowledging accomplishments is a way to show others that you care about them. *What are some other benefits of giving acknowledgements and compliments?*

How do you feel when someone thanks you for being a good friend or tells you how much he or she admires your honesty? Hearing such acknowledgements and compliments probably makes you feel good about yourself and your relationship with the person who made the comments. Expressing and receiving respect, admiration, and appreciation with grace and sincerity can help you maintain healthy relationships.

Acknowledgements and compliments take many forms. For example, you might tell a parent how much you enjoyed a meal that he or she prepared. You might also tell a friend that she is a good artist or congratulate the team that defeated yours in a play-off game. Gestures such as these can strengthen relationships and enhance your social health. It shows that you do not take the relationship for granted, and it demonstrates good sportsmanship and good character.

Lesson 2 Review

Reviewing Facts and Vocabulary

1. What are the three basic skills needed for effective communication?
2. List four ways to show that you are actively listening to another person.
3. Define the term *body language*, and give three examples of it.

Thinking Critically

4. **Contrasting.** Compare the different ways in which passive and aggressive communication interfere with the effective expression of thoughts and feelings.
5. **Applying.** List three ways to demonstrate consideration and respect for self, family, and others through communication skills.

Applying Health Skills

Refusal Skills. In a group, develop a skit that includes both dialogue and body language to show how teens can demonstrate refusal strategies in resisting pressure to take part in an unhealthful activity.

WEB SITES Use your skit to make a PSA (public service announcement) or video that is part of a Web page you develop on refusal skills. See **health.glencoe.com** for help in planning and building your own Web site.

Resolving Conflict

VOCABULARY

conflict
interpersonal
 conflicts
conflict resolution
negotiation
mediation
confidentiality
peer mediators

YOU'LL LEARN TO

- Analyze the causes of conflict.

- Analyze the relationship between the use of refusal skills and the avoidance of unsafe situations.

- Demonstrate healthful strategies for resolving conflicts, and evaluate the effectiveness of conflict resolution techniques in various situations.

QUICK START Write three things you could say or do in a tense situation that would encourage better understanding and avoid conflict.

Two drivers argue over a parking space; fans of opposing soccer teams brawl in the stadium parking lot; a shoving match occurs as students wait in line in the cafeteria. All of these events have something in common—they involve conflict. **Conflict** is *any disagreement, struggle, or fight*. Conflicts are a normal part of life. They often occur when one person's wants, needs, wishes, demands, expectations, or beliefs clash with those of another person.

▼ Unresolved conflicts can interfere with healthy relationships. *What communication skills can help teens deal with everyday conflicts?*

Understanding Conflict

The types of conflicts that impact relationships are **interpersonal conflicts**. These are *disagreements between groups of any size, from two people to entire nations.* Interpersonal conflicts can begin over minor problems, such as when siblings argue over what to watch on television. They can also affect large groups of people, such as a dispute over how to spend community funds.

As you learn more about conflict, keep in mind that disagreements are normal in healthy relationships and that not all conflicts are harmful. A beneficial result of some conflicts is that they require people to come together to work out problems. Learning to recognize how conflict builds and knowing how to deal with conflict effectively can have a direct impact on your total health and well-being.

What Causes Conflicts?

Conflicts can begin in many ways and for many reasons. Some conflicts begin innocently, such as when one person accidentally bumps another's lunch tray. Other conflicts are the result of deliberate acts or remarks that provoke another person—for example, purposely tripping someone or making a derogatory comment. In personal relationships, conflicts can occur when one person wants to control the actions, opinions, or decisions of another person. Such conflicts may be *chronic*, or ongoing. **Figure 10.4** identifies other common causes of conflicts.

Understanding the causes of conflict in relationships may help you keep conflict from developing. If you see that a conflict is building, it is often wise to walk away. Doing so may prevent the conflict from escalating, or growing, into a situation that is unhealthful or unsafe for everyone involved.

How are internal conflicts different from interpersonal conflicts?
Internal conflicts take place within an individual. For example, if a friend's birthday party and a sibling's championship soccer game occurred on the same day, you might feel conflicted about which event to attend. Using an effective decision-making model and seeking advice from parents or other trusted adults will often help you resolve these struggles in a positive, healthful way.

FIGURE **10.4**

COMMON CAUSES OF CONFLICT

Situations such as these often lead to conflict.

Power struggles
Now that he is a teen, Terrence thinks that he, rather than his parents, should decide what time he will come home at night.

Loyalty
Manuel and Fred have always been best friends. When Fred takes Julio's side in an argument with Manuel, Manuel feels betrayed.

Jealousy/Envy
Keiko feels a little envious when she does not make the softball team but her best friend Meagan does.

Property disputes
Jan gets angry when Lisa borrows her clothes without asking permission.

Territory and space
Troy gets annoyed when his brother Sam uses Troy's room to watch television and play video games.

Conflict often occurs over power, property, loyalty, territory, or issues of envy or jealousy. *What are some sources of conflict that you have observed?*

To communicate effectively:

▶ Talk about what is *really*
 troubling you.

▶ Practice being assertive. Learn
 to speak up for yourself and
 tell others how you feel.

▶ When you feel hurt or
 offended, use "I" messages
 to state your feelings clearly.

▶ Avoid keeping your feelings
 bottled up. Not stating your
 feelings can worsen the
 conflict.

Responding to Conflict

When a conflict arises, you have a choice: face the conflict or ignore it. As you decide which action to take, remember the following:

▶ Your primary concern should be your health and safety.

▶ Walking away from a potentially dangerous situation is a mature, healthful choice. It does not make you a coward. It is the smart and safe thing to do.

Minor conflicts can often be resolved by a simple compromise. If you and a sibling want to watch different television programs at the same time, for example, you might compromise by watching one program while taping the other. A compromise may be difficult to reach if the differences of opinion are strong or concern serious matters. Sometimes it can be inappropriate to compromise, such as when the compromise would go against your values or lead to harmful consequences. You must evaluate each conflict to decide whether a safe, agreeable solution can be reached or whether you should simply walk away. It is often helpful to seek the advice of a parent, guardian, teacher, or other trusted adult.

Conflict Resolution

You can learn and practice conflict resolution skills to prepare yourself for unexpected situations. **Conflict resolution** is *the process of solving a disagreement in a manner that satisfies everyone involved.* **Figure 10.5** shows some strategies for resolving conflicts peacefully.

FIGURE **10.5**

STRATEGIES FOR RESOLVING CONFLICTS

1. Take time to calm down and think over the situation.
2. When discussing the conflict, take turns explaining each person's side of the conflict without interruption. Use "I" messages.
3. Ask for clarification so that each person understands the other's position.
4. Brainstorm solutions.
5. Agree on a solution that benefits both sides.
6. Follow up to see whether the correct solution was chosen and whether that solution worked for each person.

Respect for Oneself and Others

To resolve a conflict fairly and effectively, you must show respect for yourself and others. Having respect for yourself means that you recognize that you have a right to your own opinions and values. When you respect yourself, you can stand up for your beliefs. When you respect others, you can listen to them with an open mind, consider their thoughts and feelings, and honor their values.

The views and ideals of others may be different from your own. Even though you may not agree, you can demonstrate respect and tolerance. When you are tolerant of different viewpoints or ideas, fewer conflicts arise. Therefore, tolerance is crucial to preventing conflict and promoting peace.

What Causes Conflicts to Escalate?

Conflicts can occur at any time or place. The important thing is to keep them from escalating. What are some elements that can worsen a conflict? Here are two points of view.

Viewpoint 1: Marsela W., age 15

I think most conflicts escalate because of poor communication. A lot of times, people get angry and say things without considering the consequences. When there's a conflict, people also tend to forget to practice good listening skills. They ignore signs that the conflict is getting worse because they're so busy saying their piece. If people remember to use effective communication skills, they can prevent most minor conflicts from escalating.

Viewpoint 2: Annalise D., age 16

I agree that good communication skills are important, but I think the biggest reason that conflicts escalate is because of people's attitudes and emotions. If people don't know how to deal with their feelings, it's not enough to have effective communication skills. Learning to manage emotions like anger is as important as having good speaking and listening skills. In some cases, it's even more important because emotions can prevent people from thinking before they act.

ACTIVITY

Do you think Marsela's and Annalise's viewpoints are valid? What other elements may cause conflicts to escalate? What strategies can people use to prevent conflicts from escalating?

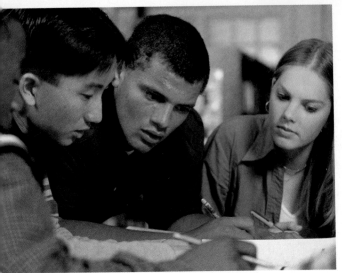

Negotiating During Conflict Resolution

Even if people demonstrate respect and tolerance, they may find it difficult to resolve their conflict. It is then necessary to try **negotiation**, *the use of communication and often compromise to settle a disagreement*. The negotiation process involves talking, listening, considering the other person's point of view, compromising if necessary, and devising a plan for working jointly to resolve the conflict.

PREPARING FOR NEGOTIATION

To prepare yourself for a successful negotiation process, keep the following points in mind:

▶ Make sure the issue is important to you.

▶ Check your facts. Make sure the disagreement is not based on incorrect information.

▶ Remind yourself that your goal is to find a solution, not to fight or prove who is "in control."

▶ Rehearse what you will say, even if you have to script it out in advance.

Ⓐ Successful negotiation requires the two parties involved to work together to find a satisfactory solution. *How did you use negotiation to resolve a recent conflict?*

STEPS TO TAKE WHEN NEGOTIATING

You can become a better negotiator through practice. Follow these steps to negotiate effectively.

▶ **Select a time and place suited to working out problems.** Arrange to meet when you are calm, not impatient or rushed. Choose a quiet meeting place.

▶ **Work together toward a solution.** Do not approach the other person as an enemy. Instead, work together to reach a solution.

▶ **Keep an open mind.** Remember that there are two sides to every story. Listen carefully to what the other person has to say.

▶ **Be flexible.** Be willing to meet the other person halfway.

▶ **Take responsibility for your role in the conflict.** Apologize if you know that you have hurt the other person.

▶ **Give the other person an "out."** If the other person seems embarrassed or uncomfortable, suggest continuing the conversation at a later time.

The Mediation Process

Even with negotiation, it's not always possible for two parties in conflict to reach an agreement. When this happens, it may be time for **mediation**, *a process in which specially trained people help others resolve their conflicts peacefully.*

Mediation sessions take place in a neutral location. During the mediation process, the mediator maintains strict **confidentiality**. This involves *respecting the privacy of both parties and keeping details secret.* The process has well-defined ground rules that are set by the mediator and explained to both sides. The mediator begins by asking each person to describe the disagreement. The mediator then summarizes each side, asking for clarification of any points that are inaccurate. Each side is then given the opportunity to talk to the other under the supervision of the mediator. The mediator may then ask the parties to sign an agreement to work out the problem within a certain time frame.

Today, many schools offer peer mediation programs for settling conflicts that take place at school. These programs have **peer mediators**, *students trained to help other students find fair resolutions to conflicts and disagreements.* You will learn more about peer mediation programs in Chapter 13.

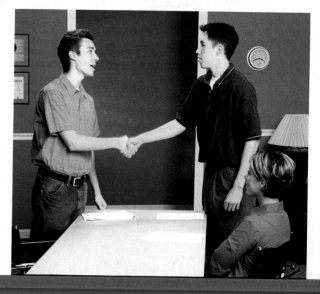

▼ Peer mediation is often effective in settling disputes and resolving conflicts. *What qualities would an effective peer mediator have?*

 Lesson 3 *Review*

Reviewing Facts and Vocabulary

1. What is an *interpersonal conflict*? What are some causes of interpersonal conflicts?

2. What are the benefits of walking away from a situation when a conflict is building?

3. What are some healthful ways of resolving conflicts?

Thinking Critically

4. **Synthesizing.** Conflicts are not always negative. Describe a situation in which a conflict can be positive. Explain why the conflict is positive.

5. **Analyzing.** Describe a conflict you have had with another person. Explain how you resolved the conflict, and evaluate the effectiveness of your conflict resolution techniques.

Applying Health Skills

Conflict Resolution. Luke wants to go to a basketball game with his friends this Saturday, but his parents want him to attend the family picnic. Write a skit in which Luke and his parents use conflict resolution techniques to solve their problem.

VIDEO PRODUCTION   Make a video of your skit. For help in planning and producing your video, see health.glencoe.com.

Internet Etiquette and Relationships

Technology such as e-mail has made it easy to keep in touch with family and friends who are far away. Like strong speaking and listening skills, strategies for effective online communication can strengthen relationships. In this activity, you will develop a list of Internet etiquette strategies that promote healthy, respectful communication.

Problems with Online Communication	Possible Solutions
Privacy issues	• Avoid sending e-mails dealing with private or sensitive issues. They can be forwarded to anyone.
Chain e-mails	• Do not send or forward such e-mails to others. • Politely ask friends and relatives not to send or forward them to you.
Viruses in attachments	• Make sure antivirus software is installed. • Do not open attachments from unknown or unreliable sources.

ACTIVITY

In a group, brainstorm potential problems with online communication and ways to resolve those problems. Use the chart above as a model, and try to come up with as many issues and solutions as possible. You might consider how traditional communication strategies (such as specific speaking and listening skills) can apply to online activities like e-mail and instant messaging. After completing your chart, use it to develop a list of Internet Etiquette Rules.

Make copies of your list, and share it with family and friends.

EXPRESS YOUR VIEWS

Write a one-page essay explaining the importance of online etiquette. Discuss how its use impacts relationships with family, friends, and peers. Your essay should promote communication strategies that maintain and strengthen healthy relationships.

CROSS-CURRICULUM CONNECTIONS

Write a Story. Conflict—that tug of war between your wishes and someone else's—arises even in the healthiest of relationships. Write a narrative about two friends who have a disagreement. Show how the characters use effective communication skills to resolve their conflict. As you write your story, consider the characters' words, tone, and body language.

Write an Essay. In the give and take of negotiating the terrain of any relationship, communication and compromise are key. Negotiation has a long history in the United States, especially the arbitration between labor unions and business management. Research and write an analytical essay on how negotiation became crucial as conflicts between workers and management grew in the early 1900s. In your essay, also consider what you can learn about negotiations that could be useful in your own relationships.

Calculate Chance. Joe wants to go to a concert, and Florence wants to go to a movie. They decide to settle the dispute amicably by flipping a coin, with the loser getting to choose the activity the next time. What are the odds that Joe will have to see a movie this time?

Research and Report. Physiologists have discovered that the primitive sections of our brains are hard-wired to protect us. The chemical activity produced by perceived threats has been called the "fight-or-flight" response. It raises blood pressure, heart rate, and respiration to increase oxygen supply and produces endorphins to fight pain. Investigate this natural response to danger, and discuss it in light of the modern need for peaceful conflict resolution.

Professional Mediator

Are you a good listener? Are you the person in your group of friends who most often helps the others reach a compromise? These skills may indicate that you are suited to a career as a professional mediator. Professional mediators often work for corporations, schools, or government agencies. They help others work together to settle disputes peacefully.

To become a professional mediator, you'll need to attend a four-year college and receive training in mediation. You can find out more about this and other health-related careers by clicking on Career Corner at **health.glencoe.com**.

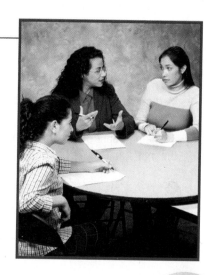

Chapter 10 *Review*

► EXPLORING HEALTH TERMS *Answer the following questions on a sheet of paper.*

Lesson 1 Match each definition with the correct term.

cooperation	citizenship
compromise	role
friendship	relationship
communication	

1. A significant relationship between two people based on caring, trust, and consideration.
2. A part you play in a relationship.
3. The ways in which you send and receive messages.
4. A process of working together for the good of all.

Lesson 2 Fill in the blanks with the correct term.

body language	constructive criticism
tolerance	"I" messages
active listening	prejudice

Tara is annoyed because Liz is late. To avoid placing blame, she uses (_5_) to let Liz know how she feels. Liz shows she is listening to Tara by using appropriate (_6_), such as nodding her head. Using (_7_) skills helps Liz understand why Tara is upset, and she apologizes for being late.

Lesson 3 Replace the underlined words with the correct term.

negotiation	peer mediators
conflict resolution	interpersonal conflict
mediation	confidentiality
conflict	

8. Any disagreement or struggle is a <u>negotiation</u>.
9. Mediation and negotiation are two processes used for <u>interpersonal conflict</u>.
10. Mediators must demonstrate <u>conflict</u>, respect for the rights and privacy of others.

► RECALLING THE FACTS *Use complete sentences to answer the following questions.*

Lesson 1

1. Name three roles you play in your relationships with others. Explain when you play each role.
2. How can compromise help strengthen a relationship?
3. What are some ways you can demonstrate the character trait of responsibility?

Lesson 2

4. How do you know when you are communicating effectively?
5. What is reflective listening?
6. How does prejudice set up a barrier to effective communication?

Lesson 3

7. List the strategies for conflict resolution.
8. What two things should you consider when deciding how to respond to conflict?
9. Define negotiation.
10. When might it be necessary to have a mediator help settle a conflict?

➤ THINKING CRITICALLY

1. **Evaluating.** Kate always decides what she and her friend Suki will do when they go out together. What trait or skill is missing in this relationship? How might the situation be changed? *(LESSON 1)*

2. **Synthesizing.** Explain how you would use reflective listening, clarifying, and encouraging techniques to demonstrate active listening skills if your friend tells you the following: "I'm sorry I missed the game last night. My mother fell and we had to take her to the hospital for stitches. It was really scary." *(LESSON 2)*

3. **Analyzing.** Making compromises is not always a good way of resolving a situation. Describe the types of situations in which you should not be willing to compromise or negotiate. *(LESSON 3)*

➤ HEALTH SKILLS APPLICATION

1. **Analyzing Influences.** Think about a relationship you have with a family member or a friend. Evaluate and describe the positive and negative effects of this relationship on each side of your health triangle. *(LESSON 1)*

2. **Communication Skills.** Imagine that you have a friend who frequently borrows things and returns them in poor condition. Explain how you could use constructive criticism to help the person change this pattern of behavior. *(LESSON 2)*

3. **Advocacy.** Write a persuasive letter to the principal of your school to advocate the use of peer mediators. In your letter, explain why peer mediation is important. Describe the steps involved in this process and the types of situations in which it might be used. *(LESSON 3)*

BEYOND
the Classroom

Parent Involvement

Advocacy. Learn more about community mediation programs. With your parents, find out how your family can become involved in raising awareness about the existence and usefulness of such programs in your community. If mediation programs do not already exist in your community, learn how you can help create one.

School and Community

Overcoming Prejudice. Speak with a law enforcement official in your community who has helped victims of hate crimes—offenses against an individual or group that are a direct or indirect result of prejudice. Ask the official what communication skills a person would need to help victims of hate crimes. Report to your class what you have learned.

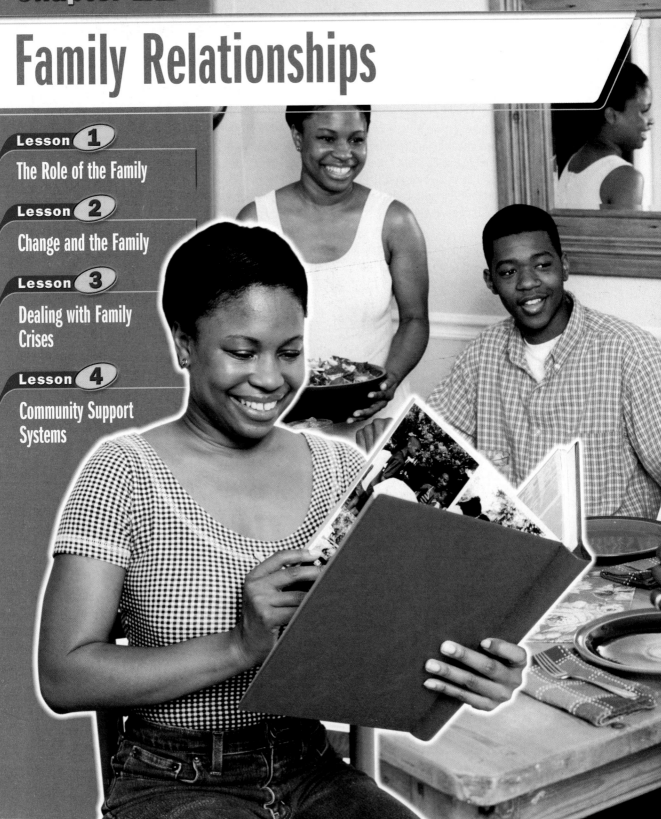

Chapter 11

Family Relationships

Changes in Family Circumstances

Changes in circumstances can also cause difficulties for families. Often, honest and open communication can help families deal with such changes in healthful ways.

Moving

When a family moves, its members may miss their old friends and the familiar surroundings of their old home. Teens may be anxious about making new friends and adjusting to a new school. If a move follows the breakup of a marriage, children may miss the parent who no longer lives with them.

When a family member becomes ill or disabled, the rest of the family assumes responsibility for his or her care. *What are some ways that teens can help in the care of a family member who is ill or disabled?*

Financial Problems

Meeting a family's financial needs is not easy. Loss of a job, medical emergencies, and overdue bills can cause anxiety about how to support family needs. Impulse buying or poor planning may also cause financial problems. *Credit card abuse,* the overuse of credit cards, can be a serious problem for those who pay the bills, and it often leads to arguments about spending habits.

Illness and Disability

A serious illness or disability can disrupt a family's normal activities. One or more family members may need to change their schedules to care for the sick or disabled person. In addition to worry and concern for the person who is ill, family members may also experience the stress of making major medical decisions about types of care or treatments. Some of this stress can be relieved if all members of the family share in the responsibility of caring for the person who is sick or disabled.

Drug and Alcohol Abuse

Substance abuse within the family threatens the health of the entire family. Without intervention and outside help, this problem can cause the family system to break down. If a family member has a substance abuse problem, seek immediate help from trusted adults, school personnel, or organizations such as Alateen. These resources can help you understand the problem and guide you in getting additional assistance.

CHARACTER CHECK

Caring. When you seek help for a problem that affects the health of the family, you are demonstrating caring. **Make a list of people you think you could approach for assistance if a family member has a substance abuse problem.**

Communication: That's What Friends Are For

"Are you okay?" Craig asked his friend Robert after school one day. "You seem down."

Robert hesitated before admitting, "My parents have decided to get a divorce. My dad's going to move across town soon. One of these days, I know that they're going to ask me who I want to live with. I feel close to both my mom and dad, and I don't want to have to choose sides. Everything is changing. I want to talk to my parents about my feelings and worries, but I'm afraid I'll add to their problems."

What Would You Do?

How would you respond if you were Craig? Finish the rest of this dialogue, incorporating effective communication skills to demonstrate how Craig shows support and empathy.

1. **Listen attentively.**
2. **Use "I" statements.**
3. **Speak in a respectful tone of voice.**
4. **Display appropriate body language.**

Coping with Family Changes

It is important to manage the stress caused by family changes. In some cases, this may be as simple as turning to a family member for help. Talking with family members can often reduce the stress and lead to a successful solution. If a parent is unavailable, find another adult who can help, such as a teacher, guidance counselor, member of the clergy, or a member of your extended family. Additional strategies for coping with family stress include the following.

▶ **Do what you can to help.** For example, if your parents are feeling stressed, you might be able to reduce their burden by taking on added chores and responsibilities. Knowing that you are helping out can make you feel better.

▶ **Read books about the subject or talk to people who have faced a similar problem.** You may find strategies for managing the problem.

▶ **Use stress-management techniques.** Engage in physical activity, get adequate sleep, eat nutritious meals, and find a way to relax, such as listening to soothing music.

hotlink

stress-management techniques To learn more about managing stress, see Chapter 8, page 209.

Effects of Abuse

Victims of domestic abuse experience feelings of shame, fear, humiliation, and guilt. They often feel powerless to change their circumstances. Long-term effects of domestic abuse may include:

▶ Inability to trust or establish healthy personal relationships

▶ Chronic physical pain

▶ Neglect of or injury to oneself, including suicide attempts

▶ Depression, anxiety, sleep disorders, and eating disorders

▶ Abuse of alcohol and other drugs

It is critical that victims of domestic violence get outside help to deal with this extremely dangerous situation. Getting to a safe place is the first priority.

Health Minute

Preventing Domestic Violence

To encourage an atmosphere of nonviolence at home:

▶ Don't provide violence-oriented toys to small children, such as toy guns or knives.

▶ Don't provide children with video games that focus on violence, such as attacks on property, people, or animals.

Breaking the Cycle of Violence

Involvement in domestic violence is often a learned behavior. A child who suffers or who witnesses abuse may view violence in the home as a normal way of life. As a result, the child may be more likely to become an adult who abuses others. In this way, domestic violence can cycle from one generation to the next. This *pattern of repeating violent or abusive behaviors from one generation to the next* is called the **cycle of violence**. The only way to break this cycle is to stop all forms of violence and abuse. **Figure 11.2** provides suggestions for breaking the cycle of violence.

FIGURE 11.2

BREAKING THE CYCLE OF VIOLENCE

You can help break the cycle of abuse. If you or someone you know is being abused . . .

• Tell a trusted adult (parent, other family member, teacher, school nurse or counselor, doctor). Ask this person to help you find a way to resolve the problem.

• Contact an abuse hot line or crisis center that can assist you in finding counselors or other forms of help.

• Report the abuse to the police. It may also be appropriate to contact child welfare or youth services.

Source: Office of Justice Programs, US Department of Justice

Avoiding Domestic Violence

There are several strategies that can help you avoid and prevent domestic abuse. You can recall these strategies by remembering the three Rs.

▶ **Recognize.** Become aware of acts that are abusive. Remember that abuse takes many forms, including physical abuse, verbal and emotional abuse, sexual abuse, and neglect.

▶ **Resist.** If anyone tries to harm you physically or abuse you in a sexual way, resist in any way you can. Be assertive and stand up for yourself. Run away from the abuser, and seek help from a trusted adult.

▶ **Report.** If someone treats you in an abusive manner, get away and tell someone about the incident as soon as you can. If you witness someone else being abused, report the abuse to the authorities or tell an adult who can help you.

 Seeking help is the first step to take when dealing with domestic violence issues. *What strategies might help individuals avoid violence within the family?*

Victims of domestic abuse need help. Their abusers also need help. Being a child victim or witness of abuse does not justify becoming an abusive adult. All forms of domestic abuse are unacceptable, and most of these acts are illegal. In the next lesson, you will learn more about sources of help for victims of abuse.

Lesson 3 *Review*

Reviewing Facts and Vocabulary

1. What are the effects of spousal abuse?
2. What is *neglect*? Explain how neglect affects each part of a child's health triangle.
3. What is the *cycle of violence*? What are some ways of breaking this cycle?

Thinking Critically

4. **Synthesizing.** One of the effects of abuse is the victim's feeling of worthlessness. How could you help a victim of abuse to feel better about himself or herself?
5. **Evaluating.** Some say that the long-term effects of abuse are worse than the short-term effects. Explain why this statement might be true for many victims.

Applying Health Skills

Advocacy. Write an article discussing the serious problem of domestic abuse. Describe the effects of abuse, and urge victims of any form of domestic violence to seek help immediately. Ask the school newspaper to print your article.

WORD PROCESSING Use a word-processing program to write your article. See **health.glencoe.com** for tips on how to get the most out of your word-processing program.

CROSS-CURRICULUM CONNECTIONS

Create a Family Tree Poem. The strong bonds of family form a foundation for a healthy, happy life. Sketch a family tree of your immediate family. Next to each family member, write a short poem describing how he or she contributes to strong, healthy family relationships. You might discuss how the person contributes to feelings of love and warmth or how he or she provides physical and emotional support for other family members. Include illustrations, sketches, or clip art to give your work an artistic look.

Analyze Family Dynamics. The impact of major historical events has shaped the American family. Through research, analyze how one of the following events or eras changed or had an effect on the American family: the Civil War, the Industrial Revolution, World War II, or the Civil Rights movement. Write an analysis in which you consider how the event or era had an impact on the family structure, how family members related to one another, and how family members took care of one another financially.

Calculate Demographics. U.S. Census figures for 1990 showed that married couples with children made up 26.3 percent of U.S. households. Figures for 2000 showed that married couples with children made up 24.1 percent of U.S. households. Assuming the same rate of decline, what percentage of U.S. households will be married couples with children in the year 2010? If the number of households in 2000 was 104,705,000, how many of those households consisted of married couples with children?

Research a Topic. There has been much debate over whether genetics or the environment has a stronger impact on an individual's development. The family unit is at the center of this "nature vs. nurture" debate. What roles do heredity and upbringing play in a child's development? Research theories on both sides of this debate, and present your findings in a report. Include your own thoughts and opinions on this topic.

Family Therapist

Depression, marital problems, and parent-child conflicts can strain family relationships. A family therapist can help families find ways to work out their problems and communicate more openly and honestly. To become a family therapist, you'll need a master's degree in couples and family therapy. Learn more about this and other health careers by clicking on Career Corner at **health.glencoe.com**.

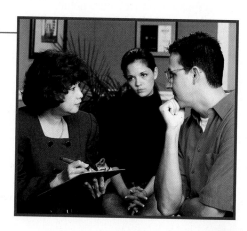

➤ EXPLORING HEALTH TERMS *Answer the following questions on a sheet of paper.*

Lesson 1 *Match each definition with the correct term.*

affirmation   family

extended family   sibling

1. A brother or sister.
2. Positive feedback that helps individuals feel appreciated and supported.
3. The basic unit of society.

Lesson 2 *Fill in the blanks with the correct term.*

custody   resiliency

divorce   separation

grief

Dan's parents fight a lot. They have considered ending their marriage through (_4_) but decided instead on a (_5_), a period in which they will live apart from each other, to see whether they can resolve their differences. During this time, Dan's mom and dad have joint (_6_), so they care for and make decisions about Dan together.

Lesson 3 *Replace the underlined words with the correct term.*

sexual abuse   emotional abuse

cycle of violence   physical abuse

domestic violence   child abuse

7. Neglect of a baby is a form of <u>spousal abuse</u>.
8. Three forms of <u>exploitation</u> are emotional, physical, and sexual abuse in the home.
9. Calling someone names or attacking his or her self-worth is <u>physical abuse</u>.

Lesson 4 *Match each definition with the correct term.*

crisis center   foster care

mediator   family counseling

10. A temporary arrangement in which a child is placed under the guidance or supervision of a family or adult not related by birth.
11. Therapy to restore healthy relationships in a family.
12. A facility that handles emergencies and provides referrals to persons who need help.

➤ RECALLING THE FACTS *Use complete sentences to answer the following questions.*

Lesson 1

1. List three ways that parents promote the physical health of their children.
2. Why is the family considered the basic unit of society?
3. List five traits of a healthy family.

Lesson 2

4. Identify three situations that may result in a change in the family structure.
5. What events may lead to a change in a family's financial situation?
6. List three ways to cope with stress within the family.

Lesson 3

7. What constitutes sexual abuse?
8. Why is a child who runs away from home to escape an abusive situation often at risk of exploitation?
9. What are the three Rs for preventing and avoiding domestic violence?

Lesson 4

10. Besides crisis centers and hot lines, list three resources to which families in crisis can turn for help.

11. What is the main difference between a support group and counseling?

12. What are three skills that mediators use to help families solve problems?

▶ THINKING CRITICALLY

1. **Analyzing.** Serena cooks dinner for her family when her parents work late. How does Serena benefit from her considerate behavior? How do the members of her family benefit? *(LESSON 1)*

2. **Synthesizing.** What stresses might a family experience when a child goes off to college? *(LESSON 2)*

3. **Applying.** Carlos frequently tries to speak with his mother about problems he is having at school, but she tells him that she doesn't have time to listen to his problems. This pattern of behavior might be a signal of what kind of family crisis? *(LESSON 3)*

4. **Synthesizing.** A teen has parents who abuse alcohol. What type of resource might best provide help to this teen? Explain your choice. *(LESSON 4)*

▶ HEALTH SKILLS APPLICATION

1. **Practicing Healthful Behaviors.** Make a list of specific actions that family members can take to strengthen their relationships with each other. Explain how these behaviors can improve family health. *(LESSON 1)*

2. **Communication Skills.** Write a skit in which one teen demonstrates active listening skills and empathy when a friend reveals that his or her parent is suffering from an illness or a disability. *(LESSON 2)*

3. **Advocacy.** Develop a poster or a PSA that can be used to make others aware of what they can do to break the cycle of abuse. *(LESSON 3)*

4. **Decision Making.** Carol thinks that her older sister has a drug problem. Use the steps of decision making to help Carol decide how to get help for her sister. *(LESSON 4)*

BEYOND the Classroom

Parent Involvement

Advocacy. With your parents, learn about shelters in your area that provide victims with a safe place to recover from abuse. Determine what needs the shelter has and what your family can do to help support the shelter's efforts. You might collect materials such as clothing, books, toys, and blankets for the shelter.

School and Community

Community Events. Identify events and programs in your community that are geared toward students and their families. Contact the organizations sponsoring the activities to find out how you, your classmates, and your family members can get involved.

Chapter 12

Peer Relationships

Derek's Story

Derek is 15. His father, who is in the military, is often transferred from one location to another. This means that Derek's family has to move every few years. The family has just moved from Alaska to Texas. For the third time, Derek is in a new school and surrounded by people he doesn't know.

"Everybody knows everyone else, except me. The people at school are polite to me, but it's difficult becoming good friends with them. They already have people to hang out with, and they don't need me. It's really tough for a new person."

Things seemed easier for Derek the last time he changed schools. "I was just a kid then. It's different now." For the first time in his life, Derek feels shy about approaching new people and making new friends.

"After spending about a month sitting by myself in the cafeteria, I decided I had to do something, so I joined the Community Service Club. I found out that a few people in the club play tennis. So do I."

Write a sentence or two describing what else Derek could do to make friends in his new school. In what ways could you help someone who is new to your school or community?

HEALTH Online

For instant feedback on your health status, go to Chapter 12 Health Inventory at **health.glencoe.com**.

Quick *Write*

Using Visuals. Write five sentences, each one beginning with the words: *A true friend is someone who* . . . Discuss your descriptions with your classmates.

Safe and Healthy Friendships

VOCABULARY

peers
friendship
platonic friendship
clique
stereotype

YOU'LL LEARN TO

- Evaluate the positive and negative effects of peers and friends on physical, mental/emotional, and social health.

- Evaluate the dynamics of peer groups.

- Demonstrate strategies for communicating needs, wants, and emotions.

- Develop management strategies to improve or maintain your health and that of peers.

⇒ QUICK START In what ways do friends contribute to your life? List as many examples as you can.

▲ You may know many classmates and peers, but only a few may be your good friends. *What qualities set a friend apart from other peers?*

During your teen years, you begin a search for a personal identity. This identity will be shaped, at least in part, by your **peers**—*people of similar age who share similar interests.* Your relationships with friends and peers not only contribute to your identity but can also affect your health and well-being.

Types of Peer Relationships

As you get older, the dynamics of your social groups change. For example, instead of attending a small local school, you may now go to a large school attended by students from many neighborhoods. Perhaps you have a part-time job or a volunteer position in which you and your peers have a work-based relationship. Such situations can benefit your social health by giving you opportunities to meet people of all ages, races, religions, and backgrounds. Interacting with diverse peers can enrich your life and contribute to personal growth. Some of the friendships you form in high school may last throughout your life.

Friendships

A **friendship** is *a significant relationship between two people.* Healthy friendships are based on caring, respect, trust, and consideration. Friends are people with whom you share hobbies, interests, and other friends. They may also become people with whom you are comfortable sharing your needs, wants, emotions, and confidences. Healthy friendships can give you a sense of belonging and help you define and reinforce your values.

Your friends probably include both males and females. A **platonic friendship** is *a friendship with a member of the opposite gender in which there is affection but the two people are not considered a couple.* Such relationships can help you understand and become comfortable with individuals of the opposite gender. In addition, such friends can be a valuable source of advice concerning dating issues. Platonic friendships help you realize that all people, regardless of gender, have similar feelings, needs, and concerns.

Friendships vary in importance and commitment. If you have a best friend, you already know that not all friendships are the same. In fact, there are several kinds of friendships.

These teens have a casual friendship based on a common interest. *What interests do you share with the peers you think of as casual friends?*

CASUAL FRIENDSHIPS

A casual friendship is a relationship between peers who share something in common. You may form a casual friendship with a classmate, a teammate, or someone who attends your place of worship. You may sit with casual friends in the cafeteria or at school events. Casual friends are usually people with whom you share some interests but are not necessarily people with whom you form deep emotional bonds.

CLOSE FRIENDSHIPS

Some casual friendships may develop into close friendships. Close friends have strong emotional ties and feel comfortable sharing their thoughts, experiences, and feelings. They trust and support each other, acting with kindness, courtesy, and loyalty. When problems arise in the relationship, close friends will try to work them out together.

True friendships have several common attributes:

▶ Similar values, interests, beliefs, and attitudes on basic issues

▶ Open and honest communication

▶ Sharing of joys, disappointments, dreams, and concerns

▶ Mutual respect, caring, and support

▶ Concern about each other's safety and well-being

Cliques

Does your school have cliques? A **clique** is *a small circle of friends, usually with similar backgrounds or tastes, who exclude people viewed as outsiders.* Clique members may share the same attitudes, wear similar clothing, meet regularly in an area identified as their "turf," or engage in other behaviors that identify them as a clique.

Conflict Resolution: When Best Friends Disagree

"Guess what?" Marissa asked excitedly when she saw her best friend, Julia. "Nicole and Dave asked us to join their group!"

"But I like the friends we have right now," Julia frowned. "Why do you want to be part of their group?"

"Because they're the most popular people in school!" Marissa answered. "It'll be great!"

"I've heard that they make fun of people who are different from them," Julia said.

"I'm sure that's just a rumor," Marissa insisted. "Come on, you never want to do anything fun."

Julia doesn't want to lose Marissa as a best friend, but she also doesn't feel comfortable joining Nicole and David's group. She wonders how to respond.

What Would You Do?
Write an ending to the scenario in which Julia and Marissa resolve their conflict in a healthful way. Use the following tips as a guideline.

1. Take turns explaining each side of the conflict without interruption.
2. Use "I" messages.
3. Listen carefully, and ask appropriate questions.
4. Brainstorm solutions.
5. Agree on a solution that benefits both sides.

Cliques can have both positive and negative influences on peers. Being part of a clique, for example, may provide members with a sense of belonging. However, cliques are a negative influence if members are discouraged from thinking for themselves or acting as individuals.

Clique membership is often limited—not everyone who wants to belong is welcome. Often, the beliefs and actions clique members use to exclude others are prejudicial and based on stereotypes. **Prejudice** is making assumptions or judgments about an individual without really knowing him or her. A **stereotype** is *an exaggerated and oversimplified belief about an entire group of people, such as an ethnic or religious group or a gender.*

hot link

prejudice For more information about prejudice, see Chapter 13, page 342.

Forming Healthy Friendships

Relationships with friends may become more complex as you begin sharing thoughts and feelings that are more serious in nature than those you experienced in childhood. Working to build and maintain healthy friendships is an important social skill to develop during the teen years.

Choosing Friends

Throughout your life you have many opportunities to choose friends. Positive people with healthy attitudes can support you emotionally, reinforce your values, and motivate you. For example, if your friends think education is important, you're likely to take education seriously and do well in school. Often, friends encourage each other to make healthy, responsible decisions. They might inspire each other to engage in more physical activity or participate in community service. They can also serve as mutual protective factors, helping each other avoid unsafe or unhealthy situations. For example, a friend may encourage you to walk away from a fight.

Some friends, however, may try to influence you to participate in risky activities or behaviors that go against your values and the values of your family. In such cases, it's probably best to end the relationship. Healthy relationships are based on mutual respect and caring. If a friendship isn't contributing to your life in a positive way, it's time to reevaluate that relationship.

Group outings with friends can provide you with a sense of belonging. *Evaluate other positive effects of friends on mental/emotional health.*

Mutual respect helps friends feel comfortable sharing their needs, wants, and emotions.

Building and Strengthening Friendships

Positive friendships are built on common values and interests. Having common values means friends won't pressure each other to engage in unhealthy risk behaviors. Having common interests gives friends something to talk about and do together. There are many ways to strengthen a healthy friendship.

▶ **Be loyal.** Friends can trust and depend on each other. They don't purposely do anything to hurt each other, and they always speak respectfully of each other.

▶ **Encourage each other.** A good friend is supportive and makes you feel good about yourself. Friends acknowledge each other's accomplishments and help each other through difficult times.

▶ **Respect each other.** Common courtesy helps keep friendships strong. Avoid taking friends for granted. Being on time and keeping your promises will let your friends know that you care about and respect them.

▶ Lesson 1 *Review*

Reviewing Facts and Vocabulary

1. What are *peers*?
2. Define *friendship*. Identify four character traits on which friendships are based.
3. List two ways to strengthen a friendship.

Thinking Critically

4. **Evaluating.** Interactions with friends and peers can have both positive and negative effects on all sides of your health triangle. Evaluate and provide examples of the positive and negative effects of peers and friends on physical, mental/emotional, and social health.

5. **Comparing and Contrasting.** Evaluate the dynamics of social groups consisting of casual friends, close friends, and platonic friends. What qualities do these groups share? How do they differ?

Applying Health Skills

Communication Skills. With a classmate, role-play two scenarios. In the first, demonstrate skills that close friends would use to communicate needs, wants, and emotions. In the second, show how peers might express disagreement about an issue while still showing respect for themselves and each other.

TECHNOLOGY *OPTION*

PRESENTATION SOFTWARE Use presentation software to develop a slide show that demonstrates strategies for communicating needs, wants, and emotions to peers. Find help in using presentation software at **health.glencoe.com**.

Peer Pressure and Refusal Skills

VOCABULARY

peer pressure
harassment
manipulation
assertive
refusal skills
passive
aggressive

YOU'LL LEARN TO

- Demonstrate refusal strategies and apply skills for making responsible decisions under pressure.

- Classify forms of communication as passive, aggressive, or assertive.

- Analyze the relationship between the use of refusal skills and the avoidance of unsafe situations.

⟶ **QUICK START** Make a two-column chart. In the left column, list examples of positive peer pressure. In the right column, list examples of negative peer pressure.

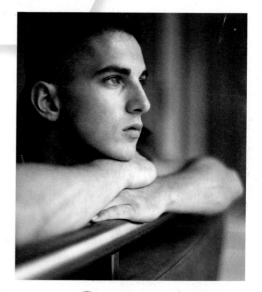

I magine that you are out with friends and someone suggests going to a party a few miles away. Most of your friends agree, but you aren't sure because you don't know the person who's throwing the party. Your friends spend the next few minutes trying to persuade you to join them. What will you do?

Peer Pressure

P erhaps you have been in a situation similar to the one above. Your peers can sometimes influence how you think, feel, and act. *The influence that people your age may have on you* is called **peer pressure**.

Peer pressure can have a positive or negative influence on your actions and behaviors. Because it can occur in many types of relationships, it is useful to learn to evaluate forms of peer pressure and develop healthful strategies for responding to it.

▲ Peer pressure may make some decisions more difficult. *What strategies can help you make healthful, responsible decisions when faced with peer pressure?*

Positive peer pressure can motivate you to try new activities that can benefit all sides of your health triangle. *What are some examples of positive peer pressure that you have experienced?*

Positive Peer Pressure

Peers can influence you in many positive ways. For example, they might encourage you to participate in a cleanup campaign to clear away trash from a roadside. Agreeing to work with your peers in this campaign benefits your social health because you have the opportunity to interact with others in positive ways. It also benefits the community by providing a cleaner environment. Volunteering to serve food at a homeless shelter or working at a Special Olympics event because a friend does so are other examples of positive peer pressure.

Positive peer pressure may also involve *not* participating in risky behaviors or activities. For instance, having friends who do not use tobacco, alcohol, or other drugs may positively influence you to avoid these harmful substances.

You can also use positive peer pressure to influence others in healthful ways. You can be a **role model** by inspiring peers to take part in a positive act or a worthwhile cause.

hot link

role model For more information about role models, see Chapter 2, page 40.

Negative Peer Pressure

Peers sometimes pressure others to take part in behaviors or accept beliefs that have negative consequences. The members of a clique, for example, may be disrespectful toward people they do not consider acceptable to their group. Such behavior may involve **harassment**, or *persistently annoying others*. Harassment may include name-calling, teasing, or bullying. Negative peer pressure may also lead some teens to engage in behaviors that go against their values. For instance, a peer might pressure a classmate to help him or her cheat on a test.

Manipulation is another way of exerting negative peer pressure on others. **Manipulation** is *an indirect, dishonest way to control or influence others*. Some examples of the ways people manipulate one another are listed in **Figure 12.1.** It's important to discourage this kind of hurtful behavior and encourage the victim to report the problem to a trusted adult.

FIGURE 12.1

COMMON METHODS OF MANIPULATION

- Mocking or teasing another person in mean or hurtful ways
- Using "guilt trips" to get desired results
- Bargaining—offering to make a deal to get what one wants
- Using flattery or praise to influence another person
- Bribing—promising money or favors if the person will do what is asked
- Making threats—promising violence or some other negative consequence if the person does not do what is asked
- Using blackmail—threatening to reveal some embarrassing or damaging information if the person does not do what is asked

Resisting Negative Peer Pressure

Peer pressure doesn't stop at the end of the teen years. Throughout your life, you may experience many instances in which peers, including friends and coworkers, make requests or demands of you. In some cases, your responses to these requests or demands will directly affect your health. For example, refusing to use tobacco, alcohol, or other drugs is a decision that will promote your overall health. At times there may be instances in which your response to peer pressure could seriously impact your life. For example, agreeing to get into a car with friends who have been drinking can place your life in danger.

One way to resist negative peer pressure is to avoid it. Develop friendships with people who share your values and interests. Friends who have respect for your health and well-being will be less likely to pressure you into doing something that goes against your values. You will find that it's much easier to resist negative peer pressure from someone else when you have friends who stand by you and support your decision.

Sometimes, however, the pressure to participate in unsafe or potentially harmful activities can be intense. When pressured by a friend, many teens worry about hurting the person's feelings or jeopardizing the relationship. Refusing to go along with a group may make some people concerned about appearing "uncool." Even though these situations may be difficult, it is important to remain firm and stay true to yourself. Remember, you have the responsibility to make decisions that have the best possible effect on your well-being. When making decisions that involve potentially risky consequences, your health and safety come first. Respect yourself, stand by your values, and be assertive in your refusal.

HEALTH Online

Review the vocabulary for this lesson. Play the Chapter 12 concentration game at **health.glencoe.com**.

Health Minute

Resisting Peer Pressure

To resist negative peer pressure:

- ► Stand your ground by stating your values and beliefs.
- ► Consider the consequences of unsafe behavior.
- ► Decide whether the source of pressure is from yourself or from others.
- ► Be assertive, and use refusal skills to say no to risky activities.
- ► Leave the scene if necessary.

Assertive Refusal

Being **assertive** means *standing up for your rights in a firm but positive way.* When you are assertive, you state your position and stand your ground while acknowledging the rights of the other individuals. This is the most effective approach when facing negative peer influences. Assertive teens are often role models for others because most people respect individuals who stay true to themselves.

REFUSAL SKILLS

An important aspect of being assertive is the ability to use appropriate refusal skills. **Refusal skills** are *techniques and strategies that help you say no effectively when faced with something that you don't want to do or that goes against your values.* Effective refusal skills involve a three-step process. Learning and practicing these steps will help prepare you for dealing with high-pressure situations.

► **Step 1: State Your Position.** The first step in resisting negative peer pressure is to say no. You need to state your position simply and firmly. Make sure your "no" sounds as though you really mean it. Combining your words with non-verbal messages, such as those shown in **Figure 12.2,** will make your statement more effective. Having said no, give an honest reason for your response. Your reason may be as simple as, "It goes against my values." Offering a legitimate reason will help strengthen your refusal.

FIGURE 12.2

BODY LANGUAGE AND ASSERTIVE REFUSAL

Reinforce the meaning of your words with appropriate body language.

Shaking your head is one way to communicate no.	Raising your hand in a "Stop" or "No way" signal tells others that you are not interested.	If the other person continues to pressure you, walk away from the situation.

Hands-On Health ACTIVITY

Assert Yourself

Learning to be assertive can help you maintain your commitment to a healthful lifestyle. By practicing assertiveness, you will find it easier to live by your values. In this activity, you will role-play assertive communication skills.

What You'll Need

- large index cards
- pen or pencil and paper

What You'll Do

1. With a partner, think of a realistic scenario in which you are being pressured by one or more peers to do something against your values.

2. Write your scenario on an index card, and swap cards with another pair of partners.

3. Role-play the scenario you've received, using the checklist shown here to make sure you have included the elements of assertive communication.

Apply and Conclude

Write a short reflective paper describing how being assertive can help protect your physical, mental/emotional, and social health.

Checklist: Assertive Communication Skills

✓	"I" messages
✓	Respectful but firm tone of voice
✓	Alternatives to the action
✓	Clear, simple statements
✓	Appropriate body language

▶ **Step 2: Suggest Alternatives.** When a peer asks you to take part in an activity with which you are uncomfortable, try suggesting another activity. For example, if a friend wants to go to a party where there is no adult supervision, you might say, "No, let's go to the movies instead." By offering an alternative, you create an opportunity for your friend to be with you in a way that makes you comfortable. Keep in mind that your suggestion is most effective if it takes you away from the dangerous or unpleasant situation.

▶ **Step 3: Stand Your Ground.** Even after you've refused, peers may continue trying to persuade you to join in. Make it clear that you mean what you've said. Use strong body language and maintain eye contact. If this doesn't work, remove yourself from the situation. Simply say, "I'm going home."

When faced with negative peer pressure, it's critical to stay true to yourself and do what's best for your health and well-being. Knowing that you made the decision to protect your safety and uphold your values will make you feel good about resisting the pressure.

Passive and Aggressive Responses

Practicing refusal skills will help you deal with negative peer pressure.

Give examples of passive, aggressive, and assertive ways to respond to peer pressure. Which method is most effective? Why?

Being assertive may take some practice. To some people, a passive response to negative peer pressure seems more natural and therefore easier. People who are **passive** have a *tendency to give up, give in, or back down without standing up for their own rights and needs.* Teens who respond passively to peer pressure may believe they are making friends by going along. However, being passive may cause others to view them as pushovers who aren't worthy of respect.

Some people may feel more comfortable with an aggressive response. **Aggressive** people are *overly forceful, pushy, hostile, or otherwise attacking in their approach.* An aggressive way of resisting peer pressure may involve yelling, shouting, shoving, or insulting others or the use of other kinds of verbal or physical force. Aggressive people may get their way, but most people react to aggressive behavior by avoiding the individual or by fighting back. Either reaction can result in emotional or physical harm to both parties.

Learning and practicing assertive responses is the most effective way to deal with peer pressure. Being assertive will help you resist negative peer pressure today, and it will also serve as a useful skill throughout your life.

Lesson 2 *Review*

Reviewing Facts and Vocabulary

1. What is *peer pressure*?
2. Identify two examples of manipulation.
3. How might a friend help you resist negative peer pressure?

Thinking Critically

4. **Analyzing.** Suppose a group of friends constantly teases a student in your school. How can you show disapproval of this inconsiderate and disrespectful behavior?
5. **Comparing and Contrasting.** Explain the differences between passive, aggressive, and assertive forms of communication.

Applying Health Skills

Refusal Skills. With a classmate, develop a scenario in which peers use pressure to try to get you to use tobacco or alcohol. Demonstrate strategies for resisting the negative peer pressure.

SPREADSHEETS Use spreadsheet software to develop a table that provides examples of how refusal skills might make use of passive, aggressive, and assertive forms of communication. Find help in using spreadsheet software at **health.glencoe.com.**

Dating and Setting Limits

VOCABULARY

infatuation
affection
curfew

YOU'LL LEARN TO

- Analyze behavior that will enhance dignity, respect, and responsibility in a dating relationship.

- Examine strategies for maintaining safe and healthy dating relationships.

QUICK START Give examples of health-related goals and limits you have set for yourself. How do the goals and limits benefit each side of your health triangle?

During adolescence it's natural to experience a change in attitude toward the opposite gender. Teens may find themselves feeling attracted to people they'd only thought of as classmates or friends before. These feelings of attraction may cause you to begin—or at least to begin thinking about—dating.

Dating teens can express their affection in healthy, respectful ways. *List three positive ways for teens to show affection for a dating partner.*

Dating

Dating can be an enjoyable learning experience. It provides opportunities to develop social skills, such as communicating and interacting with a person of the opposite gender. Dating also allows people to learn more about themselves. Through dating, some people discover new interests, reaffirm their values, and even start thinking about the type of person with whom they might like to build a future.

Sometimes when a teen is attracted to someone, an **infatuation**, or *exaggerated feelings of passion for another person*, develops. Although such feelings are natural, it is important not to mistake them for genuine affection. **Affection**, *a feeling of fondness for someone*, comes when you know another person well. Friendship and caring are essential for building an affectionate, close relationship with a dating partner. Teens who are dating can express affection by communicating with and listening to each other, holding hands, hugging, and spending quality time together.

Deciding to Date

Not everyone dates. Some teens choose not to date because they're shy around persons of the opposite gender. Others may choose not to date because they have other interests or time commitments. Still others may not date because of family traditions or values. Everyone is unique. There's no reason to let anyone pressure you into dating if you're not ready for it.

As a way of easing into dating, many teens go out with groups of friends of both genders. Being part of a group allows teens to develop and practice their social skills without having the pressure of focusing on only one person. Going out in a group takes some of the attention away from the individual, helping him or her relax and feel less self-conscious. Group dates or double dates can also relieve the pressure of being alone with someone new.

Exploring Issues

What Are the Benefits of Group Dating and Individual Dating?

There are benefits to both group dating and individual dating. What are your thoughts on these dating situations? Here are two viewpoints.

Viewpoint 1: Daphne L., age 15

I think group dating is the best choice for teens who are just beginning to date. Dating for the first time can be nerve-racking. It helps when you have the support of other friends. Going out on group dates makes the situation more comfortable and helps teens get used to dating. It's also a lot of fun.

Viewpoint 2: Ted R., age 16

Yeah, group dates can be fun, but it's hard to get to know a person better when you are surrounded by other friends. Going out in a group may make it seem less like a date. To really get comfortable with dating relationships, people need to go on individual dates. It's important to learn to communicate on a one-on-one basis with your date.

ACTIVITY

What do you think about group dating and individual dating? What other issues should teens consider before they start dating? Summarize your views in a one-page essay.

What to Do on a Date

What you decide to do on a date depends on the person you are with and your common interests. If you don't know the person well, a movie might be a good choice. Going out to dinner or to a school dance are also good options. You might also try attending a sports event such as a baseball or basketball game. When you get to know each other and have a better idea of your interests, you will probably find activities that both you and your date enjoy.

SPORTS OR ATHLETIC ACTIVITIES

If you and your date like sports, you might want to consider a date that includes athletic activities. In-line or ice skating, tennis, minia-ture golf, cycling, hiking, bowling, skiing, and horseback riding are all fun activities you can try on a date. Athletic activities such as these promote health and provide a way for dates to share and develop common interests. They also allow dates to get to know each other better in a friendly, relaxed atmosphere.

COMMUNITY ACTIVITIES

Consider going to the zoo or a local museum. If you and your date enjoy music or theater, you can attend concerts or plays being held in your community. You may also sign up for a painting, dancing, or photography class together at a local community center. Find out whether your community has any tourist attrac-tions that you have overlooked. Learn what's available by asking friends and family, reading the local newspaper, and looking through the telephone book. Then, choose an event or activity that interests both you and your date, and go explore together. For example, you might attend a community festival or a stargazing party hosted by a local astronomy club.

CHARITABLE ACTIVITIES

Volunteering together can help build strong friendships and dating relationships. You can help build a house for Habitat for Humanity, participate in a charity walk-a-thon, volunteer to maintain a local park or beach, or attend a fund-raising event. Such activities allow you and your date to contribute to the community in positive ways. Volunteering is also a great option for group dates!

 Many teens enjoy athletic activities during dates. *Why are athletic activities a good option for dating?*

What can I do to make a good impression on a first date?

- **Relax and be yourself.** You want your date to like you for who you are, not who you're pretending to be.
- **Be honest.** There are no "rules" about who calls whom or about telling someone how you feel.
- **Plan your date.** Come up with something you'll both enjoy doing.
- **Be courteous.** Be on time, and treat your date with kindness and respect.

A curfew is a limit that many parents set for their teens. *What are some other examples of limits that help keep you safe?*

Avoiding Risk Situations

Some dating situations may increase the chance of being pressured to participate in sexual activity or some other high-risk behaviors. Before you go on a date, know where you're going and what you will be doing. Find out who else will be there, and discuss with your parents what time they expect you home. If you're going to a party, for example, know where the party is being held and whether there will be adult supervision. Regardless of where you go on a date, make sure you have money with you in case something goes wrong and you need to call home for a ride.

Below are more tips for avoiding high-risk dating situations:

▶ **Avoid places where alcohol and other drugs are present.** The use of alcohol or other drugs interferes with judgment. People under the influence of these substances are more likely to engage in unsafe or high-risk behaviors. Prevent such situations by not using alcohol or other drugs and avoiding those who are using these substances.

▶ **Avoid being alone with a date at home or in an isolated place.** You may find it more difficult to maintain self-control when you are home alone or in an isolated place with a date. Being isolated from others also increases your risk of being forced into a sexual act against your will.

Dating Relationships

Some teens choose to have an ongoing dating relationship with only one person. This type of relationship may help you develop skills and behaviors that will someday prepare you for the dignity, respect, and responsibility required in a marriage. However, keep in mind that dating only one person during adolescence may limit your chances for socializing with others. This may prevent you from developing other positive relationships.

Your teen years are a time for trying many different roles and relationships. Although beginning and ending dating relationships can be difficult, such experiences help you mature emotionally. Staying in a relationship because you don't know how to leave it gracefully or clinging to a person who wishes to end the relationship are common dating problems. Honesty and open communication will help resolve such difficulties.

Setting Limits

Your parents or guardians may set limits regarding your dating relationships. Such limits are intended to protect your health and safety. For example, your parent or guardian might insist on a **curfew**, *a set time at which you must be home at night.* A curfew is a limit that many parents establish for their teens. Limits should be established ahead of time and agreed upon by both teens and their families before the date.

As you mature, you'll need to know how to set your own limits. Remember, your parents or guardians can guide and support you through this process. For example, it's a good idea to set a limit on the age of the person you date. You also need to set limits with your date regarding places you'll go, how you'll get there, and what you will do. Setting such limits and making them clear before a date helps you avoid potentially risky situations.

When you communicate your limit on sexual activity, you need to be clear and firm about your decision to practice abstinence. You can make this task easier by developing and rehearsing avoidance techniques and refusal skills—including specific actions and phrases—that you can use. You will learn more about these skills in the next lesson.

Health Minute

Healthful Dating Expectations

When in a dating relationship, remember:

▶ You deserve to be treated with consideration and respect.

▶ Your partner should recognize and respect your values.

▶ If pressured by your date, you can say no to drugs or other high-risk activities without apologizing or offering an explanation.

▶ No one has the right to force or pressure you into doing anything that goes against your values or your family's values.

 Lesson 3 *Review*

Reviewing Facts and Vocabulary

1. What is *affection*? How can teens show affection in a dating relationship without participating in sexual activity?

2. What are some ways to avoid high-risk dating situations?

3. Why is it important to set limits in a dating relationship?

Thinking Critically

4. **Synthesizing.** List the personal benefits that establishing a curfew can have for your health.

5. **Analyzing.** Explain the role that substance abuse plays in increasing the risk of unsafe behaviors such as sexual activity.

Applying Health Skills

Analyzing Influences. Watch several television programs that portray characters involved in dating relationships. Observe the interaction among the characters, and identify what message the program communicates to teens about peer pressure and sexual activity. Summarize your observations in a written report.

WORD PROCESSING Word processing can give your report a more polished look. Visit **health.glencoe.com** for tips on using your word-processing program.

Abstinence: A Responsible Decision

VOCABULARY
abstinence
sexually transmitted
   diseases (STDs)
priorities
self-control

YOU'LL LEARN TO

- Analyze the importance of abstinence from sexual activity as the preferred choice of behavior for teens.

- Discuss the legal implications regarding sexual activity as it relates to minors.

- Discuss abstinence as the only method that is 100 percent effective in preventing pregnancy and sexually transmitted diseases.

→ *QUICK START* On a sheet of paper, list several consequences of being sexually active. Explain how each consequence could affect the health of the individual and the health of his or her family members.

A These teens have chosen to make abstinence from sexual activity a priority in their relationship. *Why is abstinence the best choice for teens?*

Many of the sexual feelings teens experience are brought on by the body's release of chemicals. You don't have control over the feelings caused by your hormones, but you do have complete control over how you respond to them.

Abstinence Until Marriage

Each year, more and more teens make the safe and responsible choice of abstinence from sexual activity until marriage. **Abstinence** is *a deliberate decision to avoid high-risk behaviors, including sexual activity before marriage and the use of tobacco, alcohol, and other drugs.* Many teens choose to practice abstinence because it is the only 100 percent sure way to eliminate health risks associated with sexual activity. These risks include unplanned pregnancy and **sexually transmitted diseases (STDs)**—*infections spread from person to person through sexual contact.*

Committing to Abstinence

The teen years are a time for physical, mental/emotional, and social growth. Part of this growth process involves setting goals for the future and establishing priorities. **Priorities** are *those goals, tasks, and activities that you judge to be more important than others.* A priority for many teens, for example, is to get good grades and succeed in school. Think about your plans for the future. How might an unplanned pregnancy or a **sexually transmitted disease** (STD) affect your plans? Making abstinence from sexual activity a priority can eliminate these risks and help you achieve your goals.

Practicing abstinence requires planning and self-control. **Self-control** is *a person's ability to use responsibility to override emotions.* Use the following tips as a guide to commit to abstinence.

▶ **Establish your priorities.** Think about your goals, and set priorities that will help you reach them. Consider your values and those of your family, such as respect, honesty, integrity, and morality.

▶ **Set personal limits on how you express affection.** Base your limits on your priorities. Set your limits before you are in a situation where sexual feelings begin to build.

▶ **Share your thoughts with your partner.** One sign of a mature, responsible relationship is being able to communicate with your partner openly and honestly. Discuss your priorities, and clearly define your limits.

▶ **Talk with a trusted adult.** Parents and other trusted adults are often able to suggest safe and healthful ways for you to manage your feelings.

▶ **Avoid high-pressure situations.** When possible, go out on dates in a group. Stay away from unsupervised parties and dark rooms. Avoid parking in secluded spots.

▶ **Do not use alcohol or other drugs.** Using alcohol or other drugs interferes with the ability to think clearly. It is also wise to avoid people who are using these substances.

hot link

sexually transmitted disease For more information about specific sexually transmitted diseases, see Chapter 25, page 646.

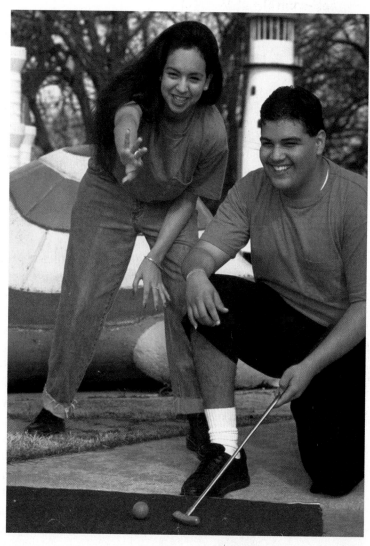

Ⓥ Choosing a safe, supervised area for a date helps you uphold your values. *What other strategies can help you maintain your commitment to abstinence?*

Reasons to Practice Abstinence

Sexual activity has many short-term and long-term consequences. In addition to having legal consequences, teen sexual activity can seriously harm an individual's physical, mental/emotional, and social health. These negative effects can disrupt a teen's life, interfere with his or her goals for the future, and complicate his or her relationships with others.

Careful consideration of the negative consequences associated with sexual activity will reinforce the decision to practice abstinence until marriage. *What are your reasons for practicing abstinence?*

hotlink

acquired immune deficiency syndrome (AIDS)
For more information on the problems associated with the AIDS epidemic, see Chapter 25, page 658.

Legal Implications

It is illegal for an adult to have sexual contact with anyone under the age of consent, which varies from state to state. In many states, it is illegal for unmarried minors to engage in sexual activity. For example, if the age of consent in a state is 18, two seventeen-year-old teens who engage in sexual activity would be breaking the law. People who are arrested for and convicted of breaking sexual laws can go to jail. Depending on the situation, they may be identified as sex offenders—a label that will follow them for the rest of their lives. This label can harm their careers and future relationships.

Effects on Physical Health

Teen sexual activity can affect the physical health of both females and males in significant ways.

UNPLANNED PREGNANCY

For many teens, unplanned pregnancy is the consequence of sexual activity. Teen pregnancy risks the health of both the teen mother and her child. Often, the body of a teen is not sufficiently mature to sustain a healthy pregnancy. This can lead to complications that threaten the lives of mother and baby.

SEXUALLY TRANSMITTED DISEASES (STDS)

Teens from 15 to 19 years of age are at the greatest risk of contracting STDs. Each year, about 3 million teens in the United States contract some form of STD. If diagnosed early, many STDs can be treated and cured. However, some of these diseases have no cure and can have lifelong consequences. For example, chlamydia can cause sterility if left untreated, making it impossible for a person ever to have a child. Other STDs, such as **acquired immune deficiency syndrome (AIDS),** can be fatal.

Abstinence Pledges: A Growing Trend

Teens who take a pledge to delay sexual activity until marriage are far less likely than their peers to become pregnant or to contract a sexually transmitted disease. How can teens strengthen their commitment to abstinence?

Abstinence Pledge

A Commitment to Myself and Others

On this day, I make a commitment to myself, my family, my friends, and to those I date, to abstain from sexual activity until marriage.

My reasons include: upholding family values, wanting to attend college, safeguarding my self-worth and self-concept, wanting to have healthy children when I marry.

People who will support me in my pledge include:

☆ my parents/guardian   ☆ my family doctor

☆ my best friend   ☆ my school counselor

I hereby sign this pledge as an indication of my personal commitment to remain abstinent until marriage.

My signature: _____

How can teens' goals be compromised by sexual activity? What are the most important reasons for you to practice abstinence?

Which people in your life can help support your decision to practice abstinence?

ACTIVITY

Work with a small group. Use your answers to the questions to create a poster advocating that high school teens practice abstinence. Communicate the importance and benefits of practicing abstinence. Make your poster persuasive and attention-getting, and include a memorable phrase or slogan.

Effects on Emotional Health

Establishing and following a strong value system leads teens to healthy feelings of self-respect. Engaging in sexual activity outside of marriage goes against the values and religious beliefs of many people. Often, the fear of being caught leads teens who engage in such activity to begin lying to parents or others about their whereabouts. This dishonesty can cause emotional distress by bringing on feelings of guilt and regret that are harmful to a teen's self-concept.

For teens facing unplanned pregnancy, the demands of being a parent can cause great emotional strain. Pregnancy followed by the birth and care of an infant is extremely demanding. Parenthood is a serious, full-time, lifelong responsibility that teens are not ready for.

Effects on Social Health

Sexually active teens risk their reputations. Being labeled by peers as "easy" can make it difficult for a teen to build new and healthy relationships. For example, to eliminate the risk of being pressured into sexual activity, some teens refuse to date those who are sexually active. Also, partners may view each other differently when a relationship involves sexual activity. In some cases, the pressure and expectations caused by sexual activity may lead to the breakup of a relationship.

Engaging in sexual activity can also harm a teen's relationship with family members. When teens decide to become sexually active, they go against their family's values. They go beyond the limits that their parents or guardians set to protect them. In failing to demonstrate responsible and healthful dating behavior, these teens break their parents' trust. Parents who discover that their teen is sexually active often feel disappointed and betrayed. Such feelings can cause tension among family members.

A Teens who choose sexual abstinence safeguard their reputations. *What are some other benefits of abstinence?*

When faced with an unplanned pregnancy, many teen parents drop out of school to support their child. By law, the teen father is required to support his child financially until the child reaches the age of 18. Frequently, teen parents sacrifice plans for college and job training. They may also give up their social lives to meet the needs of the child. Unmarried teens are not prepared to assume the responsibilities of parenthood. Committing to abstinence is the safe and healthy choice for teens.

Using Avoidance Techniques and Refusal Skills

To reduce the risk of being pressured into sexual activity, learn avoidance techniques—actions or phrases you can use to avoid risky situations. For example, if your date wants to go to a party that will not be supervised by adults, you might suggest going to a restaurant instead. If a boyfriend or girlfriend wants to come over when your parents or guardians aren't at home, you might suggest going skating or biking instead.

FIGURE **12.3**

SAYING NO TO SEXUAL ACTIVITY

If someone uses pressure lines to persuade you to break your commitment to abstinence, use refusal statements to communicate your stance firmly.

Pressure Line	Refusal Statement
• If you love me, you will. • Everyone's doing it. • Don't be such a baby. • My feelings won't change. I'll still respect you.	• If you care about me, you won't pressure me. • No, everyone's not. I'm sticking to my values. • It's the mature, responsible decision to wait. • Maybe, but I won't respect myself.

Share your commitment to abstinence with your girlfriend or boyfriend, stating your position simply but firmly. After you have discussed your decision to practice abstinence, you will find it easier to exercise self-control. If a situation seems to be getting out of control, insist on stopping. Then, back away and explain why you want to stop. If your girlfriend or boyfriend tries to pressure you, become more assertive. You might use refusal statements similar to those in **Figure 12.3.** Make sure your body language supports your verbal message. Don't be afraid of hurting the other person's feelings. It's possible to say no and still remain friends.

 Lesson 4 *Review*

Reviewing Facts and Vocabulary

1. What is *abstinence*?
2. Discuss the legal implications regarding sexual activity as it relates to minors.
3. What are effective ways to avoid being pressured into sexual activity?

Thinking Critically

4. **Evaluating.** Write a paragraph describing the short-term and long-term benefits of abstinence for the emotional and social health of both the individual and the family.
5. **Analyzing.** How can practicing abstinence benefit a teen's self-image? Explain your answer.

Applying Health Skills

Refusal Skills. With a classmate, role-play situations in which teens use refusal skills to avoid participating in sexual activity. Have classmates analyze the effectiveness of these refusal skills.

WEB SITES Create a Web page that advocates for teen abstinence. See **health.glencoe.com** for help on planning and building your own Web page.

Screenplays for Healthy Peer Relationships

Drawing from the chapter content, write a screenplay for a new teen television show that presents healthful messages about peer relationships. Use the following example as a guide for formatting your screenplay.

ACT I

SCENE 1

INT. (INTERIOR) SCHOOL CAFETERIA, NOON
TWO BEST FRIENDS, JUDY AND GREG, WALK INTO THE BUSY
CAFETERIA AND SIT DOWN AT THEIR FAVORITE TABLE.

JUDY

I think Sara is upset about something. She's been
keeping to herself all day. I wonder what's wrong.

GREG

I don't know. Do you think she and her boyfriend had
an argument about something?

SCENE 2

INT. SCHOOL HALLWAY, 3:30 PM
SARA IS AT HER LOCKER, LOOKING SAD AND DISTRACTED.

ACTIVITY

Choose one of the following scenarios, and write a screenplay with three scenes. Apply what you have learned in this chapter about healthy peer relationships.

Scenario 1: Three teen boys who have been friends for years are having a conversation about girls. Two of them are taunting the third for choosing abstinence.

Scenario 2: Four teen girls who are close friends are at a school dance.

Two of them are making fun of a classmate whom they consider overweight.

EXPRESS YOUR VIEWS

Review the healthful ways you resolved the situation in your screenplay. Using what you have learned from this chapter, write a friendship or behavior pledge that incorporates the elements of healthy friendships and positive peer pressure.

CROSS-CURRICULUM CONNECTIONS

Write a Journal Entry. Nurturing healthy friendships means taking responsibility for your actions and understanding the roles others play in your life. Brainstorm a list of important decisions you have made that were influenced by peer pressure. Write a journal entry about the decision on your list that stands out as the most significant. Describe the incident. Reflect on why it was a positive or negative experience.

Explore Dating Customs. Dating customs for teens vary from culture to culture. As a class, brainstorm a list of cultures whose dating customs you would be interested in studying. Your teacher will organize the class in teams and assign you a culture to research. Each team should report back to the class. Then, have a class discussion comparing and contrasting the different customs.

Practice Problem Solving. Bob had three friends with whom he socialized almost exclusively. When he got a job, he struck up friendships with four people at work and got invited to a party. One of his new friends brought three people that Bob liked immediately. His other three coworkers brought one friend each, but Bob didn't have anything in common with two of them. How many friends does Bob have now?

Research a Topic. Chemicals called *pheromones* contribute to the physical attraction to others that many people begin to experience during the teen years. Many animal species secrete pheromones as a means of communication. Because of the complexity of mammalian behavior, studies on pheromones have focused largely on insects. Research the ways social insects use pheromones to communicate and send messages. Summarize your findings in a one-page report.

CAREER Corner

School Social Worker

School social workers deal with a wide range of social, emotional, cultural, and economic concerns among students. They help students overcome problems that may be interfering with their education. School social workers also help improve students' decision-making skills, motivation, attendance, and self-concept.

To become a school social worker, you need a bachelor's or a master's degree in social work and a license or certificate from your state. Learn more about this and other health careers by clicking on Career Corner at **health.glencoe.com**.

Chapter 12 Review

> ## EXPLORING HEALTH TERMS *Answer the following questions on a sheet of paper.*

Lesson 1 *Match each definition with the correct term.*

clique   friendship
peers   platonic friendship
stereotype

1. A relationship with a member of the opposite gender in which there is affection but the people are not considered a couple.
2. A small circle of friends that excludes people viewed as outsiders.
3. An exaggerated or oversimplified belief about an entire group of people.

Lesson 2 *Replace the underlined words with the correct term.*

aggressive   assertive
harassment   manipulation
passive   peer pressure
refusal skills

4. <u>Harassment</u> is an indirect and dishonest way to control someone.
5. An important aspect of being assertive is to use effective <u>manipulation</u>.
6. Being overly pushy and hostile is being <u>assertive</u>.

Lesson 3 *Fill in the blanks with the correct term.*

affection   curfew
infatuation

Shane's parents worry about his (_7_), or exaggerated feelings of passion, with his girlfriend. To help Shane avoid situations that could involve him in high-risk behaviors, his parents set guidelines for him, including an early (_8_), or time by which he must be at home.

Lesson 4 *Match each definition with the correct term.*

abstinence   self-control
sexually transmitted disease   priorities

9. A risk associated with not choosing abstinence.
10. Goals, tasks, and activities you judge as more important than others.
11. A person's ability to use responsibility to override emotions.

> ## RECALLING THE FACTS *Use complete sentences to answer the following questions.*

Lesson 1

1. What is the relationship between peers and casual friendships?
2. What are the benefits of a platonic friendship?
3. Identify five attributes of a true friendship.

Lesson 2

4. What is positive peer pressure?
5. How can body language be used to communicate refusal?
6. Describe an aggressive response to peer pressure.

Lesson 3

7. What are some benefits of dating?
8. Why do some teens choose not to date?
9. What are some advantages of group dating over individual dating?

Lesson 4

10. Identify three risks associated with sexual activity during the teen years.
11. Analyze the importance of abstinence from sexual activity as the preferred choice of behavior for teens.
12. Describe a problem that can result from an unplanned teen pregnancy.

➤ THINKING CRITICALLY

1. **Evaluating.** Describe both the advantages and disadvantages of being a member of a social group such as a clique. *(LESSON 1)*

2. **Analyzing.** Suggest ways you can stand up to peers to show disapproval of inconsiderate and disrespectful behavior such as harassment of others. *(LESSON 2)*

3. **Applying.** Marriage is a long-term commitment. Getting married means that a person is deciding to spend the rest of his or her life with another person. How can the behaviors you practice in a dating relationship help prepare you for the responsibility of marriage? *(LESSON 3)*

4. **Summarizing.** Unplanned pregnancy among teens affects the teens involved, their families, and society as a whole. Write a paragraph explaining the negative consequences teen pregnancy holds for individuals, families, and society. *(LESSON 4)*

➤ HEALTH SKILLS APPLICATION

1. **Practicing Healthful Behavior.** Develop a plan for demonstrating to your friends each of the traits that characterize a healthy friendship. Over the span of a week, keep a log to describe how you demonstrated each trait. *(LESSON 1)*

2. **Analyzing Influences.** Locate a magazine or newspaper article about a teen who has set a positive example in the community. Write a brief summary of the article, and identify how the actions of that teen might be a positive influence on other teens. *(LESSON 2)*

3. **Communication Skills.** Write a skit that depicts a responsible, healthful dating relationship between two teens. The teens should demonstrate effective communication skills to show their respect for each other and their commitment to practicing abstinence. *(LESSON 3)*

4. **Advocacy.** Write a letter to the editor of your school newspaper in which you discuss abstinence from sexual activity as the only method that is 100 percent effective in preventing pregnancy, STDs, and the sexual transmission of HIV/AIDS. *(LESSON 4)*

✦ *BEYOND* the Classroom

Parent Involvement

Practicing Healthful Behaviors. Many communities have programs that provide drug-free places where teens can socialize under adult supervision. Such programs help teens avoid pressure to participate in high-risk behaviors. With your parents, learn about the programs for teens in your area. If such programs do not exist in your community, find out how one might be created.

School and Community

Stopping Harassment. Speak with a law enforcement official in your community to learn the legal definition of harassment and what penalties exist for teens found guilty of harassment. Share your findings with the class. Discuss actions that students, faculty, and community members can take to help stop harassment.

Violence Prevention

KEEP OUR COMMUNITIES SAFE

What Do You Know About Youth Violence?

Read each statement below and respond by writing *Myth* or *Fact*.

1. About one-third of teens in grades 9–12 are involved in at least one physical fight each year.

2. Teens are more likely to be victims of violence than adults are.

3. By age 13, the average American child has watched 100,000 acts of violence on TV.

4. Joining a gang is not effective protection from violence.

5. Homicide, or murder, is the leading cause of death among teens.

6. Use of alcohol and other drugs is a contributing factor in incidents of violent crime.

7. Programs intended to treat violent behavior are ineffective.

8. Nearly half of all rapes and sexual assaults are committed by acquaintances of the victim.

9. Schools can promote effective ways to prevent violence.

10. Of the industrialized nations in the world, the United States has the highest rates of homicide and firearm-related deaths among adolescents.

HEALTH Online

For instant feedback on your health status, go to Chapter 13 Health Inventory at **health.glencoe.com**.

Quick *Write*

Using Visuals. Community involvement and advocacy can contribute to safer environments for everyone. What can you do to help keep your neighborhood safe?

Personal Safety

VOCABULARY

body language
self-defense
assertive

YOU'LL LEARN TO

• Identify behaviors and strategies that enhance personal safety.

• Demonstrate ways of avoiding and reducing threatening situations.

• Examine strategies for promoting safety at home and in the community.

QUICK START On a sheet of paper, list five actions you can take to keep yourself safe. Then, write a paragraph explaining how these safety habits would help protect you.

A Being confident and not looking like a victim can help keep you safe. *How can you project self-confidence?*

The key to personal safety is to be able to recognize potentially dangerous situations and learn strategies to avoid them. In addition, simple safety habits that you practice everyday can decrease your exposure to risk. Being aware of your surroundings, not walking alone, staying away from dark or isolated areas, and looking alert and confident are all behaviors that can protect you. In this lesson, you will learn about the factors that affect your personal safety and the actions you can take to keep yourself safe.

Your Protective Factors

Although you may not be conscious of them, you already have many assets that increase your chances of staying safe. The list of personal traits and environmental conditions that reduce teens' risk of violence is shown in **Figure 13.1** on the next page. These traits and conditions are specific protective factors that can help shield you from harm. Everyone can work to strengthen his or her protective factors and help to reduce the risk of violence. Doing so will contribute to personal safety.

FIGURE 13.1

INDIVIDUAL AND SOCIAL PROTECTIVE FACTORS AGAINST VIOLENCE

These protective factors decrease the likelihood of teen violence.

Individual	Family	Peer/School	Community
• No history of aggressive behavior • Positive social skills; gets along with others • Intelligent • Antiviolence attitude • Being female	• Parents monitor child's behavior • Parents positively evaluate peers • Warm, supportive relationship with parents or other adults	• Peers and friends avoid high-risk behaviors • Commitment to school • Good attitude	• Strong economic opportunity • Involvement in community activities

Source: Youth Violence: A Report of the Surgeon General

Strategies for Staying Safe

In addition to strengthening your **protective factors,** there are behaviors you can practice to stay safe. These actions include taking precautions against risky situations and developing safety habits.

Smart Precautions

The first step in taking responsibility for your personal safety is to consider preventive behaviors that will help protect you. Many safety precautions that can prevent your becoming a victim are commonsense actions. Here are some preventive measures to follow.

▶ Avoid unsafe areas, including places with high crime rates.

▶ Don't carry your wallet or purse in a conspicuous, easy-to-grab place.

▶ Walk briskly and confidently. *Always* look as though you know where you are going and what you are doing.

▶ Avoid walking alone at night, in wooded areas, or in dark alleys. If you must walk at night, avoid doorways and walk under lights near the curb.

▶ If you drive, park your car in a well-lit area. Have your keys out and ready as you approach your parked car. Before getting into your car, look to make sure that no one is inside. Lock the doors as soon as you get in.

hotlink

protective factors For more information on protective factors, see Chapter 8, page 216.

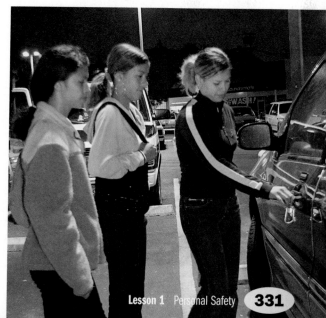

Taking safety precautions is particularly important when you are out at night. *What behaviors demonstrated by these teens help keep them safe?*

Use the Chapter 13 eFlashcards at **health.glencoe.com** to review the vocabulary for this lesson.

▶ Let your family know where you're going and when you'll return.

▶ Do not get into an elevator alone with a stranger.

▶ Get on and off buses in well-lit areas.

▶ If someone you know gives you a ride, ask the person not to leave until you have safely entered a building.

▶ Do not hitchhike or give rides to hitchhikers.

▶ Avoid the use of alcohol or other drugs. These substances impair your judgment and reduce your ability to protect yourself.

Body Language and Self-Defense

You can protect yourself from harm by communicating to others that you are worthy of being treated with respect and that you have a right to be safe and secure. You can project this information through the use of **body language**, *nonverbal communication through gestures, facial expressions, behaviors, and posture.* Making direct eye contact, using a strong voice, holding your head high, and walking with a deliberate stride demonstrate that you are in charge of your safety.

Key self-defense strategies can also protect you from becoming a victim of violence. **Self-defense** includes *any strategy for protecting oneself from harm.* Many people of all ages have taken self-defense classes to increase their sense of personal safety. A range of self-defense classes, including various martial arts courses, is available. Signing up for such a class is an effective way to enhance your confidence and sense of preparedness. Although physical strategies can be a useful part of self-defense, mental strategies are also important. In some communities, law enforcement officials teach personal safety classes on awareness and preparedness. Often, they stress the importance of projecting self-confidence and assertiveness. Being **assertive** means *standing up for your rights and beliefs in firm but positive ways.* Through words and actions, assertive people show that they are not easy targets. They are proactive in protecting their health and safety.

Taking a self-defense class can increase your sense of personal safety. *What other strategies can help protect your health and safety?*

332 **Chapter 13** Violence Prevention

Practicing Safety Strategies

Staying safe doesn't mean living in fear. It means learning and applying strategies that will reduce your risk of becoming a victim of violence. In this activity, you will role-play some strategies for staying safe.

What You'll Need

- pencil and notebook paper

What You'll Do

1. With a partner or in a small group, brainstorm several unsafe situations that teens may face. For example, a stranger in a car tells you that he is lost and asks you to approach the window to look at his map. Record your scenarios on a sheet of paper.

2. For each situation, discuss safe ways for teens to respond. If necessary, refer to the tips given in this lesson.

3. Role-play a situation from your list.

4. As a class, discuss the situations that were role-played. Which did you think were the most realistic? Why? What safety strategies might be effective?

Apply and Conclude

Using what you learned from the role-plays you observed, compose a short essay for the school paper informing teens how to stay safe in various situations. The article should include three or four safety tips and be relevant to teens in high school.

Keeping Homes Safe

A home should be a nurturing haven in which family members feel secure. The entire family can engage in responsible behaviors that will help maintain the safety of the home environment. Here are some tips for you to follow.

 Keeping your doors and windows locked can help keep you and your family safe. *What are some other strategies for keeping your home secure?*

▶ Lock doors with a bolt. All family members should make an effort to keep all doors, including sliding doors and French doors, secure and in good repair.

▶ Make sure windows have locks. Keep windows locked at night and when no one is home. Repair broken windows immediately.

▶ Never open the door to someone you don't know or trust. Don't let strangers use your phone.

▶ Do not tell unknown callers that you are home alone.

▶ Do not give out personal information over the telephone or computer.

Safety in the Community

How safe a community is has a significant impact on personal safety. Many communities have taken steps to make neighborhoods safer. Some of the strategies include:

▶ **Increased police patrol.** Some communities have increased the number of law enforcement officers on street patrol.

▶ **Neighborhood Watch programs.** Residents have joined the crime prevention effort by looking for signs of suspicious activity and reporting such incidents to the police. It is also a good idea to report suspicious vehicles in the neighborhood.

▶ **After-school programs.** Academic, cultural, or recreational programs after school provide safe environments where teens can use their time productively.

▶ **Improved lighting in parks and playgrounds.** Better lighting can discourage crime by making it more difficult to commit crimes without being seen.

By supporting and participating in efforts such as these, residents can contribute to making communities safer for everyone.

Lesson 1 *Review*

Reviewing Facts and Vocabulary

1. What is *body language*? Give three examples.
2. Define the term *assertive*, and use it in a sentence.
3. List two ways to keep your home safe.

Thinking Critically

4. **Evaluating.** Assess the value of avoiding potentially dangerous situations, even if you know how to defend yourself.
5. **Analyzing.** How can involvement in community activities serve as a protective factor against violent behavior?

Applying Health Skills

Practicing Healthful Behaviors. Develop a list of strategies that you and other members of your family can use to promote personal and family safety. Discuss these safety behaviors with your family, and put your plan into action.

TECHNOLOGY OPTION

WORD PROCESSING You can set up your plan in a word-processing program. See **health.glencoe.com** for tips on using word-processing software.

Keeping Schools Safe

VOCABULARY

violence
bullying
sexual harassment
gang
peer mediation

YOU'LL LEARN TO

• Examine factors that play a role in school violence.

• Analyze and apply strategies for avoiding school violence.

• Identify actions that individuals, schools, and communities can take to reduce violence.

⇒ **QUICK START** What are some causes of conflict that lead to violence among high school students? How do you think violence affects the students involved? How does it affect others in the school community? Write a paragraph summarizing your views.

In recent years, the media has focused attention on acts of violence in schools, including gang activities, physical attacks, and shootings. However, despite the publicity given to violent incidents, schools are generally safe places. According to the Centers for Disease Control and Prevention (CDC), the trend has been toward *less* violence in schools since 1991. For example, the number of students who participated in physical fights at school has dropped nine percentage points. During that same time, the number of students who carried weapons decreased from 26.1 to 17.4 percent.

Issues of School Safety

Although schools are generally safe, some violence may occur on or near school grounds. **Violence** is *the threatened or actual use of physical force or power to harm another person or to damage property.* The 2001 Youth Risk Behaviors Surveillance Survey found that 33.2 percent of teens in grades 9–12 had been in at least one physical fight at school in the previous year. In the same year, 8.9 percent of students were threatened or injured with a weapon at school.

Ⓐ School should be a safe place for students to learn and engage in fun, healthy activities. *How does your school help ensure the safety of students and school personnel?*

Because any violence threatens the safety of everyone in the school community, national health goals have been set to reduce physical fighting by adolescents and to reduce carrying of weapons by adolescents on school property. In order to meet these goals, it's important to look at factors that play a role in school violence. Three of these factors are bullying, sexual harassment, and involvement in gangs.

Bullies use words and physical force to seek power or attention. *What are some ways you can let bullies know that you don't approve of their actions?*

Bullying

Have you ever witnessed students teasing or taunting others? Perhaps you've seen a classmate shove another student or make offensive gestures at her or him. These activities are forms of **bullying**, *the act of seeking power or attention through the psychological, emotional, or physical abuse of another person.* Bullies come in all ages and genders, and they sometimes act in groups. Bullying may cause victims to become depressed, withdrawn, fearful, or angry. Sometimes, victims may try to strike back. Bullying is unacceptable, harmful behavior. You can take a stand against bullying by not joining in and by discouraging this kind of behavior.

Bullies often try to cause anger or fear in their victims. By walking away from a bully and encouraging others to walk away, you deny the bully this victory. In some instances, ignoring a bully can help stop the behavior. However, most cases of bullying require adult intervention. If you witness or experience bullying, report the problem to teachers, counselors, parents, or other adults. No one should tolerate bullying; witnesses can join together with school personnel to stop this behavior.

Did You Know ?

Sexual harassment occurs more frequently than many people realize. Behaviors that constitute sexual harassment include

- making sexual comments or jokes.
- writing sexual messages on notes or walls.
- spreading sexual rumors.
- spying on someone dressing or showering.
- pulling off someone's clothes.
- exposing body parts.
- inappropriate touching.

Sexual Harassment

Sexual harassment is *uninvited and unwelcome sexual conduct directed at another person.* Words, jokes, gestures, or touching of a sexual nature are all forms of sexual harassment. Harassment causes embarrassment, discomfort, and emotional pain for the victim. Federal law states that sexual harassment is illegal. Incidents of sexual harassment should be reported to school personnel at once. After a complaint has been made, school officials will investigate and take action to solve the problem.

Gangs

Some violence in schools is related to gang activity. A **gang** is *a group of people who associate with one another to take part in criminal activity.* Common gang activities include vandalism, robbery, defacing public property with graffiti, and selling drugs. Some gang activities are unpredictable and place innocent people in harm's way. Random shootings, for example, can injure or kill non-gang members. Gang members may bring weapons or drugs to school, endangering the safety of other students.

Reducing the Risk of Violence

Students and faculty have the right to feel safe at school. Being worried about personal safety in the school environment hinders the teaching and learning process. Keeping schools safe is a priority shared by communities across the nation.

Recognizing Warning Signs

Being able to recognize the warning signs of violence can help members of a school community address potentially threatening situations before they occur. **Figure 13.2** lists some common warning signs of violence. Evidence of these signs may indicate that a person is near to acting in a dangerous manner. If you observe any of these signs in a student and suspect that he or she may become violent, inform a teacher, counselor, or other faculty member immediately.

You can help keep your school safe by reporting any behaviors that may lead to violence. *What other actions can you take to contribute to school safety?*

FIGURE **13.2**

WARNING SIGNS OF VIOLENCE

- Has difficulty controlling anger
- Disobeys school rules
- Frequently engages in risk behaviors
- Creates violent artwork or writing
- Constantly talks about weapons or violence
- Vandalizes and destroys property
- Uses alcohol or other drugs
- Harms animals
- Makes threats or detailed plans to hurt others
- Brings or talks about bringing a weapon to school

What You Can Do

Making your school safe begins with building a culture of respect among all students and faculty members. You are empowered to contribute to a safe and healthy school environment. Nationwide, teens are pledging to avoid violence and are encouraging their peers to do the same. To take a stand and help keep schools safe, you can

▶ refuse to carry weapons and report people who do carry them.

▶ report any violent acts or threats of violence to school authorities or police.

▶ practice **conflict resolution** skills and help others settle disputes peacefully.

▶ use refusal skills to resist negative peer pressure and avoid unsafe situations and behaviors.

▶ choose your friends carefully. Having friends who share similar values, such as caring about school, can help protect you from violence.

▶ avoid spending time with people who show warning signs of violent behavior.

▶ tell a parent, teacher, or other adult about your fears if you suspect that your safety is in danger. Avoid being alone.

▶ join or develop a S.A.V.E. chapter (Students Against Violence Everywhere).

h⊙t link

conflict resolution For more information on conflict resolution, see Chapter 10, page 264.

Some schools use metal detectors to reduce the threat of violence. *What other measures might schools adopt to promote safety?*

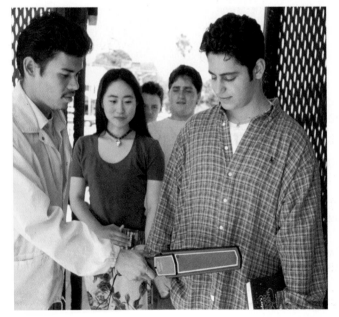

What Schools Are Doing

Schools have procedures and policies to ensure the safety of students. For example, some schools have adopted a *zero-tolerance policy,* which can require expulsion of students who participate in violence or who are found with drugs or weapons. Zero-tolerance policies apply equally to all students with no exceptions. Other efforts to reduce school violence include using metal detectors, examining students' backpacks, or searching lockers for weapons or drugs. Some schools have "closed" campuses, keeping all doors except the main entrance locked. This helps prevent unauthorized persons from coming into the school. Security guards may also be hired to patrol hallways and grounds while classes are in session.

School Safety—What Works?

Though violence in schools remains low, there is a public perception that schools need to be safer. Some schools are employing crisis drills, security guards, and metal detectors. Do these measures work? Read what two teens have to say about one such measure—metal detectors.

Viewpoint 1: Lori M., age 16

The metal detectors create more hassles than they're worth. Sometimes we get to our first class late because all our bags have to be scanned. Besides, if students want to bring in weapons, they'll find a way. I think we should use school money for something else, like classes on conflict resolution skills. Also, we could have stricter discipline policies for those students who do cause problems.

Viewpoint 2: Jason C., age 16

I feel safer with the extra security that metal detectors provide. I think they do act as a deterrent for carrying weapons, and the policy sends the message that our school does not tolerate weapons. It shows that the school cares about our safety and well-being. As far as the cost goes, anything that can save a life is worth it.

ACTIVITY

Do you think that metal detectors and other measures, such as security guards, decrease the risk of violence in schools? Are they necessary to keep schools safe? How do you think limited funds should be spent to enhance school safety? Is technology or education the answer?

PEER MEDIATION

Many schools use peer mediation to help reduce the risk of violence that may stem from unresolved conflicts. **Peer mediation** is *a process in which trained students help other students find fair ways to resolve conflict and settle their differences.* Such programs are successful because they are confidential and do not punish the students involved. Peer mediation sessions typically follow these steps:

▶ **Making introductions.** The mediator explains that he or she will remain neutral and that the session will be confidential.

▶ **Establishing ground rules.** The parties agree to the rules of the process, such as listening without interrupting, maintaining respect and honesty, and being willing to accept the adopted solutions. Then, the mediator decides who talks first.

▶ **Hearing each side.** The mediator allows each party to speak. He or she may ask questions and take notes.

▶ **Exploring solutions.** After all parties have spoken, the mediator asks for possible solutions. A list is made of the suggestions, and each one is discussed. The mediator helps the parties compromise until a solution is agreed upon.

▶ **Closing the session.** The mediator summarizes the agreement and asks participants to discuss their feelings about the process. The parties are encouraged to use these skills to solve future conflicts.

▼ These teens are holding a rally to promote safe schools in their community. *What are some ways that communities can promote school safety?*

Parent and Community Involvement

Parents can work with police officers, social workers, and business leaders to promote safety in schools. Community members can help by taking part in school events and by volunteering to monitor hallways, rest rooms, cafeterias, and other areas where students gather. Developing and supporting programs and activities that provide teens a safe place to gather can also help reduce violence.

▶ Lesson 2 *Review*

Reviewing Facts and Vocabulary

1. Define *gangs*. How might gang members endanger the safety of other students?

2. List two warning signs that a person may be close to acting in a dangerous manner.

3. Identify three policies or procedures that schools use to ensure safety for students and faculty.

Thinking Critically

4. **Analyzing.** Explain the similarities and differences between bullying and sexual harassment.

5. **Applying.** What are some ways of avoiding unsafe or threatening situations at school?

Applying Health Skills

Refusal Skills. Write a scenario in which a student applies refusal skills to avoid participation in a situation that may become violent. Include both verbal and nonverbal messages in your scenario.

TECHNOLOGY *OPTION*

WORD PROCESSING Use a word-processing program to write your scenario. See **health.glencoe.com** for tips on using word-processing software.

FIGURE 14.1

STRUCTURE OF THE SKIN

The two main layers of skin, the epidermis and the dermis, are attached to bones and muscles by the subcutaneous layer, a layer of fat and connective tissue located beneath the dermis.

- hair
- dead epidermis
- living epidermis
- sweat pore
- sebaceous gland
- hair follicle
- muscle
- duct of sweat gland
- sweat gland
- artery
- vein
- nerve
- fat tissue

Certain cells in the epidermis make a substance called *keratin*, a protein that toughens nails. These same cells also produce substances called lipids, which make your skin waterproof. This waterproofing helps the body maintain a proper balance of water and electrolytes. Other cells produce **melanin**, *a pigment that gives the skin, hair, and iris of the eyes their color*—the more melanin, the darker the skin. People with fair skin have less melanin and are at risk of damage from harmful ultraviolet (UV) radiation.

The dermis is a single thick layer composed of connective tissue, which gives the skin its elastic qualities. **Sebaceous glands**, *structures within the skin that produce an oily secretion called sebum*, are also found in the dermis. Sebum helps keep skin and hair from drying out.

Blood vessels in the dermis supply cells with oxygenated blood and nutrients and facilitate the removal of cellular wastes. These blood vessels also function in temperature regulation. When body temperature begins to rise, the blood vessels in the skin dilate. This allows heat to escape through the skin's surface. If body temperature begins to drop, the blood vessels in the skin constrict, decreasing the amount of blood and heat loss at the skin's surface. **Sweat glands**, *structures within the dermis that secrete perspiration through*

QuickWrite

Using Visuals. Many routine tasks, such as brushing and flossing your teeth or caring for your skin, are behaviors that positively affect your long-term health. What are some simple behaviors you can practice each day to protect your health?

Myth or Fact?

What Do You Know About Healthy Skin, Teeth, Eyes, and Ears?

Read each statement below and respond by writing *Myth* or *Fact* for each item.

1. There is a safe way to tan.

2. Skin cancer is never fatal.

3. As long as I brush my teeth every day, I do not need to floss.

4. Eating foods that contain vitamin A can help keep my eyes healthy.

5. Exposure to loud noises does not damage hearing.

6. Tattooing or piercing can result in serious infection transferred by nonsterile needles.

7. Regular breaks can keep your eyes from becoming fatigued when using a computer.

8. People with dry skin are more likely to develop wrinkles.

Keep your responses for review later in the chapter. When you complete the chapter, review this list of myths and facts again. If necessary, change your answers according to what you have learned.

Health Online

For instant feedback on your health status, go to Chapter 14 Health Inventory at health.glencoe.com.

Healthy Skin, Hair, and Nai[ls]

VOCABULARY

epidermis
dermis
melanin
sebaceous glands
sweat glands
melanoma
hair follicle
dandruff

YOU'LL LEARN TO

• Examine the structure of the skin.

• Identify the functions of the skin.

• Examine the effects of health behaviors on skin, hair, and

• Relate the importance of early detection of skin diseases
  healthy life.

→ **QUICK START** Divide a sheet of paper into three columns labeled "Skin," "Hair,"
and "Nails." Record how much time you spend over the course of one day on personal
grooming in these areas. How do these personal grooming habits affect your health?

**Washing your face regularly
keeps skin free of dirt,
bacteria, and perspiration.**
*How does keeping your
face and hands clean
affect your overall health?*

Beads of perspiration form on your f
exercising or when you are outside on
largest organ of your body, produces persp
keep your body cool. Skin is the main orga
system, which also includes hair, nails, an
skin. Your skin serves as a physical barri
world and your internal organs. It shields t
is the first line of defense against pathogen

Structure and Function of

The skin consists of two main layers, as
The **epidermis** is *the outer, thinner
composed of living and dead cells.* The **dermi**
*skin beneath the epidermis that is made up of a
tains blood vessels and nerves.*

The epidermis is composed of several
consists of dead cells that are constantly b
In the deeper layers of the epidermis, living
and replace dying cells, which are pushed t

**A diet rich in vitamin
A will contribute to healthy
skin.** *Which foods do you
enjoy that are a good
source of vitamin A?*

ducts to pores on the skin's surface, also are involved in temperature
regulation. Sweat glands produce perspiration on the surface of the
skin. Body heat is lost as the sweat evaporates.

Touch a hot stove, and your hand immediately pulls back. Why?
The skin is a major sense organ. Nerve cells in the dermis act as
receptors, which are stimulated by changes in the outside environment. These receptors enable you to feel sensa-
tions such as pressure, pain, hot, and cold.

Healthy Skin

Keeping your skin healthy should be an
important part of your daily routine.
Wash your face every morning and evening
with mild soap and water. Daily washing,
bathing, or showering helps remove and slow
the growth of bacteria that cause body odor.
Avoid touching your face with your hands.
This can introduce new bacteria to the skin's
surface. Carefully choose personal skin care
products, such as moisturizers, shaving cream, or
cosmetics, to help keep your skin from becoming
irritated or having an allergic reaction. Follow a well-balanced
diet that is rich in vitamins and minerals. Foods such as milk, green
and yellow vegetables, and liver are rich in vitamin A—a vitamin
that is particularly important for healthy skin.

Skin and the Sun

Understanding the effects of UV radiation on the skin and knowing some preventive behaviors can help you protect your skin now
and throughout your life. When skin is exposed to UV rays,
whether from the sun, a tanning booth, or another source, melanin
production is increased. This self-protective mechanism is the skin's
attempt to protect its cells from UV rays. Fair-skinned people whose
skin has little melanin, and thus little natural protection from UV
radiation, burn in the sun. People with more melanin will tan.

The symptoms of sunburn will disappear, and a tan will fade. The
long-term effects, however, are cumulative and the damage is permanent. UV rays damage the genetic material in skin cells and
cause it to undergo changes. These changes can eventually result in
the formation and growth of cancerous cells. Exposure to UV radiation is the leading cause of certain types of skin cancer. UV radiation
also breaks down the elastic fibers that support your skin and allow
it to be flexible yet retain its shape. The skin will become wrinkled
or hard and leathery with repeated exposure to UV radiation.

**What is UVA and
UVB radiation?**
Ultraviolet rays come in
different wavelengths—UVA
and UVB. UVB rays cause
most sunburn; thus, most
sunscreens block these rays.
However, UVA rays penetrate
the skin more deeply than
UVB, causing more damage.
Now that dermatologists
know about UVA, they
recommend sunscreens that
block both UVA and UVB rays.

CROSS-CURRICULUM CONNECTIONS

Create a Poem. Taking good care of your eyes, nose, skin, and teeth help you better appreciate your surroundings. Using a chart, make an account of details from a day you have spent at an event that appealed to your five senses. Then use some of these details to write an imagist poem, which is a poem that presents a picture in words.

Research Braille. Braille, a system using the sense of touch to read, helps visually impaired people function in the everyday world. Write a short research report on the recent progress to improve the quality of life of the visually impaired. Include information on groups such as the American Council of the Blind that have fought to improve conditions for the visually-impaired.

Measure the Speed of Sound. Your ears and brain can calculate the direction of a sound. If a man's head is 7 inches wide and the speed of sound at his location is 741.82 miles per hour, how much later, in seconds, does a sound coming from the right side reach the left ear? Hint: First convert inches to feet and miles/hour to feet/sec.

Examine Effects of Color Blindness. Research the various type of color blindness and their physiological causes. Locate illustrations depicting actual colors compared with those perceived by people with different types of color blindness to share with the class.

 CAREER Corner

Dental Hygienist

Regular dental care includes more than just seeing the dentist. Most dental offices rely on dental hygienists to provide some routine dental care. A dental hygienist can take your dental and medical history, clean your teeth, and teach you how to achieve and maintain good oral health.

To become a dental hygienist, you will need a high school diploma or its equivalent. Taking biology, chemistry, and math classes is recommended. After high school, hygienists complete a two-year training program in which they earn an Associate's degree. You can find out more about this and other health careers by clicking on Career Corner at **health.glencoe.com**.

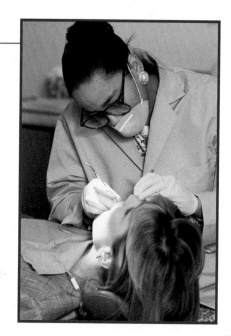

Chapter 14 *Review*

➤ EXPLORING HEALTH TERMS *Answer the following questions on a sheet of paper.*

Lesson 1 *Match each definition with the correct term.*

dermis   epidermis
dandruff   hair follicle
melanin   sebaceous glands
sweat glands   melanoma

1. A pigment that gives skin, hair, and eyes their color.
2. Structures within the skin that produce perspiration through ducts to pores on the skin's surface.
3. Structures within the skin that produce sebum.
4. A condition that can occur if the scalp becomes too dry and dead skin cells are shed as sticky, white flakes.

Lesson 2 *Replace the underlined words with the correct term.*

periodontium   pulp
tartar   plaque
periodontal disease

5. Tartar is a sticky, colorless film that acts on sugar to form acids that destroy tooth enamel and irritate gums.
6. Periodontium is completely preventable.

Lesson 3 *Fill in the blanks with the correct term.*

choroid   cornea
lacrimal gland   retina
sclera

The outer layer of the eyewall consists of the (_7_), the white part of the eye, and the (_8_), the transparent tissue in the front of the eye. The (_9_) is the inner layer of the eyewall.

Lesson 4 *Match each definition with the correct term.*

auditory ossicles   labyrinth
external auditory canal   tinnitus

10. A passageway in the outer ear that leads to the eardrum.
11. Three small bones in the middle ear.
12. Another name for the inner ear.

➤ RECALLING THE FACTS *Use complete sentences to answer the following questions.*

Lesson 1

1. Explain how the skin protects your body.
2. List three steps you can take to keep your skin healthy.
3. Why may getting a tattoo be hazardous to your health?

Lesson 2

4. Name two functions of the teeth.
5. How do the foods you eat and your eating habits affect the health of your teeth?
6. List three strategies for reducing bad breath.

Lesson 3

7. How do the lacrimal glands contribute to the health of your eye?
8. Explain how the iris and pupil regulate the amount of light entering the inner eye.
9. Describe what 20/60 vision means.

Lesson 4

10. What is the function of the eustachian tube?

11. List two actions you can take to keep your ears healthy.

12. What are three causes of hearing loss?

➤ THINKING CRITICALLY

1. **Applying.** What strategies can you use to keep track of changes in the appearance of moles on your skin? *(LESSON 1)*

2. **Analyzing.** How could having advanced stages of periodontal disease affect other areas of your life? *(LESSON 2)*

3. **Evaluating.** Resting the eyes while reading or working on the computer can help reduce eyestrain. During which other activities should you periodically rest your eyes? *(LESSON 3)*

4. **Applying.** You have developed an ear infection from swimming. Examine the effects of health behaviors on the health of the ears. What precautions could you take to prevent reinfection? *(LESSON 4)*

➤ HEALTH SKILLS APPLICATION

1. **Communicating.** A young child refuses to have a bath or wash his or her hair. How can you encourage him or her to change this behavior? *(LESSON 1)*

2. **Goal Setting.** Set a goal to brush and floss your teeth every morning and every evening. Use the goal-setting steps to help you identify behaviors that will help you meet this goal. *(LESSON 2)*

3. **Accessing Information.** Imagine that you have just been told that you need corrective lenses. Research the advantages and disadvantages of glasses and contact lenses. Make a chart that lists the pros and cons of each. Use this information along with the decision-making steps to determine which you would prefer. *(LESSON 3)*

4. **Communicating.** You suspect that a close family member is experiencing hearing loss, but he or she is not asking for help. What clues might make you think this is the case? How can you talk to this person about what is happening? *(LESSON 4)*

BEYOND the Classroom

Parent Involvement

Advocacy. With a parent or guardian, learn more about the services available for hearing-impaired individuals in your community. Are there any services that are unavailable in your community? Discuss with family members the possible reasons for this lack. What can you do to raise awareness about services for the hearing impaired?

School and Community

Volunteering. Locate an agency that works with individuals with hearing or sight impairments. Ask whether there are any opportunities for volunteer work within the agency. Report to your class on what you have learned.

Skeletal, Muscular, and Nervous Systems

Lesson 3

7. Describe the functions of the muscular system.

8. Examine the effects of health behaviors on the muscular system. Why is good posture important to the health of your muscles?

9. What is muscular dystrophy?

Lesson 4

10. What natural protective mechanisms exist in the body for the brain and spinal cord?

11. Identify and describe the three parts of the brain stem.

12. Explain the difference between the autonomic nervous system and the somatic nervous system.

Lesson 5

13. Examine the effects of health behaviors, and name three ways to prevent spinal cord injury.

14. What are some symptoms that result from neuron damage caused by Alzheimer's disease?

15. What is quadriplegia? What is paraplegia?

16. What is a degenerative disease?

17. Compare and contrast Parkinson's disease and Alzheimer's disease.

► THINKING CRITICALLY

1. **Evaluating.** Describe what lifestyle choices you can make to protect your bones and skeletal system from damage or injury. *(LESSON 1)*

2. **Analyzing.** Although some bone and joint problems, such as osteoporosis and arthritis, seldom occur until later in life, why is it important to think about these conditions now? *(LESSON 2)*

3. **Applying.** What advantage is involuntary muscle control to processes such as the contraction of the heart and the movement of food through the digestive tract? *(LESSON 3)*

4. **Synthesizing.** After you run, your heart rate slows. Which parts of your nervous system are involved in this function? *(LESSON 4)*

5. **Evaluating.** How can swelling of the brain or spinal cord result in damage to these tissues? *(LESSON 5)*

► HEALTH SKILLS APPLICATION

1. **Communicating.** Your younger brother loves to in-line skate. However, he never wears protective gear while skating. List some strategies you can use to teach him about the importance of preventing injury and encourage him to change his behavior. *(LESSON 1)*

2. **Advocacy.** Find out how often screening for scoliosis is offered in your community. To which age groups does it apply? Is there a cost? Raise community awareness by making and displaying a poster that advertises the next screening. *(LESSON 2)*

3. **Analyzing Influences.** A healthy muscular system depends on physical activity. Even when people are aware of this connection, they may fail to get the physical activity they need. List factors that may positively influence someone's decision to engage in physical activity. *(LESSON 3)*

4. **Accessing Information.** Use the Internet to find brain images made with Positron Emission Tomography (PET) scanners. Compare images of drug users' brains to those of individuals who have never used drugs. How could you use these images to explain the effects of drug use on the nervous system? *(LESSON 4)*

5. **Refusal Skills.** Alicia and her friends are exploring a lake in which they have not swum before. Someone spots a rock beneath the water's surface but suggests that it is probably safe to dive anyway. Write a dialogue between Alicia and her friends, demonstrating how she refuses to take this unnecessary risk. *(LESSON 5)*

Chapter 16

Cardiovascular and Respiratory Systems

Lesson 1

The Cardiovascular System

Lesson 2

Care and Problems of the Cardiovascular System

Lesson 3

The Respiratory System

Lesson 4

Care and Problems of the Respiratory System

What's Your Health Status?

Read each statement below and respond by writing *yes, no,* or *sometimes* for each item. Write *yes* only for items that you practice regularly.

1. I eat a well-balanced diet that is low in saturated fat, salt, and cholesterol.

2. I maintain a weight appropriate for my height.

3. I participate in aerobic physical activity at least three times a week for at least 30 minutes at a time.

4. I do not smoke or use tobacco products.

5. I eat foods that are high in iron, such as dark green leafy vegetables, dried fruits, and fortified cereals, every day.

6. I wash my hands regularly to reduce the risk of communicable disease.

7. I limit my exposure to pollutants in the air, including tobacco smoke.

8. I study, work, and exercise in well-ventilated areas.

9. I get at least eight to ten hours of sleep each night.

10. I get regular medical checkups that include monitoring the health of my cardiovascular and respiratory systems.

HEALTH Online

For instant feedback on your health status, go to Chapter 16 Health Inventory at **health.glencoe.com**.

Quick *Write*

Using Visuals. Write a short paragraph describing how the cardiovascular and respiratory systems are important for participation in active sports. How might a respiratory condition such as asthma affect a person's ability to participate?

The Cardiovascular System

VOCABULARY

plasma
hemoglobin
arteries
capillaries
veins
platelets
lymph
lymphocytes

YOU'LL LEARN TO

• Identify the functions and structures of the cardiovascular system.

• Describe the circulation of blood throughout the heart and body.

• Identify the structures and functions of the lymphatic system.

• Recognize how knowledge of the cardiovascular system is important for maintaining personal and family health.

⟶ **QUICK START** Use a digital timer or the second hand on a watch to take your pulse for 60 seconds. Use this number to calculate how many times your heart beats in 24 hours. What can cause your heart rate to increase or decrease?

When you look at a road map, you see a series of interconnected roads—some small, others large—that connect cities and towns. Vital goods are transported into and out of central areas on these roads. Similarly, your cardiovascular system consists of vessels, both large and small, that transport life-supporting materials to cells of your body. Your heart, one of the main organs of your cardiovascular system, is the central point from which these vessels branch.

Functions of the Cardiovascular System

The cardiovascular system is composed of the heart and all the blood vessels of the body. Its function is to circulate blood, thereby maintaining an internal environment in which all the cells of your body are nourished. As your heart pumps blood, blood vessels carry oxygen and nutrients to body cells. At the same time, carbon dioxide is carried, along with waste matter, from your cells. Oxygen is delivered to your lungs and waste products to the kidneys for removal from the body.

🅐 **Any physical activity that raises your heart rate will help strengthen your cardiovascular system.** *What is the main function of the cardiovascular system?*

Structure of the Cardiovascular System

The cardiovascular system consists of the heart; blood; and blood vessels, including arteries, capillaries, and veins, which transport blood throughout the body.

The Heart

The heart and the brain are perhaps the most important organs in your body. Your heart is the pump that makes the cardiovascular system work. It never rests. Most of the heart is made of muscle tissue called the myocardium, which contracts and relaxes constantly and rhythmically. Your heart rate adjusts automatically in response to an increase or decrease in physical activity. In an average life span, a person's heart beats more than 2.5 billion times.

CHAMBERS OF THE HEART

Inside the heart are four chambers. Each of the two smaller chambers is called an *atrium*. The two lower, larger chambers are called *ventricles*. A wall of tissue called the *septum* separates the right and left atria, as well as the right and left ventricles, from one another.

At the top of the right atrium is an area of muscle that acts as a natural pacemaker for the rest of the heart. Regular electrical impulses generated from this area stimulate the muscles of each atrium to contract, forcing blood into the ventricles. Within milliseconds each electrical impulse travels through the heart to an area between the two ventricles. There it stimulates the muscles of the ventricles to contract, pumping blood out of the heart.

Valves between the atria and ventricles allow blood to flow through the chambers of the heart. These valves are "one-way" valves, opening to allow blood to flow from the atria into the ventricles. When the ventricles contract, the valves close again to keep blood from flowing back into the atria. The sounds heard as the heart beats are produced by the closing of the valves.

CIRCULATION IN THE HEART

The circulation of blood through the heart and lungs is shown in **Figure 16.1** on page 418. Blood that has been depleted of oxygen but contains carbon dioxide and waste matter is carried to the heart by two large blood vessels called the *vena cava*. This deoxygenated blood enters the right atrium and is transferred to the right ventricle. The blood is then pumped to the lungs. In the lungs the blood releases carbon dioxide and picks up oxygen from inhaled air. This newly oxygenated blood is returned from the lungs to the left atrium of the heart. The left atrium pumps the oxygenated blood into the left ventricle, which then pumps the blood out of the heart to the rest of the body by way of a large artery called the aorta.

Health Minute

Get the Most from Your Physical Activity

Aerobic activities can reduce your risk of developing cardiovascular diseases later in life.

Exercising within your target heart range:

▶ Sit quietly for five minutes, and then take your pulse. This is your resting heart rate.

▶ Subtract your age from the number 220 to find your maximum heart rate.

▶ Subtract your resting heart rate from your maximum heart rate.

▶ Multiply the number you arrived at by 60 percent and again by 85 percent. Round off these numbers.

▶ Add your resting heart rate to the numbers you just calculated. These two new numbers represent your target heart range.

FIGURE **16.1**

PULMONARY CIRCULATION

The circulation of the blood between the heart and lungs is called pulmonary circulation.

right lung
pulmonary artery
superior vena cava
capillaries
pulmonary veins
right atrium
right ventricle
inferior vena cava

left lung
pulmonary artery
aorta
left atrium
left ventricle

What is blood type?

There are four blood types: A, B, AB, and O. Blood type is determined by the presence or absence of certain substances, called antigens, that stimulate an immune response. Type A has antigen A, type B has antigen B, type AB has both those antigens, and type O has neither. Most blood also carries another substance called the Rh factor. Blood that doesn't have the Rh factor is called *Rh negative.*

Blood

Blood delivers oxygen, hormones, and nutrients to the cells and carries away wastes that the cells produce. About 55 percent of total blood volume consists of **plasma**, *the fluid in which other parts of the blood are suspended.* Plasma, which is mostly water, contains nutrients, proteins, salts, and hormones. Red blood cells make up about 40 percent of blood. White blood cells and platelets together make up the remaining 5 percent of blood. One milliliter of blood contains millions of each of these types of cells.

RED BLOOD CELLS AND WHITE BLOOD CELLS

Red blood cells transport oxygen to the cells and tissues of the body. Formed in bone marrow, red blood cells contain hemoglobin. **Hemoglobin** is *the oxygen-carrying protein in blood.* Hemoglobin contains iron that binds with oxygen in the lungs and releases the oxygen in the tissues. Hemoglobin also combines with carbon dioxide, which is carried from the cells to the lungs.

The main role of white blood cells is to protect the body against infection and fight infection when it occurs. White blood cells, which are part of the body's immune system, are also produced in bone marrow. Production of these cells increases when an infection is present. Some white blood cells surround and ingest disease-causing microbes. Others are involved in allergic reactions. A third type of white blood cell forms antibodies that provide immunity.

Blood Vessels

The network of more than 60,000 miles of blood vessels that transports blood is shown in **Figure 16.2** on page 420. There are three main types of blood vessels: arteries, capillaries, and veins.

ARTERIES

The *blood vessels that carry blood away from the heart* are called **arteries**. Arteries have thick elastic walls that contain smooth muscle fibers. The elastic fibers in the walls of arteries allow them to withstand the pressure exerted by the blood as the heart beats.

Pulmonary arteries carry deoxygenated blood from the right ventricle to the lungs. Systemic arteries, such as the aorta, carry oxygenated blood from the left ventricle to all areas of the body. As arteries move away from the heart, they branch into progressively smaller vessels called *arterioles*. Arterioles deliver blood to capillaries.

CAPILLARIES

Capillaries are *small vessels that carry blood between arterioles and small vessels called venules*. Capillaries form an extensive network throughout tissues and organs in the body, reaching almost all body cells. The exchange of gases, nutrients, and wastes between blood and cells takes place through the ultra-thin walls of capillaries. Capillaries also play a role in body temperature regulation. As body temperature rises, capillaries near the skin's surface dilate, allowing heat to escape the body through the skin. If body temperature begins to drop below normal, the capillaries constrict, reducing heat loss.

 The blood regulates body temperature. *Explain how these swimmers' bodies adjust to cold water temperature.*

VEINS

The *blood vessels that return blood to the heart* are called **veins**. Although the walls of veins are thinner and less elastic than those of arteries, veins are still able to withstand the pressure exerted by blood as it flows through them. The large veins called the *vena cava* carry deoxygenated blood from the body to the right atrium of the heart. Pulmonary veins carry oxygenated blood from the lungs to the left atrium. Many veins throughout the body, especially those in the legs, have valves that help prevent the backflow of blood as it is pumped under lower pressure back to the heart. Pressure on the vessel walls from the contraction of surrounding muscles helps move blood through the veins. The venules collect blood from capillaries and empty it into larger veins.

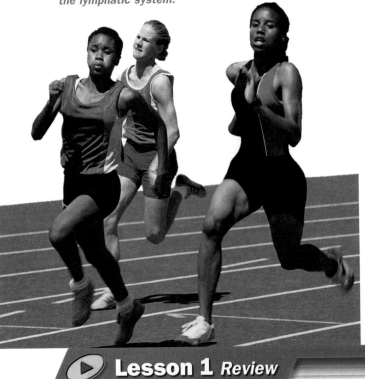

V Lymph is moved through the body by the contraction of skeletal muscles during physical activity. *Name the structures of the lymphatic system.*

Structure of the Lymphatic System

The lymphatic system consists of a network of vessels and tissues that are involved in the movement and filtering of lymph. Much like the capillaries and arterioles in the cardiovascular system, small lymph vessels collect lymph and combine to form larger vessels. Lymph is moved toward the heart both by the contraction of smooth muscles that line the walls of lymph vessels and by the contraction of surrounding skeletal muscles.

Two large lymphatic ducts empty lymph into veins close to the heart, where it is returned to the blood. As it is moved through the body, lymph is filtered by lymph nodes, small, bean-shaped organs that are found in lymph vessels. White blood cells within lymph nodes trap and destroy foreign organisms such as bacteria and viruses to keep them from spreading throughout the body. Other structures of the lymphatic system include the spleen, thymus gland, and tonsils, all of which play a role in immunity, protecting the body from infection.

▶ Lesson 1 *Review*

Reviewing Facts and Vocabulary

1. What are the functions of the cardiovascular system?
2. Describe the functions of arteries, capillaries, and veins.
3. Define *lymph* and *lymphocytes.*

Thinking Critically

4. **Comparing and Contrasting.** Compare and contrast the lymphatic and cardiovascular systems.
5. **Evaluating.** What might swollen lymph nodes indicate?

Applying Health Skills

Advocacy. Research and demonstrate knowledge about behaviors that benefit personal and family health. Examine the effects of sedentary behavior on the cardiovascular system. Create an informative brochure about the relationship between an active lifestyle and a healthy heart. Share the brochure with your family.

TECHNOLOGY *OPTION*

INTERNET RESOURCES Use information and links found at **health.glencoe.com** to help with your research.

Care and Problems of the Cardiovascular System

VOCABULARY
blood pressure
congenital
anemia
leukemia
Hodgkin's disease

YOU'LL LEARN TO
- Analyze the relationship between health promotion and the prevention of cardiovascular disease.
- Examine the effects of health behaviors on the cardiovascular and lymphatic systems.
- Relate the importance of early detection and warning signs that prompt individuals of all ages to seek health care.

QUICK START Think about the last time you were examined by a medical professional. Which parts of the examination focused on the health of your cardiovascular and lymphatic systems?

Most problems of the cardiovascular and lymphatic systems can be prevented with proper care and by healthy decisions you make during your teen years. These involve physical activity, adequate rest, proper diet, and regular medical checkups. Some problems may be hereditary. If you know that heart disease runs in your family or if you have other traits that may lead to heart disease, you need to make careful choices now to promote a lifetime of cardiovascular health.

Health Behaviors and the Cardiovascular and Lymphatic Systems

Healthful habits can help reduce many of the risk factors associated with problems of the cardiovascular and lymphatic systems. Here are some healthful behaviors that should become part of your life.

These coronary arteries are partially blocked. Blood supply to the heart is reduced if blood cannot flow through arteries. *What health behaviors will help you avoid cardiovascular system problems?*

hot link

cholesterol For more information on heart disease and cholesterol, see Chapter 26, page 675.

illegal drugs For more information about how illegal drugs can damage the cardiovascular system, see Chapter 23, page 594.

▼ **Medical professionals check your heart and blood pressure during regular medical examinations.** *What measurements are taken during blood pressure readings?*

▶ Follow a well-balanced diet that is low in saturated fats, **cholesterol,** and salt.

▶ Maintain a healthy weight to reduce stress on the heart, blood vessels, and lymph vessels.

▶ Participate in regular aerobic exercise for at least 30 minutes three to four times per week.

▶ Avoid the use of tobacco products and exposure to secondhand tobacco smoke.

▶ Avoid **illegal drugs,** including stimulants, marijuana, and Ecstasy (MDMA).

Blood Pressure

Maintaining pressure in the cardiovascular system is important for proper blood circulation. Pressure in arteries is created as the ventricles contract. As blood is forced into the arteries that exit the heart, arterial walls stretch under the increased pressure. When the ventricles relax and refill with blood, arterial pressure decreases. **Blood pressure** is *a measure of the amount of force that the blood places on the walls of blood vessels, particularly large arteries, as it is pumped through the body.*

Blood pressure can be measured with an instrument called a sphygmomanometer (sfig-mo-muh-NAH-muh-ter) and a stethoscope. A cuff is placed around the upper arm and inflated until the pressure from the cuff blocks the flow of blood. As the cuff is deflated, the health care professional listens through the stethoscope for blood flow. As your heart contracts to push blood into your arteries, the maximum pressure, called *systolic* pressure, is measured. This is recorded as the upper number of the fraction representing your blood pressure. As the ventricles relax to refill, blood pressure is at its lowest point, called the *diastolic* pressure. This is the lower number of the fraction in a blood pressure reading.

Blood pressure is an indicator of cardiovascular health. Although a healthy person's blood pressure will vary with physical activity or emotional stress, it should remain within a normal range. Blood pressure above 140/90 is considered high, and if chronic, places a strain on the heart as it pumps. Chronic high blood pressure is associated with several cardiovascular system problems including hardening of the arteries and heart attacks. Prevention of high blood pressure includes maintaining a healthy weight, staying physically active, managing stress, avoiding tobacco and drugs, and following a **healthful eating plan** that is low in salt.

hot link

healthful eating plan For more information on eating right for cardiovascular health, see Chapter 5, page 113.

Sinusitis

An inflammation of the tissues that line the sinuses, air-filled cavities above the nasal passages and throat, is called **sinusitis**. Symptoms include nasal congestion, headache, and fever. Treatment includes nasal decongestant drops or sprays and antibiotics.

Tuberculosis

Tuberculosis is *a contagious bacterial infection that usually affects the lungs.* When a person is infected with tuberculosis, the immune system surrounds the infected area and isolates it. In this inactive stage, symptoms do not appear. This stage can last for many years. If the immune system is weakened by illness or advancing age, the infection can become active. Symptoms of active tuberculosis include cough, fever, fatigue, and weight loss. Treatment involves antibiotics and hospitalization. Numbers of reported cases of tuberculosis have increased in the United States in recent years.

Emphysema

Emphysema is *a disease that progressively destroys the walls of the alveoli.* Symptoms include difficulty breathing and chronic cough. Although the symptoms of emphysema can be treated, tissue damage is irreversible. Eventually the lungs cease to function. Emphysema is almost always caused by smoking.

 Anti-inflammatory medications keep bronchial tubes open and reduce swelling to help control asthma before an attack. *What other treatment can be used to relieve symptoms during an asthma attack?*

 Lesson 4 *Review*

Reviewing Facts and Vocabulary

1. Explain the effects of smoking on the health of the respiratory system.
2. Define *bronchitis* and describe its symptoms.
3. List three things you can do to help keep your respiratory system healthy.

Thinking Critically

4. **Applying.** Your friend is having trouble with shortness of breath during everyday activities. How can you encourage him or her to be examined by a health care professional?
5. **Analyzing.** Why is early detection important in the treatment of respiratory disorders?

Applying Health Skills

Accessing Information. Analyze the relationship between health promotion and the prevention of respiratory system disorders. Draw a diagram of the respiratory system, and label each part with health behaviors that will help teens avoid respiratory problems.

INTERNET RESOURCES Find information on the Internet about smoking and its effects by visiting Web links at **health.glencoe.com.**

Healthy Hearts and Lungs Week

Health advocacy organizations use special events and the media to promote awareness of their programs. For instance, the American Heart℠ Walk, a noncompetitive walking event, promotes awareness of and raises funds for the American Heart Association. Use the activity below to explore the media outlets available in your school, and plan a variety of events for a "Healthy Hearts and Lungs Week."

ACTIVITY

As a class, brainstorm a list of the media outlets available in your school, such as a public announcement (PA) system, bulletin boards, school newspapers, and school sporting events. Work in groups to create a project or an event that promotes awareness of heart and lung health issues, using the media assigned to you. For instance, one group might write short tips on heart and lung health to be read over the PA system during morning announcements. Another group might create fact sheets on asthma and allergies and distribute them at school sporting events. Be creative in your use of the media and how you present the information.

EXPRESS YOUR VIEWS

Research local events such as the American Heart℠ Walk or the American Lung Association's Christmas Seals® program. Then write an open letter to the student body, promoting these charitable events. Include information on upcoming local events, and encourage fellow students to get involved.

CROSS-CURRICULUM CONNECTIONS

Writing a Heartbeat Poem. The steady thump of a beating heart and the rhythm of pumping lungs often take on symbolic meaning. For example, in Edgar Allan Poe's "The Tell-Tale Heart," the beating heart represents the narrator's guilty conscience. Write a poem using either a heartbeat or a breathing rhythm to symbolize something other than itself. Use rhyme or rhythm to suggest the sound of a beating heart or the illusion of someone's breathing in your poem.

Measuring Gallons of Blood. Assume that the average human heart rate is 72 beats per minute. If the average human heart pumps 4,300 gallons of blood per day, how many gallons of blood does the heart pump every time it beats?

Researching Organ Transplants. Every 27 minutes someone in the world receives an organ transplant. The first lung and heart transplants were performed in the 1960s. Research and report on the development of either heart or lung transplants over the last four decades. Include information on legislation that affects transplants, such as the National Organ Transplant Act.

Examining Sound Physics. The lungs are the primary organs used to produce sound. Whether you are whispering, singing, shouting, or humming, control of the flow of air from the lungs is essential. Research the physics of vocal sound production, and list or diagram the various muscles and body structures that produce and shape sounds.

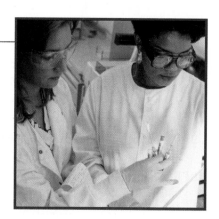

Medical Laboratory Technician

If you are interested in biology, chemistry, math, and computer science, and if you enjoy working in the laboratory, consider a career as a medical laboratory technician (MLT). MLTs discover information about a patient's health by analyzing tissue samples and using the latest laboratory technology and techniques.

To become an MLT, you need a high school diploma or its equivalent to enter a college-level course of study. Successful completion of an associate's degree program and a national certification exam are required for employment. You can find out more about this and other health careers by clicking on Career Corner at **health.glencoe.com**.

► **EXPLORING HEALTH TERMS** *Answer the following questions on a sheet of paper.*

Match each definition with the correct term.

arteries	lymphocytes
capillaries	plasma
hemoglobin	platelets
lymph	veins

1. The fluid in which other parts of the blood are suspended.
2. The oxygen-carrying protein in blood.
3. Cells that prevent the body's loss of blood.
4. Blood vessels that carry blood to the heart.

Lesson 2 *Identify each statement as True or False. If false, replace the underlined term with the correct term.*

anemia	Hodgkin's disease
blood pressure	leukemia
congenital	

5. Leukemia is a condition in which the ability of the blood to carry oxygen is reduced.
6. A congenital condition is present at birth.
7. Anemia is a type of cancer that affects the lymphatic system.

Lesson 3 *Replace the underlined words with the correct term.*

bronchi	pharynx
diaphragm	respiration
larynx	trachea

8. The exchange of gases between the body and the environment is known as bronchi.
9. The pharynx is a muscle that separates the chest from the abdominal cavity.
10. The diaphragm are airways that connect the trachea and the lungs.
11. The windpipe is also referred to as the pharynx.
12. The voice box is the trachea.

Lesson 4 *Match each definition with the correct term.*

asthma	pneumonia
bronchitis	sinusitis
emphysema	tuberculosis
pleurisy	

13. An inflammation of the lungs commonly caused by a bacterial or viral infection.
14. An inflammatory condition in which the trachea, bronchi, and bronchioles become narrowed, causing difficulty breathing.
15. An inflammation of the lining of the lungs and chest cavity.

► **RECALLING THE FACTS** *Use complete sentences to answer the following questions.*

Lesson 1

1. Compare and contrast red blood cells, white blood cells, and platelets.
2. Differentiate between B cells and T cells.
3. What is the purpose of the lymphatic system?

Lesson 2

4. What are some possible causes of congenital heart disease?
5. What causes anemia, and how can it be avoided?
6. What can cause a deficiency of the immune system?

Lesson 3

7. What is the difference between external and internal respiration?
8. Explain how the process of breathing occurs.
9. What is the function of the epiglottis?

Lesson 4

10. How is physical activity related to the health of your respiratory system?

11. What is pneumonia? What causes it?

12. What effects does emphysema have on the respiratory system?

➤ THINKING CRITICALLY

1. **Analyzing.** How would the improper functioning of the valve between the left atrium and ventricle affect the movement of blood through this area of the heart? *(LESSON 1)*

2. **Analyzing.** How could having hemophilia affect a person's everyday activities? *(LESSON 2)*

3. **Synthesizing.** Describe the process of respiration, including both internal and external respiration. Identify each body structure involved, and explain how these work together in respiration. *(LESSON 3)*

4. **Evaluating.** Review the information provided for each respiratory disease. How many of the diseases are linked to smoking? How can you use this information to persuade a family member not to smoke? *(LESSON 4)*

➤ HEALTH SKILLS APPLICATION

1. **Analyzing Influences.** Explain the effect technology has had on cardiovascular health. Evaluate both the positive and negative effects of technologies such as the automobile, elevators, and medical equipment. *(LESSON 1)*

2. **Decision Making.** You are sick with tonsillitis and your friends want you to go hiking. Your doctor has advised you to avoid physical activity and get plenty of rest. Using the steps in the decision-making process, role-play with a friend how you will make your decision. *(LESSON 2)*

3. **Accessing Information.** Find information about abdominal thrusts. Why is it important to properly perform this maneuver? What agencies in your community offer training in first aid for choking? *(LESSON 3)*

4. **Advocacy.** An antibiotic-resistant strain of tuberculosis is increasing in frequency in the United States. Find out how often testing for tuberculosis is offered in your community. For which age groups does it apply? Is there a cost? Raise community awareness by making a poster that encourages individuals to get tested. *(LESSON 4)*

BEYOND the Classroom

Parent Involvement

Practicing Healthful Behaviors.
Brainstorm with parents or guardians ways your family can practice healthful behaviors to maintain the health of your cardiovascular and respiratory systems. Find ways to incorporate low-fat, low-cholesterol foods, including fresh fruits, into your family's daily eating plan.

School and Community

A Smoke-Free Community. Find information about the Great American Smoke Out. What does your community do to participate in this event? Share the information you learn with your classmates, and brainstorm ideas about how your school can become involved with this event.

Digestive and Urinary Systems

What's Your Health Status?

Read each statement below and respond by writing *yes, no,* or *some-times* for each item. Write *yes* only for items that you are sure of.

1. I understand how hormones affect my body during adolescence and adulthood.

2. I eat a well-balanced diet.

3. I include physical activity in my daily routine.

4. I have regular medical checkups.

5. For males: I do a monthly testicular self-exam.

6. For females: I do a monthly breast self-exam.

7. I follow strategies for practicing abstinence.

8. I avoid situations that might put me at risk of contracting STDs.

9. For males: I wear a protective cup or supporter when participating in sports or a strenuous physical activity.

10. For females: I avoid the use of feminine products such as douches and sprays.

HEALTH *Online*

For instant feedback on your health status, go to Chapter 18 Health Inventory at **health.glencoe.com.**

Quick **Write**

Using Visuals. Many changes take place during the teen years. Some of these changes are controlled by hormones produced by the endocrine system. Describe how the endocrine and reproductive systems are related.

The Endocrine System

VOCABULARY

endocrine glands
hormones
thyroid gland
parathyroid glands
pancreas
pituitary gland
gonads
adrenal glands

YOU'LL LEARN TO

- Identify the glands of the endocrine system and explain the function of each.

- Examine the effects of health behaviors on the endocrine system.

- Appraise the significance of body changes during adolescence.

QUICK START *Endo* means "within" and *crine* means "to separate." How does this information help you understand one of the characteristics of the endocrine system?

When the brain recognizes a stressful situation, the endocrine system reacts by releasing the hormone adrenaline. *How do these changes help prepare the body to react under stress?*

All the cells in your body respond to messages sent by three of your major body systems—the nervous system, the immune system, and the endocrine system. These three systems work closely together to coordinate the functions of the body. The endocrine system is especially important during the teen years because one of its main functions is to regulate growth and development.

Structure of the Endocrine System

The endocrine system consists of a network of endocrine glands located throughout the body. **Endocrine glands** are *ductless—or tubeless—organs or groups of cells that secrete hormones directly into the bloodstream.* **Hormones** are *chemical substances that are produced in glands and help regulate many of your body's functions.* Hormones are secreted by the endocrine glands and then carried to their destinations in the body by the blood. These chemical messengers influence physical and mental responses. Hormones produced during puberty trigger physical changes in the body. **Figure 18.1** describes the major glands of the endocrine system and the body functions they regulate.

FIGURE 18.1

THE ENDOCRINE SYSTEM

The glands of the endocrine system are located throughout the body. Each gland has at least one particular function.

Thyroid The **thyroid gland** *produces hormones that regulate metabolism, body heat, and bone growth.* The thyroid produces thyroxine, which regulates the way cells release energy from nutrients.

Parathyroid Glands The **parathyroid glands** *produce a hormone that regulates the body's calcium and phosphorus balance.*

Testes The testes are the male reproductive glands.

Ovaries The ovaries are the female reproductive glands.

Besides playing a role in reproduction (as described in Lessons 2 and 3), the testes and ovaries control the development of secondary sex characteristics during puberty.

Hypothalamus The hypothalamus links the endocrine system with the nervous system and stimulates the pituitary gland to secrete hormones.

Pineal Gland This gland secretes melatonin, which regulates sleep cycles and is thought to affect the onset of puberty.

Pituitary Gland The pituitary regulates and controls activities of other endocrine glands.

Thymus Gland The thymus regulates development of the immune system.

Adrenal Glands These glands produce hormones that regulate the body's salt and water balance. Secretions from the adrenal cortex and the adrenal medulla control the body's emergency response.

Pancreas The **pancreas** is *a gland that serves both the digestive and the endocrine systems.* As an endocrine gland, the pancreas secretes two hormones that regulate the level of glucose in the blood—glucagon and insulin.

Pituitary Gland

The **pituitary gland** *regulates and controls the activities of all of the other endocrine glands.* The pituitary is known as the master gland. It has three sections, or lobes—anterior, intermediate, and posterior.

▶ **Anterior lobe.** The anterior, or front, lobe of the pituitary gland produces six hormones. Somatotropic, or growth, hormone stimulates normal body growth and development by altering chemical activity in body cells. Thyroid-stimulating hormone (TSH) stimulates the thyroid gland to produce hormones. Adrenocorticotropic (uh-DREE-noh-kawr-ti-koh-TROH-pik) hormone (ACTH) stimulates production of hormones in the adrenal glands.

Two hormones that stimulate production of all other sex hormones are secreted by the pituitary's anterior lobe during adolescence. Follicle-stimulating hormone (FSH) and luteinizing hormone (LH) control the growth, development, and functions of the **gonads**, another name for *the ovaries and testes*.

- In females, FSH stimulates cells in the ovaries to produce estrogen, a female sex hormone that triggers the development of ova. LH is responsible for ovulation and stimulates ovarian cells to produce progesterone. The hormone prolactin stimulates milk production in females who have given birth.

- In males LH stimulates cells in the testes to produce the male hormone testosterone. FSH controls the production of sperm.

▶ **Intermediate lobe.** The intermediate, or middle, lobe of the pituitary secretes melanocyte-stimulating hormone (MSH), which controls the darkening of the skin by stimulating skin pigments.

▶ **Posterior lobe.** The posterior, or rear, lobe of the pituitary gland secretes antidiuretic hormone (ADH), which regulates the balance of water in the body. ADH also produces oxytocin, which stimulates uterine contractions during the birth of a baby.

Adrenal Glands

The **adrenal glands** are *glands that help the body recover from stress and respond to emergencies*. They each have two parts.

▶ The **adrenal cortex** secretes a hormone that inhibits the amount of sodium excreted in urine and serves to maintain blood volume and pressure. It also secretes hormones that aid the metabolism of fats, proteins, and carbohydrates. These hormones play a role in immunity and the body's response to stress.

▶ The **adrenal medulla** is controlled by the hypothalamus and the autonomic nervous system. It secretes the hormones epinephrine (also called adrenaline) and norepinephrine. Epinephrine increases heartbeat and respiration, raises blood pressure, and suppresses the digestive process during periods of high emotion.

Problems of the Endocrine System

Factors such as stress, infection, and changes in the balance of fluid and minerals in the blood can cause hormone levels to vary. Often these situations will correct themselves. More serious problems, including those described here, may require medication.

▶ **Diabetes mellitus** is a disorder in which the pancreas produces too little or no insulin, resulting in high blood glucose levels. Symptoms include fatigue, weight loss, thirst, and frequent urination.

Ⓐ **Hormones produced by the pituitary gland play a role in determining height.**
Locate the pituitary gland in Figure 18.1. Name two other important functions of the pituitary gland.

HEALTH Online

Review the vocabulary for this lesson. Play the Chapter 18 concentration game at health.glencoe.com.

hotlink

diabetes For more information on different types of diabetes and the risk factors for this disease, see Chapter 26, page 691.

- **Graves' disease,** also called *hyperthyroidism,* is a disorder in which an overactive and enlarged thyroid gland produces excessive amounts of thyroxine. Symptoms include nervousness, weight loss, increased thirst, rapid heartbeat, and intolerance for heat. Low thyroxine production, called *hypothyroidism,* causes fatigue, dry skin, weight gain, constipation, and sensitivity to cold.

- **Cushing's disease** results from the overproduction of adrenal hormones. Symptoms include round face, humped upper back, thin and easily bruised skin, and fragile bones.

- **Goiter,** an enlargement of the thyroid gland, is caused mainly by a lack of iodine in the diet. Since the introduction of iodized salt, goiters have become rare in the United States.

- **Growth disorders** are caused by abnormal amounts of growth hormone. With early diagnosis and proper treatment, a child with a growth disorder can reach a normal height.

Care of the Endocrine System

To keep your endocrine system functioning at peak performance, take care of all of your body systems. Eat nutritious meals, get enough sleep, and avoid stress. A health care professional can perform medical tests to determine whether your endocrine function is normal.

Staying physically active is one way of reducing stress and keeping your endocrine system healthy. *What other healthy behaviors help ensure the health of this system?*

Lesson 1 *Review*

Reviewing Facts and Vocabulary

1. What is an *endocrine gland*?
2. What are the two parts of the adrenal glands, and what do they do?
3. What are the functions of FSH and LH?

Thinking Critically

4. **Evaluating.** Do you agree with the statement that the pituitary gland is the "master gland"? Explain your reasoning.
5. **Analyzing.** Which endocrine glands become more active during puberty? Name the hormones these glands produce, and appraise their effects on changes in the body during adolescence.

Applying Health Skills

Self Management. On a sheet of paper, write the names of two endocrine glands. List one important function of each gland. Then write a statement examining the effects of health behaviors on the endocrine system.

TECHNOLOGY *OPTION*

WORD PROCESSING Use the bullet feature of your word-processing program to make your list. For help with word-processing software, go to health.glencoe.com.

The Male Reproductive System

VOCABULARY

reproductive system
sperm
testosterone
testes
scrotum
penis
semen
sterility

YOU'LL LEARN TO

• Describe the parts of the male reproductive system and explain the function of each part.

• Relate the importance of early detection and warning signs that prompt males of all ages to seek health care for the male reproductive system.

• Identify situations requiring professional health services for preventive care.

• Analyze the importance of abstinence as it relates to the prevention of STDs.

 QUICK START Why is it important to protect your reproductive system? List two ways you can safeguard this system.

There are 300 million to 400 million sperm in each ejaculation, but only one can fertilize an ovum.
What is the relationship of testosterone to sperm?

An essential function of all living things is reproduction, the process by which life continues from one generation to the next. In humans, as in many other animal species, reproduction results from the union of two specialized sex cells—one from the male and one from the female. These cells are made by the **reproductive system**, *the system of organs involved in producing offspring.*

Structure and Function of the Male Reproductive System

The male reproductive system includes both external and internal organs. The two main functions of the male reproductive system are the production and storage of **sperm**, *the male reproductive cells,* and transfer of sperm to the female's body during sexual intercourse. During the early teen years, usually between the ages of 12 and 15, the male reproductive system reaches maturity.

At that time hormones produced in the pituitary gland stimulate the production of **testosterone**, *the male sex hormone*. Testosterone initiates physical changes that signal maturity, including broadening of the shoulders, development of muscles and facial and other body hair, and deepening of the voice. Testosterone also controls the production of sperm. A physically mature male is capable of producing sperm for the rest of his life.

External Male Reproductive Organs

The testes, the penis, and the scrotum are external structures involved in the process of reproduction. The **testes**, (singular, *testis*) also called testicles, are *two small glands that produce sperm*. These glands secrete testosterone. The testes are located in the **scrotum**, *an external skin sac*. The **penis** is *a tube-shaped organ that extends from the trunk of the body just above the testes*. It is composed of spongy tissue that contains many blood vessels. When blood flow to the penis increases, it becomes enlarged and erect. This normal body function is called an *erection*. Males experience erections easily and frequently during puberty. Erections can occur for no reason. Sometimes an erection results when clothing the male is wearing causes friction.

The penis releases semen. **Semen** is *a thick fluid containing sperm and other secretions from the male reproductive system*. At the height of sexual arousal, a series of muscular contractions known as *ejaculation* may occur. **Fertilization**—the joining of a male sperm cell and a female egg cell—can result if ejaculation occurs during sexual intercourse.

At birth a male has a covering of thin loose skin, called the *foreskin*, over the tip of the penis. Some parents choose *circumcision*—surgical removal of the foreskin of the penis—for their male children. Circumcision is often performed for cultural or religious reasons, but is not generally considered medically necessary today.

Sperm cannot live in temperatures higher than the normal body temperature of 98.6°F. The scrotum protects sperm by keeping the testes slightly below the normal body temperature. When body temperature rises, muscles attached to the scrotum relax, causing the testes to lower away from the body. If body temperature lowers, the muscles tighten and the testes move closer to the body for warmth. Tight clothing that holds the testes too close to the body may interfere with sperm production.

When a male begins to produce sperm, he may experience nocturnal emissions, or ejaculations that occur when sperm is released during sleep. This is a normal function that relieves the buildup of pressure as sperm begin to be produced during puberty.

Development of facial hair is one of the changes that occurs during a male's early teens. Another change is the ability to produce sperm. *Which hormone stimulates physical changes in a maturing male?*

h⊙t link

Fertilization To learn more about fertilization, see Chapter 19, page 486.

CHARACTER ✓ CHECK

Responsibility. Here are some ways a teen can show that he or she is mature and responsible.

- Demonstrate respect for yourself and others.
- Control sexual urges, and never impose them on others.
- Practice abstinence from sexual activity before marriage.

Internal Male Reproductive Organs

Although sperm are produced in the testes, which are suspended outside the body, they must travel through several structures inside the body before they are released. These structures include the vas deferens, the urethra, the seminal vesicles, and the prostate and Cowper's glands. **Figure 18.2** shows the path taken by sperm cells from the testes until they are released from the body.

FIGURE **18.2**

MALE REPRODUCTIVE SYSTEM

The internal structures of the male reproductive system play a role in the delivery of sperm.

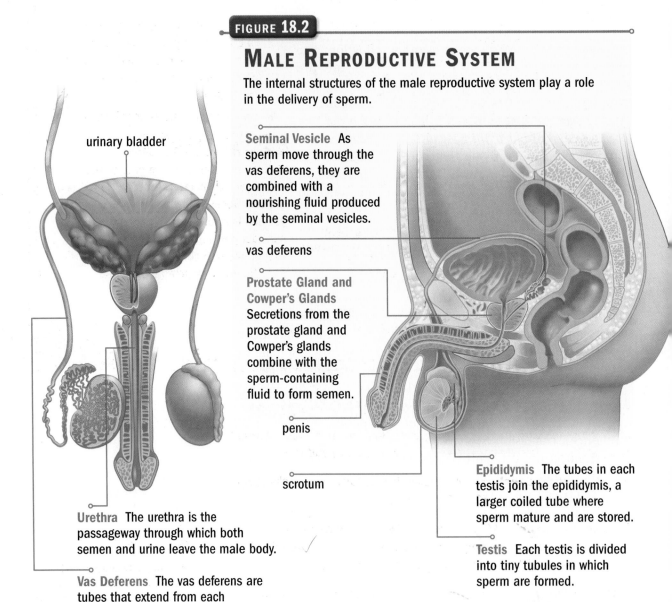

urinary bladder

Seminal Vesicle As sperm move through the vas deferens, they are combined with a nourishing fluid produced by the seminal vesicles.

vas deferens

Prostate Gland and Cowper's Glands Secretions from the prostate gland and Cowper's glands combine with the sperm-containing fluid to form semen.

penis

scrotum

Epididymis The tubes in each testis join the epididymis, a larger coiled tube where sperm mature and are stored.

Testis Each testis is divided into tiny tubules in which sperm are formed.

Urethra The urethra is the passageway through which both semen and urine leave the male body.

Vas Deferens The vas deferens are tubes that extend from each epididymis to the urethra.

Monthly TSE Reminder Card

It's important for males to do a testicular self-exam (TSE) every month. However, not all males are accustomed to performing it. In this activity you will create a reminder card for yourself or the males in your family.

What You'll Need

- paper
- colored pens
- lamination supplies (optional)

What You'll Do

1. Cut the paper into a wallet-sized card.
2. On one side of the card, write out the steps in performing a TSE (see page 472).
3. On the other side of the card, create a message that will remind and persuade you or males in your family to do a monthly exam. The exam could be scheduled for the same time each month, such as the first day of every month.
4. Laminate the card so that it will last.

Apply and Conclude

Keep the reminder card in a location where you (or males in your family) will see it often. Because the best time to examine yourself is after a warm bath or shower, consider placing the card in the bathroom. Explain the importance of taking responsibility for regularly performing a TSE.

Care of the Male Reproductive System

Caring for the male reproductive system involves medical checkups, hygiene, protection, and self-examination.

▶ **Get regular checkups.** All males should have regular checkups by a physician every 12 to 18 months.

▶ **Bathe regularly.** Males should shower or bathe daily, thoroughly cleansing the penis and scrotum. Uncircumcised males should take care to wash under the foreskin.

▶ **Wear protective equipment.** Use a protective cup or supporter during physical activities to shield external organs.

▶ **Perform regular self-examinations.** Check the scrotum and testicles for signs of cancer. Report any change to a physician.

▶ **Practice abstinence.** Abstain from sexual activity before marriage to avoid contracting **STDs.**

hot link

sexually transmitted diseases (STDs) For more information on STDs and how they affect the male reproductive system, see Chapter 25, page 652.

hot link

steroids For more information about the harmful effects of anabolic-androgenic steroids, see Chapter 23, page 601.

Sexually Transmitted Diseases (STDs)

Listed below are some of the STDs that affect the male reproductive system. More information about STDs can be found in Chapter 25. The primary means of transmission of all STDs is sexual activity. Teens who practice abstinence from sexual activity greatly reduce or even eliminate their risk of contracting these diseases:

▶ **Chlamydia** and **gonorrhea** are bacterial infections that cause discharge from the penis and burning upon urination; both conditions can damage reproductive health. Treatment includes a course of antibiotics.

▶ **Syphilis** is another bacterial infection. Initially, a painless, reddish sore appears at the site of infection. If left untreated, syphilis can spread and damage internal organs. It is treated with antibiotics.

▶ **Genital herpes** is a virus that causes periodically occurring blisterlike sores in the genital area. Medication relieves symptoms, but the virus remains in the body for life.

Problems of the Male Reproductive System

The organs of the male reproductive system can be affected by functional and structural problems. Infections from sexually transmitted diseases (STDs) also affect these organs.

Inguinal Hernia

An inguinal (IN-gwuh-nuhl) hernia is a separation of tissue that allows part of the intestine to push into the abdominal wall near the top of the scrotum. Straining the abdominal muscles or lifting heavy objects can cause a tear in this tissue. Symptoms of inguinal hernia may include a lump in the groin near the thigh, pain in the groin or, in severe cases, partial or complete blockage of the intestine. Surgery is usually necessary to repair the opening in the muscle wall.

Sterility

Sterility is *the inability to reproduce.* In males it can result from too few sperm—fewer than 20 million per milliliter of seminal fluid—or sperm of poor quality. Sterility can result from environmental hazards, including exposure to X rays or other radiation, toxic chemicals, and lead. Hormonal imbalance, certain medications, or use of drugs, including anabolic **steroids,** can damage sperm. Some diseases, including STDs, and contracting mumps as an adult also can result in sterility.

Testicular Cancer and Problems of the Prostate

Testicular cancer can affect males of any age but occurs most often in males between the ages of 14 and 40. These factors increase the risk of developing the disease: undescended testicle, abnormal testicular development, and family history of testicular cancer. A monthly testicular self-exam is recommended by the American Cancer Society. Males should see a health care professional if they notice any changes or symptoms, such as a painless lump or swelling in either testicle or pain or discomfort in a testicle or in the scrotum. With early detection most testicular cancer is treatable through surgery, radiation therapy, or chemotherapy.

The prostate gland can become enlarged as a result of an infection, a tumor, or age-related problems. An enlarged gland presses against the urethra, resulting in frequent or difficult urination. Symptoms may also indicate more serious conditions, including prostate cancer. Prostate cancer screening is usually done during routine physical exams for males over age 50. Early detection increases the chance of survival. Treatment includes surgery, radiation, and hormone therapy.

National and world champion cyclist Lance Armstrong is a survivor of testicular cancer.

Why are testicular self-exams important for male reproductive health?

 Lesson 2 *Review*

Reviewing Facts and Vocabulary

1. What is the function of the testes?
2. Describe the path that sperm follow from the time they form until they leave the body.
3. What are the symptoms of testicular cancer? Identify conditions requiring professional health services for preventive care.

Thinking Critically

4. **Analyzing.** Why would knowing the correct way to lift a heavy object be an important behavior to protect the health of the male reproductive system?
5. **Synthesizing.** Analyze the importance of abstinence as it relates to the prevention of STDs. How can problems related to STDs affect the male reproductive system?

Applying Health Skills

Practicing Healthful Behaviors. Analyze the relationship between unsafe behaviors related to drug use and the harmful effects of these substances on the male reproductive system. Write a paragraph stating how avoiding drugs, including steroids, can ensure the health of your reproductive system.

TECHNOLOGY | *OPTION*

WORD PROCESSING Word-processing software can help you record your healthy behaviors. For tips go to **health.glencoe.com**.

The Female Reproductive System

VOCABULARY

ova
uterus
ovaries
ovulation
fallopian tubes
vagina
cervix
menstruation

YOU'LL LEARN TO

• Describe the parts of the female reproductive system and explain the function of each part.

• Relate the importance of early detection and warning signs that prompt females of all ages to seek health care for the female reproductive system.

• Identify situations requiring professional health services for preventive care.

• Analyze the importance of abstinence as it relates to the prevention of STDs.

➡ **QUICK START** Write a short paragraph that contains the words *reproductive system, responsibility,* and *health.* Share these sentences with your classmates.

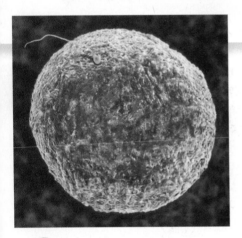

The female reproductive system stores ova that unite with sperm in the process of reproduction.
Name another function of the female reproductive system.

The female reproductive system has several functions. It produces female sex hormones and stores *female reproductive cells,* called **ova** (singular, *ovum*). The **uterus,** *a hollow, muscular, pear-shaped organ inside a female's body,* nourishes and protects the fertilized ovum from conception until birth.

Structure and Function of the Female Reproductive System

The female reproductive system includes several organs and glands. **Ovaries** are *the female sex glands that store the ova and produce female sex hormones.* At birth a female's ovaries contain more than 400,000 immature ova, or eggs. One ovum matures each month, beginning at puberty when the pituitary gland produces hormones. **Ovulation** is *the process of releasing a mature ovum into the fallopian tube each month.* The right ovary will release a mature ovum one month, and the left ovary will release one the next month.

Female Reproductive Organs

Figure 18.3 shows the structures of the female reproductive system. Notice the tube that lies next to each ovary. When a mature ovum is released from the ovary, it moves to one of the **fallopian tubes**, *a pair of tubes with fingerlike projections that draw in the ovum.*

Tiny hairlike structures called cilia work, along with muscular contractions in the fallopian tubes, to move the ovum along. Sperm from the male enter the female reproductive system through the **vagina**, *a muscular, elastic passageway that extends from the uterus to the outside of the body.*

If sperm are present in the fallopian tubes, a sperm cell may unite with an ovum, resulting in fertilization. The fertilization of an egg by a sperm produces a cell called a *zygote*. When the zygote leaves the fallopian tube, it enters the uterus. There, the zygote attaches itself to the uterine wall and begins to grow. In preparation for receiving the zygote, the uterine wall has thickened and is rich in blood, which enables the uterus to nourish the zygote. The developing fetus will remain attached to the uterine wall until **birth.**

hot link

birth For more information on prenatal development and birth, see Chapter 19, page 486.

FIGURE **18.3**

FEMALE REPRODUCTIVE SYSTEM

The female reproductive system produces sex cells called ova and provides a place for a fertilized ovum to grow.

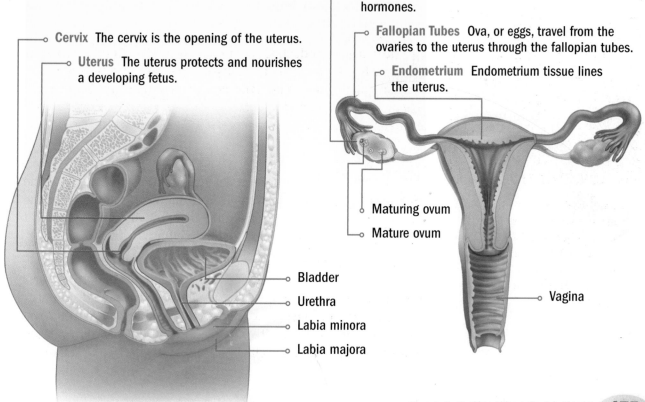

Ovaries The ovaries contain ova and produce hormones.

Fallopian Tubes Ova, or eggs, travel from the ovaries to the uterus through the fallopian tubes.

Endometrium Endometrium tissue lines the uterus.

Cervix The cervix is the opening of the uterus.

Uterus The uterus protects and nourishes a developing fetus.

Maturing ovum

Mature ovum

Bladder

Urethra

Labia minora

Labia majora

Vagina

FIGURE 18.4

THE MENSTRUAL CYCLE

Days 1–13	Day 14	Days 15–20	Days 21–28
A new egg is maturing inside the ovary.	The mature egg is released into one of the fallopian tubes.	The egg travels through the fallopian tube to the uterus.	After seven days, if the egg is not fertilized, menstruation begins.

Eating nutritious foods and avoiding caffeine can often reduce discomfort related to menstruation. *What other health behaviors will keep your reproductive system healthy?*

Menstruation

In a mature female, each month the uterus prepares for possible pregnancy. If pregnancy doesn't occur, the thickened lining of the uterus, called the *endometrium,* isn't needed, and it breaks down into blood, tissue, and fluids. These materials pass through the **cervix**, *the opening to the uterus,* and into the vagina. This *shedding of the uterine lining* is called **menstruation** and is part of the menstrual cycle, which is summarized in **Figure 18.4.** Females wear either sanitary pads or tampons to absorb the blood flow. After the menstrual period ends, usually within five to seven days, the entire cycle begins again in preparation for receiving a fertilized ovum the next month.

Most females begin their first menstrual cycle between the ages of 10 and 15. The cycle may be irregular at first. As a female grows and matures, her menstrual cycle usually becomes more predictable. Endocrine hormones control the cycle, but poor nutrition, stress, and illness can influence it.

Care of the Female Reproductive System

Good hygiene is important for maintaining the health of the female reproductive system. In a mature female, cells in the lining of the vagina are constantly being shed, causing a slight vaginal discharge. Cleanliness will help eliminate odors.

▶ **Bathe regularly.** It is especially important to shower or bathe daily during the menstrual period. During menstruation, change tampons or sanitary pads every few hours. Feminine deodorant sprays and douches are not necessary and may cause irritation or infection in the sensitive tissues around the vagina.

▶ **Practice abstinence.** Abstain from sexual activity before marriage to avoid unplanned pregnancy and STDs.

BREAST SELF-EXAM

Breast cancer is the most common cancer and the second leading cause of death, after lung cancer, for women in the United States. The American Cancer Society recommends that females examine their breasts once a month, right after the menstrual period, when breasts are not tender or swollen. Early detection is an important factor in the successful treatment of breast cancer.

▶ Lie down and place a pillow under the right shoulder. Place the right arm behind the head. Use the fingers of the left hand to feel for lumps or thickening in the right breast. Move around the breast first in a circle, then up and down, and be sure to go over the entire breast area. Repeat the procedure the same way each month. Examine the left breast with the right hand.

▶ Repeat the examination of both breasts while standing, with one arm behind the head. In the upright position, check the upper and outer parts of the breasts, toward the armpit. Standing in front of a mirror, inspect the breasts for any dimpling of the skin, changes in the nipple, redness, or swelling.

Problems of the Female Reproductive System

Several disorders can affect the female reproductive system. Problems related to menstruation can range from minor discomfort to life-threatening illness.

▶ **Menstrual cramps** sometimes occur at the beginning of a menstrual period. Light exercise or applying a heating pad to the abdominal area may help relieve symptoms. A health care professional may recommend medication for pain relief. Severe or persistent cramping, called dysmenorrhea, may be an indication that medical attention is needed.

▶ **Premenstrual syndrome (PMS)** is a disorder caused by hormonal changes. Its symptoms, which may be experienced one to two weeks before menstruation, include nervous tension, anxiety, irritability, bloating, weight gain, depression, mood swings, and fatigue. Regular physical activity and good nutrition may reduce the severity of symptoms.

▶ **Toxic shock syndrome (TSS)** is a rare but serious bacterial infection that affects the immune system and the liver, and can be fatal. To reduce the risk of TSS, use tampons with the lowest possible absorbency and change tampons often. Symptoms of TSS include fever, vomiting, diarrhea, a sunburn-like rash, red eyes, dizziness, and muscle aches. Any female with these symptoms should contact a physician immediately.

Did You Know ?

The American Cancer Society recommends that females have pelvic exams by age 18 or when recommended by their physician. A pelvic exam is not painful.

- During a pelvic exam, a health care professional checks the shape, size, and position of pelvic organs and checks for any tumors or cysts.
- An examination of cells collected from the cervix, called a *Pap test*, can detect early changes in cells that may indicate a risk of cervical cancer.
- The health care professional also may test for certain sexually transmitted diseases.

Health Skills Activity

Communication: Asking Difficult Questions

"Hello, Brooke," says Dr. Morgan, "How are you? I see we're doing a basic summer camp physical."

Brooke smiles and nods. She has been coming to Dr. Morgan for years and feels comfortable with her.

"Before we begin," Dr. Morgan continues, "do you have any questions for me? Everything okay?"

"Well," Brooke begins, "about a week before my period, I get depressed. It seems much worse than the everyday blues. Once my period starts, I'm okay."

"It's important to ask about your concerns," Dr. Morgan replies. "Many girls and women feel a little blue before their periods, but if your depression is severe, there are treatments we can try. Let's talk more about your symptoms."

What Would You Do?

How would you bring up a reproductive health topic with your parents or guardian or a health care professional? Use the following guidelines for effective communication to help you develop a dialogue.

1. Use "I" messages.
2. Speak in a respectful tone.
3. Make eye contact.
4. Show appropriate body language.
5. Express clear, organized ideas.

Problems Related to Infertility

Infertility, the inability to conceive a child, can have several causes.

▶ **Endometriosis.** This painful, chronic disease occurs when tissue that lines the uterus migrates and grows in the ovaries, fallopian tubes, the uterus, or the lining of the pelvic cavity. Treatments include pain medications, hormone therapy, and surgery.

▶ **Pelvic inflammatory disease (PID).** PID is an infection of the fallopian tubes, ovaries, and the surrounding areas of the pelvis. It can damage a female's reproductive organs. PID usually is caused by **sexually transmitted diseases (STDs).**

▶ **Sexually transmitted diseases** are the most common causes of infertility and other disorders of the reproductive system. Often symptoms of STDs are not evident in females unless a medical examination is performed. Avoiding sexual contact until marriage is the one sure way to prevent STDs.

hot link

STDs For more information on STDs and how they affect the female reproductive system, see Chapter 25, page 652.

Other Female Reproductive Disorders

Other reproductive disorders include the following:

► **Vaginitis,** caused by bacterial vaginosis, is the most common vaginal infection in women of childbearing age, and it is often accompanied by discharge, odor, pain, itching, or burning. If not treated with antibiotics, vaginitis can sometimes lead to PID.

► **Blocked fallopian tubes,** the leading cause of infertility, may result from PID, abdominal surgery, STDs, or endometriosis.

► **Ovarian cysts** are fluid-filled sacs on the ovary. Small, noncancerous cysts usually disappear on their own. Larger cysts may require surgery.

► **Cervical, uterine, and ovarian cancer** occur in the female reproductive system. Early sexual activity and STDs such as human papillomavirus (HPV) are related to an increased incidence of cervical cancer. Regular checkups and pelvic exams are important for early detection and treatment.

Did You Know

Untreated STDs put women at risk for infertility, chronic pelvic pain, and cancer.

- Chlamydia is the most common bacterial STD in the United States. Symptoms, when present, include vaginal discharge or unexpected bleeding, burning upon urination, and abdominal pain.
- HPV is probably the most common viral STD among sexually active young people. Infection with certain types of HPV can lead to cervical cancer. This STD has no known cure.

 Lesson 3 *Review*

Reviewing Facts and Vocabulary

1. How do the structures in the fallopian tubes help move the ovum from the ovaries to the uterus?
2. Explain *ovulation, fertilization,* and *menstruation.*
3. List three causes of infertility in females.

Thinking Critically

4. **Synthesizing.** Analyze the importance of abstinence as it relates to the prevention of STDs. What behaviors can female teens practice to protect the health of their reproductive systems?
5. **Analyzing.** Relate the importance of early detection and warning signs for problems of the female reproductive system. Why is it important for every female to have regular pelvic exams starting at age 18 or when recommended by her physician?

Applying Health Skills

Advocacy. Make a card reminding yourself or the females in your family to perform a monthly breast self-exam. Provide step-by-step instructions. Add a catchy phrase that will remind users of the importance of early detection, and include warning signs that should prompt females to seek professional health services.

TECHNOLOGY O P T I O N

PRESENTATION SOFTWARE You can use presentation software to combine text and graphics on your reminder card. For help in using presentation software, go to **health.glencoe.com.**

Eye ON THE Media

Gender Representation in the Media

Studies have shown that although the numbers of males and females represented in the media are becoming more equal, women continue to be less visible in news reporting and news magazine writing. For instance, women often cover human interest stories, sometimes called "soft news," while male reporters cover "hard news," such as world and local news. In this activity you will look for potential gender bias in the media by examining types of news stories presented by male and female reporters.

	Male Reporters / Writers	Female Reporters / Writers
Number of Stories/ Resource	3/television 5/newspaper 2/news magazine	1/television 3/newspaper 5/news magazine
Kinds of Stories	1. 2. 3. 4.	1. 2. 3. 4.

ACTIVITY

Use a chart similar to the one shown to survey the number of stories you see on television, in newspapers, or news magazines. Count the number of stories presented by male reporters and the number of stories presented by female reporters. Then, in each column, describe the kinds of stories that males and females present. Discuss your findings with the class.

EXPRESS YOUR VIEWS

Write a brief analysis of the results of your survey on the types of stories presented primarily by men or primarily by women. Which gender was most represented by feature or lead articles? Which was most represented by "soft news" items?

CROSS-CURRICULUM CONNECTIONS

Create a Mood Poem. During puberty both males and females experience sudden emotional changes. These fluctuations can produce intense feelings. As a class, brainstorm different emotions associated with mood swings. Pick one of these emotions and write a metaphor or simile that communicates how you feel about that emotion beyond its literal meaning. Use your metaphor or simile as the basis for a poem about that emotion.

Research Health Advances. Although many married couples can conceive a child easily, some who desire children are infertile, meaning that they cannot conceive at all. Infertility was considered an insurmountable misfortune until the development of in vitro fertilization techniques. More than 20,000 babies have been born worldwide through in vitro procedures. In a research report, trace the significant advances in reproductive health over the last few decades.

Find Percentages of Infertility. About 12 percent of all couples experience infertility. Forty percent of these cases are primarily male problems, 40 percent female, and the remaining 20 percent are the result of problems stemming from both partners. What percentage of all couples are infertile as a result of problems stemming from both partners?

Research Adrenal Gland Functions. The adrenals produce adrenaline for the "fight or flight" response and help the body recover from stress. Recent research indicates that they may play a role in memory. Research the adrenal glands and write a report explaining their many functions. Include information on adrenal disorders such as Addison's Disease.

School Nurse

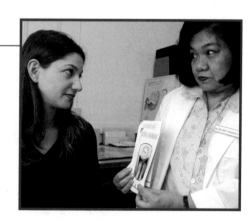

Are you caring and sympathetic, and are you concerned with the physical and mental/emotional needs of others? If so, a career as a school nurse may be right for you. School nurses perform screenings, provide emergency first aid, monitor state immunization laws, develop health-related curricula to meet the needs of students and teachers, and counsel students on personal health issues.

Nursing students need a strong background in science and mathematics. To become a registered nurse, a student must graduate from an accredited nursing school and pass a national licensing exam. For more information, click on **health.glencoe.com**.

Chapter 18 *Review*

► EXPLORING HEALTH TERMS *Answer the following questions on a sheet of paper.*

Lesson 1 *Match each definition with the correct term.*

adrenal glands	pituitary gland
endocrine glands	parathyroid glands
hormones	thyroid gland
pancreas	gonads

1. The gland that regulates activities of all the other endocrine glands.
2. The gland that produces hormones that regulate metabolism and bone growth.
3. Glands that produce a hormone that regulates the body's calcium and phosphorus balance.
4. Glands that help the body recover from stress and respond to emergencies.

Lesson 2 *Identify each statement as True or False. If false, replace the underlined term with the correct term.*

penis	sperm
reproductive system	semen
scrotum	testes
sterility	testosterone

5. <u>Semen</u> is the male reproductive cell.
6. The testes are contained in the <u>penis</u>.
7. <u>Testosterone</u> is the male sex hormone.

Lesson 3 *Fill in the blanks with the correct term.*

cervix	ovulation
fallopian tubes	ovum
menstruation	uterus
ovaries	vagina

8. Ova mature in the _____ .
9. The _____ is a muscular, elastic passageway that extends from the uterus to the outside of the body.
10. The hollow, pear-shaped organ inside a female's body where a fetus is nourished is the _____ .

► RECALLING THE FACTS *Use complete sentences to answer the following questions.*

Lesson 1

1. What is the function of hormones?
2. Why are the ovaries and testes considered endocrine glands?
3. What is epinephrine and what function does it have?
4. Why is a goiter an uncommon problem in the United States?

Lesson 2

5. What are three physical changes initiated by testosterone in the male?
6. What are three ways to care for the male reproductive system?
7. What is an inguinal hernia?
8. Relate the importance of early detection and warning signs of prostate cancer that prompt males of all ages to seek health care.

Lesson 3

9. Name and describe the two processes that are part of the menstrual cycle.
10. How can menstrual cramps be relieved?
11. Relate the importance of early warning signs for seeking health care. Why should a female with symptoms of TSS contact a health care professional immediately?
12. Identify situations requiring professional health services for preventive care. What is PID, and what usually causes it?

➤ THINKING CRITICALLY

1. **Synthesizing.** Compare and contrast the symptoms of Graves' disease, also known as hyperthyrodism, and hypothyrodism. Why might you infer that the thyroid plays a role in internal temperature regulation? *(LESSON 1)*

2. **Summarizing.** Relate the importance of early detection and warning signs that prompt males to seek health care for the reproductive system. Suppose that a friend tells you he won't perform a testicular self-exam because it is too embarrassing. What advice would you give him? *(LESSON 2)*

3. **Analyzing.** In what ways are PMS, TSS, and PID similar to and different from one another? *(LESSON 3)*

➤ HEALTH SKILLS APPLICATION

1. **Practicing Healthful Behaviors.** Excessive weight has been shown to be a contributing factor for developing diabetes mellitus. Identify three things you can do each day to help maintain a healthy weight for life. *(LESSON 1)*

2. **Accessing Information.** Some athletes use anabolic-androgenic steroids—chemicals similar to testosterone—to increase muscle size and improve overall performance. Research and list the harmful effects of steroids on the body. Then create a visual presentation that informs others of the dangers of steroid use. *(LESSON 2)*

3. **Advocacy.** Annual Pap tests are important for all women over the age of 18. Relate the importance of early detection and warning signs that prompt females to seek health care. Prepare an informative, accurate, and persuasive pamphlet to encourage women to have an annual Pap test. *(LESSON 3)*

BEYOND the Classroom

Parent Involvement

Advocacy. Share the information about breast and testicular self-exams with a parent. Work together to find a place to display the reminder cards you made. Then discuss will all family members the importance of these exams for early detection of cancers. Discuss also the warning signs that should prompt persons of any age to seek medical attention.

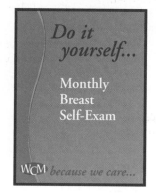

Do it yourself...

Monthly Breast Self-Exam

W©M *because we care...*

School and Community

School Health Services. Ask the school nurse to talk to your class about the importance of proper hygiene and care of the reproductive systems. Also, have the nurse describe the health services available through his or her office. How can students access these services? Which services require the approval of a parent?

Prenatal Development and Birth

What Do You Know About Prenatal Development?

Read each statement below and respond by writing *Myth* or *Fact* for each item.

1. The egg from the mother determines a baby's gender.

2. Twins result when more than one sperm fertilizes a single egg.

3. A fetus usually remains in the uterus for about nine months.

4. If a pregnant female uses tobacco, alcohol, or other drugs, these substances can harm the fetus.

5. A female should gain as much weight as possible during pregnancy.

6. Both prescription and over-the-counter drugs can harm a fetus.

7. A pregnant female should never exercise.

8. Genes carry the hereditary traits of an individual.

9. Balanced nutrition is especially important during pregnancy because the nutrients a female ingests affect her baby's development.

10. A female who wants children does not need to take special care of herself until she knows for sure that she is pregnant.

Quick Write

Using Visuals. Both parents have the responsibility to provide for the health of their unborn child. What steps can parents-to-be take to maximize the chances of having a healthy baby?

HEALTH Online

For instant feedback on your health status, go to Chapter 19 Health Inventory at **health.glencoe.com**.

The Beginning of the Life Cycle

VOCABULARY

fertilization
implantation
embryo
fetus
amniotic sac
umbilical cord
placenta
labor

YOU'LL LEARN TO

- Explain the stages of fetal development from conception through pregnancy and birth.

- Recognize how nutrients and other substances are transferred from a pregnant female to her fetus.

QUICK START A developing baby grows rapidly inside its mother's body. How is an unborn baby nourished? Write down your ideas.

A This human egg cell is surrounded by sperm. Chemical changes take place in the egg's surface so that only one sperm can fertilize it.

D id you know that your body is made of trillions of cells? These cells form the tissues and organs in your body. Yet your heart, lungs, skin, bones, and other body organs all begin as a single cell that is smaller than the period at the end of this sentence.

Conception and Implantation

T he entire complex human body begins as one microscopic cell that is formed by the union of an egg cell, or ovum, from a female and a sperm cell from a male. The *union of a male sperm cell and a female egg cell* is called **fertilization**, which is also known as *conception*. The resulting cell is called a *zygote* (ZY-goht).

Look at **Figure 19.1** on page 487. Notice that within a day after the zygote forms, it begins dividing as it travels down the fallopian tube. By the time it reaches the uterus, the zygote has divided many times to form a cluster of cells with a hollow space in the center. Within a few days, *the zygote attaches to the uterine wall* in the process called **implantation**. After this, the cluster of cells is known as an **embryo** (EM-bree-oh), *the developing child from the time of implantation until about the eighth week of development*. The *developing embryo in the uterus* is called a **fetus** (FEE-tuhs).

Embryonic Growth

As the embryo grows, its cells continue to divide, forming three tissue layers that later become various body systems. One layer becomes the respiratory and digestive systems. A second layer develops into muscles, bones, blood vessels, and skin. A third layer forms the nervous system, sense organs, and mouth.

During this time two important structures form outside the embryo:

▶ The **amniotic** (am-nee-AH-tik) **sac** is *a thin, fluid-filled membrane that surrounds and protects the developing embryo.* It also insulates the embryo from temperature changes.

▶ The **umbilical** (uhm-BIL-uh-kuhl) **cord** is *a ropelike structure that connects the embryo and the mother's placenta.* The **placenta** (pluh-SEN-tuh) is *a thick, blood-rich tissue that lines the walls of the uterus during pregnancy and nourishes the embryo.*

Although the blood supply of the mother and the developing embryo are kept separate, materials diffuse from one blood supply to the other through the umbilical cord. Nutrients and oxygen pass from the mother's blood to the embryo, and wastes from the embryo diffuse into the mother's blood. The wastes are excreted from the mother's body along with her body wastes.

Substances that are harmful to the developing embryo can pass through the umbilical cord, too. If a pregnant female uses harmful substances, such as tobacco, alcohol, or other drugs, they can cross the placenta and harm the developing embryo.

How do twins form?
Identical twins result when a single egg that has been fertilized by a single sperm divides and forms two embryos. Because they develop from the same zygote, identical twins have the same genetic information, are the same gender, and look almost exactly the same.

Fraternal twins form when a female's ovaries release two eggs. Separate sperm fertilize each egg, and two embryos develop. Each twin has a different genetic makeup, and may or may not be the same gender. Fraternal twins do not resemble each other any more than other brothers and sisters do. Fraternal twins are much more common than identical twins.

FIGURE 19.1

IMPLANTATION

Fertilization and implantation occur after an egg is released from the ovary.

Cell Division
As the zygote travels down the fallopian tube toward the uterus, it divides many times.

Fertilization
Only one sperm can fertilize an egg.

Implantation
About six days after fertilization, the zygote burrows into the lining of the uterus.

Fetal Development

The time from conception to birth is usually about nine full months. These nine months are divided into three 3-month periods called *trimesters*. Read about the changes that take place during each trimester in **Figure 19.2.** Compare the images to see the growth of the fetus in each trimester.

FIGURE 19.2

STAGES OF EMBRYONIC AND FETAL DEVELOPMENT

First Trimester (0 to 14 weeks)	Major Changes
0–4 weeks	A zygote may float freely in the uterus for 48 hours before implanting. The spinal cord grows faster than the rest of the body. The brain, ears, and arms begin to form. The heart forms and begins to beat.
5–8 weeks	The fetus is about 1 inch long at 8 weeks. The mouth, nostrils, eyelids, hands, fingers, feet, and toes begin to form. The nervous system can respond to stimuli. The cardiovascular system is fully functional.
9–14 weeks	The fetus develops a human profile. Sex organs, eyelids, fingernails, and toenails develop. By week 12 the fetus makes crying motions but no sound and may suck its thumb.

During the period of growth in the uterus, the fetus develops in preparation for living outside the mother's body. Organs develop and become ready to function on their own. The fetus grows and gains weight. After about the seventh month, fat deposits are added under the skin to help the baby maintain body heat after birth. The fetus stores nutrients and builds immunity and protection from diseases and infections.

Second Trimester (15 to 28 weeks)	Major Changes
15–20 weeks	The fetus can blink its eyes. The body begins to grow, growth of the head slows, and the limbs reach full proportion. Eyebrows and eyelashes develop. The fetus can grasp and kick and becomes more active.
21–28 weeks	The fetus can hear conversations and has a regular cycle of waking and sleeping. Weight increases rapidly. The fetus is about 12 inches long and weighs a little more than 1 pound. Fetus may survive if born after 24 weeks but will require special medical care.
Third Trimester (29 weeks to birth)	Major Changes
29–40 weeks	The fetus uses all five senses and begins to pass water from the bladder. Brain scans have shown that some fetuses dream during their periods of sleep in the eighth and ninth months of development. Approximately 266 days after conception, the baby weighs 6 to 9 pounds and is ready to be born.

Stages of Birth

In the final weeks of pregnancy, the fetus becomes more and more crowded in the uterus and puts increased demands on its mother's body. Most often the baby's head moves to the lower part of the uterus. Many females experience weak, irregular muscular contractions of the uterus for weeks or even months before the baby is born. As the time approaches for the baby to be born, however, these contractions become regular, stronger, and closer together. The stronger contractions induce **labor**, *the final stage of pregnancy in which the uterus contracts and pushes the baby out of the mother's body.* The stages of labor are summarized in **Figure 19.3.**

Real-Life Application

Fetal Ultrasound Technology

Ultrasound is a nonintrusive technology used to monitor a fetus in the uterus using the reflection of sound waves. A moving image of the developing fetus can be viewed on a monitor. Doctors can measure how the fetus is growing and whether organs such as the heart are developing properly. Ultrasound is used to determine the position of the fetus before birth.

Fetal ultrasound is harmless for the mother and child.

Only a trained specialist should interpret an ultrasound image.

In many cases gender can be determined with ultrasound.

Ultrasound can be done quickly in a doctor's office.

Ultrasound is helpful for identifying twins or other multiple births.

ACTIVITY

Access print or online sources to investigate at least two other technologies used in fetal monitoring. Tell when and why each is used, cite your sources of information, and provide the criteria you used to evaluate your sources of valid health information. Write a paragraph explaining how fetal ultrasound technology helps protect the health of the mother and unborn child.

FIGURE 19.3

LEAVING THE WOMB

A female goes through three stages of labor to deliver a baby. Labor can last from a few hours to several days.

Stage 1: Dilation	Stage 2: Passage Through Birth Canal	Stage 3: Afterbirth
The contractions of the uterus cause the cervix, the opening to the uterus, to begin to dilate, or widen. In about 95 percent of pregnancies, the baby's head is resting on the cervix. Toward the end of this stage, contractions break the amniotic sac that surrounds the baby.	When the cervix is fully dilated, the baby passes through the birth canal and emerges from the mother's body. Right after birth the baby takes its first breath and cries to clear the lungs of amniotic fluid.	The placenta is still attached to the baby by the umbilical cord. Contractions continue until the placenta, now called the *afterbirth,* is pushed from the mother's body. The umbilical cord will be cut to separate the placenta from the baby.

Lesson 1 *Review*

Reviewing Facts and Vocabulary

1. Define *fertilization* and *implantation.*
2. Explain the relationship between a zygote, an embryo, and a fetus.
3. How is a developing fetus nourished?

Thinking Critically

4. **Synthesizing.** Considering what you learned about the female reproductive system in Chapter 18, explain what would happen if the zygote did not implant in the uterus after leaving the fallopian tube.
5. **Applying.** Explain how harmful substances taken in by a pregnant female can be transferred to a developing fetus. How might fetal development be affected?

Applying Health Skills

Accessing Information. Research the changes that occur in a female's body during the nine months of pregnancy. Make an informative pamphlet that summarizes this information by trimester. Illustrate the pamphlet with pictures that show fetal development during each trimester.

TECHNOLOGY *OPTION*

PRESENTATION SOFTWARE Create a slide show that describes changes during pregnancy and fetal development. For help in making a computer slide show, see health.glencoe.com.

Prenatal Care

VOCABULARY

prenatal care
birthing center
fetal alcohol syndrome (FAS)
miscarriage
stillbirth

YOU'LL LEARN TO

- Explain the importance of prenatal care and proper nutrition in promoting optimal health for both mother and baby.

- Analyze the harmful effects of tobacco, alcohol, and other drugs on the fetus.

- Identify and analyze the effects of environmental hazards on the fetus.

- Explain why seeking prenatal care early in pregnancy is important.

➔ **QUICK START** List five positive health behaviors that a person should practice each day. Circle any that you think would also benefit a developing fetus.

▲ Regular physical activity under the guidance of a health care professional, along with good nutrition, contribute to a healthy pregnancy.

Although most pregnancies proceed with few or no complications, a female should begin prenatal care as soon as her pregnancy is confirmed. **Prenatal** (pree-NAY-tuhl) **care** refers to *steps that a pregnant female can take to provide for her own health and the health of her baby.*

Importance of Prenatal Care

One of the first decisions a pregnant female must make is who will provide her prenatal care. An *obstetrician* (ahb-stuh-TRI-shuhn) is a doctor who specializes in the care of a female and her developing child. A *certified nurse-midwife* is an advanced practice nurse who specializes in prenatal care and the delivery of babies. The mother-to-be must also decide where the birth will take place. In the United States, most births take place at a hospital, but some women may choose to have the delivery at home or in a **birthing center**, *a facility in which women with low-risk pregnancies can deliver their babies in a homelike setting.* Regardless of where the birth takes place, a doctor or certified nurse-midwife should be present.

During prenatal visits the female will have a complete physical that includes blood tests and a pelvic exam. The purpose of the exam is to identify problems so that they can be corrected or treated as early as possible. The obstetrician or nurse-midwife will monitor the mother's weight and blood pressure. Often the developing baby will be viewed with an ultrasound machine. These visits also give the parents-to-be the opportunity to ask questions and to learn about important behaviors that can help ensure the health of the baby.

Proper Nutrition During Pregnancy

An unborn baby depends on its mother for nourishment. For this reason, a pregnant female needs more nutrients than at any other time in her life. To ensure the health of the developing fetus, increased amounts of many nutrients, including those below, are needed.

▶ **Calcium** helps build strong bones and teeth and healthy nerves and muscles. It is also important in developing heart rhythm.

▶ **Protein** helps form muscle and most other tissue.

▶ **Iron** makes red blood cells and supplies oxygen to cells.

▶ **Vitamin A** aids in cell and bone growth and eye development.

▶ **Vitamin B complex** aids in forming the nervous system.

▶ **Folic acid** is a critical part of spinal fluid and helps close the tube that contains the central nervous system. This neural tube forms 17 to 30 days after conception, so neural tube defects can occur before a female knows that she is pregnant. Health care providers suggest that all females of childbearing age consume 400–600 micrograms of folic acid daily to prevent these defects.

Choosing nutritious foods such as fruits and vegetables, and drinking milk during pregnancy can ensure that a mother-to-be receives the optimal amount of nutrients. *What nutrients are especially important for proper development of the fetus?*

Although a pregnant female's nutritional requirements may increase, she must be careful not to gain too much weight. Most pregnant females need only 300 additional calories each day—about the number of calories found in two and a half cups of low-fat milk. Most health care professionals suggest that females who are at a healthy pre-pregnancy weight gain between 25 and 35 pounds during pregnancy. Excess weight can be a health risk for both mother and baby.

Weight reduction diets during pregnancy can harm the developing fetus. Such diets should be undertaken only under the guidance of an experienced health care provider.

Caffeine, present in coffee, tea, chocolate, and many cola drinks, can affect the developing fetus. A high intake of caffeine during pregnancy has been linked to an increased risk of birth defects and low birth weight.

Physical activity can be beneficial to the pregnant female and developing child. Before starting any exercise program, the expectant mother should discuss the matter with her health care provider.

The Health of the Fetus

A pregnant female must be very careful about the substances she takes into her body. Tobacco, alcohol, and other drugs can enter the body of the developing fetus and have serious effects.

Alcohol and Pregnancy

Any alcohol consumed during pregnancy quickly passes through the umbilical cord to the fetus. The fetus breaks down alcohol much more slowly than an adult does, so the alcohol level in the fetus's blood can be higher than that of the mother and remain higher for a longer period of time. An elevated alcohol level can result in permanent damage to the fetus and a condition known as **fetal alcohol syndrome (FAS)**, a *group of alcohol-related birth defects that includes both physical and mental problems*. The serious, lifelong consequences of FAS are listed at the left.

The tragedy of **FAS** is that it is entirely preventable. Because even small amounts of alcohol can be harmful, especially early in pregnancy, the safe decision for pregnant females and females considering pregnancy is not to drink any alcoholic beverages.

Tobacco and Pregnancy

Smoking during pregnancy is estimated to account for up to 30 percent of low birth weight babies, 14 percent of premature births, and 10 percent of all infant deaths. Studies suggest that a pregnant female's smoking may also affect the growth, mental development, and behavior of her child until he or she is 11 years old. The only sure way to protect the developing fetus and child from the negative effects of tobacco is not to smoke.

The responsibility to provide a smoke-free environment extends beyond the expectant mother. According to the American Lung Association, pregnant females exposed repeatedly to secondhand smoke also have an increased risk of having a low birth weight baby. Low birth weight is a leading cause of death for children under 12 months old.

A Smokers inhale nicotine and carbon monoxide, both of which reach the fetus through the umbilical cord, preventing the fetus from getting enough nutrients and oxygen. *How might this affect fetal development?*

h⊙t link

FAS For more information about alcohol and FAS, see Chapter 22, page 575.

Did You Know ?

Children with FAS suffer lifelong consequences, including

• mental retardation.
• learning disabilities.
• serious behavior problems.
• slowed growth.
• physical deformities including a small skull, abnormal facial features, and heart defects.

Medicines, Other Drugs, and Pregnancy

Using **drugs** when pregnant can have serious consequences. During pregnancy even prescription and over-the-counter **medicines** should be taken only with the approval of a doctor or other qualified health care provider.

Using illegal drugs when pregnant poses a serious health threat to both the mother and the fetus. Drug abuse can harm the mother's health and make her less able to support the pregnancy. Drugs also can directly harm fetal development. The use of certain illegal drugs during pregnancy can cause serious birth defects, premature labor, or miscarriage. In addition, a baby can be born addicted to the drugs the mother uses during pregnancy. The infant will suffer withdrawal when it no longer receives the drugs after birth. The baby may be hypersensitive and irritable and may cry for hours. It may tremble and jerk. A baby born addicted to drugs may fail to bond with its parents as normal babies do.

hotlink

drugs and **medicines** For more information about the effects of medicines and drugs on the body, see Chapter 23, page 594.

Hands-On Health ACTIVITY

Tips for a Healthy Pregnancy

In this activity you will write and design a brochure with tips to help ensure a healthy pregnancy. Keep in mind that prenatal care isn't just the responsibility of the mother-to-be. Expectant fathers, for example, can buy and prepare healthful food and accompany their wives to medical visits and childbirth classes.

What You'll Need

- construction paper
- colored markers or pens
- magazines or newspapers

What You'll Do

1. Fold the construction paper to make a three-panel pamphlet.
2. Using the information in this chapter, write at least five tips for a healthy pregnancy. Under each tip, include actions both parents should take to ensure that their baby is healthy.
3. Illustrate your pamphlet with photos from magazines or newspapers, or draw your own illustrations. Make your pamphlet persuasive, and target it to expectant parents.
4. Share your pamphlet with the class.

Apply and Conclude

As a class, combine the best features of all the pamphlets to create one pamphlet. Make copies, and give them to family members who are expecting a child or planning a family.

Environmental Hazards

Harm to the fetus can result when a pregnant female is exposed to some common substances in the environment. Being familiar with these substances can help a female avoid exposing her unborn child to their harmful effects.

► **Lead.** Lead exposure has been linked to miscarriage, low birth weight, mental disabilities, and behavior problems in children. Lead can be found in the paint of houses built before 1978 and can leach from old pipes into tap water.

► **Smog.** Recent studies have linked air pollution with birth defects, low birth weight, premature birth, stillbirth, and infant death. The greatest risk occurs during the second month of pregnancy when most organs and facial features develop.

► **Radiation.** Ionizing radiation—the type found in X rays—can affect fetal growth and cause mental retardation. Other types of radiation, such as that from video displays, color television sets, and microwave ovens, have not been shown to be harmful.

► **Cat Litter.** Cat feces may contain a parasite that can cause a disease called toxoplasmosis (tahk-suh-plaz-MOH-suhs). This disease can result in miscarriage, premature labor, and health problems in a newborn. Pregnant females should wash their hands after petting a cat, have others clean the cat litter box, and wear gloves when gardening where cats may be present.

In addition, when using household chemicals, pregnant females should read the cautions on cleaning products, wear gloves, and work in well-ventilated areas.

Although most pregnancies progress without complications, certain environmental factors can affect the healthy development of a fetus. *What steps can a mother-to-be take to protect the health of her unborn child?*

Complications During Pregnancy

Most pregnancies proceed with few problems. However, complications can arise, some of them serious. One complication is **miscarriage**, *the spontaneous expulsion of a fetus that occurs before the twentieth week of a pregnancy. A dead fetus expelled from the body after the twentieth week* is called a **stillbirth**. Women who use tobacco or drugs during pregnancy are more likely to experience a miscarriage or stillbirth than those who abstain from these substances. A miscarriage or stillbirth doesn't necessarily mean that the mother did something wrong. Receiving the proper prenatal care during pregnancy can reduce the risk or severity of any problems that do arise.

Ectopic Pregnancy

Ectopic (ek-TAH-pik) pregnancies result when the zygote implants in the fallopian tube, the abdomen, the ovary, or the cervix. Ectopic pregnancy can occur when the fertilized egg can't pass to the uterus, sometimes because of inflammation or scar tissue that has developed as a result of **sexually transmitted diseases.** The fetus can't get the nourishment it needs to grow normally. The situation is a threat to the pregnant female's life. Ectopic pregnancy is the number one cause of death of females in the first trimester of pregnancy. The treatment of ectopic pregnancy is removal of the fetus from the female's body.

Preeclampsia

Preeclampsia (pree-ee-CLAMP-see-ah), also called toxemia, can prevent the placenta from getting enough blood. The condition may result in low fetal birth weight and problems for the mother. Symptoms of preeclampsia in a pregnant female include high blood pressure, swelling, and large amounts of protein in the urine. Treatment includes reducing blood pressure through bed rest or medicines. In some cases, hospitalization is necessary.

hot link

sexually transmitted diseases Read more about STDs in Chapter 25, page 648.

Did You Know

Two to five percent of pregnant females in the United States are diagnosed with Gestational Diabetes Mellitus, or GDM. It usually disappears after the baby's birth.

 Lesson 2 *Review*

Reviewing Facts and Vocabulary

1. Explain the importance of *prenatal care* and describe what it involves.

2. Define the term *stillbirth.*

3. Analyze the effects of certain substances on the fetus. Why should pregnant females avoid drugs, alcohol, and tobacco?

Thinking Critically

4. **Evaluation.** Suppose someone told you that pregnancy is a natural process so prenatal care is not important. What information would you give such a person?

5. **Synthesizing.** Analyze the harmful effects of environmental hazards on the fetus. Over which factors that affect a developing fetus does a pregnant female have control?

Applying Health Skills

Stress Management. Pregnancy causes extra stress on the body of the mother. Along with these physical stresses come concerns about the health of the baby and about parenthood. Make a list of healthy "stress-busters" pregnant females could use. Share your list with families who are expecting a child.

INTERNET RESOURCES Use the Internet to find information on stress management techniques. See **health.glencoe.com** for links to help your research.

Heredity and Genetics

VOCABULARY

heredity
chromosomes
genes
DNA
genetic disorder
amniocentesis
chorionic villi
sampling
gene therapy

YOU'LL LEARN TO

• Explain the significance of genetics and its role in determining human traits.

• Identify common genetic disorders.

• Explain how genetic research has impacted the health status of families and those with genetic disorders.

QUICK START Fold a sheet of paper in half. Think of a family you know. Make two columns, one listing ways family members are alike and one listing ways they are different.

No two individuals are exactly alike. Even identical twins have some differences. What accounts for this variety of traits? A number of factors influence the way an individual develops. One significant factor is heredity.

▼ Family members often share a strong physical resemblance. *What inherited characteristics are visible in this family?*

Heredity

The *passing of traits from parents to their children* is called **heredity**. Examples of traits that you inherited from your parents are your eye and hair color and the shape of your earlobes. Environment can also influence inherited traits. For example, height is an inherited trait, but poor nutrition may stunt a child's growth.

Chromosomes and Genes

Most cells of your body contain a nucleus—the cell's control center. Inside each nucleus is a set of **chromosomes** (KROH-muh-sohmz), *threadlike structures found within the nucleus of a cell that carry the codes for inherited traits.* Most cells in the body contain 46 chromosomes arranged as 23 pairs.

Sections of chromosomes, called genes, carry codes for specific traits. **Genes** are *the basic units of heredity.* Like chromosomes, genes occur in pairs. One gene from each pair is inherited from each parent. You have thousands of genes in every cell of your body.

DNA

The chemical unit that makes up chromosomes is called **DNA**, or deoxyribonucleic (dee-AHK-si-REYE-boh-nyoo-KLEE-ik) acid. All living things are made of DNA. Chemical compounds, called bases, make up the structure of DNA. The arrangement of the bases along each DNA molecule differs. Because several thousand pairs of bases are in each gene, countless numbers of arrangements are possible. The order of the bases is called the *genetic code.* Cells use the genetic code to make proteins. Proteins help to build and maintain body tissues. Different kinds of proteins will result in various individual traits. All the characteristics that you have—the color of your eyes and the amount of curl in your hair—are determined by your genetic code. Unless you have an identical twin, your DNA is different from that of any other person.

Genetics and Fetal Development

Every living organism has a certain number of chromosomes. Although most human cells contain 46 chromosomes —23 pairs—sperm and egg cells have only half that amount, or 23 chromosomes. When a sperm and an egg unite, the resulting zygote will have 46 chromosomes—23 from each parent. These chromosomes carry the hereditary traits of the parents.

As you learned in Lesson 1, a zygote divides many times, producing the trillions of cells that make up the human body. Between each cell division, each chromosome in the cell nucleus duplicates itself, producing two sets of 46 chromosomes. As the cell divides, the two sets of chromosomes separate. Each new cell will contain one set of 46 chromosomes that are identical to those in the first cell of the zygote.

DNA resembles a long twisted helix, with ladder-like chains. Nitrogen bases make up the rungs of the ladder. *Give an example of a trait that is determined by genes.*

Human X and Y chromosomes determine gender. Each of the body cells in a male has an X and a Y chromosome. Each body cell of a female has two X chromosomes.

Explain why the sperm, not the ovum, determines the gender of a fetus.

Dominant and Recessive Genes

At least one pair of genes is responsible for each human trait. Some genes are *dominant,* and others are *recessive.* The traits of dominant genes generally appear in offspring whenever they are present. The traits of recessive genes usually appear only when dominant genes are not present. For example, suppose an individual receives two genes for eye color—one for brown eyes and one for blue eyes. The resulting individual will have brown eyes because the gene for brown eyes is dominant and the gene for blue eyes is recessive. An individual with blue eyes must have two recessive genes for blue eye color.

The situation is more complex than in the example above because traits that express a quantity or an extent—such as height, weight, or color—usually depend on many gene pairs, not just one.

Genes and Gender

In humans one pair of chromosomes determines the gender of an individual. If you are female, these two chromosomes look exactly alike and are called X chromosomes. If you are male, the two chromosomes differ—one is shorter than the other. The shorter chromosome is the Y chromosome. The longer one is the X chromosome.

Remember that sperm and egg cells contain only half the chromosomes of other cells, or one sex chromosome, not two. Sperm contain an X or a Y chromosome. Eggs have only an X chromosome. The gender of a child is determined by which type of sperm—X or Y—unites with an egg.

Genetic Disorders

Sometimes the genes that an individual inherits contain a *mutation,* or abnormality, in the base sequence of the genetic code. Often the mutation has little or no effect on the individual, but sometimes the mutation can result in defects or other health problems. **Genetic disorders** are *disorders caused partly or completely by a defect in genes.* Some genetic disorders, such as those that cause birth defects, are apparent right away. One example of such a defect is cleft palate. However, other genetic disorders do not show up until later in life. **Figure 19.4** gives information about some common genetic disorders.

FIGURE 19.4

COMMON HUMAN GENETIC DISORDERS

Disorder	Characteristics
Sickle-cell anemia	Red blood cells have a sickle shape and clump together; may result in severe joint and abdominal pain, weakness, kidney disease, restricted blood flow
Tay-Sachs disease	Destruction of nervous system; blindness; paralysis; death during early childhood
Cystic fibrosis	Mucus clogs many organs, including lungs, liver, and pancreas; nutritional problems; serious respiratory infections and congestion
Down syndrome	Varying degrees of mental retardation, short stature, round face with upper eyelids that cover inner corners of the eyes
Hemophilia	Failure of blood to clot

Although most genetic disorders cannot be cured, in some cases they can be treated, especially if they are diagnosed early—often before birth. Two common procedures used to test for genetic disorders are amniocentesis (am-nee-oh-sen-TEE-sis) and chorionic villi (kor-ee-ON-ik VIL-eye) sampling.

▶ **Amniocentesis** is *a procedure in which a syringe is inserted through a pregnant female's abdominal wall into the amniotic fluid surrounding the developing fetus.* Doctors can examine the chromosomes in fetal cells taken from amniotic fluid for genetic abnormalities or to determine the gender and age of the fetus. Amniocentesis is usually performed 16 to 20 weeks after fertilization.

▶ **Chorionic villi sampling**, or **CVS**, is *a procedure in which a small piece of membrane is removed from the chorion, a layer of tissue that develops into the placenta.* The tissue can be examined for genetic disorders or to determine fetal age and gender. The procedure is done around the eighth week of fetal development.

Tests for genetic disorders may also be done after a child is born. For example, many states require the testing of all newborns for phenylketonuria (PKU). If PKU is diagnosed soon after birth, a baby's diet can be altered to stop possible mental retardation caused by this genetic disorder.

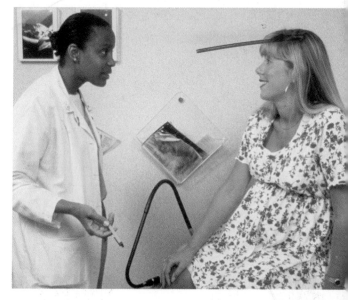

Health care professionals can check the health of a fetus using a variety of testing procedures. *How can the age of a fetus be determined?*

Should People Undergo Genetic Testing?

In the past few years, researchers have linked specific genes or gene mutations with particular diseases. People can be tested to find out whether they are genetically predisposed to those diseases. Some people feel that the disadvantages of genetic testing outweigh the advantages. Others think the opposite is true. Here are two points of view.

Viewpoint 1: Neil S., age 15

I don't think that people should undergo genetic testing. What if they have the gene for a disease for which there's no cure? They would probably worry about it all the time and not be able to do anything about it. A positive test doesn't necessarily mean that the person will develop the disease, but it could cause the person to lose his or her health insurance.

Viewpoint 2: Jan P., age 16

I think genetic testing should be available for those who want it. A person who carries the gene for a particular disease may be able to take additional precautions such as more frequent screenings to reduce the risk of developing the disease. Also, I think that having genetic testing is a personal choice. People can choose not to have it if they don't want to know.

ACTIVITIES

1. **Research some diseases or conditions for which people can undergo genetic testing.**

2. **After researching, list some legal and ethical questions to consider before having a genetic test. How do you think these issues might influence someone's decision about whether to be tested?**

Genetic Counseling

Research for diagnosing, preventing, and treating genetically related diseases has resulted in a wide variety of programs. Genetic counselors can advise families about the probability of having a child with a genetically related disease. They also can guide families of children with genetic disorders about possible treatment options.

Genetic Research to Cure Disease

Scientists have taken an important step in understanding and treating genetic disorders. The Human Genome Project is an international effort that has successfully identified the approximately 30,000 genes on the 46 human chromosomes. Gene maps can be used to diagnose genetic disorders.

Gene Therapy

Many disorders result when an individual lacks a functioning gene. Without the functioning gene, certain substances that the body needs are not produced. **Gene therapy** is *the process of inserting normal genes into human cells to correct genetic disorders.* When the defective gene is replaced with a normal one, the cells with the new gene begin to make the missing substance. Most often, viruses are the carriers used to insert the new gene into a person's cells. The practice of placing fragments of DNA from one organism into another is called *genetic engineering,* and it is considered highly experimental. Genetic diseases for which scientists are researching gene therapies include cystic fibrosis and various types of cancer.

Genetically Engineered Drugs

Genes used to treat disease aren't usually inserted directly into human beings. Instead they are placed into other organisms, causing them to produce substances that can be used to treat human diseases and disorders. Genetically produced medicines include treatments for burns and ulcers, growth defects, and for ovarian and breast cancers. Factor VIII medicines treat hemophilia. Genetic engineering also is used to produce some vaccines that prevent diseases.

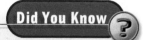

Did You Know

Two purposes of the Human Genome Project are to identify all of the genes in human DNA and to determine the sequences of the 3 billion base pairs that make up human DNA. A working draft of the entire human genome sequence was announced in June 2000. Scientists hope to use the information from the project to improve diagnosis and treatment for approximately 4,000 human genetic disorders.

 Lesson 3 *Review*

Reviewing Facts and Vocabulary

1. What is *heredity*?
2. Name three human genetic disorders.
3. Explain the difference between *amniocentesis* and *chorionic villi sampling (CVS).*

Thinking Critically

4. **Analyzing.** Explain how chromosomes, genes, and DNA are significant in determining human traits.
5. **Synthesizing.** Explain how genetic research technology has impacted the health status of families. How might a genetic counselor help a family that has just learned that their child may have inherited a genetic disorder?

Applying Health Skills

Accessing Information. Research a particular genetic disorder. Prepare a presentation that summarizes the cause, symptoms, and treatment of the disorder and the latest research being conducted. Explain how technology has impacted the health status of communities throughout the world.

TECHNOLOGY *OPTION*

PRESENTATION SOFTWARE Use presentation software to combine text, photos, and illustrations in an interesting summary of a genetic disorder. Find help in using presentation software at health.glencoe.com.

Infancy and Childhood

VOCABULARY

developmental
tasks
autonomy
scoliosis

YOU'LL LEARN TO

- Identify and explain the developmental tasks of childhood.

- Analyze the influence of laws and policies in regard to health screenings for children.

- Identify school and community health services that offer vision and hearing screenings and immunization programs for children.

→ **QUICK START** Do you or any of your friends have younger brothers or sisters? List activities and behaviors you have noticed about younger siblings. Look for patterns among children of similar ages.

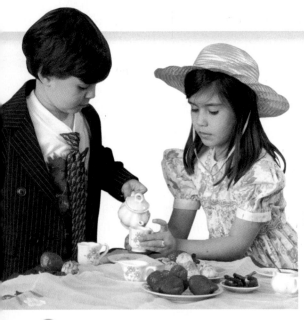

A Children often imitate the behavior of adults. *What are some examples of positive behaviors adults can display when they are around children?*

D ramatic physical and mental changes take place as an infant grows through childhood. Many scientists have studied these changes, and they have developed different theories about them. One of the most widely accepted theories of development is that of psychologist Erik Erikson.

Childhood Development

A ccording to Erikson, each individual passes through eight developmental stages during his or her life. Each stage is characterized by **developmental tasks**, *events that need to happen in order for a person to continue growing toward becoming a healthy, mature adult.* Success in each stage is dependent on an individual's experiences during that stage. Partial development at one stage can be overcome by developmental successes in following stages. The four stages that apply to infancy and childhood are summarized in **Figure 19.5**.

Infancy

Infancy is the period of fastest growth in a person's life. During this time a child's weight may triple, and his or her height may

FIGURE 19.5

STAGES OF INFANCY AND CHILDHOOD

Each stage of development is associated with a developmental task that involves a person's relationship with other people.

Stage 1	Stage 2	Stage 3	Stage 4
Infancy: Birth to 1 year	**Early Childhood: 1 to 3 years**	**Middle Childhood: 4 to 6 years**	**Late Childhood: 7 to 12 years**
Task: To develop trust	**Task:** To develop ability to do tasks for oneself	**Task:** To develop responsibility, take initiative, to create one's own play	**Task:** To develop an interest in performing activities
Description: Infant is completely dependent on others to meet his or her needs. Must be able to trust others to provide for needs.	**Description:** Child learns to walk, talk, and dress and feed himself or herself. Self-control and confidence begins to develop, and child begins a desire for independence.	**Description:** Child becomes more engaged in interactions with others. Models adult behavior by helping with household chores. Learns to control impulses.	**Description:** Child completes transition from home to school; learns to make things, use tools, and acquire skills.

increase by 50 percent. Infancy is a time of learning—how to eat solid food and how to sit, crawl, and walk. An important task for an infant is developing trust. Infants of parents who are attentive—who play with and talk to the infant and give comfort—learn to view the world as a safe place. These children see people as being dependable. If parents ignore a child's needs, the child may learn to be distrustful.

Early Childhood

Children in early childhood begin to feel proud of their accomplishments, and they become eager to learn more. During this time children develop many new skills. They learn to talk, climb, push, and pull. They increase their vocabulary and begin talking in sentences. If parents accept the child's need to do whatever he or she is capable of, the child will develop a sense of **autonomy**, *the confidence that a person can control his or her own body, impulses, and environment.* If parents are overprotective or critical of the child's behaviors, the child may develop doubts about his or her abilities.

Caring. When a child feels understood and has physical and emotional needs taken care of, he or she will thrive. Take the time to listen attentively and show that you care whenever you have a chance to help a toddler or young child. **Think of ways you demonstrate caring with younger siblings or other children.**

Middle Childhood

During middle childhood children learn to initiate play activities rather than merely following the lead of others. Children of this age display their intelligence by asking many questions. They must learn to recognize emotions and practice expressing them in appropriate ways. If parents show approval of these new abilities and encourage questions, children learn creativity, initiative, and the ability to start something on their own. Children of parents who are impatient with the child may develop a sense of guilt about self-initiated activities, resulting in low self-esteem.

Late Childhood

During late childhood school becomes an important part of a child's life. Children develop skills in reading, writing, and math.

Health Skills Activity

Decision Making: Choosing Toys

Colleen is buying a gift for her sister's second birthday. She and her friend, Amanda, are in the toy store. "What about this puzzle?" asks Amanda.

"That's cute," Colleen replies, "but it looks complicated. What if she chokes on the small pieces?"

"Maybe a ride-on toy?" Amanda suggests. "My little brother loves his tricycle."

"Those are fun," Colleen agrees. "But you have to make sure they're stable, so the child doesn't tip over. There are a lot of safety issues to consider when you get a toy for a child."

Amanda sighs. "Maybe we need to do some research to find out what two-year-olds can play with."

"The party is tomorrow," Colleen replies. "I don't have a lot of time for research."

What Would You Do?
How can Colleen find out more about age-appropriate toys? Apply the six steps of the decision-making process to Colleen's situation.

1. State the situation.
2. List the options.
3. Weigh the possible outcomes.
4. Consider values.
5. Make a decision and act.
6. Evaluate the decision.

Children learn to get along with peers, learn appropriate roles in society, and develop a conscience. If their efforts are rewarded and appreciated, their pride in their work increases. Children who are scolded for making a mess, getting in the way, or not following directions may develop feelings of self-doubt.

Health Screenings in Childhood

Vision and hearing impairments can affect a child's development as much as social factors do. Immunizations and health screenings can prevent many problems.

Vision and Hearing

According to the CDC, nearly one in every 1,000 children in the United States has low vision or is legally blind. The American Academy of Ophthalmology recommends that vision screenings be given to newborns and regularly throughout childhood. Schools often provide regular vision screenings for students.

In the United States, two to three of every 1,000 infants are born with a hearing impairment severe enough to affect a child's language development. Some states require that newborns be screened at birth for hearing loss. Schools often provide periodic screenings.

Scoliosis

Scoliosis, an *abnormal lateral, or side-to-side, curvature of the spine*, may begin in childhood and go unnoticed until the teen years. Its exact cause is unknown, though it is more common in girls. Many public schools check for scoliosis in middle school.

HEALTH Online

Take the online quiz for Chapter 19 at **health.glencoe.com**. Use the quiz to evaluate your understanding of this chapter and to find out what you may need to review.

▶ Lesson 4 *Review*

Reviewing Facts and Vocabulary

1. Define *developmental tasks.* List three developmental tasks of infancy and childhood.

2. What developmental task must be accomplished in early childhood?

3. Which health screenings are usually provided by schools?

Thinking Critically

4. **Synthesizing.** How do the actions of parents contribute to the developmental tasks of their children?

5. **Evaluating.** Do you think that all states should have laws requiring regular health screenings for children? Explain your answer.

Applying Health Skills

Accessing Information. Research where individuals in your community can get free or low-cost vision and hearing screenings or immunizations. Post your findings on a class Web site.

TECHNOLOGY *OPTION*

WEB SITES Go to health.glencoe.com for help in building your Web site.

Reading Programs for Children

Some experts suggest that children should read or be read to for at least 20 to 30 minutes each day. For school age children, reading skills are essential for achieving a sense of competence about their own abilities. For preschoolers, being read to fosters the desire to read and teaches them cooperation and listening skills. In the activity below, you will research and select print media sources for children that illustrate or reinforce the developmental tasks discussed in Lesson 4 of this chapter.

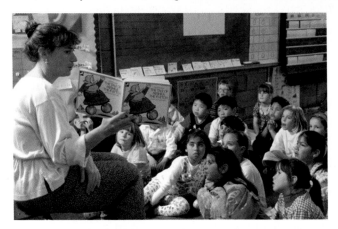

ACTIVITY

You have been asked by your local library to develop a summer reading program for children. Pick one of two age groups for your project, children ages 3 to 5 or children ages 6 to 11. For children ages 3 to 5, research and select five stories to be read aloud to the children. For children ages 6 to 11, identify five books or stories for the children to read themselves.

Using your school or local library as a resource, research and select the five stories you will recommend for your summer reading or story-telling program. For each selection you make, write a brief synopsis of the story that explains how the selection illustrates or reinforces the developmental tasks for that age group.

EXPRESS YOUR VIEWS

Research summer reading and literacy programs in your area. Write an editorial for your school newspaper that encourages teens to volunteer for these programs. Your editorial should state why reading is important, give information about local programs, and contain suggestions for how to get involved.

CROSS-CURRICULUM CONNECTIONS

Create a Futuristic Story. As a result of scientific breakthroughs in genetic research, scientists predict they can make even greater strides in treating and curing illnesses. From what you have learned about genetics, write a science fiction story of how the human genome-mapping project might further impact the future. Remember that although science fiction contains the possibilities of the imagination, the plot must reflect in some way the laws of science.

Examine Theories of Development. Understanding the physical and mental stages of human development helps parents guide their children toward adulthood. Select and study the work of a psychologist or scientist, such as Sigmund Freud, who has theorized about early childhood development. Using a Venn diagram, compare and contrast this researcher's stages to Erik Erikson's theory outlined in Lesson 4 of this chapter.

Calculate Percentage of Births and Deaths. The number of live births in the U.S. in 1999 was 3,959,417, and the total number of deaths was 2,391,399. What was the number by which births exceeded deaths? What percentage of total births does this number represent?

List Discoveries in Health. A general map of the human genetic code was completed in June 2000 through the Human Genome Project. Enormous potential exists for the correction of birth defects and the production of highly specific medications. Investigate the progress made by the Human Genome Project. Make a list of current technologies that use the information and future uses proposed.

Pediatrician

Being a physician who specializes in treating children from birth through the teen years takes patience, understanding, and a lot of education. Pediatricians get a four-year college degree and then complete four years of medical school. This is followed by three or more years of residency training in pediatrics. Some pediatricians have additional training in specialties such as neonatal care or heart diseases in children. Find out more about this and other health careers by clicking on Career Corner at **health.glencoe.com**.

Chapter 19 *Review*

➤ **EXPLORING HEALTH TERMS** *Answer the following questions on a sheet of paper.*

Lesson 1 *Replace the underlined words with the correct term.*

amniotic sac	implantation
embryo	labor
fertilization	placenta
fetus	umbilical cord

1. The final stage of pregnancy, in which the uterus contracts and pushes the baby out of the mother's body, is <u>fertilization</u>.

2. The ropelike structure that connects the embryo and the placenta is the <u>fetus</u>.

3. The <u>amniotic sac</u> is the thick, blood-rich tissue that lines the walls of the uterus and nourishes the embryo during pregnancy.

Lesson 2 *Match each definition with the correct term.*

birthing center	prenatal care
stillbirth	fetal alcohol syndrome (FAS)
miscarriage	

4. A facility in which females with low-risk pregnancies can deliver their babies in a homelike setting.

5. A group of alcohol-related birth defects.

6. The spontaneous expulsion of a fetus that occurs before the twentieth week of a pregnancy.

Lesson 3 *Fill in the blanks with the correct term.*

CVS	genetic disorder
DNA	chromosomes
genes	heredity
gene therapy	amniocentesis

7. The threadlike structures found within the nucleus of a cell that carry the codes for inherited traits are called _____.

8. The basic units of heredity are _____.

9. The chemical units that make up chromosomes are called _____.

10. A defect in genes can result in a(n) _____.

Lesson 4 *Fill in the blanks with the correct term.*

autonomy	scoliosis
developmental tasks	

11. _____ is/are a series of events that must happen in order for an individual to continue growing toward becoming a healthy, mature adult.

12. _____ is/are the confidence that a person can control his or her own body, impulses, and environment.

13. An abnormal sideways curvature of the spine is _____.

➤ **RECALLING THE FACTS** *Use complete sentences to answer the following questions.*

Lesson 1

1. From where does a zygote's DNA originate?

2. What is the function of the amniotic sac?

3. Summarize the three stages of labor.

Lesson 2

4. What happens during a prenatal visit to a doctor or certified nurse midwife?

5. Why is nutritional counseling during pregnancy important?

6. List four environmental hazards that can harm a fetus.

Lesson 3

7. Explain the role of genetics in human development. If a baby boy receives a dominant gene for brown eyes and a recessive gene for blue eyes, what color will his eyes be?

8. How does the genetic makeup of a male differ from that of a female?

Lesson 4

9. How might impatience toward someone in middle childhood affect the development of that child?

10. How soon after birth should an infant have a hearing screening?

11. When is a child commonly checked for scoliosis?

► THINKING CRITICALLY

1. **Summarizing.** Make a booklet to explain the process of fetal development to young children. Share your booklet with a young child you know. *(LESSON 1)*

2. **Synthesizing.** Suppose you observed a pregnant female drinking an alcoholic beverage. How might you inform her about the effects of her drinking on her unborn child? *(LESSON 2)*

3. **Applying.** Identify and survey occurrences of an easily observed genetic trait such as hair color. From your data, decide whether the trait you observed is dominant or recessive. Research the trait to confirm or disprove your decision. *(LESSON 3)*

4. **Evaluating.** You observe a parent interacting with a child in the grocery store. The child is pushing a mini-cart and mimicking the motions of "shopping." Periodically the child asks, "Why?" and wants to examine everything in the store. Which stage of childhood is the child displaying? What clues help you make this determination? *(LESSON 4)*

► HEALTH SKILLS APPLICATION

1. **Accessing Information.** Choose a human body system. Research its development before birth. Prepare a visual report of your findings. *(LESSON 1)*

2. **Communicating.** Research and analyze the effects of secondhand smoke on a developing fetus. Write a dialogue in which a pregnant woman uses this factual information and "I" messages to communicate her desire for a person not to smoke in her presence. *(LESSON 2)*

3. **Advocacy.** Research a genetic disorder that interests you. Find out what organizations are currently doing research on the disease and how this research is funded. Write a letter to the funding organization urging them to continue their support. *(LESSON 3)*

4. **Practicing Healthful Behaviors.** Identify screening and immunization programs in your community. What screenings and immunizations are required by your state? By your school district? Check with your parents about whether your own family's immunizations are up to date. *(LESSON 4)*

 BEYOND *the* Classroom

Parent Involvement

Analyzing Influences. Talk with a parent or other adult family member about the responsibilities of parenthood. Share Erikson's stages of infancy and early, middle, and late childhood, and discuss how your family helped you move successfully from one stage to another.

School and Community

Child Care. Invite a child psychologist to your school to discuss the developmental tasks of children. Have the person explain the positive behaviors that caregivers can use to help ensure that the children they care for become healthy, mature adults. Then use the information to prepare a pamphlet for all babysitters to read.

Chapter 20

Adolescence and the Life Cycle

CROSS-CURRICULUM CONNECTIONS

Shape a Poem. Learning to fulfill a promise to yourself, to a friend, or to your family helps you as an adolescent build toward a successful future. Make a list of the promises you have made to yourself and others. From this list, write a vertical poem using the word "promise." A vertical poem is one in which the letters of a word appear down the page, and each letter starts a line of the poem.

Calculate Life Expectancy. According to Lesson 4, page 529, the average lifespan in 1900 was 47.3 years but has risen to a current life expectancy of 77 years. Assuming that figure to be valid for the year 2004, if the life expectancy continues to rise at the same rate, how long should a person born in the year 2050 expect to live?

Debate on Change. Historians debate whether adolescence is a modern concept. They note that in medieval England, few common people lived past the age of 40, which denied them the pleasures of youth and instead forced them into apprenticeships or to begin life's work as a teen. Research and make a time line of changes that took place in the nature of adolescence in the industrialized Western culture during the twentieth century. Have a class discussion of what you learned.

Compare Self-Sufficiency. For humans, the responsibilities of caring for offspring last through adolescence and sometimes young adulthood. This is not so for many animal families. Research the development of one type of animal. Find out how soon the offspring of this animal are physically developed enough to survive on their own. Compare and contrast the self-sufficiency of human offspring with the animal you researched.

Gerontologist

If you get along well with older adults, you might want to consider a career as a gerontologist. A gerontologist often works with other professionals, such as occupational and physical therapists, dietitians, or lawyers, to improve the quality of life for older persons. Some gerontologists work in nursing homes, senior centers, and other community facilities. Still others teach or work in research facilities. Because the population of the United States is aging, the job outlook for individuals working in gerontology is excellent. Find out more about this and other careers in Career Corner at **health.glencoe.com**.

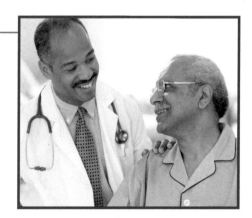

Chapter 20 *Review*

➤ **EXPLORING HEALTH TERMS** *Answer the following questions on a sheet of paper.*

Lesson 1 *Replace the underlined words with the correct term.*

adolescence	hormones
cognition	puberty
gametes	sex characteristics

1. A person begins to develop sex characteristics during <u>cognition</u>.

2. <u>Gametes</u> are produced in glands and help regulate many of the body's functions.

3. During adolescence, <u>puberty</u>, the traits related to a person's gender, develop.

Lesson 2 *Match each definition with the correct term.*

emotional intimacy	physical maturity
emotional maturity	

4. The state in which the physical body and all its organs are fully developed.

5. The state in which the mental and emotional capabilities of an individual are fully developed.

Lesson 3 *Fill in the blanks with the correct term.*

commitment	self-directed
marital adjustment	unconditional love
adoption	

6. When someone adjusts to marriage or to his or her spouse, that person makes a _____ .

7. Making decisions about behavior when adults are not present to enforce the rules is an indication that a child is _____ .

8. When parents show their child love at all times without limitation or qualification, the parents are giving _____ .

Lesson 4 *Identify each statement as True or False. If false, replace the underlined term with the correct term.*

empty-nest syndrome	transitions
integrity	

9. The critical changes that take place during adulthood are called <u>integrity</u>.

10. <u>Empty-nest syndrome</u> may result when children move from home.

➤ **RECALLING THE FACTS** *Use complete sentences to answer the following questions.*

Lesson 1

1. What are two physical changes that take place in the teen brain? How are these changes significant?

2. Why is it important for adolescents to expand their verbal skills?

3. How does the value system of an adolescent differ from that of a child?

Lesson 2

4. What are two characteristics of an emotionally mature person?

5. Why does emotional maturity take longer to achieve than physical maturity?

6. What are some ways that young adults can contribute to society?

Lesson 3

7. Why do most people marry?

8. How can couples reduce the impact of conflict on their marriage?

9. Why are teen marriages often unsuccessful?

10. How can a parent help a child become self-directed?

Lesson 4

11. How do mental activities such as reading or solving puzzles help older adults?

12. What are some ways in which older adults can use the freedom that comes from having children move away from home?

13. How has increased life expectancy affected the way people view retirement?

► THINKING CRITICALLY

1. **Synthesizing.** In a private health journal, answer each of the questions asked in the developmental tasks section of Lesson 1. Reflect on your answers and identify the areas that need attention. Determine the steps you could take to accomplish those particular tasks. *(LESSON 1)*

2. **Summarizing.** Interview three adults about their contributions to society, and make a list indicating how that contribution met a need in their lives. Write a short report summarizing your findings. *(LESSON 2)*

3. **Evaluating.** In some cultures parents arrange the marriages of their children. How do you think this would work in today's American society? *(LESSON 3)*

4. **Applying.** What advice would you give to someone who is suffering from empty-nest syndrome? Write a letter to a friend or relative with this problem. *(LESSON 4)*

► HEALTH SKILLS APPLICATION

1. **Analyzing Influences.** Adolescence is a stage marked by change. List three changes teens experience. Appraise and explain how each influences and contributes to personal growth for a healthy life. *(LESSON 1)*

2. **Refusal Skills.** You have your sights set on a career goal, but your friends want you to go against a school rule that might cause you to jeopardize that goal. Write three refusal statements that are based on your goals. *(LESSON 2)*

3. **Accessing Information.** Poll friends and acquaintances who want to get married about why they would like to do so. Identify similar reasons, and use the information to create a graph showing the number of individuals choosing each reason. *(LESSON 3)*

4. **Practicing Healthful Behaviors.** Analyze the dynamics of family roles and responsibilities relating to health behaviors. Work with an older adult in your family to identify one health behavior that you can do together.

BEYOND *the* Classroom

Parent Involvement

Advocacy. Find out about community resources available to help parents with their parenting roles and child-care options. Are there programs associated with local schools or colleges? Find out how you and your parents can become involved in such programs.

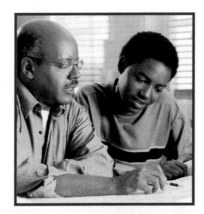

School and Community

Active Older Adults. Visit a senior center in your community. Meet some of the older adults who use the center. Find out why they visit the center and what other resources they use. If possible, volunteer at the center.

Tobacco

Make a Difference

Mike is an advocate for a smoke-free environment. He and his friends are active members of Teens Against Tobacco Use (TATU), a national peer education program sponsored by the American Lung Association. The group's goal is to help its members and others understand the dangers of tobacco and prevent its use.

Mike says, "I got involved with TATU because you get to teach young people about the harmful effects of smoking—a big health issue. We went to an elementary school and taught the facts and consequences of smoking. We used a metal bowl and a bunch of metal BBs to teach our lesson. Each BB represented a certain number of people who had died because of a specific condition, such as AIDS or car crashes. When we dropped those BBs into the bowl, they made a pretty loud sound. When we dropped the BBs representing the 450 thousand people a year, however, who die of smoking-related diseases—more than all the other causes combined—the students were stunned!

We also put on a skit, teaching refusal skills to use if someone offers them cigarettes. Helping people choose to live tobacco free has made a difference in my life and, I hope, in the lives of others."

Quick Write

Using Visuals. Using tobacco can seriously damage a person's health. What strategies can you use to prevent the use of tobacco?

HEALTH Online

For instant feedback on your health status, go to Chapter 21 Health Inventory at **health.glencoe.com**.

The Effects of Tobacco Use

VOCABULARY

addictive drug
nicotine
stimulant
carcinogen
tar
carbon monoxide
smokeless tobacco
leukoplakia

YOU'LL LEARN TO

- Describe the harmful substances contained in tobacco and in tobacco smoke.

- Examine the harmful effects of tobacco use on body systems.

- Analyze the physical, mental, social, and legal consequences of tobacco use.

➔ **QUICK START** Most people know that using tobacco is harmful. Why do you think some people continue to use tobacco products? Write your response on a sheet of paper.

▼ Tobacco products, which are made from the leaves of tobacco plants, contain nicotine. Experts say that nicotine is more addictive than heroin or cocaine. *List some harmful effects of nicotine.*

Trends in tobacco use are changing, and that's good news for public health, according to the American Lung Association. The public is becoming more aware of the health costs of tobacco use, and more individuals are making the choice to be tobacco free.

Tobacco Use—A Serious Health Risk

According to the Surgeon General, tobacco use, particularly smoking, is the number one cause of preventable disease and death in the United States. Because tobacco use has been linked to many health risks, the government requires all tobacco products to carry warning labels. Avoiding *all* forms of tobacco can prevent many serious health problems. Still, every day some teens begin to smoke, chew, or dip tobacco. Many people begin to use tobacco products thinking that they can quit whenever they want to. Once a person has formed the habit, however, it's very difficult to quit.

Nicotine

One of the reasons that tobacco users find it difficult to quit is that tobacco contains an **addictive drug**, *a substance that causes* *physiological or psychological dependence.* All tobacco products contain **nicotine**, *the addictive drug found in tobacco leaves.* Nicotine is classified as a **stimulant**—*a drug that increases the action of the central nervous system, the heart, and other organs.* Nicotine raises blood pressure, increases heart rate, and contributes to heart disease and stroke. Once addicted, people need more and more tobacco to satisfy the craving for nicotine.

Cigarette Smoke—A Toxic Mixture

Not only is tobacco addictive, but the smoke from burning tobacco is toxic. In 1992 the Environmental Protection Agency classified environmental tobacco smoke, or secondhand smoke, as a Group A carcinogen. This is the most dangerous class of carcinogen. A **carcinogen** is *a cancer-causing substance.* Other compounds in tobacco smoke are described below.

Tar and Carbon Monoxide

Cigarette smoke contains **tar**, *a thick, sticky, dark fluid produced when tobacco burns.* As tar penetrates the smoker's respiratory system, it destroys cilia, tiny hairlike structures that line the upper airways and protect against infection. Tar damages the alveoli, or air sacs, which absorb oxygen and rid the body of carbon dioxide. It also destroys lung tissue, making the lungs less able to function. Lungs damaged by smoking are more susceptible to diseases such as bronchitis, pneumonia, emphysema, and cancer.

Carbon monoxide, another compound found in cigarette smoke, is *a colorless, odorless, and poisonous gas* that is taken up more readily by the blood than oxygen is. Carbon monoxide replaces oxygen in the blood, thereby depriving the tissues and cells of oxygen. It also increases the risk of high blood pressure, heart disease, and hardening of the arteries.

Harmful Effects of Pipes and Cigars

Like smoking cigarettes, smoking pipes or cigars presents major health risks. Cigars contain significantly more nicotine and produce more tar and carbon monoxide than cigarettes do. One cigar can contain as much nicotine as a pack of cigarettes. Pipe and cigar smokers have an increased risk of developing cancers of the lip, mouth, and throat.

Cigarettes contain 43 known carcinogens, including cyanide, formaldehyde, and arsenic. They also contain poisonous chemicals used in insecticides, paint, toilet cleaners, antifreeze, and explosives. *How can you use this knowledge to help others stay tobacco free?*

(A) **Your decision not to smoke can help keep your lungs healthy.** *Compare the healthy lung (top) with the one damaged from smoking (bottom). Discuss how tar and other components in tobacco smoke affect the lungs and their function.*

Harmful Effects of Smokeless Tobacco

Smokeless tobacco is *tobacco that is sniffed through the nose, held in the mouth, or chewed.* These products are *not* a safe alternative to smoking. Like tobacco that is smoked, smokeless tobacco contains nicotine in addition to 28 carcinogens, all of which are absorbed into the blood through the mucous membranes or the digestive tract.

Because smokeless tobacco is often held in the mouth for a length of time, it delivers both nicotine and carcinogens to the body at levels that can be two to three times the amount delivered by a single cigarette. As a result, people who chew eight to ten plugs of tobacco each day take in the same amount of nicotine as a two-pack-a-day smoker. Smokeless tobacco is as addictive as smoked tobacco. In addition, it irritates the mouth's sensitive tissues, causing **leukoplakia**, or *thickened, white, leathery-looking spots on the inside of the mouth that can develop into oral cancer.* Cancers of the throat, larynx, esophagus, stomach, and pancreas are also more common among users of smokeless tobacco.

How Tobacco Affects the Body

For several decades health officials have warned the public about the health risks of tobacco. The chemicals in tobacco products can cause damage to many body systems. **Figure 21.1** on page 543 illustrates some of the effects of tobacco on the body.

Short-Term Effects of Tobacco Use

Some effects of tobacco use can occur immediately after using the product. Here are some of these short-term effects:

▶ **Changes in brain chemistry.** The addictive properties of nicotine cause the body to crave more of the drug. The user may experience withdrawal symptoms such as headaches, nervousness, and trembling as soon as 30 minutes after his or her last tobacco use.

▶ **Increased respiration and heart rate.** Breathing during physical activity becomes more difficult; and in some cases, nicotine may cause an irregular heart rate.

▶ **Dulled taste buds and reduced appetite.** Tobacco users often lose much of their ability to enjoy food.

▶ **Bad breath and smelly hair, clothes, and skin.** These unattractive effects may cause people to avoid the tobacco user.

Long-Term Effects of Tobacco Use

Over time, tobacco use takes a serious toll on many body systems, including the respiratory, cardiovascular, and digestive

FIGURE 21.1

HEALTH RISKS OF TOBACCO

Tobacco use damages several important body systems, causing severe health problems that may result in death.

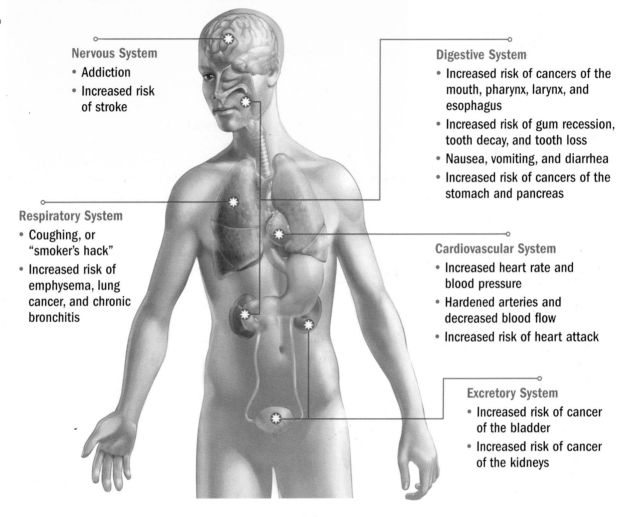

Nervous System
- Addiction
- Increased risk of stroke

Respiratory System
- Coughing, or "smoker's hack"
- Increased risk of emphysema, lung cancer, and chronic bronchitis

Digestive System
- Increased risk of cancers of the mouth, pharynx, larynx, and esophagus
- Increased risk of gum recession, tooth decay, and tooth loss
- Nausea, vomiting, and diarrhea
- Increased risk of cancers of the stomach and pancreas

Cardiovascular System
- Increased heart rate and blood pressure
- Hardened arteries and decreased blood flow
- Increased risk of heart attack

Excretory System
- Increased risk of cancer of the bladder
- Increased risk of cancer of the kidneys

systems. The immune system is weakened, making the body more vulnerable to disease. Long-term tobacco use can lead to health problems such as:

▶ **Chronic bronchitis.** Repeated tobacco use can damage the cilia in the **bronchi** until they no longer function. This leads to a buildup of tar in the lungs, causing chronic coughing and excessive mucus secretion.

▶ **Emphysema.** This is a disease that destroys the tiny air sacs in the lungs. The air sacs become less elastic, making it more difficult for the lungs to absorb oxygen. A person with advanced emphysema uses up to 80 percent of his or her energy just to breathe.

hot link

bronchi For more information about the respiratory system functions, see Chapter 16, page 428.

► **Lung cancer.** When the cilia in the bronchi are destroyed, extra mucus cannot be expelled. Cancerous cells can grow in these conditions, block the bronchi, and move to the lungs. Unless detected early, lung cancer causes death.

► **Coronary heart disease and stroke.** Nicotine constricts **blood vessels,** which cuts down on circulation, or blood flow. Nicotine also contributes to plaque buildup in the blood vessels, which can lead to hardened arteries, a condition called arteriosclerosis. Arteries may become clogged, increasing the risk of heart attack and stroke. The risk of sudden death from

hotlink

blood vessels For more information on the cardiovascular system, see Chapter 16, page 416.

Exploring Issues

Are Tobacco Warning Labels Effective?

The Canadian government requires tobacco companies to place full-color pictures and warning labels on all cigarette packages. Do you think such labels are effective in influencing people to practice healthful behaviors?

Viewpoint 1: Hillary F., age 16

I don't think that warning labels on cigarette packages are effective. People who smoke know the dangers—they've heard it all before, from newspapers, magazines, and doctors. If they haven't quit before this, a message and a

WARNING:
CIGARETTES CAUSE LUNG CANCER

85% of lung cancers are caused by smoking. 80% of lung cancer victims die within 3 years.

Health Canada

picture on a pack of cigarettes isn't going to have much influence. Labels like these lose their impact after a while anyway. Smokers get used to seeing them and eventually ignore them.

Viewpoint 2: Gary H., age 15

The labels on these cigarette packages are effective media messages. Smokers see them every time they pull a cigarette out of the pack. It will cause some of those people to think about quitting, and some will quit. Sure, smokers hear about the health risks of smoking from other sources, but that doesn't mean the labels aren't effective. Images often have a stronger impact than words.

ACTIVITIES

1. Do you think the Canadian warning labels on cigarette packs are more effective than American labels? Why or why not?

2. Do you agree that people become desensitized to labels? If so, what can health advocates do to make labels promoting healthful behaviors more effective?

heart disease is three times greater for smokers than for nonsmokers.

Other Consequences

Tobacco use brings many other serious consequences especially for teens.

► **Legal consequences.** Selling tobacco products to persons under the age of 18 is illegal in all states. Schools prohibit the use of tobacco products on school property, and a student may be suspended or expelled for breaking these rules.

► **Social consequences.** Many people find secondhand smoke and the smell of tobacco offensive, so tobacco users may be excluded from social gatherings. Having bad breath, yellowed teeth, and stained fingers may also harm a tobacco user's social life.

► **Financial consequences.** Use of tobacco products can be very expensive. Someone who smokes a pack of cigarettes a day can spend more than $2,000 each year just on cigarettes. According to a recent report, the total economic cost of tobacco use to taxpayers in the United States, including medical costs, is about $97 billion a year.

Most teens choose healthy alternatives and avoid the negative consequences of tobacco use.

 Lesson 1 *Review*

Reviewing Facts and Vocabulary

1. What is *nicotine*? Why is it harmful?
2. Explain why cigarette smoke is toxic.
3. List the short-term and long-term effects of tobacco use.

Thinking Critically

4. **Applying.** Examine the effects of tobacco use on the respiratory and cardiovascular systems.
5. **Synthesizing.** Analyze the harmful effects of teen tobacco use. Include physical, mental, social, and legal consequences.

Applying Health Skills

Advocacy. Help others recognize how tobacco use can harm body systems. Write a letter to your parents or adult members of your family explaining what damage can occur as a result of using tobacco products.

WORD PROCESSING Word processing can give your report a professional look. Learn more about using word-processing software at **health.glencoe.com**.

Choosing to Live Tobacco Free

VOCABULARY
nicotine withdrawal
nicotine substitute

YOU'LL LEARN TO

• Explain the benefits of a tobacco-free lifestyle.

• Develop strategies for preventing the use of tobacco products.

• Identify health services in the community that help prevent tobacco-related diseases and promote a tobacco-free lifestyle.

QUICK START On a sheet of paper, list all of the negative effects of tobacco use that you can recall. Then write three refusal statements you can use to avoid tobacco use.

After peaking in 1997, teen smoking has fallen sharply. *What has contributed to the drop in teen smoking in recent years?*

High school students who reported smoking a cigarette in the last 30 days

40 percent

35
30
25
20
15
10
5

'91 '93 '95 '97 '99 '01

Source: Centers for Disease Control and Prevention, 2001

K nowing the health risks of tobacco use has helped people make the healthful decision to stay tobacco free. In fact, the number of people in the United States who don't smoke, either because they never started or because they have quit, has been rising steadily.

Reduced Tobacco Use Among Teens

A ccording to the Centers for Disease Control and Prevention (CDC), smoking rates among teens have fallen sharply in recent years. Reports show that nationally 28 percent of high school students smoke. This is down from 36 percent in 1997. Some factors contributing to this ongoing trend include:

▶ **Antismoking campaigns.** In 1998, tobacco companies and 46 states reached a legal settlement that restricted tobacco advertising and promotion. Tobacco companies are now required to fund ads that discourage young people from smoking.

▶ **Financial cost.** Tobacco use is expensive. Many teens find that they would rather spend their money on healthier alternatives.

▶ **Societal pressures.** Legislative acts have limited smoking in public places. More young people are growing up in an environment that is less tolerant of secondhand smoke.

▶ **Family influence.** Many teens avoid tobacco use because their parents strongly disapprove of the use of tobacco products.

Benefits of Living Tobacco Free

People who have never used tobacco and people who have quit enjoy the many benefits of a tobacco-free lifestyle. Avoiding tobacco lowers the risk of lung cancer, heart disease, and stroke. It improves cardiovascular endurance and lung function, which increases physical fitness and enhances athletic performance.

Living tobacco free has mental, emotional, and social benefits, too. Tobacco-free people have a sense of freedom because they know that they are not dependent on an addictive substance. They experience less stress because they don't have to worry about health-related problems caused by tobacco use. A tobacco-free lifestyle will also help a person look and feel better. Having higher energy levels, healthier skin, fresher breath, and better-smelling clothes and hair will increase confidence in social situations.

A tobacco-free lifestyle improves heart and lung function, which helps your athletic performance. *List some other benefits of living tobacco free.*

Strategies for Preventing Tobacco Use

The best way to avoid the negative consequences of tobacco use is never to start using tobacco products. Nearly 90 percent of all adult smokers started when they were teens, so if you avoid tobacco use during middle school and high school, you are likely to stay tobacco free throughout your life. Below are some strategies to help you stick to your decision to live tobacco free.

▶ **Choose friends who don't use tobacco.** Being around people who share your values and beliefs will strengthen your commitment to lead a tobacco-free life.

▶ **Avoid situations where tobacco products may be used.** By staying away from such situations, you reduce the chance of being pressured to use tobacco.

▶ **Practice and use refusal skills.** Prepare in advance what you will say if someone offers you tobacco. Your refusal may be a simple "No thanks," or you may give a reason, such as, "No, I need to stay fit for the track competition." Be assertive, and leave the situation if the pressure continues.

Benefits of Quitting:

► **Within 20 minutes** blood pressure and pulse rates drop. Body temperature in limbs returns to normal.

► **Within eight hours** oxygen levels return to normal.

► **In 24 hours** the chance of heart attack begins to decrease.

► **In 48 hours** nerve endings begin to regrow. Senses of taste and smell improve.

► **In three days** breathing becomes easier as lung capacity increases.

► **Within two weeks to three months** lungs function up to 30 percent better.

► **Within one to nine months** lung cilia regrow and coughing, sinus congestion, and shortness of breath decrease.

► **In one year** the risk of coronary heart disease is cut in half.

► **In five years** the risk of lung cancer and cancers of the mouth, throat, and esophagus is reduced by 50 percent. Stroke risk is also decreased.

► **In ten years** the risk of cancer of the bladder, kidney, cervix, and pancreas decreases.

Why Some Teens Use Tobacco

In spite of the many benefits of a tobacco-free lifestyle, some teens choose not to resist the pressure to start smoking. Some teens think that smoking will help them control their weight or cope in times of stress and crisis. Other teens believe that smoking will make them seem mature and independent. These beliefs are far from the truth about tobacco use. Because smoking reduces the body's capacity for physical activity, it may actually lead to weight gain. In addition, health problems and nicotine dependency will increase the tobacco user's stress level.

Other reasons for teen tobacco use are peer pressure and media influences. Some teens try their first cigarette with a friend who already smokes. Other teens may try tobacco to imitate, or model, celebrities or other adults who smoke. Some teens are influenced by ads that depict tobacco use as glamorous and sophisticated.

Being aware of these influences and being informed about the harmful effects of tobacco can help teens resist the pressure to use tobacco products. Teens who analyze these influences realize that most people who use tobacco products suffer from health problems and wish they could quit the habit.

Reasons to Give Up Tobacco Use

Many teens who start using tobacco do decide to quit. Here are just a few of the reasons they cite:

► They begin to have health problems, such as asthma or respiratory infections.

► They have the desire, will, and commitment to stop.

► They realize how expensive the habit is.

► They realize that using tobacco can lead to other risky behaviors, such as the use of alcohol and other drugs.

► They find it difficult to purchase tobacco products because selling tobacco products to persons under the age of 18 is illegal in all 50 states.

► They realize the damaging effects of secondhand smoke and don't want to harm their families and friends.

Stopping the Addiction Cycle

Millions of people have succeeded in their effort to quit tobacco use. Overcoming nicotine addiction can be difficult, but it's not impossible. Most people who stop using tobacco will experience symptoms of **nicotine withdrawal**, *the process that occurs in the body when nicotine, an addictive drug, is no longer used.* The cravings and discomfort caused by these symptoms are temporary, and smokers trying to quit should remember that success will lead to better health.

Withdrawal

Symptoms of nicotine withdrawal include irritability, difficulty concentrating, anxiety, sleep disturbance, and cravings for tobacco. To relieve the symptoms, some people use a **nicotine substitute**, *a product that delivers small amounts of nicotine into the user's system while he or she is trying to give up the tobacco habit.* Many nicotine substitutes are available, including gum, patches, nasal sprays, and inhalers. Nicotine gum is an over-the-counter product; the other nicotine substitutes require a doctor's prescription. Users who are trying to quit should take the process one step at a time. They might begin by seeking help from a health care professional.

Real-Life Application

Help a Friend STOP Using Tobacco

Studies have shown that most people who try to quit have a greater success rate if they have support from others. Use the **STOP** approach to help someone stop using tobacco.

Show concern. Approach the person in a caring, nonjudgmental manner. Use "I" messages to let the person know that you care about his or her health.

Take time to plan. Putting a plan on paper makes it easier to set objectives. You may need to help the person create a physical activity program. Set a date to quit, locate formal tobacco cessation programs, and devise strategies to cope with tobacco cravings.

Offer support. Put the plan into action. For example, you might bring the person sugarless gum. Ride a bike, shoot hoops, or take a walk together to help him or her get physical activity. Arrange to attend a class together to learn relaxation techniques.

Promote success. Let the person know that you are proud of him or her for quitting. Celebrate each week of abstinence. If the person relapses, continue to encourage him or her. Keep in touch with the person after he or she has quit.

ACTIVITY

Write a plan that addresses each of the STOP guidelines. If you have a family member or a friend who uses tobacco, create the plan for that person, or work with a classmate who knows someone who uses tobacco. Make sure that your plan contains messages that promote the health benefits of stopping tobacco use. Consider the person, and tailor the plan to that person's needs and interests.

Getting Help—Tips for Quitting

People who are trying to give up tobacco use can try the following strategies.

▶ **Prepare for the day.** Set a target date for quitting.

▶ **Get support and encouragement.** Support from family, friends, and peers will increase a person's chance of success.

▶ **Access professional health services.** It may be necessary to seek advice from a doctor, enroll in a tobacco cessation program, or join a support group. Other helpful resources include the American Lung Association, the Centers for Disease Control and Prevention (CDC), and local hospitals.

▶ **Replace tobacco use with healthier alternatives.** Sugarless gum, carrots, and cinnamon sticks are substitutes that people can use when they feel an urge to have a cigarette.

▶ **Change daily behavior.** Avoiding other tobacco users, preparing one's environment for a tobacco-free life, and changing daily routines can also help smokers avoid their tobacco triggers.

▶ **Engage in healthful behaviors.** Physical activity, good nutrition, stress management techniques, and abstinence from alcohol and other drugs will help people through the withdrawal process.

HEALTH *Online*

Learn more about the American Lung Association's programs to help people quit smoking. Click on Web Links at **health.glencoe.com.**

 Lesson 2 *Review*

Reviewing Facts and Vocabulary

1. List three benefits of staying tobacco free.
2. List four strategies for preventing tobacco use.
3. What is *nicotine withdrawal*, and what are *nicotine substitutes*?

Thinking Critically

4. **Evaluating.** Why might tobacco advertisements target teens?
5. **Synthesizing.** Identify services in your community that help to prevent tobacco-related diseases and explain how helping people quit tobacco use promotes a healthy community.

Applying Health Skills

Refusal Skills. Make a two-column chart. In the first column, write five situations in which a teen might be pressured to use tobacco. In the second column, develop effective refusal statements and strategies the teen can use to avoid tobacco use.

TECHNOLOGY *OPTION*

SPREADSHEETS   Use a spreadsheet to draft and finalize your lists. Using this type of program makes it easy to make revisions, and it produces a product that is easy to read. See **health.glencoe.com** for tips on how to use a spreadsheet.

Promoting a Smoke-Free Environment

VOCABULARY

environmental tobacco
    smoke (ETS)
mainstream smoke
sidestream smoke

YOU'LL LEARN TO

• Analyze the harmful effects of tobacco on the health of fetuses, infants, and young children.

• Analyze the influence of laws, policies, and practices on preventing tobacco-related disease.

• Relate the nation's health goals and objectives for reducing tobacco-related illnesses to the individual, family, and community.

→ **QUICK START** Many communities encourage a smoke-free environment in which people can live, work, and play. What places in your community are smoke free? List the benefits of a smoke-free environment.

As more and more people become aware of the harmful effects of tobacco, efforts to curb tobacco use in public places are gaining ground.

The dangers of ETS have prompted some states to pass laws that prohibit all tobacco use in public buildings. *What other measures can be taken to protect the health and well-being of nonsmokers?*

Risks for Smokers and Nonsmokers

Both smokers and nonsmokers who breathe air containing tobacco smoke are at risk for health problems. **Environmental tobacco smoke (ETS)**, or secondhand smoke, is *air that has been contaminated by tobacco smoke.* Environmental tobacco smoke is composed of **mainstream smoke**, *the smoke exhaled from the lungs of a smoker,* and **sidestream smoke**, *the smoke from the burning end of a cigarette, pipe, or cigar.* Sidestream smoke is more dangerous than mainstream smoke because it has higher concentrations of carcinogens, nicotine, and tar.

Effects of Smoke on Nonsmokers

Environmental tobacco smoke from cigarettes and cigars contains more than 4,000 different chemical compounds, 43 of which are identified as carcinogens. Inhaling this smoke either by smoking or by breathing in ETS brings these carcinogens into the body. ETS affects people of all ages, causing eye irritation, headaches, ear infections, and coughing. It worsens asthma conditions and other respiratory problems. Three thousand people every year are diagnosed with lung cancer caused by secondhand smoke.

Effects of Smoke on Unborn Children and Infants

Choosing to live tobacco free is one of the best things a pregnant woman can do to make sure that her baby will be born healthy. Smoking during pregnancy can seriously harm the developing fetus. Nicotine passes through the placenta, constricting the blood vessels of the fetus. Carbon monoxide reduces the oxygen levels in the mother's and the fetus's blood. These negative effects increase the risk of impaired fetal growth, miscarriage, prenatal death, premature delivery, low birth weight, deformities, and stillbirths. The infant may also suffer from growth and developmental problems throughout early childhood.

Babies of smokers are two and a half times more likely to die of sudden infant death syndrome (SIDS). One study found that nearly 60 percent of all SIDS cases could be prevented if babies and pregnant females were protected from tobacco smoke. Infants exposed to ETS have an increased risk of asthma, tonsillitis, and respiratory tract infections.

Effects of Smoke on Young Children

Young children are also particularly sensitive to environmental tobacco smoke. Children of smokers are nearly twice as likely to be in poor health as those of nonsmokers. Consider these facts:

▶ Children of smokers tend to have a higher incidence of sore throats, ear infections, and upper respiratory problems than children of nonsmokers.

▶ Children who live with smokers have double the risk of developing lung cancer than children of nonsmokers.

Because children learn by example, it's not surprising that children of smokers are nearly three times as likely to smoke as children of nonsmokers. Being a positive role model is another good reason to make the choice to be tobacco free.

Parents protect the health of their children by staying tobacco free. *What specific healthful behaviors should pregnant females practice?*

Reducing Your Risks

What can you do to protect yourself from ETS? If you and your family want your home to be smoke free, politely ask visitors to refrain from smoking inside. If someone in your household smokes, open windows to allow fresh air to circulate and request that certain rooms remain smoke free. Consider using air cleaners to help remove contaminants from the air. If you are visiting a home in which someone smokes, go outside or to another room. Ask to open the window slightly to provide fresh air. Suggest meeting elsewhere, such as in your home or at a library. In restaurants and other public places, request seating in a nonsmoking area. If no smoke-free area is available, go to another restaurant.

Health Skills Activity

Communication: Avoiding Environmental Tobacco Smoke

You can protect your health and the health of others by asking smokers not to light up in your presence. Read the scenarios below, and practice communication skills by stating polite requests for a smoke-free environment.

Situation 1

You are at a wedding rehearsal dinner with relatives. Your favorite cousin, whom you haven't seen for a long time, is seated next to you. As you begin catching up on family news, your cousin lights a cigarette.

Situation 2

You and your friends have been waiting for 30 minutes to be seated in a restaurant. A table becomes available in the smoking section, where several people are smoking heavily. Your friends want to take it.

What Would You Do?

Using the communication skills you have learned, write a response to each scenario. Be prepared to role-play your response for the class.

1. Use "I" statements.
2. Keep your tone respectful.
3. Maintain appropriate body language.
4. Give reasons for your request.

Toward a Smoke-Free Society

A s people realize that smoking causes diseases and harms not only their own health but also the health of others, the drive to become a smoke-free society increases. Many states have taken steps to prohibit smoking in all public buildings and private workplaces. In the past the law required only that "no smoking" areas be available to those who wished to avoid ETS. Now, however, many people are promoting laws that would ban smoking and eliminate ETS in public places such as restaurants, civic buildings, business offices, and lobbies. Laws prohibiting the sale of tobacco products to minors are being strictly enforced. Tobacco licenses are being revoked when stores sell tobacco products to people under the age of 18.

Hands-On Health ACTIVITY

Smoking Out Underage Tobacco Sales

Federal law prohibits the sale of tobacco products to all persons under 18. In some states, buyers must be 21. The easier it is to buy tobacco products, the more likely it is that teens will experiment with tobacco and become addicted. Promote health in your community by reminding peers that it's illegal for stores to sell tobacco products to minors.

What You'll Need

- information provided by your teacher
- poster board • masking tape
- markers

What You'll Do

1. In a small group, use the information your teacher has provided on tobacco control in your state to answer these questions:
   - What is the legal age to purchase tobacco products?
   - What is the penalty for minors who use or possess tobacco products?
   - What are the penalties for merchants who sell tobacco to minors?
   - What is your state doing to curb underage tobacco sales?

2. With your group, discuss your findings. Recall signs you have seen that explain store policies regarding the sale of tobacco products. How do you think these signs affect teens who wish to purchase tobacco products?

Apply and Conclude

With your group, create a poster that is targeted at teens who wish to purchase tobacco products even though it is against the law. Include the responses to at least two of the questions you answered in the activity. Your poster should be attention-getting, persuasive, and accurate. Ask a local merchant to display your poster.

Increasingly, the law is taking into consideration the rights of the nonsmoker. Certain states have successfully sued tobacco companies to recover the cost of treating tobacco-related diseases. The money awarded in these cases is often used to fund statewide antismoking campaigns or to offset the medical costs related to tobacco use.

Working Toward National Health Goals

The Department of Health and Human Services has launched a program, called *Healthy People 2010*, to promote health and prevent disease nationwide. One of the goals of *Healthy People 2010* is to reduce the number of people who use tobacco and the number of deaths associated with tobacco use. Decreasing tobacco use and reducing exposure to secondhand smoke are important steps in increasing the years of healthy life among people in the United States.

You, your family, and your community can join in the national effort to take a stand against tobacco. Become involved in activities that promote a healthy lifestyle, and encourage others to practice healthful behaviors, too. You can start a tobacco prevention program at school or join a youth group campaigning for stricter government control of tobacco and its availability.

These teens are asking the storeowner to remove a tobacco ad because their state prohibits such ads from appearing within 1,000 feet of a school. *What other actions can teens take to promote health in their community?*

 Lesson 3 *Review*

Reviewing Facts and Vocabulary

1. Define *mainstream smoke* and *sidestream smoke*. Explain what they have in common.

2. Explain how the tobacco settlement money helps disease prevention and health promotion.

3. What strategies can you use to limit the amount of ETS you breathe?

Thinking Critically

4. **Evaluating.** Analyze the influence of laws on teen tobacco use and explain how this influence relates to prevention of disease.

5. **Analyzing.** Analyze the harmful effects of environmental tobacco smoke on fetuses, infants, and young children.

Applying Health Skills

Advocacy. You can help others make the decision to stay tobacco free. Using the goals of *Healthy People 2010*, create a pamphlet that will educate people about the harmful effects of tobacco use and secondhand smoke. Relate the nation's health goals and objectives for reducing tobacco-related illnesses in your pamphlet.

WEB SITES Instead of a pamphlet, create a Web site advocating a tobacco-free lifestyle and a smoke-free environment. See **health.glencoe.com** for help in planning and building your Web site.

Which Antismoking Ads Are Most Effective with Teens?

Studies show that antismoking ads aimed at teen audiences are effective in helping teens make the healthful decision to avoid tobacco use. Antismoking advertisements may be sponsored by health organizations, by nonprofit companies, or by tobacco companies. Some ads use satire or humor while others give hard facts about the health risks of tobacco use. Use the activity below to help you identify different techniques in antismoking ads and analyze the effectiveness of these ads on teens.

ACTIVITY

Read the script of the television ad. Using the Internet and your library as resources, find an antismoking advertisement created by a tobacco company. Compare the tobacco company ad with the ad pictured above.

1. How do the messages of each ad differ?

2. What techniques are used in each ad? Does either ad use satire or humor? Does either ad use dramatic visuals to convey its message?

3. Does each ad contain credible information? How do you know it is credible?

4. How does each ad explain or show the harmful effects of smoking?

EXPRESS YOUR VIEWS

Write a letter to the editor of your local newspaper advocating for citizens to take action to promote a tobacco-free society. Include your views on which antismoking ads you find most effective for teens and why.

CROSS-CURRICULUM CONNECTIONS

Write a Story. Tobacco ads once used cartoon characters intended to be appealing to young people. Relying on the same appeal, work with a group to write a story in which the main character, the wily coyote, tricks another character into quitting tobacco use, and teaches him an important life lesson. Personify a cigarette, making it the villain of your story and the target of the trick.

Warnings Against Tobacco. Opposition to tobacco use dates back to its early cultivation. For example, in 1604 King James I of England pronounced in his "Counterblast to Tobacco" that smoking was "loathsome to the eye, hatefull to the Nose, harmfull to the brain, [and] dangerous to the lungs." Research and write a report on the fight against tobacco, citing warnings throughout history. Show how similarities in these warnings support medical evidence about the health risks of tobacco use.

Lung Cancer Deaths. From 1995 to 2000, a community averaged 1,126.7 deaths per 100,000 people. Lung cancer accounted for an average of 115.3 of those deaths. What percent of all deaths was the result of lung cancer?

Diagram the Lungs. All the blood in your body passes through the lungs. This allows the red blood cells to absorb oxygen and release carbon dioxide. The lungs are made up of a number of structures that allow the exchange of gases and prevent infection. Diagram the lungs, and show the various parts and their functions. Demonstrate how inhalation of tobacco smoke affects each function, and explain how this might affect related systems, particularly circulation.

CAREER Corner

Respiratory Therapist

Do you enjoy interacting with people of all ages? Are you interested in working in a medical field? A respiratory therapist works with patients who need respiratory care. Therapists may provide temporary relief to patients suffering from asthma or emphysema or provide emergency care to patients who are suffering from a heart attack, stroke, drowning, or shock.

Formal training is required to enter this profession. Training programs vary in length and in the credentials or degrees awarded. Find out more about this and other health careers by clicking on Career Corner at **health.glencoe.com**.

➤ EXPLORING HEALTH TERMS *Answer the following questions on a sheet of paper.*

Lesson 1 *Match each definition with the correct term.*

stimulant   carcinogen
addictive drug   smokeless tobacco
carbon monoxide   nicotine
tar   leukoplakia

1. The addictive drug in tobacco.
2. A drug that increases the action of the central nervous system, the heart, and other organs.
3. A cancer-causing substance.
4. A thick, sticky, dark fluid produced when tobacco burns.

Lesson 2 *Fill in the blanks with the correct term.*

nicotine withdrawal
nicotine substitute

(**_5_**) is the process that occurs in the body when nicotine is no longer used. A (**_6_**) can be used to ease the side effects associated with this process.

Lesson 3 *Replace the underlined words with the correct term.*

mainstream smoke
sidestream smoke
environmental tobacco smoke (ETS)

7. <u>Sidestream smoke</u> is another name for secondhand smoke.
8. <u>Environmental tobacco smoke</u> is the smoke exhaled from the lungs of a smoker.
9. <u>Mainstream smoke</u> is tobacco smoke from the burning end of a cigarette, pipe, or cigar.

➤ RECALLING THE FACTS *Use complete sentences to answer the following questions.*

Lesson 1

1. What effect does tar in cigarette smoke have on the respiratory system?
2. What effect does carbon monoxide have on the body?
3. How does tobacco use harm the digestive and excretory systems?
4. How does smoking lead to lung cancer?

Lesson 2

5. How do tobacco companies encourage teen tobacco use?
6. List two refusal skills you can use to say no to tobacco.
7. What are some reasons why teens stop using tobacco?
8. Identify three sources of help for people who want to quit tobacco use.

Lesson 3

9. List three health problems associated with environmental tobacco smoke.
10. How does ETS harm infants and young children?
11. How do state laws discourage teen smoking?
12. Describe the goals of *Healthy People 2010* that relate to tobacco use.

➤ THINKING CRITICALLY

1. **Explaining.** Why would a smoker tend to inhale more deeply and smoke more cigarettes when he or she switches to low-nicotine cigarettes? *(LESSON 1)*

2. **Analyzing.** What factors influence a teen's decision to use tobacco? *(LESSON 2)*

3. **Evaluating.** How do laws that prohibit smoking in specified areas contribute to community health? *(LESSON 3)*

4. **Synthesizing.** Relate the nation's health goals for reducing tobacco-related illness in your community. Explain how smoke-free zones in your community support *Healthy People 2010*. *(LESSON 3)*

➤ HEALTH SKILLS APPLICATION

1. **Decision Making.** What would you do if a close friend wanted to use tobacco to relieve stress? Use the six steps of decision making to form a plan of action. *(LESSON 1)*

2. **Accessing Information.** Conduct research to identify, describe, and assess health services in the community that provide tobacco cessation programs to prevent disease. Make a list of resources that will provide help for tobacco users who want to quit. *(LESSON 2)*

3. **Communication Skills.** What would you say to a pregnant female to encourage her to live tobacco free? *(LESSON 3)*

4. **Advocacy.** Write a letter to a state or local official expressing your opinions on what the government should do to promote the health of its citizens. Include in your letter information on the benefits of a smoke-free environment for all people. *(LESSON 3)*

BEYOND the Classroom

Parent Involvement

Advocacy. With your parents, brainstorm ways your family can help promote a smoke-free environment in your community. What actions can you take to contribute to a healthy environment for all people in your community?

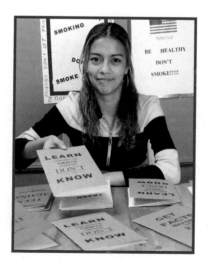

School and Community

Antitobacco Programs. Work with classmates, teachers, and administrators to start a Teens Against Tobacco Use (TATU) program at your school. As a group, design a plan for promoting health in your school and community by reducing tobacco use. Ask members of the community to support your goals.

Alcohol

Noon Concert

Sponsored by: Students Against Alcohol Use

Do You Know Which Is a Myth and Which Is a Fact About Alcohol?

Read each statement below and respond by writing *Myth* or *Fact* for each item.

1. Alcohol has the same chemical and physical effects on everyone who drinks.

2. Someone who doesn't act drunk isn't drunk.

3. When a person is intoxicated, coffee, a cold shower, or fresh air will sober him or her up.

4. Alcohol impairs judgment and social behaviors.

5. People can get into serious health, legal, and social problems *anytime* they use alcohol.

6. Drinking alcohol on weekends or once in a while is not harmful.

7. No amount of alcohol is safe for a pregnant woman to drink.

8. Binge drinking has no long-term effects.

HEALTH Online

For instant feedback on your health status, go to Chapter 22 Health Inventory at **health.glencoe.com**.

Quick*Write*

Using Visuals. Teens who make the decision to avoid the use of alcohol enjoy safe and healthy activities. How can you and your peers make a statement about your decision to stay alcohol free?

Choosing to Be Alcohol Free

VOCABULARY

ethanol
fermentation
depressant
intoxication
alcohol abuse

YOU'LL LEARN TO

- Identify factors, such as the media, that influence decisions about alcohol use and your health.

- Analyze the physical, mental, social, and legal consequences of alcohol use.

- Explain the relationship between alcohol use by adolescents and the role alcohol plays in unsafe situations.

- Develop strategies for preventing the use of alcohol.

- Demonstrate refusal strategies regarding alcohol use and the benefits of choosing to be alcohol free.

QUICK START Fold a sheet of paper in half. On the left side of the paper, list reasons why drinking alcohol is risky for teens. On the right side, list alternatives to alcohol use.

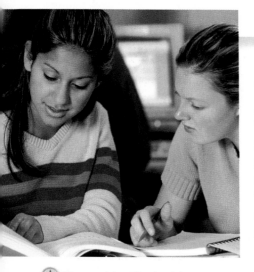

Recognizing the health risks of alcohol will help you make the decision to stay alcohol free. *How can avoiding alcohol use help you succeed in school?*

For many people the image is a familiar one: energetic young adults playing sports, cooking out, living life to the fullest. The purpose of this attractive advertisement scene is to promote and sell a drug—alcohol—that is addictive, physically damaging, and often an entry into other drug use. In reality, alcohol is a lethal drug with harmful physical, mental, social, and legal consequences. These consequences can result in serious health problems to the drinker and those around him or her and even death caused by disease, violence, or vehicle crashes.

The Facts About Alcohol

Alcohol, or, more accurately, **ethanol**—*the type of alcohol in alcoholic beverages*—is a powerful and addictive drug. Ethanol can be produced synthetically or naturally through the fermentation of fruits, vegetables, and grains. **Fermentation** is *the chemical* *action of yeast on sugars.* Water, flavoring, and minerals are mixed with ethanol to produce a variety of beverages, such as beer and wine. Alcohol also can be processed to create spirits, or liquors, such as whiskey, rye, and vodka.

Immediate Effects of Alcohol Consumption

At first drinking alcohol may provide a kind of energy "rush." This initial reaction masks alcohol's true effects as a **depressant**, *a drug that slows the central nervous system.* Alcohol quickly affects a person's motor skills by slowing reaction time and impairing vision. Clear thinking and good judgment also diminish. A variety of factors, including a person's body size and stomach contents, determines alcohol's effect. For this reason, the amount of alcohol that leads to intoxication varies from person to person. **Intoxication** is *the state in which the body is poisoned by alcohol or another substance and the person's physical and mental control is significantly reduced.*

A Your family, friends, and peers influence your decisions about avoiding the use of alcohol. *How does your family support you in your healthy choice to be alcohol free?*

Factors That Influence Alcohol Use

Despite the many problems associated with alcohol use, many teenagers still choose to drink. Why? Several reasons influence teens in their choice to use—or not use—alcohol:

▶ **Peer pressure.** It's normal for teens to want to feel accepted within a group. The desire to fit in is strong. Teens who choose friends who avoid alcohol use are more likely to be alcohol free than teens whose friends accept alcohol use.

▶ **Family.** Family members can help teens be alcohol free. Parents who discourage and avoid the use of alcohol are more likely to have teens who do the same. In fact, teens cite parental disapproval as the number one reason for not using alcohol.

▶ **Media messages.** Many media messages on TV and radio and in movies make alcohol use appear exciting, attractive, and fun. Many of these messages feature elements targeted to a teen audience, such as young, attractive people engaging in problem-free drinking in a partylike atmosphere. The message of many ads is "To fit in, drink alcohol." However, teens who recognize these messages and their meanings are more likely to resist negative influences.

Did You Know ?

Through the media teens are exposed to alcohol use in many forms.

- By the time teens reach ninth grade, most will have seen more ads for beer or wine than for any other product.
- A recent study found that 93 percent of the 200 most popular movie rentals depicted alcohol use.
- A review of top-selling rap recordings found alcohol mentioned in 47 percent of the songs.

Advertising Techniques

Companies that produce alcoholic beverages spend billions of dollars each year and use various strategies to advertise and sell their products. Advertisements appear on billboards, can be seen or heard on television and radio, and fill magazines and newspapers. Alcohol companies sponsor sporting events, music concerts, art festivals, exhibits, and other community events. They do this to

Real-Life Application

Seeing Through Alcohol Advertising

What media images come to mind when you think of advertisements for alcohol? Many advertisers appeal to emotions and desires to influence people to buy their products. By understanding the ways in which advertisers market alcohol, teens can make the informed choice to avoid using it.

JOIN THE FUN!

ACTIVITY

Use a critical eye when looking at advertisements in magazines and news-papers and on billboards, television, and the Internet. Select three examples of alcohol advertising. For each example, ask yourself these questions:

1. **What is really being advertised?** Write a paragraph that analyzes how the ad appeals to an emotion or a desire in a particular audience.

2. **What is the hidden message?** Create a caption that describes what the advertisers want the intended audience to believe about drinking alcohol.

3. **What is the truth?** Explain why the ad is misleading, using at least three facts about alcohol use that the ad does not mention.

Demonstrate what you have learned from your analysis by writing a statement on the truthfulness of alcohol advertising.

What is really being advertised?
The ad is "selling" physical attractiveness. It appeals to an internal influence that most people share: the desire to be among friends who enjoy being together.

What is the hidden message?
"You need our beer to have fun with your friends."

What is the truth?
Drinking beer is not the reason people are enjoying the party. This picture is staged. In fact, drinking alcohol impairs coordination; the ability to play volleyball would be affected. None of the risks of alcohol use are shown.

associate their products with attractive and healthy people having fun. It is important to thoroughly analyze and interpret media messages that encourage the consumption of alcohol.

Avoid Alcohol: Avoid Unsafe Situations

Alcohol use can be dangerous and even deadly. Alcohol-related traffic collisions are the number one cause of death and disability among teens. Alcohol use also is linked with deaths by drowning, fire, suicide, and homicide. Even if you are not drinking but are around people who are, you have an increased risk of being seriously injured, involved in a vehicle crash, or affected by violence. Alcohol-related incidents can be damaging to the health and safety of the user and those associated with the user.

Alcohol and the Law

If you are under 21, it is illegal to buy, possess, or consume alcohol. For teens who break the law, the costs can be very high. Teens can be arrested, fined, and sentenced to a youth detention center. By breaking the law, the offender risks both damaging his or her reputation and losing the trust and respect of friends and family members.

Alcohol, Violence, and Sexual Activity

Teens can protect their health by avoiding situations where alcohol is present. Teens who drink alcohol are more likely to be victims or perpetrators of violent crimes such as rape, aggravated assault, and robbery. They are also more likely to become involved in fights, resulting in school or police action.

Alcohol use and sexual activity are a dangerous mixture. Alcohol impairs a person's judgment, lowers his or her inhibitions, and compromises his or her moral standards. Teens who use alcohol are more likely to become sexually active at earlier ages, to engage in sexual activity more often, and to engage in unprotected sexual activity more often than teens who do not use alcohol. Such careless sexual activity can lead to unplanned pregnancy, sexually transmitted diseases, and emotional scars that don't heal easily.

Alcohol Abuse

Most young people do not live in families in which alcohol abuse is a problem. However, it is estimated that 25 percent of all youth *are* exposed to family **alcohol abuse**—*the excessive use of alcohol*— at some time before they reach the age of 18. Young people who live in a household in which a family member abuses alcohol are at a high risk for neglect, abuse, economic hardship, and social isolation. Sometimes, these problems can lead a young person to try alcohol

Did You Know ?

Alcohol use is a serious matter. It is a key factor in

- 33 percent of suicides.
- 50 percent of homicides.
- 62 percent of assaults.
- 68 percent of manslaughter cases.
- 50 percent of head injuries.
- 41 percent of traffic fatalities.
- Alcohol also plays a major role in domestic abuse and injury, child abuse and neglect, and workplace injuries.
- More than half of all people who drown have consumed alcohol before entering the water.

Health Skills Activity

Refusal Skills: Avoiding Alcohol

Chantelle has been invited to a party at her friend Natasha's house. When Chantelle arrives, she is surprised to see people drinking alcoholic beverages. Natasha's parents are not at home.

Chantelle walks over to Natasha. "What kind of party is this?" she asks.

"It's a *high-school* party," Natasha says. "Here, have a beer."

"No, thanks," Chantelle responds. "Won't your parents be upset if they see this?"

"Don't worry," Natasha says. "They won't be home for hours. Here, have a drink. It'll loosen you up."

Chantelle knows she needs to communicate her refusal and leave the party. What should she do?

What Would You Do?

Apply the following refusal skills to write a response for Chantelle.

1. Say no in a firm voice.
2. Explain why you are refusing.
3. Suggest alternatives to the proposed activity.
4. Back up your words with body language.
5. Leave if necessary.

---

as an escape. However, drinking only makes the situation worse. Studies indicate that a person who begins drinking as a teen is four times more likely to develop alcohol dependence than an adult is.

Alcohol and Extracurricular Activities

The negative consequences of alcohol use for teens can extend to their eligibility for participation in extracurricular activities, including athletics. Most schools have adopted a zero-tolerance policy for students found using alcohol. If caught, students may become ineligible to participate or may be suspended from their activities or from school. A student's future college and job prospects could be damaged.

Being Alcohol Free

Deciding to be alcohol free is an important step in achieving a healthy lifestyle. Many people, especially teens, make the commitment to stay alcohol free. This commitment helps you:

Choosing to be alcohol free allows you to reach your potential and achieve your goals.

- ▶ **Maintain a healthy body.** Avoiding alcohol use protects body organs from damage and decreases the chance of injury.

- ▶ **Make responsible decisions.** Having a clear head helps you make decisions to protect your health and the health of others.

- ▶ **Avoid risky behavior.** Teens who avoid alcohol reduce their risk of participating in unsafe behaviors such as sexual activity or drinking and driving, and of being a victim or perpetrator of a violent crime.

- ▶ **Avoid illegal activities.** Purchasing or possessing alcohol is against the law for anyone under the age of 21. You can avoid arrest and legal problems by being alcohol free.

Call home for a ride if you find yourself in a situation where alcohol is present. *What other strategies can you use to avoid unsafe situations?*

Refusing Alcohol

Even if the pressure to use alcohol becomes intense, saying no is much easier when you're prepared. If you find yourself in a situation in which alcohol is present, be assertive: refuse to drink, leave the situation quickly, and call for a ride home. Remember that your best defense is to avoid situations in which alcohol is present. Avoid parties where alcohol is served. Practice refusal skills at home to build confidence when you are with peers.

 Lesson 1 *Review*

Reviewing Facts and Vocabulary

1. Define the terms *alcohol*, *depressant*, and *intoxication*.

2. Identify and explain ways families can have a positive influence on teens' decisions about alcohol use.

3. Describe two effective refusal strategies for avoiding the use of alcohol.

Thinking Critically

4. **Analyzing.** Explain the depressant effects of alcohol. How might alcohol affect your ability to make healthful decisions?

5. **Synthesizing.** Explain why refusing alcohol will help you avoid unsafe situations such as sexual assault and violence. In what ways will you also be avoiding the risk of exposure to STDs?

Applying Health Skills

Advocacy. Prepare a pamphlet or an article for your school newspaper that advocates an alcohol-free lifestyle. Describe the risks and consequences of alcohol use. Be sure to explain the benefits of being alcohol free and to include examples of effective communication skills when avoiding alcohol use.

TECHNOLOGY OPTION

WORD PROCESSING Give your pamphlet or article a professional look by using word-processing software. See **health.glencoe.com** for tips on using different features of most word-processing programs.

Harmful Effects of Alcohol Use

VOCABULARY

metabolism
blood alcohol
   concentration
binge drinking
alcohol poisoning

YOU'LL LEARN TO

- Examine the short-term effects of alcohol use.
- Apply responsible decision making by associating the risks and consequences of drinking and driving.
- Recognize the dangers of alcohol-drug interactions.
- Demonstrate refusal strategies concerning alcohol use.

➡️ **QUICK START**   Make a list of all the organs in the body you can think of that are affected by alcohol use. Make a word web of your ideas with the term "alcohol use" in the center.

(A) **Many over-the-counter and prescription drugs carry warning labels about alcohol interactions.** *Analyze how these warnings help protect users from health risks.*

S tatistics confirm that drinking alcohol is a high-risk behavior. Nevertheless, some teens feel pressured to drink alcohol. Finding out about the physical effects alcohol has on the body can help you strengthen your commitment to staying alcohol free.

Short-Term Effects of Drinking

T he short-term effects of alcohol are different for each individual. Many of these effects are described in **Figure 22.1.** Some factors that influence the onset of these effects include:

▶ **Body size and gender.** A small person feels the effect of the same amount of alcohol faster than a large person does. In general, alcohol moves into the bloodstream faster in females.

▶ **Food.** Food in the stomach slows down the passage of alcohol into the bloodstream.

▶ **Amount and rate of intake.** As the amount of alcohol consumed increases, the level of alcohol in the bloodstream also rises. When a person drinks alcohol faster than the liver can break it down, intoxication results. When blood alcohol levels become too high, alcohol poisoning can occur.

Alcohol and Drug Interactions

lcohol and medications or any other drugs don't mix. Interactions between medications and alcohol can lead to illness, injury, or even death. In fact, alcohol-drug interactions are a factor in about one-fourth of all emergency room admissions. To understand why these interactions occur, you must understand how the body works. When a drug enters the body, it travels through the bloodstream to its target organ or tissue. Over time, the body metabolizes the drug. **Metabolism** is *the process by which the body breaks down substances.* Alcohol travels through the bloodstream to the brain. At the same time, the liver metabolizes the alcohol in the bloodstream and makes it less active. Then the kidneys filter the neutralized particles and other waste products from the blood and produce urine, which is excreted.

The presence of both alcohol and medication or another drug within a person's body can be dangerous. This is because alcohol combined with medicines or other drugs can result in a *multiplier effect*, in which the medication has a greater or different effect than if it were taken alone. Both prescription drugs and over-the-counter medicines, such as aspirin, can alter the way in which alcohol affects the body. Labels on medicines that might cause reactions warn against combining them with alcoholic beverages.

FIGURE 22.1

SHORT-TERM EFFECTS OF ALCOHOL

Physical and mental impairment begin with the first drink of alcohol and increase as more alcohol is consumed.

Nervous System	Cardiovascular System	Digestive System	Respiratory System
• **Brain.** The brain becomes less able to control the body. Movement, speech, and vision may be affected. • **Memory.** Thought processes are disorganized, and memory and concentration are dulled. • **Judgment.** Judgment is altered and coordination is impaired.	• **Heart.** With a low intake, alcohol causes an increase in heart rate and blood pressure. At higher intake levels, heart rate and blood pressure decrease and heart rhythm becomes irregular. Risk of cardiac arrest increases. • **Blood Vessels.** Alcohol causes the blood vessels to expand. The increased surface area of the blood vessels allows body heat to escape and the body's temperature to drop.	• **Stomach.** Some alcohol passes quickly from the stomach into the bloodstream. Stomach acid production increases and often results in nausea and vomiting. • **Liver.** Toxic chemicals are released as the liver metabolizes alcohol. These chemicals cause inflammation and scarring. • **Kidneys.** Alcohol causes the kidneys to increase urine output, which can lead to dehydration.	• **Lungs.** Carbon dioxide formed by the liver is released from the body through the lungs. • **Breathing.** Alcohol depresses nerves that control involuntary functions such as breathing. If an excessive amount of alcohol is consumed, breathing may slow, become irregular, or stop.

These are some typical alcohol-drug interactions.

▶ Alcohol may slow down a drug's absorption by the body. This increases the length of time that the alcohol or drug is in the body and increases the risk of harmful side effects from the drug.

▶ Frequent drinking may increase the number of metabolizing enzymes in the body. This can cause medications to be broken down faster than normal, decreasing their effectiveness.

▶ Metabolizing enzymes can change some medications into chemicals that can damage the liver or other organs. For example, when taken with alcohol, acetaminophen, a common painkiller and fever reducer, can cause serious liver damage even when it is used in small amounts.

▶ Alcohol can increase the effects of some drugs. For example, antihistamines, which are taken for colds or allergies, react with alcohol and cause excessive dizziness and sleepiness. This effect is especially dangerous if you are operating machinery or driving.

HEALTH Online

To investigate what Mothers Against Drunk Driving (MADD) is doing about reducing drunk driving crashes, use Web Links at **health.glencoe.com**.

Driving Under the Influence

Drinking alcohol impairs vision, reaction time, and coordination. When drinking is mixed with driving, the results can be disastrous or even deadly. In fact, *driving while intoxicated* (DWI), also known as *driving under the influence* (DUI), is the leading cause of death among teens. A person is said to be intoxicated when his or her blood alcohol concentration exceeds the state's legal limit. **Blood alcohol concentration (BAC)** is *the amount of alcohol in a person's blood, expressed as a percentage.* In most states driving while intoxicated is defined as having a 0.1 percent BAC, although in some states the figure is 0.08. However, signs of intoxication can begin to appear at BACs as low as 0.02. **Figure 22.2** on the next page illustrates the alcohol content of some common alcoholic beverages. Remember that for anyone under 21, there is no acceptable BAC percentage. Medical researchers have found that drinking of any sort

▶ slows reflexes.

▶ reduces a person's ability to judge distances and speeds.

▶ increases risk-taking behaviors.

▶ reduces a person's concentration while increasing forgetfulness.

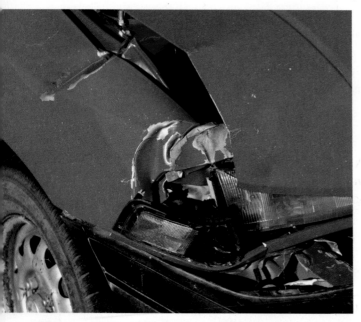

Alcohol-related vehicle fatalities are a leading cause of death for teens. *What effect does alcohol have on a person's ability to control a vehicle?*

Consequences of DWI

When a person is stopped for drinking and driving, a police officer will administer a field sobriety test before the person is given a breathalyzer test to measure BAC. The consequences for a teen caught driving while intoxicated or driving under the influence may include

▶ harm to the driver and others.

▶ severely restricted driving privileges and/or immediate confiscation of a driver's license.

▶ alcohol-related injuries, property damage, and death.

▶ living with regret and remorse from these consequences.

▶ loss of parental trust and respect.

▶ arrest, jail time, court appearance, and a heavy fine or bail.

▶ a police record and possible lawsuits.

▶ higher insurance rates—up to three times higher than those for nondrinking peers.

Like drinking and driving, riding in a vehicle with a driver who has been drinking is also a serious matter. Every day at least a dozen teens are killed in alcohol-related crashes. Never ride in a vehicle with a driver who has been drinking. If you are faced with this situation, find a ride with someone who has not been drinking or call home to have someone come to get you.

Binge Drinking

Recent studies show that **binge drinking**, *drinking five or more alcoholic drinks at one sitting,* is a serious problem among young people. Rapid binge drinking (sometimes done on a bet or dare) is especially dangerous because it is possible to consume a fatal dose of alcohol. Binge drinking can cause alcohol poisoning.

Alcohol Poisoning

It is very dangerous, and can be deadly, to drink a large amount of alcohol. **Alcohol poisoning** is *a severe and potentially fatal physical reaction to an alcohol overdose.* Alcohol acts as a depressant and shuts down involuntary actions such as breathing and the gag reflex that prevents choking. A fatal dose of alcohol will eventually stop these involuntary actions. It's common for a person who has consumed too much alcohol to vomit because alcohol is a stomach irritant. If the involuntary actions are shut down, a person can choke and be asphyxiated by his or her own vomit.

FIGURE 22.2

COMPARING BEER, WINE, AND SPIRITS

Each of these beverages contains the same amount of pure alcohol—about 0.5 ounces.

Drink	Alcohol by Volume	Alcohol Content
Beer 12 oz.	4%	0.5 oz.
Wine 5 oz.	10%	0.5 oz.
Vodka or Whiskey 1.25 oz.	40%	0.5 oz.

Hands-On Health ACTIVITY

Saying No to a Driver Who Has Been Drinking

You've heard the statement "Don't drink and drive." It's also dangerous to ride in a car if you suspect the driver has been drinking. Here are some ways to refuse that ride.

- Make a firm commitment to yourself not to ride with someone who has been drinking. If you know that alcohol will be available at a party, don't go.
- When you suspect a driver has been drinking, be prepared to make the right choice for your health and safety. Be strong. Find another way home.

Direct Statements: "I am not riding with you. You have been drinking."

Excuses: "I forgot to tell you—my dad is picking me up."

Insults: "You are really crazy to drive after drinking."

Humor: "I'm not getting in that car with you; I value my life."

Alternate suggestion: "Give me the keys; I'll drive."

What You'll Need

- 1 index card per student
- colored pencils or markers
- hole punch
- scissors

What You'll Do

1. Working with a small group, brainstorm a list of refusal strategies a teen can use to avoid riding in a car with a driver who has been drinking.

2. Write and present a skit that has dialogue showing one or more successful refusal skills. Be sure that every group member has a part.

3. Act out your skit for the class. Analyze each skit for the dialogue you think is most effective. Remember and practice these statements so that you'll be prepared if a drinking driver offers you a ride.

Apply and Conclude

On your own, cut a $3'' \times 5''$ index card in half so that you have a $3'' \times 2\frac{1}{2}''$ card. Punch a hole in one corner. Write "Don't Ride with a Drunk Driver" on the card. Then write at least two statements you can use to refuse such a ride. Use markers to make the card eye-catching. After your teacher laminates the card, place it on your key ring.

Effects of Alcohol Poisoning

Passing out is a common effect of drinking too much alcohol. Alcohol doesn't stop entering a person's bloodstream after he or she passes out, however. Instead, alcohol in the stomach and intestines continues to enter the bloodstream, and blood alcohol concentration continues to rise. For this reason, it's dangerous to assume that a person who has consumed a lot of alcohol will be fine if left to "sleep it off."

Symptoms that indicate alcohol poisoning include

► mental confusion, stupor, coma, inability to be roused, vomiting, and seizures.

► slow respiration—10 seconds between breaths or fewer than 8 breaths a minute.

► irregular heartbeat.

► hypothermia or low body temperature—pale or bluish skin color.

► severe dehydration from vomiting.

A person who exhibits any of these signs or has passed out may die if left untreated. If you suspect that a person has alcohol poisoning, call 911 immediately.

The consequences of binge drinking can have serious effects on a person's health. *What should you do if you suspect someone has alcohol poisoning?*

 Lesson 2 *Review*

Reviewing Facts and Vocabulary

1. Define *blood alcohol concentration* and *metabolism.*

2. Examine the short-term effects of alcohol use. List three ways alcohol impairs the functioning of the nervous system.

3. What are the signs of alcohol poisoning?

Thinking Critically

4. **Analyzing.** Explain why it's dangerous to mix alcohol and medications or other drugs.

5. **Synthesizing.** Describe the legal and financial consequences of operating a motor vehicle while under the influence of alcohol. Explain why these are only a few of the risks faced by a person driving under the influence.

Applying Health Skills

Advocacy. Prepare a public service announcement to get the word out about the health risks of binge drinking. Include facts about alcohol's effects on the body, as well as the risks involved with rapid binge drinking and how it can cause alcohol poisoning. Demonstrate effective refusal strategies to avoid these risks.

WORD PROCESSING Word processing can help you organize and present your information. See **health.glencoe.com** for tips on how to get the most out of your word-processing program.

Alcohol, the Individual, and Society

VOCABULARY

**fetal alcohol
    syndrome (FAS)**
alcoholism
alcoholic
recovery
detoxification
sobriety

YOU'LL LEARN TO

- Relate the nation's health goals in *Healthy People 2010* to reducing injury, death, and disease caused by alcohol-related influences.

- Examine the effects of alcohol use on body systems and the risk of disease caused by alcohol use.

- Analyze the harmful effects of alcohol on a fetus.

- Identify and assess community health services for the prevention and treatment of alcoholism and alcohol use.

*QUICK
START*   Fold a sheet of paper into three sections. Label the sections "physical," "mental/emotional," and "social." Then list the ways that alcohol use affects each part of the health triangle.

Ⓐ **Compare the healthy liver (top) with the liver that has been damaged by alcohol use.** *Explain the relationship between a healthy liver and an alcohol-free lifestyle.*

The costs of alcohol use are far-reaching and involve individuals, families, and society. One goal of *Healthy People 2010* is to reduce a number of risk behaviors associated with alcohol. This includes reducing the amount of average annual alcohol consumption, binge drinking, and the total number of alcohol-related deaths and deaths due to alcohol-related vehicle crashes.

Long-Term Effects of Alcohol on the Body

Alcohol use has long-term effects on the user and on others as well. In teens alcohol use can interfere with growth and development. Excessive alcohol use over a prolonged period of time can damage most body systems. These effects are more severe on the body of a young person. **Figure 22.3** shows some of the long-term effects of alcohol abuse.

FIGURE 22.3

LONG-TERM EFFECTS OF ALCOHOL USE

Alcohol affects many of the major organs in the body, and long-term drinking can cause death. The worst damage occurs after years of abuse, but some damage occurs with only moderate drinking.

Changes to the Brain

- **Addiction**—inability to stop drinking.
- **Loss of brain functions**—loss of verbal skills, visual and spatial skills, and memory.
- **Brain damage**—long-term excessive use of alcohol can lead to major brain damage and even to a reduction of brain size. Moderate drinking can destroy brain cells; however, the brain can regain some of its lost abilities over time if a person stops drinking.

Cardiovascular Changes

- **Heart**—damage to heart muscle.
- **Enlarged heart**—from increased workload caused by alcohol.
- **High blood pressure**—damages the heart and can cause heart attack and stroke.

Liver Problems

- **Fatty liver**—fats build up in the liver and cannot be broken down; excess fat blocks the flow of blood to liver cells, leading to cell death.
- **Alcoholic hepatitis**—inflammation or infection of the liver.
- **Cirrhosis**—liver tissue is replaced with useless scar tissue; the disease can lead to liver failure and death unless a liver transplant is performed.

Digestive System Problems

- **Irritation**—digestive lining is damaged; can lead to stomach ulcers and cancer of the stomach and esophagus.

Pancreas Problems

- **Lining of the pancreas**—swells to block the passage from the pancreas to the small intestine. Chemicals the small intestine needed for digestion can't pass through the blocked area. The chemicals begin to destroy the pancreas itself, causing pain and vomiting. A severe case can lead to death.

Alcohol During Pregnancy

When a pregnant female drinks, so, in effect, does her fetus. Alcohol passes from the mother's body into the bloodstream of the fetus. Unlike the adult liver, the fetus's liver is not developed enough to process the alcohol. As a result, a pregnant female who drinks during pregnancy risks permanent damage to the fetus.

hot link

fetal alcohol syndrome
For more information on fetal development, see Chapter 19, pages 488–489.

Drinking during the first few weeks of pregnancy—when many women do not yet realize they are pregnant—can be especially harmful to a baby's central nervous system. Infants born to mothers who drink during pregnancy may be at risk of **fetal alcohol syndrome (FAS)**, *a group of alcohol-related birth defects that include physical and mental problems.*

Effects of Fetal Alcohol Syndrome (FAS)

The effects of fetal alcohol syndrome are both severe and lasting. An FAS baby may be born with a small head and deformities of the face, hands, or feet. Heart, liver, and kidney defects, as well as vision and hearing problems, are common. FAS babies experience slow growth and coordination and have difficulties with learning, attention, memory, and problem solving.

FAS is the leading known cause of mental retardation in the United States. The good news is that it's totally preventable—provided that expectant mothers understand two things: there is no safe amount of alcohol to drink and no safe time in which to drink it. Even small amounts of alcohol can harm a fetus.

Alcoholism

One of the most devastating effects of alcohol use is **alcoholism**, *a disease in which a person has a physical or psychological dependence on drinks that contain alcohol.* Alcoholism is characterized by an impaired ability to study, work, or socialize normally.

Alcoholics

An **alcoholic** is *an addict who is dependent on alcohol.* Some alcoholics may display harmful behaviors such as drunken driving and violent or aggressive actions. Others may become quiet and withdrawn. Alcoholism isn't limited to any age, race, ethnic, or socioeconomic group. Alcoholics may be middle-aged business people or high-school athletes. Regardless of background, alcoholics can develop serious health problems, such as cirrhosis of the liver and brain damage. An alcoholic might display these symptoms:

▶ **Craving.** An alcoholic has a compulsion, or strong need, to drink; he or she cannot manage tension or stress without drinking.

▶ **Loss of control.** An alcoholic cannot limit his or her drinking and is preoccupied with alcohol.

GOVERNMENT WARNING: (1) ACCORDING TO THE SURGEON GENERAL, WOMEN SHOULD NOT DRINK ALCOHOLIC BEVERAGES DURING PREGNANCY BECAUSE OF THE RISK OF BIRTH DEFECTS. (2) CONSUMPTION OF ALCOHOLIC BEVERAGES IMPAIRS YOUR ABILITY TO DRIVE A CAR OR OPERATE MACHINERY AND MAY CAUSE HEALTH PROBLEMS.

(A) Avoiding tobacco, alcohol, and other drugs is an important decision a female can take toward a healthy pregnancy. *What other steps can an expectant mother take to protect the health of her unborn child?*

- **Physical dependence.** When not drinking, an alcoholic may experience withdrawal symptoms, such as nausea, sweating, shakiness, and anxiety.

- **Tolerance.** An alcoholic experiences a need to drink increasingly greater amounts of alcohol in order to feel its effects.

- **Health, family, and legal problems.** An alcoholic often suffers repeated injuries, receives multiple drunk driving citations, and has frequent arguments and generally poor relationships with family members.

Factors Affecting Alcoholics

Growing scientific evidence suggests a genetic link to alcoholism. In fact, the American Academy of Child and Adolescent Psychiatry reports that children of alcoholics are four times more likely than other children to become alcoholics. However, this does not necessarily mean that a person with such a genetic predisposition will become an alcoholic. Other environmental factors, such as family, friends, culture, peer pressure, availability of alcohol, and stress, also put a person at risk for alcoholism. There is, however, one guarantee: You can protect yourself against this disease by making the healthy choice to stay alcohol free.

Stages of Alcoholism

According to the American Medical Association, alcoholism develops in three stages. All alcoholics do not experience each stage equally.

- **Stage 1—Abuse.** Typically, alcoholism begins with social drinking in an attempt to relax. Over time, a physical and psychological dependence on alcohol to manage stress develops. At this point a person begins to drink and become intoxicated regularly, which can result in blackouts and memory loss. Often, a person begins to lie or make excuses about his or her drinking. The person needs to consume more alcohol to feel the desired effect. He or she may be a problem drinker.

- **Stage 2—Dependence.** The person reaches a point where he or she cannot stop drinking and is physically dependent on the drug. Alcohol becomes the person's central focus. The drinker tries to hide the problem, but performance on the job, at school, or at home soon suffers. The drinker makes excuses and blames others for problems.

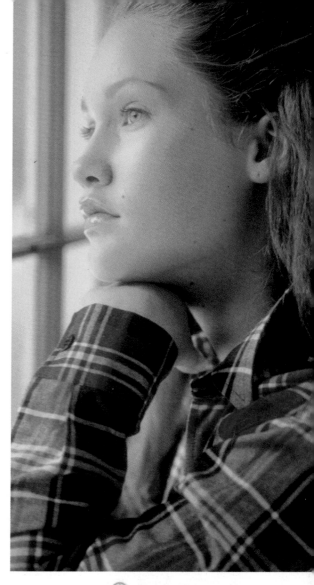

Family members of alcoholics also experience the negative effects of alcoholism. *List ways a person can avoid the risks of alcoholism.*

▶ **Stage 3—Addiction.** In the final stage of alcoholism, drinking is the *most* important thing in a person's life. The person is addicted to the drug and his or her life is out of control, although frequently he or she does not realize or acknowledge this fact. Because liver damage is common at this stage, less alcohol may be required to produce intoxication. If the alcoholic stopped drinking, he or she would experience severe withdrawal symptoms.

Effects on Family and Society

There are an estimated 14 million alcoholics in the United States. Alcohol use is a major factor in the four leading causes of accidental death—car accidents, falls, drownings, and house fires. Alcohol also plays a major role in violent crimes, such as homicide, forcible rape, and robbery. For example:

▶ About 40 percent of violent crimes, totaling about 3 million annually, are alcohol-related.

▶ Two-thirds of victims who encounter **domestic violence** report that alcohol was a factor in the crime.

▶ Nearly half of all homicide victims have alcohol in their bloodstreams.

Often, alcoholism has indirect, as well as direct, effects on people associated with alcoholics. These people may be involved in a process known as *codependency.* Codependents learn to ignore their own needs and focus their energy and emotions on the needs of the alcoholic. In the process codependents lose their trust in others, their self-esteem, and, at times, their own health.

Treatment for Alcohol Abuse

Although alcoholism cannot be cured, it *can* be treated. *The process of learning to live an alcohol-free life* is called **recovery**. As many as two-thirds of all alcoholics who try to recover do so with proper treatment. The goal of treatment programs is to stop or control the intake of alcohol. Counseling and medication can help an alcohol user set goals to deal with problems of alcohol abuse. **Sobriety**, *living without alcohol*, is a lifelong commitment. Many resources are available to help people who have a drinking problem. Help is also available for the families and friends of a problem drinker. Some of these programs are described in **Figure 22.4.**

hot link

domestic violence For more information on dealing with family crises, see Chapter 11, page 286.

STEPS TO RECOVERY

Step 1: Admission
The person admits to having a drinking problem and asks for help.

Step 2: Detoxification
The person goes through **detoxification,** *a process in which the body adjusts to functioning without alcohol.*

Step 3: Counseling
The person receives counseling to help him or her learn to live without alcohol.

Step 4: Recovery
The person takes responsibility for his or her own life.

FIGURE 22.4

WHERE TO GET HELP FOR ALCOHOL ABUSE

There are many places to get information about treatment for alcohol dependency. The goal of these programs is to provide support for alcoholics, family members, and friends affected by alcoholism.

Al-Anon/ Alateen	Alcoholics Anonymous	National Association for Children of Alcoholics	National Clearinghouse for Alcohol and Drug Information	National Drug and Treatment Referral Routing Service
helps families and friends of alcoholics deal with and recover from the effects of living with an alcoholic	provides help for alcohol users of all ages	provides help for children of alcoholics	provides information about alcohol and other drugs	provides treatment referral and information about treatment facilities

It's Not Your Fault!

Lesson 3 *Review*

Reviewing Facts and Vocabulary

1. Identify three serious effects of alcohol abuse.

2. Define *sobriety*. Explain why sobriety is a lifelong commitment.

3. What steps must an alcoholic take during the recovery process?

Thinking Critically

4. **Analyzing.** Explain how damage can occur in the body of the developing fetus when a pregnant woman drinks alcohol.

5. **Synthesizing.** Alcoholism can have devastating effects on people associated with an alcoholic. Explain ways that these individuals can be affected, and tell how and where those living with an alcoholic can get help.

Applying Health Skills

Accessing Information. Consult your school counselor or use the phone book to identify community resources for families with alcohol-related problems. Research the availability of family counseling. Explain why these sources are valid. Share your information in a flyer or pamphlet.

TECHNOLOGY OPTION

PRESENTATION SOFTWARE Use presentation software to show the results of your research on community resources to your family and friends. See health.glencoe.com for tips on using presentation software.

Researching Alcohol Issues on the Internet

A variety of Internet resources exist that provide information regarding alcohol-related issues. These Web resources may be from a nonprofit advocacy organization, a government institution, a journalist, or even a business. In this activity, you will learn to evaluate Internet resources regarding teen drinking and driving and validate the information contained in those resources.

Criteria

- **Who is the author?** Is the page created by an individual, news organization, or charitable organization?
- **Who is the audience?** Is the page intended for a particular age group or other specific demographic group?
- **How current is the information contained in the source?** What date appears on the page? Can you verify the date from other sources?
- **Is the information provided factual?** Research the source of any statistics, check any references or other sources listed on the page, and check all facts against other sources you know to be reliable.
- **What is the purpose of the page?** Is there a particular viewpoint on the subject matter? If so, what is that viewpoint?

ACTIVITY

Suppose you have been assigned to write a research paper on the subject of teen drinking and driving. Using Web Links at **health.glencoe.com**, choose one Web site or article on the Internet that contains information on the topic of teen drinking and driving. Evaluate the information found in your Web resource by answering the questions in the grid above.

EXPRESS YOUR VIEWS

Working in groups of three or four, create a storyboard for a Web site dedicated to warning teenagers of the dangers of drinking and driving. A storyboard is a mock-up of what each page of your Web site would look like. Include information from the research activity above. Use persuasive language and graphics to illustrate your points. Also, include a list of resources where teens can find further information on the subject.

CROSS-CURRICULUM CONNECTIONS

Create a Campaign. Use your peer pressure in a positive way by organizing an anti-drinking campaign, which will culminate in a class rally. First, put your writing skills to work to appeal to other teens not to use alcohol. Your teacher will divide you into teams and assign each team a different task. Write speeches and skits, create slogans for placards, posters, and bumper stickers. Write a special pledge for students to sign. Devise games to show teens that there are fun alternatives to drinking. Share your final products during the class rally.

Research Alateen. Alcoholics Anonymous, or AA, has helped alcoholics worldwide by introducing them to the 12-step program. Write a short research report on the story of Bill W., who founded the organization in the 1930s, as well as how the organization developed. Then investigate the creation of related groups such as Alateen.

Calculate BAC. The average person's body contains 4 quarts of blood. The standard BAC for intoxication is 0.1 percent. How many ounces of pure alcohol must the average person have in his or her blood to be considered intoxicated?

Find Out More About Addiction. Alcoholism is addiction to alcohol. Recent research has shown that the process of becoming addicted is similar regardless of the substance or activity that is misused. Regular use of the substance alters the neural pathways in the brain. Research the connection between the concentration of neurotransmitters, such as serotonin and dopamine, and addiction to drugs and alcohol.

Substance Abuse Counselor

Do you like helping friends with their problems? Would you enjoy counseling people who need to find help for alcohol abuse problems in their families? As a substance abuse counselor, you would assess and treat people with substance problems and help those who live with alcoholics or substance abusers.

More than half of all counselors in the United States have a master's degree. Most states require some form of credentials, certification, license, or registry before someone can become a counselor. Find out more about this and other health careers by clicking on Career Corner at **health.glencoe.com.**

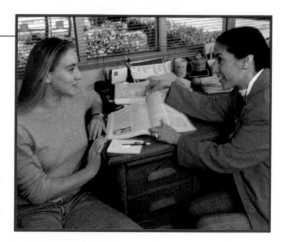

Chapter 22 *Review*

➤ EXPLORING HEALTH TERMS *Answer the following questions on a sheet of paper.*

Lesson 1 *Fill in the blanks with the correct term.*

alcohol abuse	**fermentation**
depressant	**intoxication**
ethanol	

Drinks that contain (_**1**_) act as a (_**2**_) on the central nervous system. Drinking alcohol can lead to physical and mental impairment that is called (_**3**_). (_**4**_) puts family members at risk for neglect, physical abuse, or economic hardship.

Lesson 2 *Match each definition with the correct term.*

blood alcohol concentration	**metabolism**
	alcohol poisoning
binge drinking	

5. The process by which the body breaks down substances.

6. Drinking five or more alcoholic drinks at one sitting.

7. The amount of alcohol in a person's blood expressed as a percentage.

8. A severe and potentially fatal physical reaction to an alcohol overdose.

Lesson 3 *Fill in the blanks with the correct term.*

alcoholism	**alcoholic**
detoxification	**fetal alcohol syndrome**
sobriety	**recovery**

9. _____ is a condition in which a fetus has been adversely affected mentally and physically by the mother's alcohol use during pregnancy.

10. A(n) _____ has an addiction to alcohol.

11. _____ is a process in which the body adjusts to functioning without alcohol.

➤ RECALLING THE FACTS *Use complete sentences to answer the following questions.*

Lesson 1

1. List three factors that influence alcohol use.

2. What are some of the risks of alcohol use?

3. Describe the effects that alcohol has on the body.

4. What impact can alcohol use have on a teen's education and career goals?

Lesson 2

5. Describe one typical alcohol-drug interaction.

6. What are some factors that affect an individual's short-term reaction to alcohol?

7. What are some consequences of driving while intoxicated or driving under the influence?

8. Explain how alcohol poisoning can cause a person's blood alcohol concentration to continue to rise even after the person stops consuming alcohol.

Lesson 3

9. What are some specific goals of *Healthy People 2010* for reducing ways in which alcohol affects the family and society?

10. What is a safe amount of alcohol that a mother can drink during pregnancy?

11. Describe the symptoms an alcoholic might display.

12. Describe two programs that offer help to alcoholics and their families. Explain the services they provide.

➤ THINKING CRITICALLY

1. **Analyzing.** What are some strategies alcohol companies use to target teens in their advertising? *(LESSON 1)*

2. **Synthesizing.** Consider the short-term effects of alcohol on major body systems. How might the organs in the digestive and respiratory systems be damaged by alcohol use over a long period of time? *(LESSON 2)*

3. **Analyzing.** Describe an effective strategy for locating appropriate help and resources available to an alcoholic and his or her family members. *(LESSON 3)*

➤ HEALTH SKILLS APPLICATION

1. **Practicing Healthful Behaviors.** What consequences are faced by students who are caught using or possessing alcohol? *(LESSON 1)*

2. **Communication Skills.** Suppose a friend who has been drinking is going to drive himself or herself and others home. How would you respond to this situation? *(LESSON 2)*

3. **Advocacy.** Find out about groups at your school that advocate for an alcohol-free lifestyle. Get involved with a group, using what you have learned about the consequences of drinking to get local stores to advocate for less advertising of alcohol products. *(LESSON 3)*

 BEYOND the Classroom

Parent Involvement

Advocacy. With your parents or guardians, learn more about SADD—Students Against Destructive Decisions. Learn when, where, and why it was founded, what its mission is, and how you and your family can get involved. Draw up a contract for all family members to sign that includes a commitment never to drink and drive and never to ride with any driver who has been drinking— even a family member.

School and Community

Support Programs. Locate an alcohol treatment program in your community. Contact the agency and find out how the program works, what is required of participants, and how people are supported during the recovery process. Report to your class what you have learned.

Chapter 23

Medicines and Drugs

What's Your Health Status?

Respond by writing *yes*, *no*, or *sometimes* for each item. Write *yes* only for items that you practice regularly.

1. I take medicines as prescribed by my doctor, am careful to follow directions, and never abuse or combine medicines.

2. I use over-the-counter drugs carefully and only as they are intended.

3. I avoid all illegal drug use.

4. I choose friends who avoid using drugs.

5. I would feel comfortable saying no to peers and friends if they offered me drugs.

6. I stay away from areas and events where I know illegal drugs are likely to be used or sold.

7. I never cover for a friend or peer who abuses drugs.

8. I don't attend parties if I know drugs will be used.

9. I know of resources to get help for drug problems and would feel comfortable passing the information along to someone who needed it.

10. I understand the dangers of drugs and am committed to avoiding high-risk situations.

HEALTH Online

For instant feedback on your health status, go to Chapter 23 Health Inventory at **health.glencoe.com**.

Quick *Write*

Using Visuals. Illegal drugs can seriously damage a person's physical, mental/emotional, and social health. In what specific ways can drugs impact an athlete's life?

The Role of Medicines

VOCABULARY

medicines
drugs
vaccine
analgesics
side effects
additive interaction
synergistic effect
antagonistic interaction

YOU'LL LEARN TO

- Analyze ways that medicines promote health and prevent disease.

- Describe the difference between prescription and over-the-counter medicines.

- Analyze how laws, policies, and practices influence safe use of medicines.

QUICK START What precautions do you take when you are about to use a medicine? On a separate sheet of paper, write three types of medicine with which you are familiar, tell why each is taken, and explain what you know about proper use of that medicine.

Medicines are taken for many different reasons. A person may sustain a painful injury while playing a sport or perhaps develop a chest cold accompanied by a hacking cough. To help overcome these ailments and regain their health, people often take medicines.

▲ Medicines are taken to fight illness, promote health, prevent disease, or reduce pain. *When was the last time you needed to use some type of medication?*

Classification of Medicines

There are countless medicines that treat a wide range of health problems. **Medicines** are *drugs that are used to treat or prevent disease or other conditions.* **Drugs** are *substances other than food that change the structure or function of the body or mind.* All medicines are drugs, but not all drugs are medicines. Medicines can be sorted into four broad categories: medicines that

▶ help prevent disease.

▶ fight pathogens, or infectious agents that cause disease.

▶ relieve pain.

▶ help maintain or restore health and regulate the body's systems.

Medicines That Prevent Disease

One main purpose of medicines is to prevent diseases before they occur. There are two main types of preventive medicines:

▶ **Vaccines.** A **vaccine** is *a preparation introduced into the body to stimulate an immune response.* These medicines contain weakened or dead pathogens that stimulate your body to produce specific **antibodies** against those pathogens. Once the antibodies are produced, they give your body long-lasting protection against these specific pathogens in the future.

▶ **Antitoxins.** These extracts of blood fluids contain antibodies and act more quickly than vaccines. They are produced by inoculating animals, such as sheep, horses, or rabbits, with specific toxins that stimulate the animal's immune system to produce antibodies. In humans, the injection of antitoxins neutralizes the effect of toxins, such as those that cause tetanus and diphtheria.

hot link

antibodies For more information on antibodies and vaccines, see Chapter 24, page 633.

Medicines That Fight Pathogens

Antibiotics are a class of chemical agents that destroy disease-causing microorganisms while leaving the patient unharmed. Antibiotics work either by killing harmful bacteria in the body or by preventing bacteria from reproducing. The chemical composition of each antibiotic is effective against a particular range of bacteria.

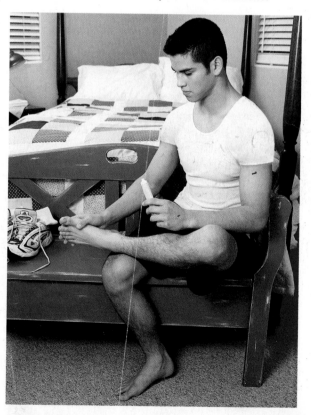

▼ **Athlete's foot can be controlled with antifungal medicines.** *Why is it important to use the correct medicine for a particular treatment?*

In recent years, strains of bacteria have emerged that are resistant to penicillin and other antibiotics. This drug resistance occurs when a bacterial strain undergoes a change in genetic structure as a result of overexposure to an antibiotic, making the bacterium "immune" to the medicine. For example, a bacteria called *pneumococcus* that causes ear and sinus infections and pneumonia is now resistant to penicillin. The overuse of antibiotics and failure to finish a prescription medication are two reasons why bacteria develop resistance. A new generation of broad-spectrum antibiotics has been developed that kill a wide variety of bacteria, including some penicillin-resistant strains.

ANTIVIRALS AND ANTIFUNGALS

Antibiotics have no effect on viruses. However, a new group of drugs called antivirals has been developed to treat some viral illnesses. Antiviral medicines often only suppress the virus; they don't kill it. Antifungals can cure or suppress infections such as athlete's foot and ringworm.

Medicines help many people with conditions such as asthma and diabetes live active, normal lives. *How are these diseases kept under control?*

Medicines That Relieve Pain

Probably the most common medicines are **analgesics**, or *pain relievers*. Analgesics range from comparatively mild medicines such as aspirin to strong narcotics, such as the opium-based morphine and codeine. Aspirin contains acetylsalicylic (uh-SEE-tuhl-sal-uh-SIL-ik) acid. Aspirin is used to relieve pain, reduce fever, and to treat arthritis.

Because of its widespread use, many people don't realize that aspirin can be dangerous. Even small amounts can irritate the stomach, especially when it's empty. Aspirin can cause dizziness and ringing in the ears. Children who take aspirin are at risk of developing Reye's syndrome, a potentially life-threatening illness of the brain and liver. Aspirin, therefore, should not be given to anyone under the age of 20 unless a health care professional directs otherwise. Some people who are sensitive to aspirin take acetaminophen (uh-see-tuh-MIH-nuh-fuhn) or ibuprofen (eye-byoo-PRO-fuhn) instead. Acetaminophen is the recommended analgesic for children.

Medicines That Promote Health

Medicines that maintain or restore health enable many people with chronic disease to function at increased level of wellness. Such medicines include these:

▶ **Allergy medicines.** Many people rely on antihistamines and other medications to reduce the sneezing, itchy or watery eyes, and runny nose that often accompany allergies.

▶ **Body regulating medicines.** Some medicines maintain health by regulating body chemistry. Insulin is used to treat diabetes. Asthma sufferers use inhalers to relieve the swelling of bronchial tubes. Cardiovascular medicines are taken to regulate blood pressure, normalize irregular heartbeats, or regulate other functions of the cardiovascular system.

▶ **Antidepressant and antipsychotic medicines.** These medicines help normalize brain chemistry. For example, mood stabilizers are often used in the treatment of mood disorders, depression, and schizophrenia. Proper medication can help people with these problems live healthy, productive lives.

▶ **Cancer treatment medicines.** These medicines reduce rapid cell growth and help stop the spread of cancer cells. For instance, chemotherapy is used to kill fast-growing cancer cells. This medication, either applied to the skin or injected, results in serious side effects that usually disappear after treatment stops.

Medicines and the Body

Medicines can have a variety of effects on individuals, or can cause different reactions. A person's reaction to a given medicine depends on how that medicine mixes with the chemicals in his or her body. Most medicines cause **side effects**, *reactions to medicine other than the one intended*. It's important to be aware of your reactions to medicines and report these to your health care provider. Patients should always tell their doctors about any medicines they are already taking when a new medicine is prescribed.

When medicines are taken together or when a medication is taken in combination with certain foods, the combination may produce different effects. In some cases, physicians make use of interactions to increase the effectiveness of a treatment. Other interactions may be harmful.

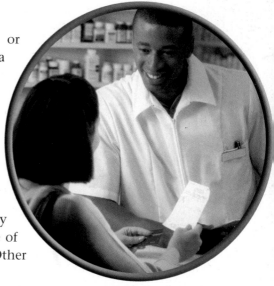

▶ **Additive interaction** occurs when *medicines work together in a positive way*. For example, both an anti-inflammatory and a muscle relaxant may be prescribed to treat joint pain.

▶ **Synergistic effect** is an *interaction of two or more medicines that results in a greater effect than when the medicines are taken alone*—one medicine increases the strength of the other. One medicine may boost the rate of digestion, for example, enabling a second medicine to be absorbed faster.

▶ **Antagonistic interaction** occurs when *the effect of one medicine is canceled or reduced when taken with another medicine*. For example, someone who receives an organ transplant must take antirejection medicines. If the person is diabetic and takes insulin, the antirejection medicine may decrease the effectiveness of the insulin.

In addition to your health care provider, your local pharmacist is a person who can answer questions about medications. *What questions should you ask your pharmacist before taking a new medication?*

Other Problems

A person may experience other problems when taking medicines:

▶ **Tolerance** is a condition in which the body becomes used to the effect of a medicine. The body then requires increasingly larger doses of the medicine to produce the same effect. Sometimes a person will experience "reverse tolerance." In this condition, the body requires less of the substance to produce the desired effect.

▶ **Withdrawal** occurs when a person stops using a medicine on which he or she has a chemical dependence. For example, medicines containing codeine can lead to dependence. Symptoms of withdrawal, which include nervousness, insomnia, severe headaches, vomiting, chills, and cramps, gradually ease over time. Withdrawal sometimes requires medical intervention.

Reduce the risk of inappropriate use of medications by following these tips.

Guidelines for safe medicine use:

► Keep medicine in the container in which it was originally packaged.

► Store medicines in a safe place that is out of the reach of children.

► Never disable or replace the child-resistant cap on a medicine container.

► Flush down the toilet any medicines that have passed their expiration date.

Medicine Safety

To minimize risks to the public, the federal government has established laws and policies for testing and approving new medicines. In the United States, all medicines must meet standards set by the Food and Drug Administration (FDA) before being approved and made available for sale. The FDA requires manufacturers to supply information about a medicine's chemical composition, intended use, effects, and possible side effects. One practice of the FDA is to determine how medicine should be released to the public.

► **Prescription medicines.** The FDA has ruled that certain medicines cannot be used without the written approval of a licensed physician. These prescription medicines are available only by means of a doctor's written instructions and can be dispensed only by a licensed pharmacist. **Figure 23.1** shows the information that must appear on every prescription medicine label.

► **Over-the-counter (OTC) medicines.** This group includes a wide variety of medicines that you can buy without a prescription. Although the FDA considers it safe to use these

---

FIGURE 23.1

PRESCRIPTION MEDICINE LABEL

Prescription labels must carry certain information about the medicine. In order to use a medicine safely, always read the label carefully and talk to your doctor or pharmacist if you have any questions.

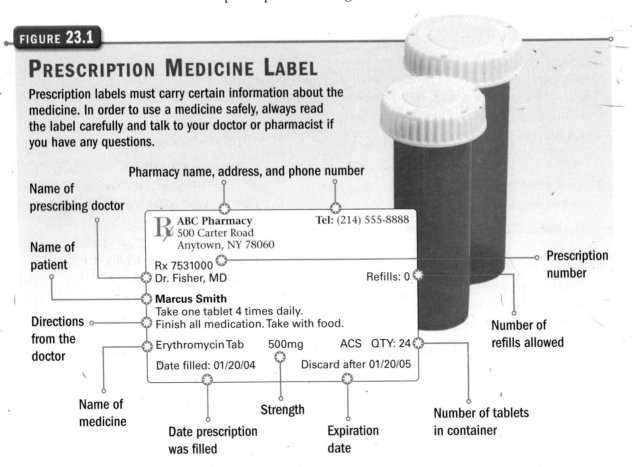

Name of prescribing doctor

Pharmacy name, address, and phone number

Name of patient

℞ ABC Pharmacy
500 Carter Road
Anytown, NY 78060

Tel: (214) 555-8888

Rx 7531000
Dr. Fisher, MD

Refills: 0

Marcus Smith
Take one tablet 4 times daily.
Finish all medication. Take with food.

Directions from the doctor

Erythromycin Tab   500mg   ACS   QTY: 24

Date filled: 01/20/04   Discard after 01/20/05

Prescription number

Number of refills allowed

Name of medicine

Date prescription was filled

Strength

Expiration date

Number of tablets in container

medications without medical supervision, any drugs can be harmful if not used properly.

When the FDA approves a medicine, it is saying that the medicine is safe when used as directed. FDA approval also means that a medicine is effective in treating the condition for which it is prescribed.

Medicine Misuse

Medicines can help maintain or improve health, but it is the responsibility of individuals and families to use medicines and supplements as they are prescribed or intended. All medicines are packaged with instructions for use. Failing to follow these instructions is one example of medicine misuse that can have serious health consequences. Other examples include

▶ giving a prescription medicine to a person for whom it was not prescribed or taking another person's medicine.

▶ taking too much or too little of a medicine or taking a medicine for a longer or shorter period than prescribed.

▶ discontinuing use of a medicine without informing the health care professional.

▶ mixing medicines.

Lesson 1 *Review*

Reviewing Facts and Vocabulary

1. What are the four broad categories of medicines?
2. What government organization tests and approves all new medications?
3. List three specific examples of medicine misuse.

Thinking Critically

4. **Synthesizing.** Analyze the influence of laws, policies, and practices on the public release of medicine in the United States.
5. **Evaluating.** Analyze the relationship and use of medicines that promote health and those that prevent disease. Give two examples.

Applying Health Skills

Accessing Information. Using reliable resources, research the known benefits and risks of aspirin. Integrate the information you have found into a poster about safe aspirin use. Make sure your poster explains why dosages vary for infants, children, adults, and the elderly.

TECHNOLOGY OPTION

SPREADSHEETS Use a spreadsheet to organize information for your poster. See **health.glencoe.com** for tips on how to use spreadsheets.

Drug Use–A High-Risk Behavior

VOCABULARY

substance abuse
illegal drugs
illicit drug use
overdose
psychological dependence
physiological dependence
addiction

YOU'LL LEARN TO

- Define substance abuse and recognize the health risks involved.

- Analyze the harmful effects of drugs on the fetus.

- Analyze the harmful physical, mental/emotional, social, and legal consequences of drug use.

⟶ **QUICK START** Substance abuse has effects both on individuals and on society as a whole. List as many of the dangerous effects of drugs as you can think of that affect the user, the user's family and friends, and the rest of society.

Substance abuse harms concentration and coordination. You cannot do your best if your body and mind are not functioning properly. *How will you protect your health and avoid substance abuse?*

No one starts using drugs with the intention of causing a drug-related injury or getting hooked on the drug. Substance abuse is a high-risk behavior. Recognizing the difference between drug misuse and substance abuse will help you avoid the risks associated with these potentially dangerous substances.

What Is Substance Abuse?

As you learned in Lesson 1, medicine misuse occurs when people use medicines carelessly or in an improper way. However, some people misuse medicines intentionally to achieve a "high." This is **substance abuse**, *any unnecessary or improper use of chemical substances for nonmedical purposes.* Substance abuse includes overuse or multiple use of a drug, use of an illegal drug, and use of a drug in combination with alcohol or other drugs.

Not all abused substances are medicines. Many are **illegal drugs**, or street drugs, *chemical substances that people of any age may not lawfully manufacture, possess, buy, or sell.* People who use illegal drugs are guilty of a crime called **illicit drug use**, *the use or sale of any substance that is illegal or otherwise not permitted.* This includes the selling of prescription drugs on the street.

Factors That Influence Decisions About Drugs

All teens are faced with choices about drug abuse. Many factors influence a teen's response to the opportunities to experiment with drugs, including the following:

▶ **Peer pressure** is the control and urging of friends or social groups to take a particular action. Teens whose friends and acquaintances avoid drug use can say no to drugs more easily than teens whose friends accept and even encourage drug use.

Real-Life Application

Analyzing Trends: Drug Prevention Programs

According to findings by a recent National Household Survey on Drug Abuse (NHSDA) more and more teens are getting involved in drug prevention programs. What effect do you think this has on teens making the decision to avoid drug use?

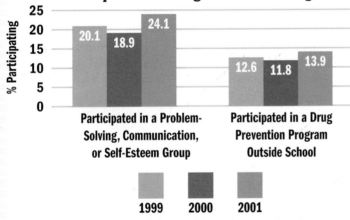

Youth Participation in Drug Prevention Programs

1999 2000 2001

Source: Substance Abuse and Mental Health Services Administration: NHSDA Survey, 2001

- In 2001, 24.1 percent of youths surveyed participated in a problem-solving, communication, or self-esteem group. The percentage of students who had participated in a drug prevention program outside of school was 13.9 percent.

- According to results of this survey, teens reporting an increase in the use of illicit drugs did not participate in such a program. What does this indicate about the influence drug prevention programs can have on a teen's decision to avoid drugs?

- Survey results also showed 55.9 percent of youths aged 12 to 17 indicated that they had talked with a parent in the past year about the dangers of alcohol and drug use. What effect do you think support from parents has on teens' participating in drug prevention programs?

ACTIVITY

Write a newspaper article that describes factors that influence teens' choices about whether to use drugs. Include internal and external influences. How can teens benefit from participating in drug prevention programs and influence others in a positive and healthful way?

▶ **Family members** can help teens resist drugs. Parents and other adults who avoid drug use and who discourage drug experimentation influence their teens to abstain from drugs.

▶ **Role models** are people you admire and want to imitate. Teens who look up to coaches, athletes, actors, and professionals who avoid and discourage drug use have an advantage in resisting drugs.

▶ **Media messages** can influence your impression of drug use. Messages from TV, digital media, film, and music, for example, may be misleading about the harmful effects of drugs.

▶ **Perceptions** of society's drug behavior are often inaccurate. According to the 2001 Youth Risk Behavior Survey, nearly 70 percent of high school students do not use drugs.

A strong, supportive system of family and friends can help a teen make the healthful decision to avoid drugs. *What other factors help you remain drug free?*

h⊙t link

hepatitis B and **HIV** For more information on hepatitis B and HIV, see Chapters 24 and 25, pages 638 and 662.

The Health Risks of Drug Use

Illegal drugs have serious side effects that can range from minor to deadly. Unlike medicines, these substances are not monitored for quality, purity, or strength. The effects of such drugs is unpredictable. Drug abuse affects all sides of the health triangle.

▶ **Physical health.** Once a drug enters the bloodstream, it can harm a user's brain, heart, lungs, and other vital organs. A serious danger of drug abuse is the risk of overdosing. An **overdose** is *a strong, sometimes fatal reaction to taking a large amount of a drug.* Some drug use involves injecting substances through a needle, which can increase the risk of contracting diseases such as **hepatitis B** and **HIV.**

▶ **Mental health.** Drugs cloud reasoning and thinking, and users lose control of their behavior. As shown in **Figure 23.2** on page 595, the drug Ecstasy alters the brain's structure and function. People who experiment with drugs often lose sight of their values. While under the influence of drugs, teens may no longer recall the positive beliefs, values, and ideals they have used to guide their own conduct.

▶ **Social health.** Even people who are "just experimenting" with drugs do and say things they later regret. Substance abuse can have a negative effect on relationships with friends and family members. It can cause teens to be expelled from school or dropped from a school team, and it often has legal consequences. Substance abuse is a major factor in many crimes, suicides, and unintentional injuries.

FIGURE 23.2

DRUG USE AND THE BRAIN

Ecstasy, a stimulant drug that speeds up the nervous system, affects parts of the brain controlling thinking, mood, memory, and perception.

neocortex — basal ganglia — amygdala — hippocampus — hypothalamus

Understanding the Addiction Cycle

Teens who experiment with drugs will experience side effects, or unwanted reactions. The side effects can range from nausea and headaches to a loss of consciousness and even death, and can occur with a teen's first use of a drug. What may begin as a seemingly harmless pastime results in serious consequences. These consequences include:

▶ **Tolerance.** The body of the substance abuser needs more and more of the drug to get the same effect.

▶ **Psychological dependence.** *A condition in which a person believes that a drug is needed in order to feel good or to function normally,* **psychological dependence** develops over time. The user has a continuing desire to take the drug for its effect.

▶ **Physiological dependence.** A person who experiences the severe effects of withdrawal when he or she stops taking a drug has a **physiological dependence,** *a condition in which the user has a chemical need for the drug.* Symptoms of withdrawal can include nervousness, insomnia, severe nausea, headaches, vomiting, chills, and cramps. In some cases, death can result.

▶ **Addiction.** Anyone who takes drugs risks one of the most frightening side effects: **addiction,** *a physiological or psychological dependence on a drug.* Addiction causes persistent, compulsive use of a substance known by the user to be harmful. People who are addicted to a substance have great difficulty in stopping without professional intervention.

hotlink

addiction For more information on addiction, see Chapter 22, page 578.

hot link

STDs For more information about STDs, see Chapter 25, page 646.

Experimenting even once with a drug can quickly lead to a harmful and damaging addiction. *What consequences of drug use affect family and friends?*

Other Consequences of Drug Use

In addition to the physical risks to a person's health, substance abuse can damage a teen's performance in school, in sports, in relationships with friends, and in family life. The abuse of drugs adds pressure and stress to a period of life that is already filled with both.

Consequences to the Individual

Drug use affects all aspects of a person's health. Mental and physical health suffer as tolerance, dependence, and addiction develop. The effects of drug use also influence emotional health. People who experiment with drugs tend to lose control more readily than those who do not. This tendency can lead to violence. Substance abuse is also a major factor in violent crimes, suicides, and both unintentional and intentional deaths. Drug use can lead to a relaxing of inhibitions. As a result, drug users are at risk for engaging in sexual activity, which can lead to unintended pregnancy or exposure to **STDs.**

LEGAL CONSEQUENCES

Teens possessing, using, manufacturing, or selling drugs are committing the crime of illicit drug use. Being arrested leads to court fines and legal fees. Some states automatically suspend the driving privileges of minors convicted of a drug offense. Suspension from school, jail time, or probation also are consequences of arrest and conviction.

Consequences for Family and Friends

Some people believe that their decision about drug use is their business and doesn't involve anyone else. That is not true. When an individual chooses to abuse drugs, the decision affects everyone in the user's life. Teens who become involved with drugs lose their interest in healthy activities and have little time for friends who value a drug-free lifestyle. Family members have a responsibility to be aware of the warning signs of drug use and encourage the individual to seek professional help.

Consequences for Babies and Children

Substance abuse can cause considerable harm to developing fetuses, infants, and children of drug users. A pregnant female who uses drugs passes the drug through the placenta to her unborn child. The baby may be spontaneously aborted or born with birth defects, behavioral problems, or an addiction. If either parent is using injected drugs, the baby may be born with HIV caused by the sharing of infected needles by one or both parents. A nursing mother who uses drugs passes these substances through breast milk to her child. Babies born to mothers who used depressants or other drugs during pregnancy may be physically dependent on drugs and show severe withdrawal symptoms at birth.

Children of drug users are often neglected and abused because their addicted parents cannot properly care for them. These children may suffer a lifetime of physical and emotional problems and may need to seek help from health professionals later in life.

Costs to Society

Drug abuse has consequences beyond the individual and family. One of the biggest burdens placed on society is a rise in drug-related crime and violence because the use of drugs decreases inhibitions, increases aggressiveness, and clouds judgment. Driving under the influence of an illegal substance can result in vehicle collisions and cause countless injuries and deaths.

Drug abuse also affects the nation's economy. According to a recent study by the Office of National Drug Control Policy, illegal drugs cost the American economy $160 billion per year. The costs result from lost work hours and productivity caused by drug-related illnesses, jail time, accidents, and deaths; health costs and legal fees resulting from illegal drug use; and law enforcement costs and insurance costs from drug-related damages, injuries, and deaths.

The consequences of drug abuse—physical, mental, social, and legal—are 100 percent preventable. By choosing a drug-free lifestyle, you avoid these consequences.

These teens recognize that using illegal drugs results in suspension or expulsion from school as well as legal consequences. *How can these consequences interfere with a teen's goals?*

 Lesson 2 *Review*

Reviewing Facts and Vocabulary

1. What are *substance abuse* and *illegal drugs*?
2. What are the factors that influence a teen's decision about substance abuse?
3. Analyze and explain the harmful effects of drugs on the fetus.

Thinking Critically

4. **Synthesizing.** List three costs of drug use to society, and give examples of how each of these costs might affect you.
5. **Evaluating.** What are some of the reasons that a substance abuser may have difficulties in achieving long-term goals?

Applying Health Skills

Advocacy. With classmates, analyze the physical, mental, social, and legal consequences of drug use. Put your ideas in the form of a video or public service announcement to advocate a drug-free lifestyle.

PRESENTATION SOFTWARE

Presentation software can help give your antidrug message a professional look. Find help in using presentation software at **health.glencoe.com**.

Marijuana, Inhalants, and Steroids

VOCABULARY

marijuana
paranoia
inhalants
anabolic-androgenic
   steroids

YOU'LL LEARN TO

• Analyze the physical, mental, social, and legal consequences of using marijuana, steroids, and inhalants.

• Analyze and apply strategies for avoiding the use of marijuana, inhalants, and steroids.

• Explain the negative effects of combining alcohol use with marijuana use.

QUICK START Knowing the risks of substance abuse can help you stay drug free. Write three reasons for saying no to drugs. Then, modify these reasons into effective refusal statements that you could use if someone offered you drugs.

A Marijuana is an illegal drug. It affects your memory, concentration, coordination, and reaction time. *What strategies do you have for avoiding marijuana use?*

Suppose that someone dared you to go into your school's chemistry lab and swallow a mixture of unfamiliar chemicals. You'd think the idea was pretty crazy, wouldn't you? Yet, this is exactly what people do when they experiment with illegal drugs. No government agency inspects these substances, as is done with medicines, to make sure they're safe or pure. People who take illegal drugs are gambling with their lives.

Marijuana

Marijuana, the common name for the Indian hemp plant Cannabis, is *a plant whose leaves, buds, and flowers are smoked for their intoxicating effects.* It is one of the most widely used illegal drugs, and is also known as grass, weed, or pot. It is often the first drug teens experiment with after alcohol. Hashish, or hash, is a stronger form of marijuana. Studies have shown that an individual who uses marijuana is 17 times more likely to use cocaine than one who has never used marijuana. Contrary to popular opinion, this drug is not harmless. All forms of marijuana are mind altering and can damage the user's health. When combined with other drugs, marijuana can be deadly.

Marijuana and Addiction

As with other mood-altering drugs, marijuana raises levels of a brain chemical called dopamine. This chemical produces a pleasurable feeling. In some users, the drug triggers the release of so much dopamine that a feeling of intense well-being or elation is reached. When the drug wears off, however, the pleasure sensation stops, often dramatically. This abrupt letdown is called a "crash." Marijuana contains *more* cancer-causing chemicals than tobacco smoke and carries the same health risks as smoking tobacco. Marijuana also interferes with the immune system, so the user becomes more susceptible to infections. Many of the physical effects of marijuana use are summarized in **Figure 23.3**.

Did You Know

Marijuana contains 421 different chemicals, including d-alpha-tetrahydrocannabinol (THC), the main psychoactive ingredient in marijuana. THC is stored in body fat, and traces of it can be present in the blood for as long as a month. It has a lasting effect on the brain. This means that a marijuana user can fail a drug test weeks after using the drug.

FIGURE 23.3

THE HEALTH RISKS OF MARIJUANA

The effects of marijuana use vary from person to person and can be influenced by an individual's mood and surroundings. In all cases, however, marijuana poses serious health risks.

- Hallucinations and paranoia
- Impaired short-term memory, reaction time, concentration, and coordination
- Distorted sense of time, sight, touch, and sound
- Decreased initiative and ambition
- Bloodshot eyes
- Dry mouth

- Lung irritation, coughing
- Heart and lung damage
- Increased risk of lung cancer
- Weakened immunity; increased susceptibility to colds, flu, and viral infections

- Increased appetite, leading to weight gain
- In pregnant females, increased risk of stillbirth and birth defects
- Changed hormone levels, affecting normal body development in teens
- In females, increased testosterone levels and risk of infertility
- In males, lowered sperm count and testosterone levels

Risks to Mental/Emotional Health

Marijuana users experience slow mental reflexes and suffer sudden feelings of anxiety and **paranoia**, *an irrational suspiciousness or distrust of others.* The user may feel dizzy, have trouble walking, and have difficulty remembering events that just happened. Because short-term memory is adversely affected, problems at school and at work may develop. Users often experience distorted perception, loss of coordination, and trouble with thinking and problem solving.

hotlink

reproductive organs For more information on keeping the reproductive organs healthy, see Chapter 18, pages 470 and 475.

Risks to Growth and Development

For teens, marijuana poses physical risks to the **reproductive organs.** In males, regular use interferes with sperm production and lowers levels of testosterone, the hormone responsible for the development of adult male characteristics such as voice change, growth of body hair, and broadened shoulders. Females experience the opposite effect—an increase in testosterone levels. This may result in unwanted facial hair and can lead to infertility.

Risks and Consequences of Driving Under the Influence

Driving under the influence of marijuana can be as dangerous as driving under the influence of alcohol because marijuana interferes with depth perception, impairs judgment, and slows reflexes. The penalties and legal consequences of driving under the influence of any drug, including marijuana, are strict. These include suspension of a driver's license, a fine, and often a jail term. Insurance premiums are increased when the driver's license is restored. If injury or death results from a drug-related accident, the impaired driver may face serious legal prosecution.

Driving under the influence of marijuana can be dangerous. *What are some effects of marijuana use that could impair a person's ability to drive safely?*

Inhalants

Inhalants are *substances whose fumes are sniffed and inhaled to achieve a mind-altering effect.* Most inhalants go immediately to the brain, causing damage and actually killing brain cells that will never be replaced. Inhalants include solvents and aerosols such as glues, spray paints, gasoline, and varnishes. They also include nitrates and nitrous oxides, which have medical uses. All inhalants are extremely dangerous, and many are labeled as poisons. These substances were never designed to be taken into the body and cause permanent nervous system and brain damage.

Most inhalants depress the central nervous system and produce effects that include a glassy stare, slurred speech, and impaired judgment. Inhalant use or huffing, inhaling the fumes from aerosol cans, can cause sudden death by increasing heart rate that results in cardiac arrest, or death by suffocation.

Anabolic-Androgenic Steroids

Anabolic-androgenic steroids are *synthetic substances that are similar to the male sex hormone testosterone. Anabolic* refers to muscle building and *androgenic* refers to increased male characteristics. When used under a doctor's guidance, these substances help build muscles in patients with chronic diseases. Steroid use

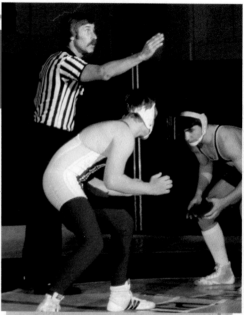

Refusal Skills: No Means No!

At a recent wrestling competition, Chris lost to an opponent he had beaten several times before.

Afterward, his teammate Josh pulled him aside and said, "You know, that guy has been getting help to build muscles. You need steroids to make State."

Josh held out a pill. Chris shook his head. "No way!"

"You'll definitely take home the title if you just help yourself to a few of these pills," Josh said.

Chris repeated, "I said no and I mean no."

Josh persisted, "If you don't, you won't make State."

"The title is not so important that I should risk my health," Chris reasoned.

"It would just be for this season," Josh continued.

Chris changed the subject, "Hey, look. Jason's match is on. I'm going to check it out." Then Chris walked away.

What Would You Do?

Write your own dialogue for this situation. Analyze and apply at least four refusal strategies for avoiding drugs.

Successful Refusal Techniques:
1. Say no in a firm voice.
2. Explain why you are refusing.
3. Suggest alternatives.
4. Back up your words by using body language.
5. Leave if necessary.

Improving athletic performance through hard work and practice shows that you are a healthful, responsible person.
How could use of steroids harm rather than help an athlete's career?

can cause mood swings; impaired judgment resulting from feelings of invincibility; and paranoia.

Legal and Social Consequences of Steroid Use

All steroid use other than that prescribed by a licensed physician is illegal and dangerous. Although steroids can increase muscle strength, the associated tendons and ligaments don't get stronger. This discrepancy can result in injuries that take a long time to heal and can end an athlete's career. In addition to causing health problems, steroid users often turn to other illegal, addictive drugs to combat the side effects of steroids. Abusers may take anabolic steroids as pills or by injection. If needles are shared or contaminated, steroid users run the risk of exposure to disease-causing bacteria and viruses, including HIV.

Serious health risks are not the only consequences of steroid use. According to the Anabolic Steroids Control Act of 1990, the nonmedical use of steroids is illegal for people of all ages in the United States. As drug testing for athletes becomes more prevalent, athletes who fail a drug test for steroids can face exclusion from an event, expulsion from the team, monetary fines, and jail time.

▶ Lesson 3 *Review*

Reviewing Facts and Vocabulary

1. Explain the relationship between marijuana use and alcohol use.
2. How does marijuana interfere with driving ability?
3. Analyze and examine the harmful effects of inhalants and steroids on body systems.

Thinking Critically

4. **Analyzing.** Analyze the physical, mental, social, and legal consequences of using marijuana. What effect can use of this drug have on a teen's future?
5. **Synthesizing.** Why are younger students especially at risk for inhalant use? What can you do to help prevent younger students from trying inhalants?

Applying Health Skills

Practicing Healthful Behaviors. Write a short story in which a teen is being pressured to use one of the drugs discussed in this lesson. Your story should show how the teen effectively analyzes and applies strategies to avoid the dangers associated with drug use.

TECHNOLOGY *OPTION*

PRESENTATION SOFTWARE   You can use presentation software to incorporate appropriate art and graphics to illustrate your story. Find help in using presentation software at **health.glencoe.com**.

Psychoactive Drugs

VOCABULARY

psychoactive drugs
stimulants
euphoria
depressants
narcotics
hallucinogens
designer drugs

YOU'LL LEARN TO

• Examine the harmful effects of psychoactive drugs on body systems.

• Explain the role psychoactive drugs play in putting teens in unsafe situations that include the risk of HIV, STDs, or unplanned pregnancies.

• Analyze the importance of alternatives to drug use.

• Analyze and apply strategies for avoiding psychoactive drugs.

QUICK START Teens have the opportunity to live healthy lives—to be the healthiest they can be. The best way to make the most of that opportunity is to make wise choices that have a positive effect on your health. On a sheet of paper, write three ways you can safeguard your health and avoid the harmful effects of drug use.

The central nervous system (CNS), which includes the brain and the spinal cord, is an amazingly complex part of the body. Every form of activity, from bending a finger to solving abstract problems, involves the central nervous system. **Psychoactive drugs**, *chemicals that affect the central nervous system and alter activity in the brain,* change the functioning of the CNS.

Classification of Psychoactive Drugs

There are four main groups of psychoactive drugs: stimulants, depressants, narcotics, and hallucinogens (huh-LOO-suhn-uh-juhnz). Some of these drugs have medicinal value when properly used. However, even under a doctor's supervision, they carry risks. When psychoactive drugs are misused or abused, a person's health and the proper function of all body systems are seriously affected. **Figure 23.4** on page 604 shows the health risks of these drugs on body systems. The effects on the developing brain and body of a teen can be especially damaging.

Your decision to stay healthy and drug free will help you succeed in school.

FIGURE 23.4

HEALTH RISKS OF PSYCHOACTIVE DRUGS

Types of Drugs	Consequences to Your Health
STIMULANTS	
Cocaine	• Nausea, abdominal pain, malnutrition • Chest pain, respiratory failure, death • Headache, stroke, seizure, heart attack, death • Exposure to HIV through contaminated needles
Crack	• Extreme addiction, with the same effects as pure cocaine • Rapid increase in heart rate and blood pressure can cause death
Amphetamines	• Decreased appetite, weight loss, and malnutrition • High blood pressure, rapid heartbeat, heart failure, death • Loss of muscle coordination, delirium, panic • Aggressiveness, increased tolerance, addiction
Methamphetamine	• Memory loss, heart and nerve damage • Increased tolerance, addiction
DEPRESSANTS	
Barbiturates	• Reduced heart rate and blood pressure • Fatigue, confusion, impaired muscle coordination • Impaired memory, loss of judgment • Reduced respiratory function, respiratory arrest, death
Tranquilizers	• Depression, unusual excitement, fever, irritability • Loss of judgment, dizziness
Rohypnol	• Confusion, inability to remember what happened • Decreased blood pressure, drowsiness, gastrointestinal disturbances
GHB	• Drowsiness, nausea, vomiting, loss of consciousness • Impaired breathing, coma, death
NARCOTICS	
Opium	• Nausea, constipation
Morphine	• Rapid onset of tolerance, addiction
Heroin	• Confusion, sedation, unconsciousness, coma
Codeine	• Reduced respiratory function, respiratory arrest, death • Exposure to HIV through contaminated needles
HALLUCINOGENS	
PCP	• Loss of appetite, depression • Panic, aggression, violent actions • Increased heart and respiratory function
LSD	• Delusions, illusions, hallucinations, flashbacks, convulsions, coma, and death
Ecstasy (MDMA)	• Confusion, depression, paranoia, muscle breakdown
Ketamine	• Kidney and cardiovascular system failure, death • Memory loss, numbness, impaired motor function • Nausea, high blood pressure, fatal respiratory reaction

Health Risks of Stimulants

Stimulants are *drugs that speed up the central nervous system.* Some foods, such as coffee, tea, and cola, contain small amounts of a stimulant called caffeine. The **nicotine** in tobacco products is also a stimulant. Sometimes, stimulants are prescribed for specific medical conditions, for example, the medication used to treat hyperactivity. Although some stimulants have medical uses, many of these substances are used illegally. The most dangerous of the illegal stimulants are cocaine, amphetamines (am-FE-tuh-meenz), and methamphetamine (me-tham-FE-tuh-meen).

hot link

nicotine For more information on nicotine and tobacco products, see Chapter 21, page 540.

Cocaine

Cocaine is a rapid-acting, powerful, highly addictive stimulant that interrupts normal functioning of the central nervous system. The purchase and possession of cocaine is illegal everywhere in the United States. Cocaine is a white powder extracted from the leaves of the coca plant. Cocaine users can experience a surge of self-confidence and **euphoria**, *a feeling of intense well-being or elation.* Effects of cocaine use can last from 20 minutes to several hours.

The feeling of confidence induced by cocaine use is followed by an emotional letdown. Regular use can lead to depression, fatigue, paranoia, and physiological dependence. Cocaine use can cause malnutrition and, especially among teens, cardiac problems. When cocaine is snorted, it shrinks the tiny blood vessels in the nose. Repeated use can lead to collapse of the nasal septum, the wall dividing the two halves of the nose. When users inject cocaine, they risk contracting HIV or hepatitis B from infected needles. Overdosing can result in cardiac arrest, respiratory failure, seizures, and death.

Crack

An even more dangerous form of cocaine is crack. Also known as crack cocaine, rock, or freebase rock, crack is one of the most deadly drugs available. It is a very pure form of cocaine that reaches the brain seconds after being smoked or injected. Once in the blood, it causes heart rate and blood pressure to soar to dangerous levels. Death may result from cardiac or respiratory failure. Mixing cocaine and alcohol is extremely dangerous. These substances are combined in the liver, increasing the risk of death from liver failure.

▼ Crack cocaine is a concentrated form of cocaine that can cause death. *What are the dangers of mixing cocaine with other drugs, such as alcohol?*

Amphetamines

Amphetamines are stimulants used in prescription medicines to reduce fatigue and drowsiness or to suppress the appetite. However, some people use amphetamines illegally to stay awake and alert, to improve athletic performance, or to lose weight. The easily developed tolerance to amphetamines causes a user to ingest more of the substance. Regular use of amphetamines can result in twitching, irregular heartbeat, paranoia, and heart and blood vessel damage.

Methamphetamine

Methamphetamine, or meth, is a stimulant used in treating certain diseases, including Parkinson's disease and obesity. It is a white, odorless powder that easily dissolves in alcohol or water.

Source: National Institute on
Drug Abuse

Because it is produced in makeshift labs, the drug is readily available, but its quality is uncertain. In recent years, this drug has been identified as one of the many dangerous and illegal substances called "club drugs," drugs associated with concerts and all-night parties called raves. Meth may provide a short-term feeling of euphoria. Often the use of this drug results in depression, paranoia, damage to the central nervous system, increased heart rate and blood pressure, and damage to brain cells. It can also cause death.

 The red areas in the
normal brain scan (top)
show memory and motor
skill control. The brain
scan on the bottom,
taken one month after
the subject's use of
methamphetamine,
indicates loss of memory
and motor control.

Health Risks of Depressants

Depressants, or sedatives, are *drugs that tend to slow down the central nervous system.* Depressant drugs relax muscles, relieve feelings of tension and worry, and cause drowsiness. They can be dangerous because they slow the heart rate, lower blood pressure to dangerous levels, and interrupt the normal rate of breathing. One of the most commonly used depressants is alcohol. Two types of sedative medications are barbiturates (bar-BICH-uh-ruhts) and tranquilizers. Other widely-used depressants include Rohypnol and GHB. Combining depressants, even in small amounts, produces a *synergistic* effect. For example, a user combining alcohol and tranquilizers can overdose, causing shallow breathing, weak and rapid pulse, coma, and even death.

What's Your Health Status?

Read each statement below and respond by writing *yes, no,* or *sometimes* for each item. Write *yes* only for items that you practice regularly.

1. I keep my immunizations up to date.

2. I avoid close contact with people who have a cold or the flu.

3. I wash my hands after using the bathroom, before handling food, before meals, and after I blow my nose.

4. I follow a nutritious eating plan.

5. I get at least eight to ten hours of sleep each night.

6. I take precautions to avoid bites from insects and ticks.

7. I prepare and store food in a safe manner.

8. I cover my nose and mouth when I cough or sneeze.

9. I don't use tobacco, alcohol, or other drugs.

10. I get plenty of rest and fluids when I have a cold or the flu.

HEALTH Online

For instant feedback on your health status, go to Chapter 24 Health Inventory at **health.glencoe.com.**

Quick *Write*

Using Visuals. To avoid spreading disease, rest, drink plenty of fluids, and stay home when you are ill. What other measures can you take to prevent communicable diseases?

What Are Communicable Diseases?

VOCABULARY

communicable disease
pathogen
infection
viruses
bacteria
toxin
vector

YOU'LL LEARN TO

- Identify the types of pathogens that cause communicable diseases.

- Analyze the relationship between healthful behaviors and the ways that communicable diseases are spread.

- Develop and analyze strategies for preventing communicable diseases.

QUICK START   Write about the last time you had a cold. Include a list of the symptoms you experienced. Explain how you think you caught the cold and what you did to treat it.

▲ The HIV virus (top), pneumonia virus, and cold virus (bottom), are pathogens.

Most of us don't spend much time thinking about micro-organisms, but they often impact our lives. Although most microorganisms—living things too small to be seen without a microscope—are harmless, a few, such as the viruses shown on this page, can cause communicable diseases. A **communicable disease** is *a disease that is spread from one living thing to another or through the environment.* Knowing how communicable diseases spread can help you choose behaviors to reduce your risk of getting them.

Causes of Communicable Diseases

An *organism that causes disease* is called a **pathogen**. Common pathogens include certain viruses, bacteria, fungi, protozoans, and rickettsias (rik-ET-see-uhz). **Figure 24.1** lists some of the diseases caused by pathogens. An **infection** is *a condition that occurs when pathogens enter the body, multiply, and damage body cells.* If the body is not able to fight off the infection, a disease develops.

Viruses

You're already familiar with two diseases caused by viruses—the common cold and influenza, or the flu. **Viruses** are *pieces of genetic material surrounded by a protein coat.* By themselves they are inactive. They need living cells to reproduce. Viruses invade all known forms of life—mammals, birds, reptiles, insects, plants, and even bacteria.

After a virus penetrates a cell, called the host cell, the virus takes control of the cell to manufacture more viruses. The new viruses burst from the cell, usually killing it, and take over other cells. Like other pathogens, viruses usually run their course and eventually are killed by the immune system. Antibiotics do not work against viruses.

Bacteria

Bacteria are *single-celled microorganisms* that live almost everywhere on earth. Most bacteria are harmless, and many types are essential for life. For example, bacteria in your digestive system help digest food and make some of the vitamins you need. When bacteria enter the body, they multiply through cell division. Some bacterial pathogens, such as the ones that cause tetanus, produce a **toxin**, a *substance that kills cells or interferes with their functions.* Like most other microorganisms that enter the body of a healthy individual, bacteria are usually destroyed by the immune system. Most bacterial diseases can be treated with **antibiotics.**

Did You Know ❓

In 1993 four children were killed and hundreds of others sickened by undercooked hamburger from a fast-food restaurant. The culprit was *E. coli O157:H7.* This bacteria causes severe damage to the cells lining the human intestines and can lead to kidney failure and death.

Common sources of the bacteria are undercooked, contaminated ground beef and unpasteurized milk and apple cider.

hotlink

antibiotics For more information about antibiotics, see Chapter 23, page 587.

FIGURE 24.1

DISEASES BY TYPE OF PATHOGEN

Viruses	Bacteria	Fungi	Protozoans	Rickettsias
• common cold • influenza (flu) • viral pneumonia • viral hepatitis • polio • mononucleosis • measles • AIDS • viral meningitis • chicken pox • herpes • rabies • smallpox	• bacterial foodborne illness • strep throat • tuberculosis • diptheria • gonorrhea • Lyme disease • bacterial pinkeye • bacterial pneumonia • bacterial meningitis	• athlete's foot • ringworm • vaginal yeast infection	• malaria • amoebic dysentery • sleeping sickness	• typhus • Rocky Mountain spotted fever

Other Types of Pathogens

Other types of organisms also can cause communicable diseases.

▶ **Fungi** are plantlike organisms, such as molds and yeasts. Some types can cause diseases of the skin, such as athlete's foot; diseases of the mucous membranes; or of the lungs.

▶ **Protozoans** are single-celled organisms that are larger and more complex than bacteria. Most are harmless, but some can cause disease, especially in people with weakened immune systems.

▶ **Rickettsias** are pathogens that resemble bacteria. Like viruses, they multiply by invading the cells of another life form. Often these organisms enter humans through the bites of insects such as fleas or lice. Rocky Mountain spotted fever is the most frequently reported illness spread by rickettsias.

How Communicable Diseases Are Transmitted

There are several means of transmission, or the spreading, of pathogens. Transmission can occur through direct or indirect contact or through breathing contaminated air. Some diseases can be transmitted in more than one way. If you know how they are spread you can take precautions and avoid infection.

Direct Contact

Many pathogens are transmitted by direct contact with an infected person or animal or with something in the environment. Direct contact includes touching, biting, kissing, and sexual contact. Sneezing and coughing can spray infectious droplets of saliva or mucus onto a nearby person's eyes, nose, or mouth. A pregnant woman may also transmit an infection to her unborn child through the placenta. A person can get tetanus from a puncture wound by a rusty nail.

Indirect Contact

Some communicable diseases can be transmitted indirectly, without being close to an infected person. The following are ways diseases can be transmitted through indirect contact:

▶ **Contaminated objects.** Inanimate objects can become contaminated with infectious discharges or secretions. Suppose that a person with a cold sneezes onto a table or into his or her hand and then touches the table. The cold viruses can be transmitted to you if you touch the table and then touch your nose or eyes. Use proper handwashing techniques to avoid transmitting infections.

Try to reduce your risk of infection when you participate in outdoor activities where vectors are common. *How is this teen protecting himself from deer ticks?*

CHARACTER ✎ CHECK

Respect. One simple action can demonstrate your respect for your own health and the health of others. Every time you wash your hands properly you reduce the risk of spreading potential pathogens, especially when you prepare food or when you touch objects that others may put in their mouths. **What other safe food handling habits can you practice?**

▶ **Vectors.** An *organism, usually an arthropod, such as a tick, that carries and transmits pathogens to humans or other animals* is known as a **vector**. For example, a mosquito may take in pathogens when it feeds on an infected person. The mosquito then injects some of those pathogens into the next person it bites, thus spreading the disease. Common vectors include flies, mosquitoes, and ticks. Lyme disease and malaria are spread by vectors.

▶ **Water and food.** Careless handling and storage of food are major sources of contamination and illness. For example, salmonella (sal-muh-NE-luh) bacteria in undercooked poultry can cause food poisoning. Water supplies that become contaminated with human or animal feces can cause illnesses such as hepatitis A.

Airborne Transmission

Pathogens from a sneeze or a cough may float in the air for a long time and travel long distances. Airborne transmission is different from direct contact because the pathogens don't settle quickly on surfaces. You don't have to be close to an infected person to inhale the pathogens. Diseases that are transmitted this way include chicken pox, tuberculosis, and influenza. A person can get inhalation anthrax by inhaling soil containing the bacteria.

Preventing the Spread of Disease

Reducing your risk of communicable diseases isn't complicated. Practicing healthful behaviors based on good hygiene and common sense will help you avoid infection.

Washing Hands

Handwashing is the single most effective way to prevent the spread of disease. Wash your hands before you prepare food, before you eat, and after you use the bathroom. Clean hands carefully before inserting contact lenses or putting on makeup. After handling animals, especially reptiles, or animal wastes, make it a habit to wash your hands. When someone in your home is ill, keep hands clean to prevent the spread of pathogens.

Handling Food Properly

Foodborne illness occurs in places where food is handled improperly. Always wash your hands before you handle food. Use paper towels, not dishcloths or sponges, to keep surfaces and equipment clean. Separate raw meat from other foods. Cook food to its proper temperature. Chill cold and leftover foods quickly to the proper temperature.

Health Minute

Strategies for Avoiding Diseases Transmitted by Vectors

Use these strategies where mosquitoes or ticks are common:

▶ Wear long-sleeved shirts, long pants, socks, and hats.

▶ Tuck shirts in at the waist, and tuck pants into socks.

▶ Wear boots, not sandals.

▶ Apply repellents to clothing, boots, socks, and all exposed skin.

▶ Check yourself and your clothing frequently. Wearing light-colored clothing can help you spot ticks and mosquitoes.

hot link

foodborne illness For more information about foodborne illness and proper food preparation, see Chapter 5, page 134.

Handwashing is important since your hands easily pick up and transfer bacteria. *List other strategies you can use to avoid the spread of disease.*

Other Prevention Measures

Here are some other strategies that will help you reduce your risk of getting or spreading communicable diseases.

▶ Eat a balanced diet. Participate in regular physical activity. Avoid the use of tobacco, alcohol, and other drugs.

▶ Avoid sharing eating utensils, makeup, combs and brushes, and other personal items.

▶ Prepare and store food safely—keep hot foods hot and cold foods refrigerated or on ice.

▶ Avoid unnecessary contact with people who are ill.

▶ Take care of yourself when you're ill. Cover your mouth when you cough or sneeze. Wash your hands after using a tissue.

▶ Be sure you are vaccinated against particular diseases as recommended by your physician.

▶ Practice abstinence from sexual activity.

▶ Learn to manage stress. Stress makes you vulnerable to illness if you do not find ways to manage it effectively.

▶ Lesson 1 *Review*

Reviewing Facts and Vocabulary

1. List five types of common pathogens, and identify one disease each type of pathogen causes.
2. Describe three ways in which pathogens spread and three healthful behaviors to limit their spread.
3. What are five ways you can reduce your risk of getting a communicable disease?

Thinking Critically

4. **Applying.** The fungus that causes athlete's foot lives in warm, moist places. What can you do to prevent getting this pathogen when you use gym or other common showers?
5. **Analyzing.** You wake up one morning with a headache, body aches, and a fever. You think you might be coming down with something. Analyze the relationship between healthful behaviors you can practice and the ways that communicable diseases are spread. What should you do?

Applying Health Skills

Practicing Healthful Behaviors. Work with a family member to identify ways in which you can reduce your risk of contracting a foodborne illness at home. Explain to family members how you will apply strategies to prevent the spread of food poisoning.

PRESENTATION SOFTWARE You've probably heard the saying, "a picture is worth a thousand words." Use presentation software to show your plan for reducing the spread of foodborne illness. For tips on using presentation software, see **health.glencoe.com**.

Preventing Communicable Diseases

VOCABULARY

immune system
inflammatory
   response
phagocyte
antigen
immunity
lymphocyte
antibody
vaccine

YOU'LL LEARN TO

- Examine how the body protects itself against invading pathogens.

- Apply strategies for caring for your immune system and preventing disease.

- Explain how technology has impacted the health status of individuals, families, communities, and the world in the prevention of communicable disease.

- Identify community health services that provide vaccines and information on disease prevention.

QUICK START   Have you ever had a small cut or other injury that became red or painful or developed pus? Write a few paragraphs describing what the area of injury looked like over several days.

You can't see it, but the teen in the picture is waging a battle. The battle is not against other players who are trying to score a point. It's a battle to fight off the pathogens that constantly attack his body. Every day, 24 hours a day, your body is exposed to millions of pathogens. Most of the time, your body manages to stay free of infection because of your immune system. The **immune system** is *a network of cells, tissues, organs, and chemicals that fights off pathogens.*

▲ Compare the protective equipment worn by this goalie to your physical and chemical barriers. *How might behaviors such as wearing appropriate safety equipment help protect you from pathogens?*

Physical and Chemical Barriers

Physical and chemical barriers make up your body's first line of defense, as shown in **Figure 24.2** on page 628. They protect against a wide variety of invaders. Physical barriers, such as skin and mucous membranes, block pathogens from invading your body. Chemical barriers, such as enzymes in tears, destroy pathogens.

The Immune System

The immune system has two major defense strategies. The inflammatory response is general, or nonspecific; it works against all types of pathogens. Specific defenses work against particular pathogens. Together, these defenses work to prevent disease.

The Inflammatory Response

The **inflammatory response** is *a reaction to tissue damage caused by injury or infection.* Its purpose is to prevent further tissue injury and to halt invading pathogens. Suppose that a splinter enters your finger. Your body immediately reacts to the damage caused by the splinter and to any pathogens on the splinter. If you've ever had the area around an injury become hot, swollen, red, and painful, you've experienced the inflammatory response.

FIGURE 24.2

PHYSICAL AND CHEMICAL BARRIERS— THE BODY'S FIRST LINE OF DEFENSE

These elements work together as your body's first line of defense to prevent pathogens from entering and causing disease.

Skin is the first line of defense against many pathogens. Few pathogens can pass through the tough layer of dead skin cells that surrounds the body.

Tears and saliva contain enzymes that destroy or disable many pathogens.

Mucous membranes line many parts of the body, including your mouth, nose, and bronchial tubes. Cells in these membranes produce *mucus*, a sticky substance that traps pathogens. The mucus then carries the trapped pathogens to other areas of the body for disposal.

Cilia, the hairlike projections that line parts of the respiratory system, sweep mucus and pathogens to the throat, where they can be swallowed or coughed out.

Gastric juice in the stomach destroys many pathogens that enter the body through the nose and mouth.

In response to invasion by microorganisms or to tissue damage, blood vessels near the site of an injury expand to allow more blood flow to the area. As blood vessels expand, fluid and cells from the bloodstream leak into the area. The collection of fluid and white blood cells causes swelling and pain because of pressure on nerve endings. One type of cell that responds to injury is called a **phagocyte** (FA-guh-site), *a white blood cell that attacks invading pathogens*. Phagocytes engulf pathogens and then destroy them with chemicals. Pus, a collection of dead white blood cells and damaged tissue, may collect at the site of inflammation as a response to bacteria. After the pathogens are killed and tissue damage is under control, tissue repair can begin. However, regardless of whether pathogens survive the inflammatory response, specific defenses are activated. This activation is an effort to prevent this same infection from occurring again.

Injury and infection caused by this splinter may trigger an inflammatory response. *What immediately happens in the body as a response to injury?*

Health Skills Activity

Decision Making: Caring for Your Immune System

Aaron has been getting a lot of colds lately. Today he woke up with a bad sore throat. Aaron knows that he should stay home and rest, both for his own health and to avoid infecting others at school. However, Aaron plays the lead saxophone in the marching band, and today is the last band practice before the big game. This practice will even be a full-dress rehearsal to make sure everything goes right for the half-time show.

Saturday's game will be the playoff, and everyone is sure the school will win. If Aaron doesn't show up, he thinks he will be letting the band down. Besides, he doesn't want to admit that he is getting sick because then he won't be there on Saturday when the team wins.

Aaron wonders what he should do.

What Would You Do?
Apply the six steps of the decision-making model to Aaron's situation.
1. State the situation.
2. List the options.
3. Weigh the possible outcomes.
4. Consider values.
5. Make a decision and act.
6. Evaluate the decision.

Specific Defenses

Specific defenses react to invasion as a result of the body's ability to recognize certain pathogens and destroy them. The process by which this happens, the immune response, is described in **Figure 24.3.** During the immune response, certain types of white blood cells react to antigens. An **antigen** is *a substance that is capable of triggering an immune response.* Antigens are found on the surfaces of pathogens and in toxins. Macrophages are a type of phagocyte that destroys pathogens by making antigens recognizable to white blood cells. The result of the immune response is **immunity**, *the state of being protected against a particular disease.*

Lymphocytes

A **lymphocyte** (LIMP-fuh-site) is *a specialized white blood cell that coordinates and performs many of the functions of specific immunity.* There are two types of lymphocytes: T cells and B cells.

T CELLS AND B CELLS

There are different types of T cells with different functions. They all work together to protect against infection.

▶ *Helper T cells* trigger the production of B cells and killer T cells.

▶ *Killer T cells* attack and destroy infected body cells. Killer T cells don't attack the pathogens themselves, only the infected cells.

FIGURE 24.3

THE IMMUNE RESPONSE

The immune response is a complex interaction between your body and an invading pathogen. It can be broken down into eight distinct stages.

1. Pathogens invade the body.
2. Macrophages engulf the pathogen.
3. Macrophages digest the pathogen and T cells recognize antigens of the pathogen as an invader.
4. T cells bind to the antigens.
5. B cells bind to antigens and helper T cells.
6. B cells divide to produce plasma cells.
7. Plasma cells release antibodies into the bloodstream.
8. Antibodies bind to antigens to help other cells identify and destroy the pathogens.

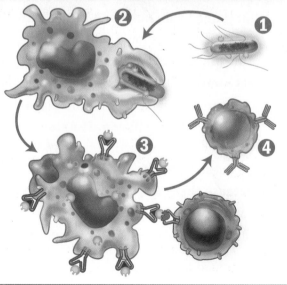

▶ *Suppressor T cells* coordinate the activities of other T cells. They "turn off" or suppress helper T cells when the infection has been cleared.

In conjunction with the work of T cells, lymphocytes called B cells produce antibodies. An **antibody** is a *protein that acts against a specific antigen.* Each B cell is programmed to make one type of antibody, specific to a particular pathogen. Some antibodies attach to foreign antigens to mark them for destruction. Some destroy invading pathogens. Others block viruses from entering body cells.

The Role of Memory Lymphocytes

Your immune system actually has a "memory." Some T cells and B cells that have been activated by antigens become *memory cells.* These memory cells circulate in your bloodstream and through the lymphatic system, shown in **Figure 24.4** on page 632. When memory cells recognize a former invader, the immune system uses antibodies and killer T cells in a quick defense to stop it. For example, if you have had measles or an immunization against measles, your immune system remembers the antigens for the measles virus. If it enters your body again, antibodies will attack the virus immediately, protecting you from becoming ill.

Active Immunity

The immunity your body develops to protect you from measles or from other diseases is called *active immunity.* Naturally acquired active immunity develops when your body is exposed to antigens from invading pathogens. Artificially acquired active immunity develops in response to a **vaccine**, a *preparation of dead or weakened pathogens that are introduced into the body to stimulate an immune response.* In this way vaccines cause your body to produce antibodies without actually causing the disease. Today, more than 20 serious human diseases can be prevented by vaccination. Active immunity to many diseases can last a lifetime, but some immunizations need to be repeated to maintain immunity.

Passive Immunity

In active immunity your body produces its own antibodies. You also can be protected from pathogens by *passive immunity*—receiving antibodies from another person or an animal. This immunity is short-lived; it usually lasts only weeks to months. Natural passive immunity occurs when antibodies pass from mother to child during pregnancy or while nursing. Artificial passive immunity results from the injection of antibodies produced by an animal or a human who is immune to the disease.

Is there a vaccine to prevent colds?
Developing a vaccine to prevent colds is difficult. More than 200 different viruses can cause the common cold. This means that more than 200 different vaccines would have to be developed to prevent this illness.

FIGURE 24.4

IMMUNITY AND THE LYMPHATIC SYSTEM

The lymphatic system circulates antibodies to give you protection against many diseases. This protection can last throughout your life.

The **lymphatic system** is part of your immune system. It includes your tonsils, lymph nodes, and a network of vessels, similar to blood vessels, that transport lymph, or tissue fluid.

Lymph nodes can become enlarged when your body is fighting an infection because of the increased number of lymphocytes. If swelling lasts for three days, see your health care professional.

Lymphocytes are produced by lymph nodes. These nodes occur in groups and are concentrated in the head and neck, armpits, chest, abdomen, and groin.

Care of the Immune System

Your health behaviors can greatly reduce your chance of contracting a disease or getting an infection. When you keep your body strong and healthy, your immune system is better able to fight off pathogens. Taking positive steps in every area of your health will give you the boost needed to reduce your chance of illness.

▶ Follow a sensible eating plan to maintain your overall health and keep your immune system strong. Include whole grains and nutrient-dense foods such as fruits and vegetables, and reduce intake of fats, sugar, and salt. Drink six to eight 8-ounce glasses of water each day.

▶ Get plenty of rest. Fatigue reduces the effectiveness of the immune system. To function at their best, teens should average nine hours of restful sleep each night.

- Get about an hour of physical activity each day. This is especially important to relieve stress.

- Avoid sharing personal items such as towels, toothbrushes, hairbrushes, or makeup.

- Avoid tobacco, alcohol, and other drugs.

- Avoid sexual contact. Some **STDs,** such as HIV, actually destroy the immune system.

- Keep your immunizations up to date.

h⊙t link

STDs For more information on sexually transmitted diseases, including HIV/AIDS, see Chapter 25, page 646.

Vaccines to Aid the Body's Defenses

When a new disease emerges or a familiar one becomes a greater health threat than in the past, health care workers begin to look for ways to prevent the disease. Research and advances in medical technology have allowed scientists to develop vaccines. Today, vaccines prevent diseases that once claimed millions of lives. Vaccines can be one of four types.

- **Live-virus vaccines** are made from pathogens grown under special laboratory conditions to make them lose most of their disease-causing properties. Although weakened, the organism can still stimulate the production of antibodies. The vaccines for measles, mumps, and rubella (MMR) and for chicken pox are produced in this way.

- **Killed-virus vaccines** use inactivated pathogens. Even though they are dead, the organism still stimulates an immune response and antibodies are produced. Flu shots, the Salk vaccine for polio, and the vaccines for hepatitis A, rabies, cholera, and plague are all killed-virus vaccines.

- **Toxoids** are inactivated toxins from pathogens. They are used to stimulate the production of antibodies. Though many pathogens are not harmful themselves, the toxins they produce cause sickness. Toxoids can be used to protect the body against such illnesses. Both tetanus and diphtheria immunizations use toxoids.

- **New and second-generation vaccines** are being developed by scientists using new technologies. An example is the vaccine for hepatitis B, which is made by genetically altered yeast cells.

These and many other common diseases can be prevented with vaccines:
- **Chicken pox**
- **Hepatitis B**
- **Measles**
- **Mumps**
- **Whooping cough (pertussis)**
- **Tetanus**
- **Diphtheria**
- **Polio**
- **Rubella**

Check with your parents or your health care professional to find out how many of these diseases you have been vaccinated against.

Immunization for All

Vaccines benefit more people than just those who receive them. If you are vaccinated against a particular disease, you can't spread that disease to others. In this way vaccination not only protects you but also helps protect those around you, especially your family and friends. One exception is tetanus, which is transmitted through the environment, not from person to person. The tetanus vaccine protects only the individual who receives it.

You should have up-to-date immunizations, including those for tetanus, diphtheria, measles, mumps, rubella, and hepatitis B. Vaccination against chicken pox is recommended if you have not had this disease. Some vaccines require more than one dose over time, or "booster shots." Your family physician or your local health department can advise you on the immunizations you need and provide them for you. Most high schools and colleges require that students show proof of current immunizations before admission. Each state has its own laws governing immunizations and school attendance. Some schools may have additional requirements.

 Lesson 2 *Review*

Reviewing Facts and Vocabulary

1. List three physical and chemical barriers that pathogens encounter when they try to enter the human body.

2. What is the difference between active immunity and passive immunity?

3. Where can you go to find out which immunizations you need?

Thinking Critically

4. **Analyzing.** How do you think the development of vaccines for more than 20 communicable diseases has affected the average human life span in areas where these vaccines are available?

5. **Evaluating.** What would you say to someone who says that he or she is careful never to come into contact with pathogens and therefore will not become ill?

Applying Health Skills

Accessing Information. Research those vaccinations suggested for someone your age, and make a table of this information. Work with a parent or guardian to determine which of your immunizations are current, and fill in the information on the table. Plan to get any immunizations you lack. Use this table to track when you should update your immunizations.

TECHNOLOGY *OPTION*

SPREADSHEETS Use spreadsheet software to create a chart showing the immunizations suggested for different age groups. You might also include a column listing facilities in the area that offer these vaccinations. See health.glencoe.com for information on how to create a spreadsheet.

Common Communicable Diseases

YOU'LL LEARN TO

- Identify the causes, transmission, symptoms, and treatment of several communicable diseases.

- Analyze strategies to reduce the risk of contracting some communicable diseases.

- Explain how technology impacts world health status.

QUICK START Make a two-column chart. In the first column, list communicable diseases with which you are familiar and write one fact about each. In the second column, list communicable diseases you have heard of but know little about.

You probably have experienced a fever or the stuffy or runny nose of a cold. In this lesson you'll learn about some common communicable diseases, their symptoms, and how they are treated. Most important, you will learn ways to reduce your risk of contracting these diseases.

Respiratory Infections

The most common communicable diseases are those of the respiratory tract. These infections can occur anywhere from the nose to the alveoli of the lungs. Most are caused by viruses or bacteria. You can reduce your risk of most respiratory illnesses by avoiding close contact with people who are infected, washing your hands often, keeping your hands away from your eyes and nose, and keeping your immune system healthy. Smoking can contribute to illness by damaging cilia and irritating respiratory passages. In addition, symptoms of these diseases may be more severe in smokers. Smoking has also been shown to suppress the immune system.

▲ When you have a cold, the best thing to do is rest, eat nutritious foods, and drink plenty of fluids such as water or fruit juice. *How might these strategies help your body fight cold viruses?*

Common Cold

The common cold is a viral infection that causes inflammation of the mucous membranes that line the nose and throat. Symptoms include a runny nose, sneezing, and sore throat. The most common way of getting a cold is from rubbing your eyes or nose after picking up the virus directly through hand-to-hand contact or indirectly by handling a contaminated object.

There is no cure for the common cold. Treatment is for relief of symptoms, and most colds clear up in a week or so. Often treatment includes the use of **analgesics.** It's important to note that anyone under 20 years of age should avoid use of medications containing salicylates, such as aspirin. Such use is linked to Reye's syndrome, a condition that can be fatal. Avoid these products no matter what disease you might have. Use acetaminophen or ibuprofen instead.

Influenza

Influenza, or the flu, is a viral infection of the respiratory tract. It is most often spread through airborne transmission but also may spread through direct or indirect contact. Symptoms of flu include high fever, fatigue, headache, muscle aches, and cough. The flu can lead to **pneumonia**, (noo-MOH-nyah) *an infection of the lungs in which the air sacs fill with pus and other liquid.* This is a serious disease that is more likely to occur in the elderly and people with lung and heart problems.

Antiviral drugs for treatment of the flu are available but need to be given as soon as the illness arises. Persons who have the flu should get proper nutrition and plenty of rest and fluids. Older adults and persons of any age with chronic health problems should get a flu shot every year. However, anyone who wants to avoid the flu can be given the vaccine.

Pneumonia

Along with influenza, pneumonia is one of the top ten causes of death in the United States. Viral pneumonia is relatively short-lived and produces symptoms similar to those of influenza. Antiviral drugs are used in some cases. Bacterial pneumonia can be treated with antibiotics if diagnosed early. The bacteria that cause pneumonia are often present in healthy throats. When body defenses are weakened in some way, the bacteria can get into the lungs and multiply. For example, if a person is elderly or has influenza, he or she may be more at risk for complications leading to pneumonia.

hot link

analgesics For more information about analgesics, see Chapter 23, page 588.

Health Minute

Is It a Cold or the Flu?

Cold symptoms include:

► Runny or stuffy nose
► Sneezing
► Sore throat
► Headache

Flu symptoms include:

► High fever
► Chills
► Dry cough
► Muscle and joint pain
► Runny nose
► Sore throat
► Extreme fatigue

Strep Throat

Strep throat is a bacterial infection spread by direct contact, often through droplets that are coughed or sneezed into the air. Symptoms of strep throat include a sore throat, fever, and enlarged lymph nodes in the neck. Untreated, strep throat can lead to serious complications, including inflammation of the kidneys and rheumatic fever, which can cause permanent heart damage. Strep throat can be treated with antibiotics. A doctor cannot always diagnose strep by examination. If a sore throat lasts more than three days, a culture is taken to identify the bacteria.

Tuberculosis

Tuberculosis, or TB, is a bacterial disease that usually attacks the lungs. TB is spread through the air when a person with the disease coughs or sneezes. Most people who are infected carry the bacteria in their lungs but never develop the disease because the body's defenses prevent the bacteria from multiplying and spreading to others. People with weakened immune systems are more likely to develop the active disease with symptoms that include fatigue, coughing (sometimes coughing up blood), fever, night sweats, and weight loss. People with the active disease can spread TB. Prolonged or repeated exposure is usually required for infection. Some strains have developed resistance to antibiotics. Physicians may have to prescribe several antibiotics at one time until tests are conducted to determine which are effective for a particular person.

Hepatitis

Hepatitis is inflammation of the liver and can be caused by chemicals, including drugs or alcohol, or by many different pathogens. The hepatitis A, B, and C viruses are some of the most common causes of this type of liver damage, and there is no cure for them. However, vaccines for hepatitis A and B are available.

Hepatitis A

Hepatitis A is another of the top ten communicable diseases reported in the United States. About 1.5 million people worldwide are newly infected each year. The hepatitis A virus is most commonly spread through contact with feces of an infected person. Infected persons who do not wash their hands properly may contaminate inanimate objects or food or spread the virus through direct contact.

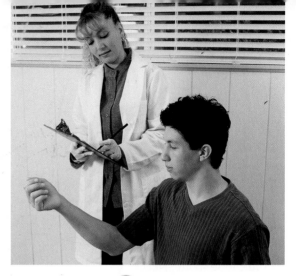

A **Many employers in the health care industry require applicants to show proof of a negative TB test.** *Why may patients in hospitals or in long-term care facilities be at increased risk for tuberculosis?*

Did You Know **?**

Many people mistakenly believe that tuberculosis is no longer a problem, but experts estimate that about 10 million people in the United States are currently infected with TB bacteria and that about 10 percent of these people will develop the disease.

TB is increasingly a worldwide problem. In 1999, 2 million deaths were attributed to TB; 100,000 of those deaths were among children. The CDC estimates that by 2020 nearly 1 billion people worldwide will become infected with tuberculosis.

Symptoms of hepatitis A are generally mild and may include fever, nausea, vomiting, fatigue, abdominal pain, and **jaundice**, a *yellowing of the skin and eyes*. Most infected individuals recover completely. Chronic, or long-lasting, infection is rare. The best way to reduce your risk of hepatitis A is to practice careful handwashing and avoid close contact with people who are infected.

About 30 to 40 percent of people with hepatitis B don't know how they got the infection. *How can you protect yourself from exposure to hepatitis B?*

Hepatitis B

Hepatitis B is a more serious disease than hepatitis A. The hepatitis B virus (HBV) is found in most bodily fluids of an infected person, especially blood. It is most often transmitted through sexual contact. It also can be transmitted through needles shared by infected drug users. Though most people who are infected never experience symptoms, the hepatitis B virus frequently causes severe liver damage, including liver failure and cirrhosis, or scarring, of the liver. Hepatitis B may be responsible for up to 80 percent of all cases of liver cancer worldwide. More than two billion people worldwide have been infected with HBV. About 1.25 million people in the United States have chronic HBV infection.

You can reduce your risk of hepatitis B by practicing abstinence from sexual contact and from illegal drug use. Do not share personal items, such as toothbrushes or razors, which could have trace amounts of saliva or blood. Body piercing and tattooing using contaminated needles can spread the disease. The CDC recommends that all children and teens receive the hepatitis B vaccine.

Hepatitis C

Hepatitis C is the most common chronic blood-borne infection in the United States; about four million Americans are infected. It is most often transmitted by direct contact with infected blood through contaminated needles shared by drug users. Hepatitis C can lead to chronic liver disease, liver cancer, or liver failure. It is the leading reason for liver transplants in the United States. Up to 90 percent of those infected with the hepatitis C virus (HCV) don't realize they have the disease until years later when routine tests show liver damage. You can reduce your risk of hepatitis C by practicing abstinence from illegal drug use. In addition, don't share personal care items, such as razors and toothbrushes. As with other viral infections, there is no cure for hepatitis. Treatment includes rest, proper nutrition, and drinking plenty of fluids.

Other Diseases

Several other communicable diseases are common among adolescents and young adults. **Figure 24.5** on page 640 provides a summary of these diseases.

Emerging Infections

Some diseases have been effectively controlled with the help of modern technology such as antibiotics and vaccines. Yet new diseases, such as AIDS and Lyme disease, are constantly appearing. Others, such as malaria and tuberculosis, are occurring in forms

Real-Life Application

Reducing Your Risk of Lyme Disease

In 1982 fewer than 1,000 cases of Lyme disease were reported in the United States. Today, more than 16,000 cases are reported each year. Lyme disease is transmitted to humans by the bite of an infected deer tick. Ticks favor a moist, shaded environment, such as forests. Coastal ticks thrive in areas of high rainfall. Ticks are most active in the spring and summer. Study the graph to help you analyze the environmental and geographical factors that influence the distribution and rate of disease in the United States. Use this information to develop a plan to reduce your risk.

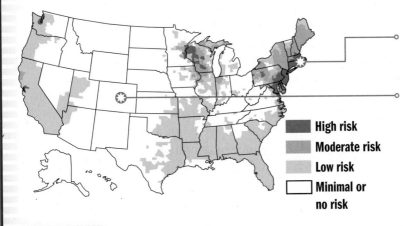

High risk
Moderate risk
Low risk
Minimal or no risk

What does the concentration of cases here tell you about the environment in which ticks live?

What is different about this part of the country that could account for the lower incidence of Lyme disease?

What human activities (leisure and industrial) could have influenced the increase in cases from 1982 to the present?

ACTIVITY

Work with a small group of students. Together, analyze the graph and discuss the questions. Use what you've learned to develop an action plan to decrease your risk of contracting Lyme disease. Include specific steps to protect yourself. Consider clothing, insect repellents, where you live or travel, and the time of year.

FIGURE 24.5

OTHER COMMON COMMUNICABLE DISEASES

Disease	Cause/Transmission	Symptoms	Treatment/Prevention
Mononucleosis	Virus attacks lymphocytes; spreads through direct contact, including sharing eating utensils and kissing	Chills, fever, sore throat, fatigue, and swollen lymph nodes	Rest if tired
Measles	Virus spreads when an infected person coughs, sneezes, or talks; highly contagious	High fever, red eyes, runny nose, cough, bumpy red rash usually starting on head or face	No definite treatment; vaccine for prevention
Encephalitis	A virus usually carried by mosquitoes; causes inflammation of the brain	Headache; fever; hallucinations; confusion; paralysis; and disturbances of speech, memory, behavior, and eye movement	If caused by herpes simplex virus, antiviral medicine; if caused by another virus, no known treatment
Meningitis	Virus or bacteria cause inflammation of the membranes that cover the brain	Fever, severe headache, nausea, vomiting, sensitivity to light, stiff neck	Viral meningitis: antiviral medicine if severe; bacterial meningitis: antibiotics; vaccine is available

that are resistant to drug treatments. These diseases are known as "emerging." An **emerging infection** is a *communicable disease whose incidence in humans has increased within the past two decades or threatens to increase in the near future.* Many factors are contributing to the development of emerging infections:

▶ **Transport across borders.** Infected people and animals carry pathogens from region to region, often to places where those pathogens previously were not a problem. Two examples of this are the appearance of dengue fever and West Nile encephalitis which is caused by West Nile virus. Dengue fever is found mostly in South and Central America and parts of Asia, and has appeared in the southwestern United States. West Nile encephalitis appears in Asia, Africa, and Europe and is now expanding across the Western Hemisphere, including parts of the United States. Both diseases are carried by mosquitoes.

▶ **Population movement.** A factor in the increase in Lyme disease is the movement of people into heavily wooded areas where ticks are prevalent. Symptoms include a rash, fatigue, fever, headache, stiff neck, sore muscles, and joint pain. Lyme disease can be treated with antibiotics.

▶ **Resistance to antibiotics.** The widespread use of antibiotics has resulted in pathogens that have become resistant. The pathogens that cause tuberculosis, gonorrhea (a sexually transmitted disease), and a type of pneumonia all have developed resistance to one or more antibiotics.

▶ **Changes in food technology.** Mass production and distribution of food increases the chance that contaminated food will infect a great number of people. *E. coli* has been responsible for outbreaks affecting thousands.

▶ **Agents of bioterrorism.** Because of the ease and frequency of travel, a contagious bioterrorist agent such as smallpox can spread rapidly from country to country.

Public health officials in the United States are addressing infectious diseases elsewhere in the world because pathogens can emerge in one region and spread. Information on emerging diseases is widely available—on the Internet, in books and magazines, and through news reports. With health information readily available, individuals can become more proactive and responsible for reducing their risk of communicable diseases, including emerging infections.

Health Minute
What You Can Do

Precautions to avoid emerging or reemerging infections:

▶ Take all of the antibiotics prescribed by your doctor.

▶ Eat only fully cooked eggs.

▶ Avoid swallowing water at water parks.

▶ Take precautions to prevent bites by vectors such as ticks and mosquitoes.

Lesson 3 *Review*

Reviewing Facts and Vocabulary

1. Compare and contrast the common cold and the flu.

2. What are three ways you can reduce your risk of getting influenza?

3. What are emerging infections?

Thinking Critically

4. **Synthesizing.** What healthful behaviors can students in your class practice to reduce everyone's risk of respiratory infection?

5. **Analyzing.** Why might emerging infections be an important area to receive funding for research? How can technology impact the reduction of diseases worldwide?

Applying Health Skills

Advocacy. Choose one emerging infection to research. Prepare a script for a public service announcement describing this disease. Be sure to include information on how the disease is transmitted and what the symptoms are. Urge individuals who suspect they may be infected to seek medical attention immediately. Share your script with the class.

PRESENTATION SOFTWARE Use presentation software to present the information you found on the disease you chose to investigate. Find help in using presentation software at **health.glencoe.com**.

Eye ON THE Media

Media Messages on Emerging Infections

Government agencies such as the Centers for Disease Control and Prevention (CDC) are responsible for getting important health information to the public. A particular challenge for these agencies is alerting the public to information about emerging infections, such as dengue fever, West Nile virus, and anthrax. These agencies use press releases as part of a media campaign to pass this information to as many people as possible.

—— DESIGN A LOGO FOR YOUR TEAM AND PLACE HERE

PRESS RELEASE   for immediate release

INCLUDE THE DATE HERE

Name of your City

Your PRESS RELEASE should include all the important information you want people to know about the disease.

—————— WHOM TO CONTACT IF A REPORTER HAS QUESTIONS
OR WANTS TO INTERVIEW SOMEONE SHOULD GO HERE

—————— INCLUDE A PHONE NUMBER

ACTIVITY

Research one of the emerging diseases that recently have been identified in the United States. Pretend you are on a communications team at the CDC whose job it is to let as many people as possible know about that disease. Begin with a press release, following the example shown above. Design a media campaign to notify the public about the health risks of the disease, what causes the disease, how it is transmitted, and how the disease is treated or prevented.

EXPRESS YOUR VIEWS

Write to your local health department, and ask about its role in responding to the emerging disease you've researched. Find out whether there is a community program that provides information about the disease and whether there is something you and your classmates can do to help spread the word.

CROSS-CURRICULUM CONNECTIONS

Tell a Story. Develop a story that is suitable for retelling aloud and is based on your own experience with one of the common childhood diseases mentioned in this chapter (flu, strep throat, chicken pox, measles, or the common cold). Use the story as a means of teaching your audience about how they can help prevent the spread of such diseases.

Calculate Bacteria Growth. Bacteria can grow rapidly under the right conditions. Some can duplicate themselves every 20 minutes. Calculate how many bacteria would be produced in four hours if a single bacterium reproduced at this rate.

Write a Report. Plague is a communicable disease that had a significant impact on world history, especially European history during the fourteenth century. Using reliable resources, research this disease and its impact during this period of history. Include the plague's causes, symptoms, and effects on society. Be sure to explain how the disease changed people's attitudes and became part of Renaissance folklore.

Create a Visual Display. Choose a vector-borne disease and find out about the life cycle of the pathogen that causes it. Create a display that illustrates the life cycle. Include information about how it is transmitted from host to host. Post the display in your classroom.

Epidemiologist

Did you ever wonder why and how diseases move the way they do? Why is the incidence of a particular disease suddenly on the increase? If these questions interest you, consider a career as an epidemiologist.

Epidemiology is a branch of medical science that deals with the incidence, distribution, and control of disease. Epidemiologists complete at least six years of college, studying science, human behavior, and biostatistics. They usually work in a university, research facility, or public health department. People who want to become epidemiologists should be logical, patient, organized, and curious. Find out more about epidemiology and other health careers by clicking on Career Corner at **health.glencoe.com**.

Chapter 24 Review

► EXPLORING HEALTH TERMS *Answer the following questions on a sheet of paper.*

Lesson 1 *Match each definition with the correct term.*

communicable disease	pathogen
toxin	vector
viruses	bacteria

1. A microscopic organism that causes disease.
2. A substance that kills cells or interferes with their function.
3. An organism that carries and transmits pathogens to humans or other animals.

Lesson 2 *Fill in the blanks with the correct term.*

antibody	antigen
immune system	immunity
inflammatory response	lymphocyte
phagocyte	vaccine

4. The swelling and pain that accompanies an injury such as a splinter is part of the body's _____ .
5. A white blood cell that attacks an invading pathogens is a(n) _____ .
6. The state of being protected against a particular disease is _____ .

Lesson 3 *Identify each sentence as True or False. If false, replace the underlined term with the correct term.*

emerging infection	jaundice
pneumonia	

7. <u>Jaundice</u> can be a complication of the flu.
8. A person with <u>pneumonia</u> will have skin and eyes that are slightly yellow.
9. An <u>emerging infection</u> is an infectious disease that has become more common within the past two decades or that threatens to increase in the near future.

► RECALLING THE FACTS *Use complete sentences to answer the following questions.*

Lesson 1

1. What is one way that some bacteria are helpful to the human body? How do some bacteria harm the body?
2. How do pathogens spread when a person sneezes?
3. Analyze how handwashing can help prevent communicable diseases from spreading.

Lesson 2

4. How do mucous membranes help fight pathogens?
5. How are antibodies and antigens related?
6. Describe how vaccines work, and evaluate their impact on disease prevention.
7. Explain how technology, such as the development of vaccines, has impacted the health status of individuals, families, communities, and the world in the prevention of communicable disease.

Lesson 3

8. With what do the air sacs in the lungs fill in a person infected with pneumonia?
9. What healthful behaviors will reduce your risk of contracting hepatitis A, B, and C?
10. Identify three emerging infections.

► THINKING CRITICALLY

1. **Applying.** Imagine that you are a pathogen living in the lungs of an infected person. Write a story about your journey as you leave your host through a sneeze. Tell what happens to you and your fellow pathogens as you travel through the air and land on another individual. *(LESSON 1)*

2. **Analyzing.** Compare and contrast the function of phagocytes in the inflammatory response with the function of specific lymphocytes in the immune response. *(LESSON 2)*

3. **Synthesizing.** Suppose that several people in a community have a disease that is spreading rapidly. If you were a public health worker assigned the task of finding out how the disease is being transmitted, what might you do to find the cause? *(LESSON 3)*

► HEALTH SKILLS APPLICATION

1. **Goal Setting.** Identify three things you can do to lower your risk of contracting a communicable disease. Make a plan to incorporate these strategies into your daily life. Prepare a "Staying Healthy" checklist that gives strategies you can use to reduce the number of infections. *(LESSON 1)*

2. **Advocacy.** Check with state and local governments to find out what immunizations are required for admission to schools at various levels from preschool through college. Use this information to create a public service pamphlet that explains why immunizations are important. *(LESSON 2)*

3. **Accessing Information.** Visit **health.glencoe.com** to link to a site on communicable diseases. Choose one of the diseases to research, and create a poster on your chosen disease. Be sure to include information about what symptoms accompany the disease, how it is transmitted, what lasting effects it can have on the body, what the trends are, who is most at risk, and whether a cure or an effective treatment is available. If a vaccination is under development for this disease, include information on that as well. You should also include a section with tips on protecting yourself against this disease. *(LESSON 3)*

BEYOND the Classroom

Parent Involvement

Advocacy. Many diseases and emerging infections are spread by vectors. Contact a state or local health department to determine which vector-borne diseases occur most often in the state in which you live. Choose one of these diseases, and interview a local public health official about precautions that can be taken to avoid infection. Be sure to ask what treatments are available to an infected person. Prepare a fact sheet with this information, including a picture of the vector.

School and Community

Vaccine clinics. Gather information about clinics and other public sites where free or low-cost flu vaccines are offered. Prepare a flyer that explains the need for this immunization. Include the dates, times, and locations for these vaccination opportunities.

Chapter 25

Sexually Transmitted Infections and HIV/AIDS

Lesson 1
The Risks of STIs

Lesson 2
Common STIs

Lesson 3
HIV and AIDS

Lesson 4
Treatment for HIV and AIDS

AIDS Ride

Quick Write

Using Visuals. HIV/AIDS awareness and understanding the dangers of STDs can help prevent the spread of these infections. What can you do to participate in fund-raisers and awareness campaigns for HIV/AIDS research?

Myth or Fact?

Read each statement below and respond by writing myth or fact for each item.

1. A person can get an STD only through sexual activity with many people.

2. Abstinence from sexual activity is 100 percent effective in preventing STDs and the sexual transmission of HIV and hepatitis B.

3. All STDs can be cured with antibiotics.

4. Anyone with an STD will have symptoms.

5. Many cases of HIV/AIDS go unreported.

6. A person can have only one type of STD at a time.

7. After a person has been treated for an STD, he or she can't get it again.

8. Untreated STDs can lead to difficulty in having children.

9. Some STDs, including HIV/AIDS, can be fatal.

10. Nationwide, STDs are on the rise among teens.

Keep your responses for review later in the chapter. When you complete the chapter, review this list of myths and facts again. If necessary, change your answers according to what you have learned.

For instant feedback on your health status, go to Chapter 25 Health Inventory at **health.glencoe.com**.

The Risks of STIs

YOU'LL LEARN TO

• Explain the relationship between alcohol and other drugs used by adolescents and the role these substances play in STDs.

• Analyze the importance and benefits of abstinence as it relates to the prevention of STDs.

• Discuss abstinence from sexual activity as the only method that is 100 percent effective in preventing STDs.

• Develop and analyze strategies related to the prevention of STDs.

QUICK START Your health is affected by the decisions you make regarding risk behaviors. What strategies do you use to help you make responsible decisions?

▲ STDs are the most common communicable diseases in the United States. *Why do you think this has been called the hidden epidemic?*

Some communicable diseases, such as the cold or flu, can be transmitted through actions as simple as shaking hands. Other communicable diseases are not so easily spread. **Sexually transmitted diseases (STDs)**, also referred to as **sexually transmitted infections (STIs)**, are *infectious diseases spread from person to person through sexual contact*. A person can have an infection, and pass the infection to others, without necessarily having the disease.

STDs: The Hidden Epidemic

Throughout history people have been faced with **epidemics**, *occurrences of diseases in which many people in the same place at the same time are affected*. Today in the United States, we are now facing another epidemic—an epidemic of STDs. An estimated 65 million people in the United States are living with an incurable STD. Many of these cases go undiagnosed and untreated. Why?

▶ Many people with STDs are asymptomatic—without symptoms. They do not seek treatment because they don't know they are infected. Individuals who don't know that they are infected can continue to transmit STDs. Some people who suspect they have an STD may be too embarrassed to seek treatment.

▶ Even when STDs are diagnosed, they may not be reported to health departments so that contacts can be notified and treated. These contacts can continue to unknowingly transmit the disease to others.

High-Risk Behavior and STDs

In the United States teens make up one quarter of the estimated 15 million new cases of STDs each year. That's more than 10,000 young people infected every day. Why are teens at particularly high risk for infection from STDs? Teens who are sexually active are likely to engage in one or more of the following high-risk behaviors:

▶ **Being sexually active with more than one person.** This includes having a series of sexual relationships with one person at a time. However, being sexually active with even one partner puts a person at risk. Most teens are unaware of a partner's past behavior and whether he or she already has an STD.

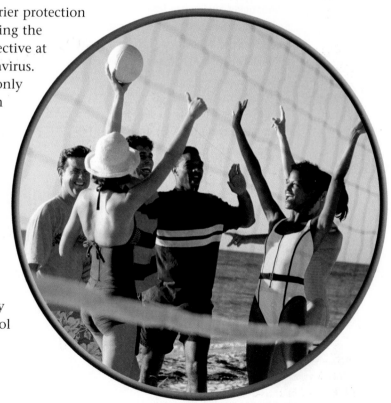

Avoid high-risk behaviors by forming friendships with people who share your commitment to abstinence.

▶ **Engaging in unprotected sex.** Barrier protection is not 100 percent effective in preventing the transmission of STDs, and it is not effective at all against HPV—the human papillomavirus. Abstinence from sexual activity is the only method that is 100 percent effective in preventing STDs.

▶ **Selecting high-risk partners.** Such partners include those with a history of being sexually active with more than one person and those who have injected illegal drugs.

▶ **Using alcohol and other drugs.** Alcohol use can lower inhibitions. In a recent survey, more than 25 percent of teens who engaged in sexual activity had been under the influence of alcohol or drug use.

The Consequences of STDs

Most people, including teens, are not fully aware of the consequences of STDs. These are serious infections that can dramatically change the course of a person's life.

▶ **Some STDs are incurable.** The pathogens that cause these STDs cannot be eliminated from the body by medical treatment, such as antibiotics. The viruses that cause genital herpes and AIDS (the human immunodeficiency virus, or HIV), for example, remain in the body for life.

▶ **Some STDs cause cancer.** The hepatitis B virus can cause cancer of the liver. The human papillomavirus (HPV) can cause cancer of the cervix. These STDs also cannot be cured and may last a lifetime.

Hands-On Health ACTIVITY

The Benefits of Abstinence

Practicing abstinence from sexual activity can benefit you in many ways. By encouraging your friends to abstain, you can be a positive influence on their health and well-being.

What You'll Need

- paper and pencil
- number cube (one for each group)
- paper cup (one for each group)
- construction paper
- markers

What You'll Do

1. Roll the cube from the cup onto your desk five times and record each number. Complete the following steps at your teacher's instruction.

2. Stand if you rolled one 5. Imagine that you have just found out that you have an STD. Tell how this will affect your life now and in the future.

3. Stand if you rolled a 5 more than once. Tell what you think and how you feel about having more than one STD.

4. As a class, brainstorm reasons for practicing abstinence.

5. Work in small groups to cut out a sheet of construction paper as your teacher instructs.

6. Write a different reason to practice abstinence on each of the six sides of the paper. Target the message to teens and be persuasive.

7. Fold and tape the paper to form a cube, then hang the cube from the ceiling.

Apply and Conclude

Imagine how you want your life to be in five years. Write it down. Be specific. Add how practicing abstinence now can help you achieve the life you want.

▶ **Some STDs can cause complications that affect the ability to reproduce.** Females can develop pelvic inflammatory disease (PID), which damages reproductive organs and can cause sterility.

▶ **Some STDs can be passed from an infected female to her child before, during, or after birth.** STDs can damage the bones, nervous system, and brain of a fetus. Premature births can result, and infants infected with STDs at delivery may become blind or develop pneumonia and some may die.

Preventing STDs Through Abstinence

You may have experienced how an action that has a result demonstrates a cause-and-effect relationship. Touching a hot stove, for example, is the *cause* of sustaining a burn, which is the *result*.

A clear cause-and-effect relationship exists between sexual intercourse in any form and sexually transmitted infection. If you have sexual contact with an infected person, you put yourself at risk of being infected with an STD. Sexual activity is the cause—an STD is the effect.

Prevent exposure to STDs by practicing **abstinence**, *the deliberate decision to avoid harmful behaviors, including sexual activity before marriage and the use of tobacco, alcohol, and other drugs.* Use refusal skills to avoid situations in which you may be at risk. Choose friends who are abstinent and who support your decision to abstain.

HEALTH *Online*

Investigate facts about the rise in hepatitis B in an article from Health Updates at **health.glencoe.com.**

hot link

abstinence For more information on abstinence, see Chapter 12, page 318.

▶ Lesson 1 *Review*

Reviewing Facts and Vocabulary

1. Identify three reasons why teens are at high risk for getting an STD.

2. Explain the relationship between alcohol use as a high-risk behavior in regard to sexual activity and the risk of STDs.

3. How are refusal skills related to the prevention of STDs?

Thinking Critically

4. **Analyzing.** Analyze, discuss, and communicate the importance and benefits of abstinence as it relates to the prevention of STDs.

5. **Evaluating.** Explain and discuss why abstinence from sexual activity is the only method that is 100 percent effective in preventing STDs.

Applying Health Skills

Advocacy. Write an article for your school newspaper to inform students about the STD epidemic. Include the negative consequences that can affect a person's life, as well as strategies for avoiding STDs.

TECHNOLOGY *OPTION*

WEB SITES Use the article you wrote as the basis for a Web page. See **health.glencoe.com** for help in planning and building your own Web site.

Common STIs

YOU'LL LEARN TO

- Identify symptoms and treatments for some common STDs.

- Identify community health services for getting help with prevention and treatment of STDs.

- Analyze the influence of public health policies and practices on the prevention and treatment of STDs.

- Analyze the harmful effects of STDs on the developing fetus.

QUICK START   Suppose you received a letter from a friend telling you that she may have a sexually transmitted disease. Your friend asks your advice as to whether she should tell her boyfriend. Write a short response to the letter.

Learning about STDs can help you avoid the behaviors that lead to infection. *In addition to having accurate information, what else should you know or do to avoid infection from STDs?*

You have already learned why STDs are referred to as a hidden epidemic in the United States, which has the highest rates of STDs in the industrialized world. The Centers for Disease Control and Prevention (CDC) reports that STDs account for more than 85 percent of the most common communicable diseases in the United States. The estimated incidence and prevalence of STDs is shown in **Figure 25.1.** The most important fact to remember is this: The primary means of transmission of STDs is sexual activity. Teens who practice abstinence from sexual activity greatly reduce their risk of contracting STDs.

Human Papillomavirus

The **human papillomavirus**, or HPV, is *a virus that can cause genital warts or asymptomatic infection.* HPV is considered the most common STD in the United States. The CDC estimates that 50 to 75 percent of sexually active males and females acquire HPV infection at some time during their lives. About 30 different types of HPV can infect the genital area.

Most types of HPV infections are asymptomatic. A **Pap test** and other medical examinations may detect changes associated with HPV. There is no treatment. However, most asymptomatic HPV infections appear to be temporary and are probably cleared by the immune system. Almost all cases of cervical cancer are caused by certain types of HPV. HPV also can cause cancers of the penis and anus.

Genital Warts

Genital warts are pink or reddish warts with cauliflowerlike tops that appear on the genitals, the vagina, or the cervix one to three months after infection from HPV. Genital warts are highly contagious, and are spread by any form of sexual contact with an infected person. It may take up to three months for warts to appear, but they often disappear, even without treatment. Diagnosis is determined by a health care worker by examination of the warts. If a person suspects he or she has been infected, examination and treatment are essential, because once infected, a person has the virus for the rest of his or her life. Treatments can rid the body of the warts but not the virus. Complications of HPV and genital warts can result in cervical cancer and cancer of the penis. Infants born to females infected with HPV may develop warts in their throats, obstructing the breathing passages, which can be life-threatening.

hot link

Pap test For more information about the Pap test and the health of the reproductive systems, see Chapter 18, page 477.

FIGURE 25.1

ESTIMATED INCIDENCE AND PREVALENCE OF STDS IN THE UNITED STATES

STD	Incidence (Estimated number of new cases every year)	Prevalence (Estimated number of people currently infected)
Human Papillomavirus (HPV)	5.5 million	20 million
Chlamydia	3 million	2 million
Genital Herpes	1 million	45 million
Gonorrhea	650,000	Not Available
Trichomoniasis	5 million	Not Available
Syphilis	70,000	Not Available
Hepatitis B	120,000	417,000

Source: CDC, Tracking the Hidden Epidemics. Trends in STDs in the United States 2000

Chlamydia

Chlamydia is *a bacterial infection that affects the reproductive organs of both males and females.* Forty percent of cases are reported in teens 15 to 19 years old. Chlamydia is asymptomatic, meaning there are no visible symptoms, in 75 percent of infected females and 50 percent of infected males. When symptoms are present, males may experience a discharge from the penis and burning upon urination. Females may have vaginal discharge, burning upon urination, or abdominal pain. Chlamydia is diagnosed by laboratory examination of secretions from the cervix in females or from the **urethra** in males. It can be treated with antibiotics, but no immunity develops, so a person can become infected again.

Because chlamydia is usually asymptomatic, it often goes undetected until serious complications occur. In females who are untreated, the infection can cause pelvic inflammatory disease (PID) and lead to chronic (long-term) pelvic pain or infertility. Untreated chlamydia also can lead to infertility in males. Chlamydia can cause premature birth, and infants born to infected females may develop eye disease or pneumonia.

Genital Herpes

Genital herpes is *an STD caused by the herpes simplex virus (HSV).* There are two types of HSV:

▶ Type 1 usually causes cold sores.

▶ Type 2 usually causes genital sores.

However, both types can infect the mouth and the genitals. Nationwide, about 20 percent of the total adolescent population is infected with the virus. Genital herpes is twice as common in adults from 20 to 29 years old today as it was 20 years ago.

Most individuals who have genital herpes are asymptomatic and are not aware that they are infected. Those who do show symptoms typically have blisterlike sores in the genital area that occur periodically. It is not true that the virus can be spread only when blisters are present; the virus can spread in the absence of symptoms. Diagnosis is made through laboratory tests on the fluid from the blisters. Medication can relieve the symptoms, but cannot cure herpes infection—once contracted, the virus remains in the body for life.

The herpes virus is potentially fatal for infants who contract the virus from their mothers at the time of delivery. The virus may also play a major role in the spread of HIV by making people who are infected with herpes more capable of transmitting or acquiring HIV.

hot link

urethra For more information about the male reproductive system, see Chapter 18, page 470.

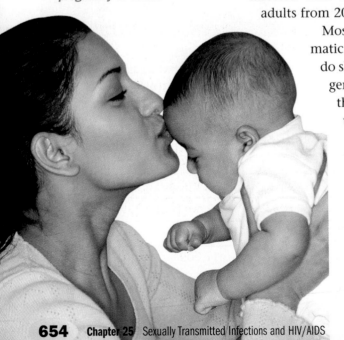

Ⓥ Mothers have a responsibility to protect their infants from exposure to STDs during pregnancy as well as during breast-feeding. *Which STDs can be transmitted from a mother to her child during pregnancy or birth?*

Gonorrhea

Gonorrhea is *a bacterial STD that usually affects mucous membranes.* The highest rates of gonorrhea infection are found in females from 15 to 19 years old and in males from 20 to 24 years old. Symptoms in males include a discharge from the penis and painful urination. Diagnosis in males is made by staining and examining the discharge under a microscope. Approximately 50 percent of females with gonorrhea have no symptoms. Those who do may experience a vaginal discharge and pain or burning upon urination. Diagnosis in females is made by swabbing the cervix and growing the organisms in a laboratory. Gonorrhea can be treated with antibiotics. However, increased resistance to antibiotics can complicate treatment. A person can be reinfected if exposed again to the bacteria. If untreated, gonorrhea can lead to infertility in both males and females. The bacteria can also spread to the bloodstream and cause permanent damage to the joints. Females can pass the infection to their babies during childbirth. Infants born to mothers with gonorrhea can contract eye infections that cause blindness.

Trichomoniasis

Trichomoniasis is *an STD caused by a microscopic protozoan that results in infections of the vagina, urethra, and bladder.* About five million new cases of this disease are estimated to occur every year in the United States. Females may have no symptoms, however the disease may result in **vaginitis,** an inflammation of the vagina characterized by discharge, odor, irritation, and itching. In females trichomoniasis is diagnosed by microscopic examination of the discharge. The organisms can sometimes be seen in a Pap test. Males usually show no symptoms. When symptoms do occur in males, they include mild urethral itching or discharge and burning after urination. Since the disease is difficult to diagnose in males, they are usually treated without laboratory testing if their partners are infected.

Syphilis

Syphilis is *an STD that attacks many parts of the body and is caused by a small bacterium called a spirochete.* The first sign of infection is a painless reddish sore, called a chancre (SHAN-kuhr), at the site of infection. The sore will heal on its own, but if the infection is not treated, it spreads through the blood to other parts of the body. Eventually, the disease can damage internal organs, including the heart, liver, nervous system, and kidneys. If left untreated, the person is at risk of paralysis, convulsions, blindness, and heart disease. Syphilis can be transmitted from a pregnant female to her fetus. An infant infected with syphilis may have a damaged nervous system and can die from the effects.

h⊙t link

vaginitis For more information on diseases of the female reproductive system, see Chapter 18, page 479.

 STDs are caused by bacteria, viruses, and other pathogens. This single-celled protozoan causes trichomoniasis. *Why is it important for people to get tested if they think they may have an STD?*

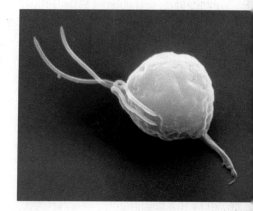

FIGURE 25.2

OTHER COMMON STDS

Disease (cause)	Symptoms	Treatment	What Could Happen
Chancroid (bacteria)	Sores or bumps on the genitals	Antibiotics	Infection of lymph glands in groin area, and sores
Bacterial vaginosis (bacteria)	Abnormal vaginal discharge, odor, pain, itching, or burning during urination	Antibiotics	In most cases no complications; can lead to PID and premature birth; risk of HIV and STDs
Hepatitis B (virus)	90% of victims are asymptomatic; nausea, vomiting, jaundice, loss of appetite	Antiviral drugs in some cases, but no cure	Chronic infection, cirrhosis of the liver, cancer of the liver
Hepatitis C (blood borne infection)	Often asymptomatic	Antivirual drugs, but no cure	Liver damage, liver disease
Pubic lice (small insects)	Itching, presence of lice and eggs in pubic hair	Medicated soaps; washing all bedding, towels, and clothes	No lasting effects

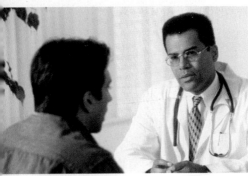

Early detection of STDs is important to avoid serious illness and further spread of the disease.
Why is it important for people not to treat an STD on their own?

Seeking Treatment

Prevention of STDs is every individual's responsibility. Treatment is also an important personal responsibility. **Figure 25.2** above lists other common STDs, along with their symptoms and the treatment that is usually prescribed for each. As you have read, STDs can cause severe, long-term health problems. Being embarrassed should not stop a person who thinks that he or she may have been exposed to an STD from visiting a private physician or a public health clinic. By law, information about these diseases is kept confidential. Only a health care professional can prescribe the correct treatment, including antibiotics for some STDs.

Individuals also have a social obligation to prevent the spread of infection. Public health clinics sometimes help with contacting current and past partners to make sure they get any needed treatment. Ultimately, however, it is the responsibility of any person infected with an STD to notify everyone with whom he or she has had sexual contact. Informing someone else about the possibility of having an STD could save someone's life.

Health Skills Activity

Refusal Skills: Lines of Defense

Juliana has been dating Kyle for several months. She has already explained to Kyle that she wants to remain abstinent, and until now he has respected her decision.

Kyle says, "Hey, Jules, let's skip the movie tonight and check out the party at my buddy's house. His folks are gone, and I hear there's going to be a band!"

Juliana responds, "It sounds like fun, but I don't know your buddy and it's pretty far away."

"No problem, I'll protect you!" Kyle laughs. "In fact, we'll finally have a chance to spend some time alone."

Juliana is worried about what might happen.

What Would You Do?

Apply the following refusal skills to write a response to Kyle. Use each refusal skill.

1. Say no in a firm voice.
2. Explain why you are refusing.
3. Suggest alternatives to the proposed activity.
4. Back up your words with body language.
5. Leave if necessary.

 Lesson 2 *Review*

Reviewing Facts and Vocabulary

1. Which STDs might not present noticeable symptoms?
2. Analyze and explain the harmful effects of two common STDs on fetuses and infants.
3. Where can a person go for treatment of an STD?

Thinking Critically

4. **Compare and Contrast.** Describe symptoms of gonorrhea and genital herpes for males and females.
5. **Analyzing.** Public policies enable health officials to locate and contact sexual partners of people who have been diagnosed with an STD. How do these policies help with the prevention and treatment of STDs?

Applying Health Skills

Refusal Skills. Construct a table similar to the one on page 656. Use this table to list reasons to say no to pressure to engage in sexual activity.

SPREADSHEETS Using spreadsheet software, create a chart to organize the material in your table. See **health.glencoe.com** for information on how to use a spreadsheet.

HIV and AIDS

VOCABULARY

acquired immune deficiency
   syndrome (AIDS)
human immunodeficiency
   virus (HIV)
opportunistic infection

YOU'LL LEARN TO

- Explain how HIV affects and destroys the immune system.

- Identify behaviors known to transmit HIV.

- Analyze the relationship between unsafe behaviors, refusal skills, and the risk of HIV.

QUICK START AIDS is a disease that attacks the immune system. Write two ways that your immune system protects your body from disease.

Health care workers wear goggles and disposable gloves whenever they may come in contact with body fluids. *Why are these precautions taken with all patients, not just those known to be infected with HIV?*

In July 1981, an outbreak of a rare form of skin cancer known as Kaposi's (KAY-puh-seez) sarcoma was reported. At the same time, doctors began seeing unusual infections among otherwise healthy individuals. About a year later, the CDC labeled the disease **acquired immune deficiency syndrome** or **AIDS**, *a disease in which the immune system of the patient is weakened.* That year more than 1,600 cases were reported and almost 700 deaths resulted from the newly identified disease. In 1983 the **human immunodeficiency virus**, or **HIV**, *a virus that attacks the immune system,* was confirmed as the cause. In 2000, AIDS was the fifth leading cause of death among adults from 25 to 44 years old.

Teens at Risk

In the United States the overall rate of new cases of HIV infection has fallen slightly since 1985, and new drug therapies help AIDS patients live longer. As a result, some people have a false sense that AIDS is no longer the problem it once was. However, data indicates that although new AIDS cases are declining among the population as a whole, there has been no decline in the number of diagnosed HIV infections among youth from 13 to 24 years old. In fact, teens have one of the fastest growing rates of HIV infection. Many young adults who are currently dying from AIDS were infected in their teens.

$1,000 a month. Worldwide, many infected individuals do not have access to treatment because of high costs and lack of availability. The time line shown in **Figure 25.4** summarizes some of the developments in HIV/AIDS research and treatment.

HIV/AIDS—A Continuing Problem

The number of newly reported AIDS cases in the industrialized world is decreasing. Much of this decrease in AIDS cases results from the success of drug cocktails—combinations of drugs—that slow the progression of HIV infection. This success has brought complacency about the need for HIV prevention. However, this is a false security. Research has identified new, drug-resistant strains of HIV. These strains do not respond to the drug cocktails currently used in the fight against AIDS. The combination of drug resistance and high-risk behaviors could result in HIV strains that are transmitted and spread even more widely. Despite the progress that has been made in development of treatment options, HIV/AIDS is still a fatal disease for which there is no cure.

HIV/AIDS: THE GLOBAL PICTURE

At the end of 2001, an estimated 40 million people worldwide were infected with HIV/AIDS. This statistic means that HIV is now **pandemic**—*a global outbreak of infectious disease.* The number of people living with HIV is growing. It is estimated that in 2001 alone, 5 million people became infected with HIV/AIDS worldwide.

CHARACTER CHECK

Responsibility. Each individual can play a role in curbing the spread of HIV by staying informed and spreading the word about this disease. **Take the time to read articles about HIV/AIDS. Share information with family and friends about recent developments in treatment and research to find a cure.**

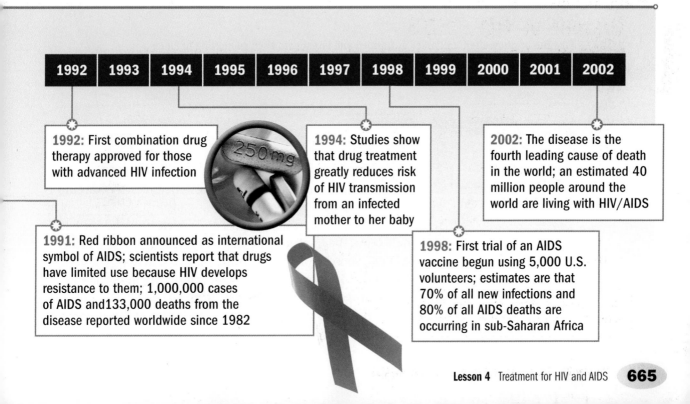

| 1992 | 1993 | 1994 | 1995 | 1996 | 1997 | 1998 | 1999 | 2000 | 2001 | 2002 |

1992: First combination drug therapy approved for those with advanced HIV infection

1994: Studies show that drug treatment greatly reduces risk of HIV transmission from an infected mother to her baby

2002: The disease is the fourth leading cause of death in the world; an estimated 40 million people around the world are living with HIV/AIDS

1991: Red ribbon announced as international symbol of AIDS; scientists report that drugs have limited use because HIV develops resistance to them; 1,000,000 cases of AIDS and 133,000 deaths from the disease reported worldwide since 1982

1998: First trial of an AIDS vaccine begun using 5,000 U.S. volunteers; estimates are that 70% of all new infections and 80% of all AIDS deaths are occurring in sub-Saharan Africa

Should More Money Be Spent on AIDS Research and Treatment?

In 1996 the National Institutes of Health (NIH) spent an average of $1,160 on research for every heart disease death, $4,700 on research for every cancer death, and $43,000 on research for every AIDS death. Do you think that more money should be spent on AIDS research and treatment? Here are two points of view.

Viewpoint 1: Parker T., age 17

I don't have a problem with the current level of NIH research money going to AIDS; I know it's a serious disease. I just wish more money were spent researching heart disease, cancer, and other conditions that affect more people. For example, in the last 20 years, 14 million Americans died of heart disease. That's 30 times more than the number who died of AIDS in the same period.

Viewpoint 2: Carmen S., age 16

I agree that heart disease, cancer, and the other diseases should get more funding for research. Unfortunately, however, AIDS is a potentially fatal disease that affects persons of all ages. You can't just look at number of deaths alone. The amount of life-years lost because of AIDS is nearly the same as cancer because many of the people who die of AIDS are young. Also, AIDS is communicable and much of the money spent is to prevent transmission. The preventive measures for AIDS also prevent other STDs, so much of the research money is going toward many diseases, not just AIDS.

ACTIVITY

Take the position of either Parker or Carmen and investigate each supporting argument. Gather additional information to support your point of view using online or print resources and present your viewpoint to the class.

STAYING INFORMED ABOUT HIV/AIDS

Because neither a cure for AIDS nor an effective HIV vaccine is available, knowledge is the first defense against infection. New research can be found in newspapers and magazines and on television, radio, and the Internet. The CDC and state health departments are excellent sources of information. Teachers, school counselors, and physicians can provide guidance on how to find information. By avoiding high-risk behaviors, staying informed, and making responsible decisions, you can protect yourself and others from infection.

Abstinence and HIV/AIDS

During your teen years, you may feel pressure to experiment with new behaviors, such as engaging in sexual activity or using drugs. Consider that your actions today can change the entire course of your life. Choosing to remain abstinent shows that you are taking an active role in caring for your own health and acting responsibly by not jeopardizing the well-being of others. These strategies will help you avoid pressure to engage in sexual activity and use drugs:

▶ Avoid situations and events where drug use or the pressure to engage in sexual activity is likely to occur. If you are at a party where things are getting out of control, leave immediately.

▶ Practice refusal skills. Be firm when you refuse to take part in drug use or sexual activity. Use body language as well as words to get your message across.

▶ Choose your relationships carefully. Avoid forming a dating relationship with someone whom you know to be sexually active. Avoid known drug users or people who approve of drug use.

 Each of the more than 44,000 colorful panels in the AIDS Memorial Quilt memorializes the life of a person who died from AIDS. When the entire quilt was in Washington, D.C., it covered the National Mall. *How does the AIDS quilt help educate the public about HIV/AIDS?*

▶ Lesson 4 *Review*

Reviewing Facts and Vocabulary

1. What is asymptomatic HIV infection?
2. When is a Western blot test performed?
3. Explain how technologies such as new drug treatments have impacted the health status of people with HIV infection as well as people's attitudes toward the AIDS epidemic.

Thinking Critically

4. **Evaluating.** Why might people in the United States have better access to AIDS treatment than people in developing nations?
5. **Analyzing.** What strategies can you use to resist pressure to engage in sexual activity or drug use and in doing so reduce your risk of HIV infection?

Applying Health Skills

Accessing Information. Research new vaccines that are being developed for HIV/AIDS. Use several different sources of information in your search, such as Web sites, books, and newspaper or magazine articles. Evaluate the validity of your sources to make sure they are reliable and accurate. Then prepare a presentation describing the promise of the new vaccines.

PRESENTATION SOFTWARE Use presentation software to present one of the treatments you researched to your class. Find help in using presentation software at **health.glencoe.com.**

Mock Radio Call-In Program

According to the National Association of Broadcasters, people over the age of 12 listen to the radio an average of three hours each day. One of today's popular formats is the radio call-in program. Radio call-in programs are one method of disseminating information to the public and often have a host who invites expert panelists to answer questions from listeners. In the following class activity, you and your classmates will stage a mock radio call-in program to talk about how to prevent the spread of STDs.

ACTIVITY

Group 1 will become the expert panel that answers callers' questions. The panel should consist of:

- **a public health official.** This person should have knowledge of current statistics on STD occurrences and information on prevention and treatment options.

- **a member of a health care organization.** This person provides services and information on community resources for STD diagnosis and treatment.

- **a member of an advocacy group.** This person campaigns for effective methods for control and prevention of STDs.

Group 2 will be the radio show's callers. Each student in Group 2 will research and compose one question for each kind of panelist. Select one person to become the host of the radio call-in show. This person will introduce the panelists and facilitate the discussion by calling on students.

EXPRESS YOUR VIEWS

Compose a short statement for a call-in radio program that promotes abstinence for youth as an effective defense against STDs. Your statement should be persuasive and should contain supporting facts.

CROSS-CURRICULUM CONNECTIONS

Prepare a Speech. Making healthy decisions is the key to preventing yourself from being infected with a sexually transmitted disease. Abstinence from sexual activity before marriage and following a drug-free lifestyle are your best choices to avoid the consequences of STDs. Using the facts you have learned in this chapter, plan a short speech on why these lifestyle choices are important for a happy and healthy future.

Research Epidemics. In the 1980s, the HIV/AIDS crisis reached epidemic levels in the United States, and the epidemic continues to heighten worldwide. Throughout history, there have been various diseases that have spread to this dangerous point. For example, in 1918 an influenza outbreak killed 30 million people. Work in groups and choose a major epidemic or plague from history to research.

Calculate AIDS Death Rates. In one recent year, the United States population reached 281,421,906. If there were 14,802 AIDS deaths during that year, what was the rate of death due to AIDS per 100,000 of population?

Investigate Viruses. A master of disguise, the HIV virus keeps changing to evade each new treatment that comes along. Research another type of virus to find out about its structure, life cycle, and characteristics. Create a poster showing how a virus infects cells. Demonstrate how the transmission of the virus can be slowed or prevented.

CAREER Corner

Health Advocate

Do you like working with people? Can you synthesize information from a variety of sources to come up with innovative solutions to complex problems? If so, you may be interested in a career as a health advocate.

Health advocates work in a wide range of settings. Some are patient representatives and administrators in large health care facilities or at consumer health agencies; others serve on ethics committees and medical policy boards. A community health advocate often provides education and information as a member of a health care team working in clinics and community centers where access to health care is limited. All health advocates work toward one goal: finding innovative ways to improve the delivery of health services.

Health advocates have several levels of certification. Two-year courses are available at some community colleges. Others become advocates through a Master of Arts program following college graduation. Find out more about this and other health careers by clicking on Career Corner at **health.glencoe.com**.

Chapter 25 *Review*

➤ **EXPLORING HEALTH TERMS** *Answer the following questions on a sheet of paper.*

Lesson 1 *Fill in the blanks with the correct term.*

abstinence	sexually transmitted disease (STD)
epidemic	sexually transmitted infection (STI)

1. An infection that spreads from person to person through sexual contact is called a(n) _____ or a(n) _____ .

2. When a community has a number of cases of an infectious disease larger than would be generally expected, the community is experiencing a(n) _____ .

3. The only 100 percent effective way to avoid STDs is to practice _____ .

Lesson 2 *Replace the underlined words with the correct term.*

chlamydia	syphilis
genital herpes	trichomoniasis
gonorrhea	human papillomavirus (HPV)

4. <u>Gonorrhea</u> can lead to pelvic pain and infertility.

5. <u>HPV</u> is an STD caused by the herpes simplex virus.

6. A bacterial STD that usually affects mucous membranes is <u>chlamydia</u>.

7. The first sign of <u>trichomoniasis</u> infection is a chancre at the site of infection.

Lesson 3 *Identify each statement as True or False. If false, replace the underlined term with the correct term.*

HIV	AIDS
opportunistic infection	

8. <u>AIDS</u> is the virus that attacks the immune system.

9. Being infected with <u>AIDS</u> does not necessarily mean a person has <u>HIV</u>.

10. <u>Opportunistic infections</u> are rare in a person with a normal immune system, but they easily invade the body of a person with a weakened immune system.

Lesson 4 *Match each definition with the correct term.*

EIA	asymptomatic stage
Western blot	symptomatic stage
pandemic	

11. A period of time during which a person infected with HIV has no symptoms.

12. The first test usually performed to screen for HIV antibodies in the blood.

13. The most common confirmation test for HIV in the United States.

➤ **RECALLING THE FACTS** *Use complete sentences to answer the following questions.*

Lesson 1

1. Why are STDs in the United States considered a hidden epidemic?

2. Explain the relationship between alcohol and other drugs used by adolescents and the role these substances play in STDs.

3. What is the only method that is 100 percent effective in preventing STDs?

Lesson 2

4. Which STDs stay in the body for life?

5. Why is early treatment of STDs important?

6. Explain why an individual diagnosed with an STD should notify contacts.

Lesson 3

7. Why is the risk of HIV infection low for a person whose coworker has tested positive for HIV?

8. Why does having multiple sexual contacts increase the risk of HIV infection?

Lesson 4

9. List and describe the stages of HIV infection.

10. Relate the importance of tests to detect HIV and why early detection is important.

➤ THINKING CRITICALLY

1. **Analyzing.** Suppose a friend tells you that he or she is considering having a sexual relationship with a girlfriend or boyfriend. Write a letter to your friend explaining the benefits of abstinence as it relates to the prevention of STDs. *(LESSON 1)*

2. **Evaluating.** Some states have laws that require couples who apply for marriage licenses to be tested for particular STDs. Analyze the influence of this public health policy on the prevention and treatment of STDs. *(LESSON 2)*

3. **Synthesizing.** State facts that support this statement: Fighting HIV infection is everyone's responsibility. *(LESSON 3)*

4. **Analyzing.** What makes opportunistic illnesses more dangerous for individuals who are infected with HIV than for those who are not infected? *(LESSON 4)*

➤ HEALTH SKILLS APPLICATION

1. **Advocacy.** Research groups that advocate teen abstinence from sexual activity. Find out what services these groups offer and how you can volunteer to help them. *(LESSON 1)*

2. **Accessing Information.** Identify community health services that help with prevention and treatment of STDs. Discover the types of educational materials they have for educating teens about the risks of STDs. Share your findings with the class. *(LESSON 2)*

3. **Advocacy.** Develop an HIV prevention program aimed at teens entering high school. Emphasize the relationship between unsafe behaviors, such as sexual contact and drug use, and the risk of HIV infection. *(LESSON 3)*

4. **Refusal Skills.** List two suggestions for practicing abstinence when pressured to engage in sexual activity or to use drugs. *(LESSON 4)*

BEYOND the Classroom

Parent Involvement

Advocacy. With your parents, research ways that parents can help their children avoid risky behaviors that might lead to STDs. Work together with your parent or guardian to organize your research, and create guidelines for other parents. If you have access to the Internet, post the guidelines on a Web site.

School and Community

Finding resources. Learn the names of organizations in your community that help people infected with HIV/AIDS. Make a list of these organizations, and describe the services each provides. Create a pamphlet containing the information you have gathered. Make the pamphlet available through the school health office.

Noncommunicable Diseases and Disabilities

affects the heart or blood vessels. Approximately 61 million Americans have some form of the disease. CVDs are responsible for more than 40 percent of all deaths in the United States, killing almost a million Americans each year.

Types of Cardiovascular Disease

The heart, blood, and blood vessels are the main parts of the circulatory system. When the parts work together properly, the cardiovascular system runs efficiently. When a problem affects one part, the entire system is threatened. As you read the description of each type of CVD, keep in mind that you can reduce your risk by avoiding tobacco; getting plenty of physical activity; maintaining a healthful weight; and following an eating plan low in saturated fat, cholesterol, and sodium.

Hypertension

Blood pressure is the force of blood created by the heart's contractions and the resistance of the vessel walls. Normal blood pressure varies with age, height, weight, and other factors. **Hypertension** is *high blood pressure*—pressure that is continually above the normal range for a particular person. If high blood pressure continues over a long period, the heart, blood vessels, and other body organs will be damaged. Hypertension is a major risk factor for other types of CVDs. Hypertension can occur at any age, but it is more common among people over the age of 35. Of Americans aged 20–74, 23 percent have hypertension. CVD, considered a "silent killer," often has no symptoms in its early stages, so it's important to get your blood pressure checked regularly. High blood pressure can be lowered with medication, weight management, adequate physical activity, and proper nutrition.

Atherosclerosis

At birth, the lining of blood vessels is smooth and elastic. Over time, factors such as tobacco smoke, high blood pressure, or high cholesterol levels can damage the inner lining of the arteries. Fatty substances in the blood, called plaques, can build up on the artery walls, causing the arteries to thicken and lose their elasticity. *The process in which plaques accumulate on artery walls* is called **atherosclerosis** (a-thuh-roh-skluh-ROH-sis). This buildup is due mainly to food choices—specifically, a high intake of saturated fats and cholesterol. Sometimes, a blood clot forms in the area of plaque. The clot grows until it blocks the artery. If the affected artery feeds the heart or the brain, a heart attack or stroke may result.

A The artery on the left is healthy. The one on the right shows evidence of atherosclerosis. *What dietary choices can you make to lower your risk of atherosclerosis?*

hot link

heart For more information about the structure of the heart and the cardiovascular system, see Chapter 16, page 417.

Diseases of the Heart

Your **heart** pumps about 100,000 times a day *every* day to move blood to all parts of your body. Just like every other organ, your heart needs the oxygen from blood to function. When the blood supply to the heart is insufficient to provide enough oxygen, the result can be pain, damage to the heart muscle, or even sudden death. Methods for diagnosing and treating diseases of the heart and other CVDs are summarized in **Figure 26.1.**

FIGURE **26.1**

DIAGNOSTIC TOOLS

EKG	MRI	Radionuclide Imaging	Angiography
An electrocardiogram produces a graph of the electrical activity of the heart. It helps detect the nature of a heart attack and shows heart function.	Magnetic resonance imaging uses powerful magnets to produce images of internal body organs. The images are used to identify heart damage and heart defects.	Radionuclides injected into the blood can be observed on a computer screen as they pass through the heart. This procedure is used to assess the heart's blood supply and to show heart function.	A thin, flexible tube is guided through blood vessels to the heart. Dye is injected and motion X rays are taken to look for heart obstructions.

TREATMENT OPTIONS

Coronary Bypass	Angioplasty	Medications	Pacemaker
Often a healthy vein is removed from the leg or chest and placed elsewhere to create a detour around a blocked artery.	A tube with a balloon is inserted into a blocked artery. The balloon is inflated against the artery walls. Then it is deflated and removed. A metal structure may remain to keep the artery open.	A variety of medications are used to treat CVDs. These include diuretics to aid with the body's fluid balance, cholesterol-lowering drugs, and drugs that slow the blood's clotting mechanisms in order to reduce risk of stroke.	Pacemakers are used to treat an irregular heartbeat. The small device sends steady electrical impulses to the heart to make it beat regularly.

ANGINA PECTORIS

Angina pectoris (an-JY-nuh PEK-tuh-ruhs) is *chest pain that results when the heart does not get enough oxygen.* This pain, which usually lasts a few seconds to minutes, is a signal that the heart is temporarily not getting enough blood. The most common cause of angina is atherosclerosis. Angina seldom causes permanent heart damage and sometimes can be treated with medication.

ARRHYTHMIAS

Arrhythmia is a change in the regular beat of the heart. The heart may seem to skip a beat or beat irregularly, very quickly, or very slowly. **Arrhythmias** or *irregular heartbeats,* are common. They occur in millions of people who do not have underlying heart disease, and they usually don't cause problems. However, certain types of arrhythmias are serious. In one type of arrhythmia, called *ventricular fibrillation,* the electrical impulses regulating heart rhythm become rapid or irregular. This is the most common cause of sudden cardiac arrest, in which the heart stops beating without warning. Without immediate emergency help, death follows within minutes.

HEART ATTACK

Each year in the United States, there are more than one million cases of heart attack, and more than 40 percent of those affected die. A heart attack is damage to the heart muscle caused by a reduced or blocked blood supply, usually because of atherosclerosis. Often, ventricular fibrillation occurs seconds to hours or even days following a heart attack and can cause sudden death.

Many heart attacks are sudden and cause intense chest pain, but one in four produces no symptoms and is detected only when routine tests are done later. Most heart attacks start slowly with mild pain or discomfort, which is often mistaken for indigestion. Immediate response to warning signs can often mean the difference between life and death.

CONGESTIVE HEART FAILURE

A heart attack is an immediate response to stress on the heart. Sometimes, however, the heart gradually weakens to the point that it cannot maintain its regular pumping rate and force. The result is a condition called congestive heart failure. This condition can be a result of high blood pressure, atherosclerosis, a heart valve defect, or other factors. Illegal drug use can also bring on this condition by increasing heart rate. Congestive heart failure can be managed with medication and the establishment of healthy lifestyle behaviors, such as a good nutrition and adequate physical activity.

Health Minute

Heart Attack Warnings

These warning **signs** indicate that a heart attack may be happening and immediate medical attention is needed.

The warning signs of heart attack:

► Pressure, fullness, squeezing, or aching in the chest area

► Discomfort spreading to the arms, neck, jaw, upper abdomen, and back

► Chest discomfort with shortness of breath, lightheadedness, sweating, nausea, and vomiting

▼ **In many cases sudden cardiac arrest can be reversed if CPR or electric shock using a defibrillator is applied.** *Why is it important to have defibrillators available in many different public places?*

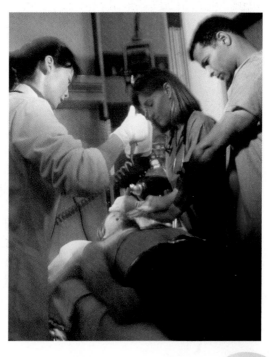

Hands-On Health ACTIVITY

Start a Healthy Habit

Working prevention strategies into your everyday life is the best way to reduce your risk of cardiovascular diseases. Take the quiz, and then complete the activity.

What You'll Need

- pen or pencil
- paper

What You'll Do

Number a sheet of paper from 1 to 10. Read each statement and write "always," "most of the time," "once in a while," or "never" for each item.

1. I avoid tobacco products and secondhand smoke.
2. I get 60 minutes of physical activity five or more days per week.
3. I get at least 30 minutes of moderate or 20 minutes of vigorous aerobic exercise at least three times a week.
4. I eat plenty of fruits, vegetables, and whole-grain foods.
5. I limit foods that are high in fat and cholesterol.
6. I limit my intake of salt and sodium.
7. I choose nutritious snacks.
8. I maintain a healthful weight.
9. I practice anger-management skills.
10. I practice stress-management skills.

Choose two habits you need to improve. In small groups, brainstorm a list of specific actions to help you practice these habits. Develop strategies to incorporate at least three healthy habits into your routine. Write a paragraph in which you describe your plan. After two weeks, evaluate what obstacles you faced, and what you are doing to improve.

Apply and Conclude

As a group, report on your successes in improving your lifestyle behaviors. Explain why the behaviors are healthful.

Stroke

When arterial blockage interrupts the flow of blood to the brain, a stroke may occur. Stroke can affect different parts of the body, depending on the part of the brain that is deprived of oxygen. Stroke also can occur as a result of a *cerebral hemorrhage*, a condition in which a blood vessel in the brain bursts, causing blood to spread into surrounding brain tissue.

Why Teens Are at Risk

The behaviors established during your teen years and early adult life determine, in large part, your risk of developing CVD. Even though the symptoms of CVD often don't show up until adulthood, the disease itself starts to develop in childhood, according to the American Heart Association. Autopsy results of adolescents who died from causes other than CVD have revealed that one in six already had evidence of CVD. Those who had a history of known risk factors, such as smoking or diabetes, were more likely to have blood-vessel damage. The health behaviors you practice *now* are affecting your cardiovascular system.

Risk Factors for Cardiovascular Disease

The American Heart Association has identified several factors, such as those in **Figure 26.2,** that increase the risk of cardiovascular disease. The more risk factors you have, the greater your chance of developing cardiovascular disease.

FIGURE 26.2

RISK FACTORS FOR CVDS YOU CAN CONTROL

Although you cannot control all risk factors, the ones listed below are the result of the daily decisions you make about your health and health habits.

Tobacco Use	• **Avoid the use of tobacco.** About 20 percent of the deaths from cardiovascular disease are smoking-related. Tobacco use is the biggest risk factor for teens. • **Avoid secondhand smoke.** Constant exposure to other people's smoke increases the risk of cardiovascular disease even for nonsmokers. About 40,000 nonsmokers exposed to environmental tobacco smoke die from CVDs each year.
High Blood Pressure	• **Have your blood pressure checked periodically.** Maintain normal blood pressure through a healthful diet, regular exercise, and proper weight. If your blood pressure is above normal, follow the advice of your physician to lower it.
High Cholesterol	• **Eat less high-fat foods.** High blood cholesterol can usually be controlled with medication and by practicing healthful lifestyle behaviors. Eat a diet low in cholesterol and saturated fats, and get regular physical activity. These behaviors help keep plaque from forming in your arteries.
Physical Inactivity	• **Get enough physical activity.** Physical inactivity can be a risk factor even if you aren't overweight. Get at least 30 to 60 minutes of physical activity each day. Regular physical activity strengthens your heart and helps you maintain a healthy weight.
Excess Weight	• **Maintain a healthy weight.** Excess weight increases the strain on the heart. It also raises blood pressure and the levels of blood cholesterol.
Stress	• **Reduce stress.** Constant stress can raise blood pressure. Practice stress-management techniques.
Drug and Alcohol Use	• **Avoid the use of alcohol and other drugs.** Drinking too much alcohol can raise blood pressure and cause heart failure or irregular heart beat. Some illegal drugs increase the heart rate and blood pressure and can result in sudden death from heart failure.

Some risk factors for cardiovascular disease are out of your control, but you should be aware of them and know how they influence your health. These factors include:

hot link

heredity To learn more about heredity and genetics, see Chapter 19, page 498.

▶ **Heredity.** Children whose parents have cardiovascular disease are more likely to develop CVD themselves.

▶ **Gender.** Men have a greater risk of developing cardiovascular disease earlier in life and a greater risk of having a heart attack than women do. However, research indicates that older women are less likely to survive a heart attack than men of the same age.

▶ **Age.** As people become older, they become more likely to develop CVD, as the risk increases with age. About 80 percent of people who die of cardiovascular disease are 65 or older.

Knowing the risk factors you can't control can help you make healthful decisions that protect your cardiovascular system. For example, if you have a family history of hypertension, you should be particularly careful to get the proper medical screenings and to practice preventive strategies, such as maintaining a healthful weight.

Lesson 1 *Review*

Reviewing Facts and Vocabulary

1. What is *atherosclerosis*? How does it contribute to heart attacks?

2. Define *cardiovascular disease*. How does regular physical activity help prevent CVD?

3. What are five risk factors for CVD that you can control?

Thinking Critically

4. **Evaluating.** Which of the treatments in Figure 26.1 would most likely be used to treat atherosclerosis?

5. **Synthesizing.** How can practicing healthy lifestyle behaviors now help you avoid cardiovascular disease in the future?

Applying Health Skills

Practicing Healthful Behaviors. On a sheet of paper, design a table that lists five of your favorite snacks, and find out which ones are "heart-healthy." For each of the others, think of healthier alternatives that you would enjoy. Enter the alternatives in your table.

TECHNOLOGY *OPTION*

SPREADSHEETS Using spreadsheet software to create your table will help you organize and display your thoughts. See **health.glencoe.com** for tips on how to get the most out of your spreadsheet program.

Cancer

VOCABULARY

cancer
tumor
benign
malignant
metastasis
carcinogen
biopsy
remission

YOU'LL LEARN TO

- Examine the causes and types of and treatments for cancer.

- Relate the importance of early detection and warning signs of cancer that prompt individuals to seek health care.

- Examine the effects of health behaviors that put you at risk for developing cancer.

- Develop, analyze, and apply strategies related to the prevention of cancer.

QUICK START   Make a list of any factors or behaviors you know of that can put a person at risk for developing cancer.

The body's cells are constantly growing and dividing. Most new cells are normal, but some are not. Sometimes these abnormal cells reproduce rapidly and uncontrollably, forming masses of abnormal cells inside otherwise normal tissue. This *uncontrollable growth of abnormal cells* is called **cancer**.

How Cancer Harms the Body

An abnormal mass of tissue that has no natural role in the body is called a **tumor**. Some tumors are **benign**, or *noncancerous*. Benign tumors grow slowly and are surrounded by membranes that prevent them from spreading from the original site. Although noncancerous tumors don't spread, they can be dangerous if they interfere with normal body functions. For example, a benign brain tumor may block the brain's blood supply.

Tumors that are **malignant**, or *cancerous,* spread to neighboring tissues and through the blood or lymph to other parts of the body. *The spread of cancer from the point where it originated to other parts of the body* is called **metastasis**. As cancer cells spread throughout the body, they divide and form new tumors.

Reduce your risk of skin cancer by protecting yourself from the sun's ultraviolet (UV) rays and reducing the amount of time you spend in the sun. *How does each item in the picture help protect you from UV rays?*

Many cancers harm the body because they kill normal cells when they compete with them for nutrients. Tumors put pressure on surrounding tissues and organs, interfering with body function. They can also block arteries, veins, and other passages in the body.

Types of Cancer

Cancer can develop in almost any part of the body and in different tissues of each part. **Figure 26.3** shows some types of cancers, grouped according to the body organs where they first develop. Cancers also can be classified according to the tissues they affect.

▶ *Lymphomas* are cancers of the **immune system.**

▶ *Leukemias* are cancers of the blood-forming organs.

▶ *Carcinomas* are cancers of the glands and body linings, including the skin and the linings of the digestive tract and lungs.

▶ *Sarcomas* are cancers of connective tissue, including bones, ligaments, and muscle.

Risk Factors for Cancer

Abnormal cells that have the potential to become cancer cells are produced every day and the immune system destroys most of them. If the immune system becomes weakened or the number of cancer cells becomes overwhelming, cancer may develop. In some cases normal cells change by themselves. In others a faulty gene may have been inherited; between 5 to 10 percent of cancers are hereditary.

The majority of cancers are caused by exposure to certain factors that increase the risk of cell damage. One factor is a **carcinogen** (car-SIN-uh-juhn), *a cancer-causing substance.* Examples of carcinogens are cigarette smoke and ultraviolet light. Several major risk factors for cancer are associated with lifestyle behaviors. It is estimated that about 60 percent of all cancers can be prevented through healthy lifestyle choices.

Tobacco Use

Tobacco use is the major cause of cancer deaths in the United States and the most preventable. Recent studies attribute nearly one in five deaths to smoking or exposure to **secondhand smoke.** About 87 percent of lung cancer deaths are caused by smoking. An additional 25 percent of females who smoke will die of other smoking-related diseases. Tobacco use also increases the risk of bladder, pancreas, and kidney cancers. At least 43 different carcinogens have been identified in tobacco and tobacco smoke.

hot link

immune system For more information about the immune system, see Chapter 24, page 628.

hot link

tobacco use For more information on the harmful effects of tobacco and **secondhand smoke,** see Chapter 21, page 538.

FIGURE 26.3

TYPES OF CANCER

Organ Affected (new cases/year)	Some Risk Factors	Symptoms	Screening and Early Detection Methods
Skin (1 million) Most common type of cancer in the United States	Exposure to ultraviolet radiation from the sun, tanning beds, sun lamps, or other sources	Change on the skin, especially a new growth, a mole or freckle that changes, or a sore that won't heal	physical exam, biopsies
Breast (205,000) Second leading cause of cancer death for women	Genetic factors, obesity, alcohol use, physical inactivity	Unusual lump; nipple that thickens, changes shape, dimples, or has discharge	self-exam, mammogram
Prostate (189,000) Found mostly in men over age 55	Possible hereditary link, possible link to high-fat diet	Frequent or painful urination; inability to urinate; weak or interrupted flow of urine; blood in urine or semen; pain in lower back, hips or upper thighs	blood test
Lung (169,400) Leading cause of cancer deaths in the United States	Exposure to cigarette smoke, radon, or asbestos	No initial symptoms; later symptoms include cough, shortness of breath, wheezing, coughing up blood, hoarseness	chest X ray
Colon/Rectum (148,000) Second leading cause of cancer deaths in the United States	Risk increases with age; close relative with colorectal cancer	Often no initial symptoms; later, blood in feces; frequent pain, aches, or cramps in stomach; change in bowel habits; weight loss	test for blood in the stool, sigmoidoscopy, colonoscopy
Mouth (30,000) Occurs mostly in people over 40	Use of tobacco, chewing tobacco, or alcohol	Sore or lump on mouth that doesn't heal; unusual bleeding; pain or numbness on lip, mouth, tongue, or throat; feeling that something is caught in the throat; pain with chewing or swallowing; change in voice	dental/oral exam
Cervix (15,000)	History of infection with HPV (human papilloma-virus)	Usually no symptoms in early stages; later, abnormal vaginal bleeding, increased vaginal discharge	Pap test
Testicle (7,000) Most common cancer in men ages 15 to 34	Undescended testicle; family history of testicular cancer	Small, hard painless lump on testicle; sudden accumulation of fluid in scrotum, pain in region between scrotum and anus	self-exam

Smokeless tobacco use is a major risk factor in the development of oral cancer, which affects the lips, mouth, and throat. Oral cancer kills roughly one person every hour. You can greatly reduce your risk of cancer by avoiding all forms of tobacco as well as secondhand smoke.

Sexually Transmitted Diseases

Some viruses, such as the human papillomavirus (HPV) and the **hepatitis B** virus, cause cervical and liver cancers, respectively. The risk of acquiring these pathogens can be reduced by abstinence from sexual activity and from injecting drugs through infected needles.

Dietary Factors

Approximately 30 percent of all cancer deaths are caused by dietary risk factors. A diet that is high in fat and low in fiber is often linked with cancer. Fats make colon cells more susceptible to carcinogens. Colon cells divide more rapidly if the diet is high in fat, increasing the chance that abnormal cells will form. Choosing foods low in fat and high in fiber reduces the risk of colon, breast, and prostate cancers. Dietary fiber speeds the movement of waste through the intestines, so carcinogens have less time to act on cells.

hot link

HPV and **hepatitis B** For more information on STDs that can cause cancer, see Chapter 25, page 648.
Skin cancer For more information on skin cancer warning signs, see Chapter 14, page 358.

Radiation

Ultraviolet (UV) radiation from the sun is the main cause of **skin cancer.** Tanning beds and sunlamps also emit UV radiation, which is just as damaging as the sun's rays. A "tan" is the body's response to being injured by UV rays.

About 80 percent of skin cancers can be prevented. Reduce your exposure to UV light by avoiding tanning beds and sunlamps. Limit your time in the sun, especially between 10:00 A.M. and 4:00 P.M. When you must be in the sun, wear protective clothing and use a sunscreen with an SPF (Sun Protection Factor) of at least 15 and that blocks all types of UV radiation. Pay attention to changes in moles on your skin, one of the seven warning signs of cancer, listed in **Figure 26.4.**

FIGURE 26.4

A WORD OF CAUTION ABOUT CANCER

The American Cancer Society recommends that every individual should be alert to the seven warning signs of cancer. Note that their first letters, when combined, spell the word *caution.*

C hange in bowel habits (either loose stools or constipation)

A sore that does not heal

U nusual bleeding or discharge (as from the uterus, bladder, bowels, nipple, or with coughing)

T hickening or a lump in the breast or elsewhere (Let your health care provider decide what the lump means.)

I ndigestion or difficulty swallowing

O bvious change in a wart or mole

N agging cough or hoarseness

Other symptoms include fatigue and unexplained weight loss. The presence of these signs do not necessarily mean a person has cancer. If you experience any of these symptoms, contact a health care professional.

Reducing Your Risk

You can't control some risk factors for cancer, such as heredity, but you can reduce your risk by practicing the healthful behaviors listed in **Figure 26.5.**

FIGURE 26.5

HOW YOU CAN REDUCE YOUR RISK OF CANCER

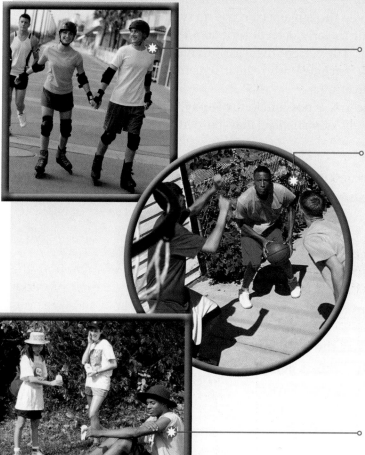

Practice abstinence from sexual activity to reduce the risk of sexually transmitted diseases. Hepatitis B can cause liver cancer, and HPV can cause cancers of the reproductive organs.

Be physically active.

Maintain a healthy weight.

Eat nutritious foods. Include 2–4 serving of fruits and 3–5 servings of vegetables every day. These foods are good sources of fiber, and some contain compounds that act against carcinogens.

Follow an eating plan that is low in saturated fat and high in fiber.

Protect your skin from ultraviolet radiation.

Avoid tobacco and alcohol. Tobacco is the single major cause of cancer death in the United States. Excess alcohol increases the risk of several types of cancer, including mouth and throat cancer.

Recognize the warning signs of cancer. Do regular self-exams to detect cancer early.

Detecting and Treating Cancer

Many advances have been made in the detection and treatment of cancer, and many more people are successfully living with the disease than ever before. The survival rate for those with cancer depends on the type of cancer and how early it is detected.

Early detection is the most critical factor in successful cancer treatment. Many types of cancer can be detected through self-examination of the **breast, testes,** and skin.

Screening for cancer is examination or testing for early signs of cancer even though a person has no symptoms. Medical screenings can result in early detection of about half of all new cancer cases each year. The current five-year survival rate with early detection is about 80 percent. With regular screenings, the rate could increase to 95 percent.

If cancer is a possibility, a **biopsy**, *the removal of a small piece of tissue for examination*, may be performed. A biopsy is usually

h⊙t link

testes and **breast** For information on testicular and breast self-exams, see Chapter 18, pages 472 and 477.

Health Skills Activity

Decision Making: Being Sun Smart

Amber rushes to meet her friends at the boat dock. "Sorry I'm late," she says breathlessly. "This is going to be great. I love to water-ski. Hey, does anyone have any sunscreen? I was in such a hurry that I forgot mine."

"I never use it. I don't burn," Taylor replies.

"I don't use it either. I like looking tan and healthy," Denise chimes in.

Amber knows that tan skin isn't healthy—it's damaged. "I always wear sunscreen," she says firmly. "I'll just run up the hill to that little corner store and buy some."

"Amber, the boat's in the water. We're ready to go," Denise protests.

What should Amber do?

What Would You Do?

Apply the six steps of the decision-making process to help Amber make a health-enhancing decision.

1. State the situation.
2. List the options.
3. Weigh the possible outcomes.
4. Consider values.
5. Make a decision and act.
6. Evaluate the decision.

necessary to determine whether cancer is present. X rays and other imaging techniques help determine a tumor's location and size.

Treating Cancer

The methods used to treat cancer depend on several factors, such as the type of cancer, whether the tumor has spread, and the patient's age and health. Treatment might include one or more of the following:

▶ **Surgery** removes some or all of the cancerous masses from the body.

▶ **Radiation therapy** aims rays from radioactive substances at cancerous cells. The radiation kills the cells and shrinks the cancerous mass.

▶ **Chemotherapy** uses chemicals to destroy cancer cells.

▶ **Immunotherapy** activates a person's immune system to recognize specific cancers and destroy them.

▶ **Hormone therapy** involves using medicines that interfere with the production of hormones. These treatments kill cancer cells or slow their growth.

Cancer that responds to treatment or is under control is said to be in **remission**, *a period of time when symptoms disappear.* Cancer in remission is not always cured; it can recur, sometimes years later.

HEALTH Online

Link to the American Cancer Society to discover the latest in cancer research in Web Links at **health.glencoe.com.**

 Lesson 2 *Review*

Reviewing Facts and Vocabulary

1. Define *cancer.* Name four risk factors for cancer.

2. What is the difference between a benign tumor and one that is malignant?

3. What are two important means of early cancer detection?

Thinking Critically

4. **Analyzing.** The physician of an adult family member has suggested that the person undergo a certain cancer screening procedure as part of a routine exam. The family member is afraid to have this procedure done. What would you tell this person?

5. **Evaluating.** Why do you think skin cancer is the most common cancer in the United States?

Applying Health Skills

Advocacy. Develop a cancer-awareness booklet that analyzes healthful strategies to reduce cancer risk and encourages people to develop these habits. Include information on technology and new treatments that impact the health status of people with cancer.

TECHNOLOGY *OPTION*

WORD PROCESSING Use word-processing software to create your booklet. Use special formats, borders, and art. Click on **health.glencoe.com** for help using word-processing software.

Allergies, Asthma, Diabetes, and Arthritis

VOCABULARY

allergy
histamines
asthma
diabetes
autoimmune disease
arthritis
osteoarthritis
rheumatoid arthritis

YOU'LL LEARN TO

• Examine the characteristics, symptoms, causes, and treatments of noncommunicable diseases.

• Describe the importance of taking responsibility for health maintenance to prevent or manage noncommunicable diseases.

• Develop and analyze strategies related to the prevention and management of noncommunicable diseases.

QUICK START Think of a family member or someone you know who has one of the diseases discussed in this lesson. What does this person do to manage the disease or its symptoms?

(A) An allergy to pollen, called hay fever, is one of the most common chronic diseases in the United States. Experts estimate that 35 million people suffer from hay fever.

Cardiovascular diseases and cancer are two of the most deadly noncommunicable diseases. Other noncommunicable diseases are chronic, meaning that they are present continuously or recur frequently over a long period time. Allergies, asthma, diabetes, and arthritis are chronic diseases that affect millions of people. Some, such as allergies, asthma, and certain types of diabetes, are caused by a response of the immune system. Others, such as osteoarthritis (ahs-tee-oh-ahr-THRY-tus), cause the breakdown of body cells and tissues.

Allergies

The sneezing and runny nose often associated with a cold are sometimes a response to substances in the air. An **allergy** is *a specific reaction of the immune system to a foreign and frequently harmless substance.* Allergies are among the common causes of illness and disability in the United States, affecting 40 to 50 million people.

Pollen, foods, dust, mold spores, chemicals, insect venom, and medicines are some of the more common *allergens*, substances that cause allergies. The body treats these allergens as foreign invaders. Antigens on the surface of allergens bind to special immune cells in the linings of the nasal passages. These cells release **histamines**, *chemicals that can stimulate mucus and fluid production in an area.*

Histamines produce the sneezing, itchy eyes, runny nose, and other symptoms that make a person with allergies uncomfortable. Some people have an allergic reaction that produces hives—itchy raised bumps on the skin. Others have serious reactions to allergens that can sometimes be life threatening. Severe symptoms include hives, itching or swelling of the stung area or the mouth, difficulty breathing or swallowing. Other severe symptoms might be a raspy voice or swelling of the tongue, or a sharp drop in blood pressure, which can cause dizziness.

If someone you know experiences any of these symptoms after eating foods such as peanuts or shellfish or after being stung by a bee or wasp, seek medical attention immediately.

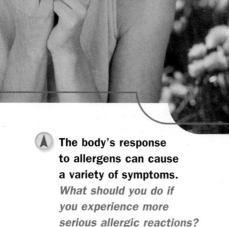

The body's response to allergens can cause a variety of symptoms. *What should you do if you experience more serious allergic reactions?*

Diagnosing Allergies

Sometimes you can diagnose an allergy yourself. You may notice that when you are near certain kinds of plants you sneeze or that eating particular foods makes you break out in a rash. In some cases tests are required to determine the cause. Three common methods are used to identify the source of an allergic reaction—a blood test, a food elimination diet, and a skin test. During a skin test, the skin is scratched and small amounts of possible allergens are applied. If a person is allergic to any of the allergens, the skin in the area of the scratch swells and turns red because of the **inflammatory response.**

Treating Allergies

Sometimes allergy treatment can be as simple as avoiding the allergen. This is the best treatment for severe food and insect sting allergies. When avoidance is not possible, medicines, including *antihistamines* that help control the symptoms triggered by histamines, may be suggested. People with long-lasting or severe allergies should seek medical attention. Allergies can irritate the respiratory tract and lead to other health problems, such as asthma. People with severe allergies may receive *immunotherapy*, a series of shots that contain small amounts of the allergen to which the person is sensitive. The injections cause the immune system to become less sensitive to the allergens.

hot link

inflammatory response
For more information about the inflammatory response, see Chapter 24, page 628.

Experiencing an unpleasant reaction to something you eat does not necessarily mean that you have a food allergy. For instance, lactose intolerance is not an allergy. Because symptoms are similar, this is a common misconception. In reality, only a very small percentage of people actually have proven food allergies. For those who do, the main method of treatment is avoiding the food that causes the allergic reaction. This usually requires diligently reading ingredient lists.

Asthma

Some allergic reactions can lead to **asthma**, *an inflammatory condition in which the small airways in the lungs become narrowed, causing difficulty in breathing.* More than 17 million people in the United States have asthma, and each year more than 5,000 Americans die of this disease. Asthma can develop at any age; however, about one-third of those with asthma are under the age of 18.

The bronchial tubes of people with asthma are sensitive to certain substances called *triggers*. Common asthma triggers include air pollution, pet dander, and tobacco smoke, as well as microscopic mold, pollen, and dust mites, shown on this page. In an asthma attack, the asthma triggers cause the muscles of the bronchial walls to tighten and produce extra mucus. The respiratory passages narrow. The result can range from minor wheezing—breathing with a whistling sound—to severe difficulty breathing. In some cases the condition becomes life threatening.

Managing Asthma

Although asthma has no cure, most people with the condition can lead normal lives by behavior changes and the proper use of medication. People with asthma can lead normal, active lives with proper management that includes the following strategies:

▶ **Monitor the condition.** Recognize the warning signs of an attack: shortness of breath, chest tightness or pain, coughing or sneezing. Treating these symptoms quickly can help prevent attacks or keep an attack from worsening.

▶ **Manage the environment.** Reduce asthma triggers in the environment. Avoid exposure to tobacco smoke, eliminate carpets and rugs when possible, and wash bedding frequently.

▶ **Manage stress.** Stress can trigger an asthma attack. Relaxation and stress-management techniques can be helpful.

▶ **Take medication.** Medications can be used to relieve symptoms, prevent flare-ups, and make air passages less sensitive to asthma triggers. *Bronchodilators* are a type of medication, taken with an inhaler, that relaxes and widens respiratory passages.

People with asthma can be active if they manage the disease and use proper precautions. *What precautions should a person with asthma take to avoid an attack?*

Diabetes

Diabetes is *a chronic disease that affects the way body cells convert food into energy.* Each year approximately one million new cases are diagnosed. There is no cure for diabetes.

In a person with diabetes, the pancreas produces too little or no insulin, a hormone that helps glucose enter the body's cells. In some diabetics adequate insulin is produced, but cells don't respond normally to it. For the cells in the body to function, they need a constant source of energy—glucose—from foods. If glucose is not converted to energy, it builds up in the blood, and cells do not get the glucose they need to function. The only way to diagnose diabetes is through a blood test. Early detection of diabetes can prevent serious side effects, such as blindness. Diabetes is the main cause of kidney failure, limb amputations, and blindness in adults, as well as a major cause of heart disease and stroke. These effects, however, are not inevitable. If diagnosed, the disease can be successfully managed with medication, a healthful diet, and regular moderate exercise. In many cases, diabetes is preventable.

Type 1 Diabetes

Type 1 diabetes, which accounts for 5 to 10 percent of all diabetes cases, appears suddenly and progresses quickly. The body does not produce insulin, and glucose builds up in the blood, starving cells of the energy they need. Over time, the high blood-sugar level can cause damage to the eyes, kidneys, nerves, and heart.

The cause of type 1 diabetes is not clear. Some scientists suspect an environmental trigger—perhaps an as yet unidentified virus—that stimulates an immune response, destroying the insulin-producing cells of the pancreas in some individuals. For this reason, type 1 diabetes is known as an **autoimmune disease**, *a condition in which the immune system mistakenly attacks itself, targeting the cells, tissues, and organs of a person's own body.* People with type 1 diabetes must take daily doses of insulin, either through injections or through a special pump that is attached to the body by tubing or that is surgically implanted. Today, because of advanced treatment methods, many people with diabetes are able to live near-normal lives.

Type 2 Diabetes

Type 2 diabetes accounts for 90 to 95 percent of all cases of this disease. It most often appears after age 40. However, type 2 diabetes is now being found at younger ages and is even being diagnosed among children and teens. In this form of diabetes, the body is unable to make enough insulin or to use insulin properly. Buildup of glucose in the blood causes many of the same symptoms as type 1 diabetes.

Symptoms of Diabetes

According to the American Diabetes Association, of the estimated 17 million people in the United States who have diabetes, almost 6 million of them don't know it.

Symptoms of diabetes include:

► Frequent urination
► Excessive thirst
► Unexplained weight loss
► Extreme hunger
► Sudden vision changes
► Tingling in hands or feet
► Frequent fatigue
► Very dry skin
► Sores that are slow to heal
► More infections than usual

People with diabetes need to work closely with health care professionals to manage their condition. *Why is early detection of diabetes important?*

Type 2 diabetes is nearing epidemic proportions in the United States because of an increased number of older individuals in the population and a greater prevalence of obesity and inactive lifestyles. A diet high in fat, calories, and cholesterol increases the risk of diabetes. Thus, choosing lower-fat, lower-calorie alternatives can help reduce the risk of this disease. Increased physical activity also reduces risk because it helps control weight and lower blood cholesterol levels.

Treatment of type 2 diabetes includes weight management and regular physical activity. Individuals with this disease must

Real-Life Application

Raising Teen Awareness of Diabetes

Over the last decade, diabetes and obesity have increased dramatically in both adults and teens. Examine the graph and answer the questions. Then use this information to create an advocacy message to encourage others to practice healthful behaviors to control their weight and reduce their risk of diabetes.

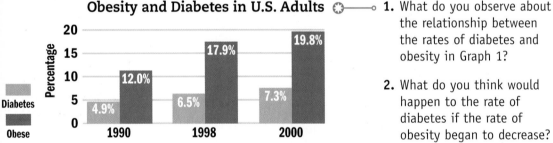

Obesity and Diabetes in U.S. Adults

Diabetes / Obese

	1990	1998	2000
Diabetes	4.9%	6.5%	7.3%
Obese	12.0%	17.9%	19.8%

1. What do you observe about the relationship between the rates of diabetes and obesity in Graph 1?

2. What do you think would happen to the rate of diabetes if the rate of obesity began to decrease?

Prevalence of Overweight Among U.S. Adolescents

1963-70	1971-74	1976-80	1988-94	1999
4	4	5	11	13

Source: CDC, Behavioral Risk Factor Surveillance System (1991–2000)

3. Look at Graph 2. What can you infer about the rate of diabetes in teens?

4. Why are healthful eating habits and physical activity lifestyle behaviors that reduce the risk of diabetes?

ACTIVITY

In small groups, generate a list of lifestyle behaviors that people can practice to maintain a healthful weight and reduce their risk of diabetes. Create a 60-second public service announcement (PSA) to persuade teens to start good health habits early in life. Include at least one fact about diabetes and one lifestyle behavior that can reduce the risk of diabetes.

carefully monitor their diet in order to control their blood-sugar levels. In some cases oral medications or injections of insulin are required to manage the disease.

Arthritis

Arthritis is *a group of more than 100 different diseases that cause pain and loss of movement in the joints.* It is one of the most common medical problems in the world and the number one cause of disability in the United States—more than one in six people suffer from the disease. Arthritis is more common in older people, but it can affect anyone, including children and teens. In fact, 8.4 million people between the ages of 18 and 44 have arthritis and millions of others are at risk for it.

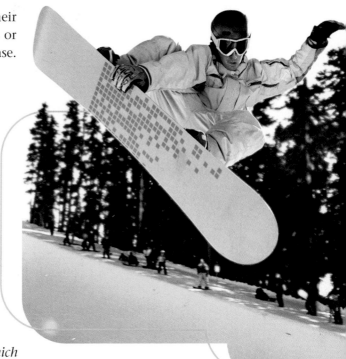

Osteoarthritis

Osteoarthritis is *a disease of the joints in which cartilage breaks down.* Cartilage is the strong, flexible tissue that provides cushioning at the joints. In this disease the cartilage becomes pitted and frayed. In time it may wear away completely, and bones may rub against each other. Although osteoarthritis affects primarily the weight-bearing joints of the knees and hips, it can affect any joint—including in the fingers, lower back, and feet—causing aches and soreness, especially when moving.

 According to the Arthritis Foundation, an arthritis epidemic may result from the number of people who participate in adventure sports. *What can you do to reduce your risk of developing osteoarthritis?*

Osteoarthritis is one of the most common types of arthritis; in fact, it accounts for half of all arthritis cases. It affects about 20 million people in the United States and is most common in women and in people over the age of 45. Many people think that arthritis is an inevitable part of aging. However, several strategies reduce the risk of osteoarthritis:

▶ **Controlling weight.** Maintaining an appropriate weight reduces stress on joints by lessening wear and tear on cartilage.

▶ **Preventing sports injuries.** Warming up before exercising, adding strength training to your physical activities, and using appropriate equipment (including wrist guards and knee pads when necessary) help avoid joint injuries and damage to ligaments and cartilage, thus decreasing the risk of osteo-arthritis. Let injuries heal completely before playing again.

▶ **Protecting against Lyme disease.** Lyme disease (which is spread by the bite of infected deer ticks) if left untreated, can result in a rare form of osteoarthritis. Using insect repellents, wearing long-sleeved shirts and pants when walking outdoors or in wooded areas, and being educated on tick recognition and removal can help reduce this risk factor.

Rheumatoid Arthritis

Did You Know **?**

Arthritis is the leading cause of disability among people age 15 and older. Arthritis and rheumatoid arthritis account for more than 15 percent of all disabilities in the United States.

Rheumatoid arthritis affects about 2.5 million people in the United States. It is three times more common in women than in men. Symptoms usually first appear between the ages of 20 and 50, but the disease also can affect young children. Juvenile rheumatoid arthritis is the most common form of arthritis in children.

Rheumatoid arthritis is *a disease characterized by the debilitating destruction of the joints due to inflammation*. Like type 1 diabetes, this type of arthritis is caused by an autoimmune disease for which there is no cure. Sufferers are likely to experience joint pain, inflammation, swelling, and stiffness. Eventually the joints may become deformed and cease to function normally. Rheumatoid arthritis affects mainly the joints in the hand, foot, elbow, shoulder, neck, knee, hip, and ankle. Other effects include fever, fatigue, and swollen lymph glands. The effects of this disease are usually symmetrical—both sides of the body develop the same symptoms at the same time and in the same pattern.

Early diagnosis of rheumatoid arthritis is crucial. With the use of medication, in many cases the effects of the disease can be controlled. Treatment methods focus on relieving pain, reducing inflammation and swelling, and keeping the joints moving as normally as possible. A combination of exercise, rest, joint protection, and physical and occupational therapy also can help manage the disease.

Lesson 3 *Review*

Reviewing Facts and Vocabulary

1. What are *histamines*, and what role do they play in allergies?
2. Define *asthma*. What are two strategies for managing this condition?
3. What is *osteoarthritis*? List two ways to reduce the risk of osteoarthritis.

Thinking Critically

4. **Synthesizing.** Why is it difficult to avoid many allergens?
5. **Analyzing.** Why is it important for people with diabetes to take responsibility for managing their condition?

Applying Health Skills

Practicing Healthful Behaviors. Make a table. In the first column, write the names of the noncommunicable diseases in this lesson. In the second column, identify risk factors for each disease. In the third column, describe and analyze strategies for healthful lifestyle behaviors that will reduce your risk for the disease.

SPREADSHEETS Using a spreadsheet can help you organize and edit your table. For help using spreadsheets, go to **health.glencoe.com**.

Lesson 4

Physical and Mental Challenges

VOCABULARY
disability
profound deafness
mental retardation
Americans with
   Disabilities Act

YOU'LL LEARN TO

- Identify and recognize the challenges of individuals with disabilities.

- Discuss health-related social issues, and determine ways in which progress has been made to better integrate individuals with disabilities into society.

⇒ *QUICK START* Make a word web with the word *disability* in the center. List the types of disabilities you know of around it. Add to your web as you study this lesson.

D oes your school have ramps and special rest room facilities to accommodate people in wheelchairs? Are there telephones for people who are hearing or vision impaired? Have you ever seen a closed-captioned television program? All these devices are designed to offset a **disability**, *any physical or mental impairment that limits normal activities, including seeing, hearing, walking, or speaking.* According to the latest U.S. Census Bureau statistics, almost 20 percent of the adult population had some type of disability. People with disabilities sometimes have difficulty doing things that others take for granted. The challenge may be physical, such as climbing stairs, seeing a sign, hearing a conversation, or holding a package, or it may be mental, such as understanding simple instructions.

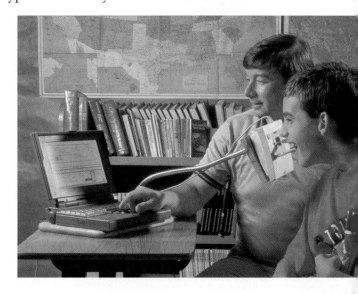

▼ **Computers are one of many devices that people with disabilities can use to meet their physical challenges.** *List other assistive technologies that help people who have disabilities.*

Physical Challenges

T he most common types of physical challenges affect a person's senses or the ability to move and get around easily. Most physical challenges can be classified as sight impairment, hearing impairment, or motor impairment.

Sight Impairment

Like other disabilities, sight impairment can be moderate, as for the more than 5 million Americans who are vision-impaired, or it can be severe, as for the 1.3 million people who are legally blind. In addition, an estimated 1.8 million people in the United States are unable to see words and letters in ordinary print even when wearing glasses or contact lenses. Although visual impairment is more common among older adults, nearly 1 in every 1,000 children has partial vision loss or is legally blind.

The leading cause of blindness is the result of complications of diabetes. Three other common causes of blindness are

▶ **macular degeneration,** a disease in which the retina degenerates. It is the leading cause of blindness in individuals over 55.

▶ **glaucoma,** a disease that damages the optic nerve of the eye.

▶ **cataracts,** a clouding of the lens of the eye.

Regular eye exams are important for people of all ages. The early diagnosis of many conditions can help prevent blindness or slow its progress.

Hearing Impairment

About 20 million adults in the United States have disabilities that affect their ability to hear, and as many as 2 in every 1,000 children have a significant hearing impairment in both ears. Like sight impairment, hearing problems can range from minor to severe. **Profound deafness** is *a hearing loss so severe that a person affected cannot benefit from mechanical amplification, such as a hearing aid.*

One cause of deafness is heredity. Other causes are injury, disease, or obstructions, which can prevent sound waves from traveling to the inner ear. Obstructions may be caused by a buildup of wax, bone blockage, or something stuck in the ear. Some individuals are born with an inherited abnormal bone growth in the inner ear that may cause obstruction. Obstruction usually affects only one ear. Surgery can cure many of these cases.

Hearing impairments caused by nerve damage often occur with age, but also can be the result of repeated exposure to loud noises—such as stereos, traffic, video games, and some machines. Going to one loud concert or blasting the stereo occasionally probably won't hurt your ears, but prolonged exposure to loud music can cause hearing loss. In fact, some experts think that hearing loss is occurring much earlier than it did just 30 years ago possibly because of the increase in environmental noise. This type of hearing impairment can be gradual, so if you have noticed that your hearing has changed, it may be time to visit an audiologist, a specialist in hearing problems.

Sign language enables many individuals with hearing impairments to enjoy concerts, plays, and other public events.

Motor Impairment

Tasks that are simple for most people—tying a shoe, climbing the stairs, opening a jar, lifting a glass—can be a challenge for someone with a motor impairment. Motor impairments result when the body's range of motion and coordination are affected by an injury to the brain or a disorder of the nervous system.

Physical therapy often is used to help those with motor impairment. Through physical therapy, the joints are kept flexible and the muscles stretched, improving the individual's ability to move around. Physical therapists can teach people to use assistive devices. For example, people with limb amputations can be fitted with *prosthetics*, or artificial limbs. Motorized wheelchairs allow many people with motor impairments to get around without assistance. Computers can be adapted in many ways, such as mouth sticks or head sticks for those unable to use their hands or arms.

Mental Challenges

Some challenges affect a person's ability to live independently in society. One such challenge is **mental retardation**, *the below-average intellectual ability present from birth or early childhood and associated with difficulties in learning and social adaptation.* This disability affects about 3 percent of the population, but many of those with this challenge are only mildly affected. Such individuals, who make up 75 percent of the mentally retarded population, cannot be outwardly distinguished from nonretarded people.

Several factors have been found to cause mental retardation, including injury, disease, or a brain abnormality. Some factors are related to **genetic disorders** such as Down syndrome, PKU, Tay-Sachs, and Fragile X syndrome, the most common cause of genetically-inherited developmental disability. Behaviors during pregnancy are another important factor. Pregnant women who use alcohol or other drugs greatly increase the risk that their babies will be born with mental retardation, low birth weight, or conditions such as **fetal alcohol syndrome.** Another preventable risk factor during pregnancy is infection with rubella. Immunization against this disease either during childhood or within three months of becoming pregnant reduces the risk. A restricted supply of oxygen during birth can cause mental retardation. In older children, it can result from a head injury, stroke, or certain infections such as meningitis.

Advances in technology have benefited people who use assistive devices to perform daily activities. *Name one way your community is improving access and services for individuals with disabilities.*

hotlink

genetic disorders Learn more about genetic disorders in Chapter 19, page 500.
fetal alcohol syndrome Learn more about the effects of alcohol use during pregnancy in Chapter 22, page 576.

Accommodating Differences

People with physical and mental challenges have the same needs and interests as do the rest of the population. They also have many of the same abilities. Historically people with disabilities have been viewed as a separate population. Fortunately, in recent decades strides have been made toward eliminating the barriers of stereotyping and prejudices. The recent trends have resulted from advocacy efforts by individuals with physical and mental challenges and their supporters who have worked to establish the following important principles:

► Society should make certain changes, such as requiring wheelchair access to public transportation and building entrances that allow people with physical and mental disabilities to take part more readily in business and social activities.

► People should be evaluated on the basis of individual merit, not on stereotyped assumptions about disabilities.

► To the extent that each is able, people with disabilities should have the same opportunities as people who do not have physical or mental challenges.

How can I show courtesy when I interact with a person who is disabled?

Treating others as you would like to be treated is the best guide for interacting with people, whether or not they are disabled. Speak directly to the person, not to his or her companion. If an individual has a working animal, such as a companion dog, don't call to the animal or pet it—remember, the animal is at work. Distracting the animal may cause it to make mistakes that endanger its handler.

 Guide dogs are trained to assist the visually impaired by safely navigating around obstacles such as curbs. *Why should you avoid touching or calling a working guide dog?*

A major action toward achieving these goals was the passage by Congress in 1990 of the **Americans with Disabilities Act**, *a law prohibiting discrimination against people with physical or mental disabilities in the workplace, transportation, public accommodations, and telecommunications.* Some provisions of the act require:

▶ employers with 15 or more employees to provide qualified individuals with disabilities an equal opportunity to benefit from of employment-related opportunities available to others.

▶ state and local governments to follow specific architectural standards in the new construction and alteration of their buildings. They also must provide access in inaccessible older buildings and communicate effectively with people who have hearing, vision, or speech disabilities.

▶ telephone companies to establish telecommunications relay services (TRS) that enable callers with hearing and speech disabilities to communicate through a third-party communications assistant.

In addition, the Workforce Investment Act of 1998 ensures that any information posted to a Web site by a government agency must meet certain standards for accessibility by those who are disabled.

This ramp is just one of the many federally required accommodations for people who are disabled. *What other accommodations exist to help those with disabilities?*

Lesson 4 *Review*

Reviewing Facts and Vocabulary

1. What is a *disability*?
2. List three common causes of blindness.
3. Discuss health-related issues and list two laws that help integrate people with disabilities into society.

Thinking Critically

4. **Analyzing.** Identify several different ways that you use the senses of sight and hearing each day. For each item, identify challenges that might be associated with each task for someone with an impairment.
5. **Evaluating.** What loud noises are you subjected to each day? What might you do to reduce your exposure to the noise?

Applying Health Skills

Accessing Information. Go to **health.glencoe.com** to find a link to the Americans with Disabilities Act Web site. Prepare a display showing a summary of the provisions of the act.

TECHNOLOGY *OPTION*

PRESENTATION SOFTWARE Make your display professional looking with presentation software. For help with presentation software, access **health.glencoe.com.**

Lesson 4 Physical and Mental Challenges **699**

Prescription Drug Advertising

The Federal Drug Administration (FDA) has rules regarding advertisements for prescription drugs used to manage chronic noncommunicable diseases. Yet, every month, the FDA issues warning letters to a number of pharmaceutical companies for violations against the rules for drug advertising. Use the activity that follows to help you identify the effects that might result from misinformation found in prescription drug advertising.

Name of Drug and what it is prescribed for	Violation (in your own words)	Possible effects of violation (health effects, effects on the perception of the medical condition or the use of the drug)
ephedrine	synthetic source, not plant-derived	no evidence that it's safe or effective

ACTIVITY

Working in groups of three or four, research at least four of the warning letters available at the FDA Web site found in the Web links at **health.glencoe.com**. Use the table to help you determine the types of violations against the FDA's prescription drug advertising policies. List the name of the drug, describe the violation, and note possible effects on a person's health if the drug is used.

EXPRESS YOUR VIEWS

Create a one-page paper discussing the rules and regulations that control information in advertisements for prescription drug products. Explain how effective these rules are in protecting the health of individuals who use these products. Consider these questions: How many warnings are issued each month? Can the effects of these violations be life threatening?

CROSS-CURRICULUM CONNECTIONS

Create a Heart Poem. Cardiovascular diseases, including hypertension and atherosclerosis, are diseases that can often be avoided through changes in lifestyle behaviors. Using information from this chapter, write a poem to communicate to teens the importance of maintaining a healthy heart. Include in your poem examples from the list of risk factors that can be controlled. If you wish, create a rap song or put your poem to music to send a positive health message to teens.

Create a Time Line. Although the passage of the Americans with Disabilities Act and other laws in recent years are victories for those with physical and mental challenges, it took years of effort on the legal and social fronts to break down barriers. Research and create a time line focusing on important legislation and events that have moved this cause forward over the decades. Also, include people who have made contributions throughout history—for example, Helen Keller and President Franklin Delano Roosevelt.

Calculate Cancer Deaths. The text states that 87 percent of lung cancer deaths are caused by smoking, and that there are 169,400 new cases of lung cancer every year. How many of these are from causes other than smoking?

Investigate New Technologies. Scientists are constantly researching techniques that will allow doctors to diagnose illnesses more accurately, deliver medication to the exact site of the problem and, in some cases, eliminate the need for surgery. Investigate and report on research programs sponsored by the National Institutes of Health and the National Cancer Institute. Discuss the progress in research for treating diseases such as diabetes and cancer.

Oncologist

Are you interested in helping people who have cancer? If so, you might consider a career as an oncologist, a doctor who studies, diagnoses, and treats cancers. A person who wants to become an oncologist should be ready to deal with the emotional and psychological challenges associated with patients who may be terminally ill. Becoming an oncologist takes many years of formal training: a four-year college degree, a medical degree, a one-year internship, a four-year residency, and a fellowship in oncology. Find out about this and other careers in Career Corner at **health.glencoe.com**.

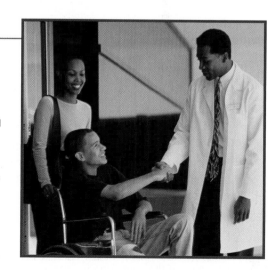

Chapter 26 *Review*

> **EXPLORING HEALTH TERMS** *Answer the following questions on a sheet of paper.*

Lesson 1 *Match each definition with the correct term.*

angina pectoris   cardiovascular disease
atherosclerosis   hypertension
arrhythmias   noncommunicable disease

1. Chest pain that results when the heart doesn't get enough oxygen.
2. A disease that is not transmitted by another person, or a vector, nor from the environment.
3. High blood pressure.
4. Irregular heartbeats.

Lesson 2 *Fill in the blank with the correct term.*

benign   malignant
biopsy   metastasis
cancer   remission
carcinogen   tumor

5. An abnormal mass of tissue that has no natural role in the body is a _____ .
6. The spread of cancer from where it originates is called _____ .
7. Cigarette smoke and UV radiation are two examples of a _____ .
8. A laboratory analysis of a section of tissue taken from a site where abnormal cell growth is suspected is a _____ .

Lesson 3 *Match each definition with the correct term.*

allergy   diabetes
autoimmune disease   histamines
arthritis   osteoarthritis
asthma   rheumatoid arthritis

9. A specific reaction of the immune system to a foreign and frequently harmless substance.
10. A chronic disease that affects the way body cells convert food into energy.
11. A disease characterized by the debilitating destruction of the joints due to inflammation.

Lesson 4 *Replace the underlined words with the correct term.*

Americans with Disabilities Act
disability
mental retardation
profound deafness

12. <u>Disability</u> is hearing loss so severe that a hearing aid doesn't help.
13. <u>Profound deafness</u> is the below-average intellectual ability present from birth or early childhood.
14. <u>Mental retardation</u> is a law prohibiting discrimination against people with physical or mental disabilities.

> **RECALLING THE FACTS** *Use complete sentences to answer the following questions.*

Lesson 1

1. Why is hypertension considered a "silent killer"?
2. How does plaque affect arteries?
3. What are the warning signs of a heart attack?
4. List four ways to prevent cardiovascular diseases.

Lesson 2

5. Which type of cancer is most common in the United States? How can the risk of this cancer be reduced?
6. How does a high-fat diet increase the risk of cancer?
7. What kind of therapy produces antibodies to activate a person's immune system?

Lesson 3

8. Why should people with long-lasting or severe allergies seek medical attention?
9. Why is managing stress important for a person who has asthma?
10. What are two major ways that people can reduce the risk of type 2 diabetes?
11. How does an autoimmune disease harm the body?

Lesson 4

12. What are some challenges a person with disabilities might face?

13. What kind of disability would someone with Down syndrome have?

14. What are two of the provisions of the Americans with Disabilities Act?

▶ THINKING CRITICALLY

1. Evaluating. What effect does physical activity have on the cardiovascular system? How does this information affect the goals you set for maintaining health? *(LESSON 1)*

2. Synthesizing. Suppose a friend tells you that she wants to get a tan because people with tans look healthier. What would you tell her? *(LESSON 2)*

3. Summarizing. Type 2 diabetes is becoming more common among children and teens. Write a letter directed to parents of young children that explains how parents can help their children avoid developing the disease. *(LESSON 3)*

4. Analyzing. In the past many people have had misconceptions about individuals with physical and mental challenges. What factors do you think contributed to negative attitudes toward people with disabilities? *(LESSON 4)*

▶ HEALTH SKILLS APPLICATION

1. Practicing Healthful Behaviors. Ask your parents about the history of cardiovascular disease in their families. Use this information to identify any potential risks you might have for developing cardiovascular disease. What steps can you take to reduce your risk? *(LESSON 1)*

2. Analyzing Influences. Look at product ads in a variety of magazines. Identify pictures that show people involved in behaviors that increase the risk of developing cancer. Describe how each of these behaviors puts a person at risk of developing cancer. Summarize your findings and report them to the class. *(LESSON 2)*

3. Accessing Information. Find out about the most common pollen allergens in your community. Gather information about when they are most prevalent and where you can get information about daily pollen counts. Display the information in the classroom. *(LESSON 3)*

4. Advocacy. Survey a local business to see how it might be made more accessible for individuals who have disabilities. Write a letter to the owner of the business making suggestions for improvement. *(LESSON 4)*

BEYOND *the* Classroom

Parent Involvement

Advocacy. Find out about health fairs or other events in your community that support cancer education. Contact local chapters of the American Cancer Society for information. See how you and your parents can become involved.

School and Community

CPR Classes. Locate agencies in your community that teach CPR. Arrange for someone from the agency to teach CPR at your school. Help organize the event and prepare posters or flyers to let people know about it.

Injury Prevention and Safe Behaviors

Personal Health Inventory

How Do You Rate?

Read each statement below and respond by writing *yes*, *no*, or *sometimes* for each item. Write *yes* only for items that you practice regularly.

1. I do not use an electrical appliance if the floor is wet or if I am near a tub or sink that contains water.

2. I keep all cleaning products and other chemicals in their original containers.

3. I stay within my abilities and limits when taking part in sports and recreational activities.

4. I use a step stool when I need to reach items on high shelves.

5. I don't risk my health or the health of others to show off.

6. I read and follow labels when using cleaning products or other chemicals.

7. I follow traffic guidelines when I drive a vehicle or ride a bike.

8. I follow posted speed limits and other traffic signs and signals when driving.

9. I wear a safety belt.

10. I wear the proper safety equipment when bike riding, skating, and skateboarding.

For instant feedback on your health status, go to Chapter 27 Health Inventory at **health.glencoe.com**.

Safety at Home and at Work

VOCABULARY

unintentional injury
accident chain
smoke alarm
fire extinguisher
Occupational Safety and Health Administration (OSHA)

YOU'LL LEARN TO

• Analyze strategies for preventing unintentional injuries.

• Examine how proper training at work can prevent unintentional injuries.

• Demonstrate knowledge of strategies to prevent unintentional injuries at home and at work.

QUICK START List five safety precautions that can help reduce the risk of unintentional injuries at home.

▲ Many unintentional injuries can be prevented by taking precautions such as wiping up spills. *How can this behavior help prevent an unintentional injury?*

Every year thousands of people are injured as a result of accidents in the home. In fact, the National Safety Council reports that a fatal home injury occurs every 18 minutes and a disabling home injury occurs every 4 seconds. One goal of *Healthy People 2010* is to reduce the number of deaths caused by unintentional injuries.

Unintentional Injuries

There are two types of injuries—intentional and unintentional. An intentional injury is the result of a deliberate attempt to cause harm. An **unintentional injury** is *an injury resulting from an unexpected event, or accident.* There are many actions you can take to prevent unintentional injuries.

Preventing Unintentional Injuries

Although unintentional injuries often seem to be random events, experts have observed an **accident chain**, or *a sequence of events that leads to an unintentional injury.* Most unintentional injuries include five steps that are connected, much like the links in a chain. **Figure 27.1** shows these steps.

FIGURE 27.1

PREVENTING UNINTENTIONAL INJURIES: THE ACCIDENT CHAIN

1. The Situation. Mark has overslept and has to rush to get ready for school.

2. The Unsafe Habit. Mark often leaves his books on the stairs.

3. The Unsafe Action. Mark isn't looking where he is going as he races down the stairs.

4. The Accident. Mark trips over his books and falls down the stairs.

5. The Result. When he falls, Mark sprains his wrist. He's also late for school.

Safety at Home

Taking precautions and planning ahead can help prevent injuries from fire, falls, electrical shock, and poisonings.

Preventing Fires

Most household fires are caused by heating equipment, appliances, electrical wiring, and smoking. Three elements—fuel, heat, and oxygen—must be present for a fire to occur. Fuel can be carelessly stored rags, wood, gasoline, or paper. A heat source can be a lighted match, a damaged electrical wire, a smoldering cigarette, or a pilot light. The oxygen in the air feeds and fans the flames. Removing one element will prevent a fire from starting. To avoid unintentional fire injuries:

▶ Never leave a candle burning unattended.

▶ Store matches and lighters out of the reach of children.

▶ Make sure that a person doesn't fall asleep while smoking.

▶ Keep stoves and ovens clean.

▶ Replace frayed electrical cords.

Hands-On Health ACTIVITY

Creating a Fire Safety Plan

In this activity you will create a home fire safety plan with a poster showing escape routes.

What You'll Need

- ruler (optional)
- poster paper and art supplies

What You'll Do

1. Draw a floor plan of your home on poster paper, including doors, hallways, windows, and stairways.

2. Use arrows to point out the fastest way to escape from every room.

3. Identify an alternate escape route for each room in case the first route is blocked by flames or smoke.

4. Indicate the location of smoke alarms and fire extinguishers.

5. Designate a place for your family to meet outside your home and mark it on the escape plan.

6. At the bottom of your plan, write:
   - When escaping, stay low to the floor.
   - Call 911 or the fire department.
   - Never go back inside to retrieve something.

Apply and Conclude

Share the plan with your family and post it in a prominent place in your home. Schedule a home fire drill at least once a month with all family members.

FIRE SAFETY EQUIPMENT

To increase your chances of survival in case of fire, here are two life-saving devices that should be present in every home.

▶ A **smoke alarm** is *an alarm that is triggered by the presence of smoke.* Safety experts recommend that one smoke alarm be located on every floor of a home, preferably outside a sleeping area and near the kitchen. They also advise that the alarm be tested once a month and that batteries be replaced at least once a year.

▶ A **fire extinguisher** is *a portable device that puts out small fires by ejecting fire-extinguishing chemicals.* If your home has a fire extinguisher, check the dial on the equipment periodically to ensure that it still has enough pressure to work in an emergency. When using an extinguisher, stand away from the flames; aim at the source of the fire, not at the flames; and move the spray from side to side. If you are unsure of your ability to put out the fire, forget the extinguisher, get out of the house, and call the fire department.

Preventing Falls

According to the National Safety Council, one-fifth of injuries that require treatment in an emergency room are the result of falls. A few simple precautions can help reduce the risk of injuries from falls:

▶ Keep stairways well lit, in good repair, free of clutter, and equipped with sturdy handrails and nonskid stair strips.

▶ Keep the floor clean. Mop up any spills immediately.

▶ Use nonskid throw rugs, or place nonskid mats under rugs.

▶ Make sure bathtubs and showers have safety rails and nonskid mats.

▶ Do not run electrical or telephone cords across areas where people walk.

▶ If there are small children in the home, install adjustable safety latches so that windows will open only a few inches. This is especially important for windows above the first floor. Make sure the windows can be opened in case of fire or other emergency.

▶ Use a sturdy step stool when reaching for items in high places.

Preventing Electrical Shock

Electricity can be dangerous if not used correctly. Improper use or maintenance of electrical appliances, wiring, or outlets can cause severe electrical shock. Follow these safety precautions when using electrical appliances to help reduce the risk of injury:

▶ Unplug an electrical appliance immediately if anything seems to be wrong. Always pull on the plug, not the cord.

▶ Inspect cords periodically for signs of cracked insulation. If the cord is frayed, replace it immediately.

▶ Do not run cords under carpets or rugs; they can be damaged when walked on.

▶ Never use an electrical appliance or power tool if your body, clothing, or the floor is wet.

▶ Check outlets and extension cords to make sure they aren't overloaded.

▶ In homes with small children, cover unused outlets with plastic protectors.

 Prevent electrical shocks by using extension cords and electrical outlets correctly. *Why might an overloaded outlet cause a problem?*

CHARACTER ✏ CHECK

Citizenship. Keep your eyes open for potential safety hazards at school. Notice any frayed electrical wires, overloaded outlets, or extension cords stretched across areas where people walk. **Do your part to help make your school a safe environment—report any unsafe situation to the custodian or a teacher.**

Preventing Poisoning

According to the Centers for Disease Control and Prevention (CDC), nearly 900,000 emergency room visits each year are associated with poisonings. About 90 percent of poisonings occur in the home, and more than half involve children under six years of age. Most potentially poisonous products—detergents, disinfectants, paints, polishes, and insecticides—are typically found in the kitchen, bathroom, utility closet, basement, and garage. Here are a few guidelines for preventing poisoning:

▶ Keep medications and other potentially poisonous substances in childproof containers. Store out of the reach of children. Dispose of any expired medications.

▶ Store all household chemicals in their original containers. Never store them in food or drink containers.

▶ Never mix household chemicals. Many household cleaners contain ammonia or bleach, which give off toxic gases when combined.

▶ Use products that give off fumes, such as ammonia, bleach, petroleum products, and paints, in well-ventilated areas.

▶ Make sure there is adequate ventilation when using fuel-burning appliances. These appliances give off carbon monoxide gas while in use. Inhaling this poisonous gas can damage body tissues and cause death from lack of oxygen.

Figure 27.2 summarizes strategies for staying safe in and around your home. Putting these strategies into practice will decrease the likelihood of unintentional injuries.

Firearm Safety

Up to 40 percent of homes in the United States contain firearms. Firearm injuries are one of the top ten causes of death in the United States, and the number of nonfatal firearm injuries is considerable—over 200,000 per year. Following these recommendations can help reduce the risk of injury from firearms.

▶ Never point a firearm at anyone for any reason.

▶ Treat all firearms as if they are loaded. If you find a firearm, leave the area and tell an adult.

▶ Store firearms unloaded and store the ammunition separately. Both should be in locked cabinets that are well out of the reach of children.

Use proper safety precautions for storing household chemicals and medicines, especially if there are small children in the home. *How should medications be stored?*

FIGURE 27.2

SAFETY AT HOME

Follow these safety practices to help prevent injuries at home.

Test smoke alarms once a month and change the batteries at least once a year.

Make sure your body and the floor are dry before using electrical appliances such as hair dryers or curling irons.

Be sure stairs and hallways are well lit.

Store gasoline and other flammable liquids away from hot water heaters or other sources of flames or sparks.

Store household products in a secure place, out of the reach of children.

Always turn the handles of pots and pans away from the front of the stove so that they cannot be accidentally knocked or pulled off.

Make sure there is good ventilation when you use chemical products to avoid being overcome by fumes.

Store propane cylinders outdoors to prevent an explosion or a fire.

Computer and Video Game Safety

Computer tasks often require you to sit in one place for long periods of time and make repetitive motions while staring at the screen. This can cause eyestrain and sore muscles and may even lead to wrist, hand, or arm injuries. To help reduce the risk of injury, take a 10-minute break every hour or so. If you are working intensely for a long period of time, occasionally give your eyes a rest by looking up and focusing on objects that are far away.

Your work area should be a comfortable and healthy place to work. **Figure 27.3** shows the correct way to sit at a computer. Determine whether your computer and chair are adjusted correctly. Here are some other things to consider when setting up a work area:

▶ **Lighting.** Lighting for a computer should be indirect and not too bright. Avoid creating a glare on your computer screen.

▶ **Adjustability.** Chairs, computer monitors, and desks or other work surfaces should be adjustable for the comfort of each user. This is especially important if people of different heights use the same work area.

FIGURE 27.3

COMPUTER WORKSTATION DESIGN

Making your workstation comfortable will reduce fatigue; eyestrain; blurred vision; headaches; and back, neck, and arm cramps.

Use indirect lighting to avoid glare. Arrange the computer so that it is at right angles to windows or other light sources.

Adjust your chair to keep your back straight. This will help keep your body aligned, which reduces muscle strain.

Adjust the height and angle of the monitor so that it is at or slightly lower than eye level. The distance between your eyes and the monitor should be 18–30 inches.

Adjust the chair so that your feet can rest flat on the floor. Use a foot rest if the chair is not adjustable. Your forearms, wrists, and hands should be straight when you are using the mouse or keyboard.

Adjust the height of the computer table so that the keyboard is comfortable, usually slightly higher than waist level. Your forearms should be parallel to the floor when you are using the keyboard.

Safety on the Job

Many teens have part-time or full-time jobs. In fact, the U.S. Department of Labor says that more than 3 million teens earn paychecks during summer vacations alone; others work part-time jobs during the school year. Unfortunately, about 500 of these workers are injured every day. Many of these unintentional injuries could have been avoided if training had been provided before machinery and equipment were used. Teens are permitted to perform certain tasks on the job, but are prohibited from performing others. The Department of Labor prohibits anyone under 18 from doing certain jobs, including roofing or construction work, demolition, driving a forklift or any vehicle, operating power-driven machinery, and handling explosives or radioactive materials.

Both employees and employers must follow safety rules issued by the **Occupational Safety and Health Administration (OSHA)**, *the agency in the federal government that is responsible for promoting safe and healthful conditions in the workplace.* Because many people spend about one third of the day on the job, it's everyone's responsibility to take steps to ensure a healthful and injury-free workplace.

The U.S. Department of Labor regulates the types of tasks that teens are allowed to perform on the job. *List two types of jobs that the Department of Labor prohibits teens under 18 from doing.*

 Lesson 1 *Review*

Reviewing Facts and Vocabulary

1. What are the five steps in the accident chain?
2. What three elements must be present for a fire to start?
3. Define the term *smoke alarm.*

Thinking Critically

4. **Analyzing.** Why should people always treat a firearm as though it were loaded?
5. **Synthesizing.** Think of a specific job that a teen might have. Analyze strategies for preventing unintentional injuries on that job, and develop a checklist that features these strategies.

Applying Health Skills

Advocacy. Make a poster that encourages family members to practice safety habits. Your poster should include specific safety precautions that family members can take to stay safe in the home. Display your poster at home and discuss with your family any steps that might be taken to improve safety.

PRESENTATION SOFTWARE Use presentation software to illustrate graphically the safety precautions described on your poster. Find help in using presentation software at **health.glencoe.com**.

Recreation and Water Safety

VOCABULARY
heat exhaustion
hypothermia

YOU'LL LEARN TO

• Analyze strategies for preventing accidental injuries that occur during recreational activities.

• Associate risk-taking during recreational activities with consequences such as unintentional injury.

→ **QUICK START** If you were planning a day at the beach or lake, what supplies would you need for a safe and healthy outing? List five specific items that you would take.

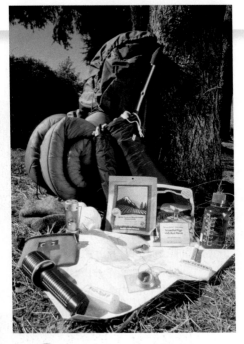

▲ Packing the right supplies will help guarantee that outdoor activities are safe and fun.

Recreational activities are fun, but they can be accompanied by the unexpected. Common sense and caution can minimize the risk of unintentional injuries during recreational activities.

Recreational Safety

Outdoor activities are enjoyable and can help you stay fit. To stay healthy and safe during outdoor activities:

▶ **Know your limits.** Stick with tasks that match your level of ability. For example, stay on beginner slopes until you gain experience as a skier.

▶ **Bring supplies.** Take plenty of safe drinking water with you. Never drink from a lake, river, or stream—these bodies of water may contain illness-causing pathogens. Plan simple meals and take any supplies, including coolers and plenty of ice to store foods safely.

▶ **Wear protective clothing.** The proper clothing can protect against the weather and poisonous plants and insects.

▶ **Tell people your plans.** Let them know where you're going and when you plan to return. If possible, carry a cell phone in case of emergencies.

▶ **Plan ahead for the weather.** Warm days may turn into cold nights and storms may occur suddenly. To avoid heat exhaustion, stay in the shade in hot weather and drink plenty of water. **Heat exhaustion** is *an overheating of the body that results in cold, clammy skin and symptoms of shock.* Use sunscreen to protect the skin from UV rays.

hot link

heat exhaustion For more information about heat exhaustion, see Chapter 4, page 99.

Safety While Camping and Hiking

To prevent injuries when camping and hiking:

▶ Stay in specified campsites, and hike only in approved areas. Never hike or camp alone.

▶ Be knowledgeable about poisonous plants, insects, and snakes. If you'll be in grassy areas, wear socks and long pants tucked into socks or boots to help protect against ticks and mosquitoes.

▶ Be cautious around wildlife. Do not store food in your tent. Store food where animals cannot get to it, such as in a vehicle or suspended from a high tree branch.

▶ Be careful around campfires and observe fire safety rules. Tie back long hair and secure loose clothing. Never cook inside a tent. Smother all campfires with dirt and water.

▶ Never drink water from lakes, rivers, or streams; it may contain disease-causing pathogens.

▼ Safe participation in winter sports requires proper clothing and equipment. *How can dressing in layers help you stay safe during cold-weather activities?*

Winter Sport Safety

When skiing, snowboarding, or participating in other winter sports, dress in layers. Air trapped between layers of clothing helps insulate you from the cold. This can prevent **hypothermia**, *a condition in which body temperature becomes dangerously low.* Make sure the outermost layer is waterproof, and wear a hat. Don't forget to put on sunscreen, especially in high elevations. Always wear the appropriate safety equipment, and make sure it's in good working order and is sized correctly for you.

Real-Life Application

Breaking the Accident Chain

Local Teen Injured in Diving Accident

A Summitville teen is in critical condition after he was recovered from the bottom of a pool Saturday night. Jon Franklin was at the party of a friend where more than 30 people were present. Franklin was found in about six feet of water. The pool had no depth indicators and the area was poorly lit. No one present had training in water safety. Witnesses say alcohol may have been a factor in the accident. A hospital spokesperson has confirmed that Franklin suffered a severe spinal cord injury and that his prognosis is uncertain.

Diving accidents cause more than 850 spinal cord injuries each year. Many of these injuries result in the paralysis of all four limbs. Read the article, and answer the questions below to increase your understanding of how "links" in the accident chain lead to injuries:

- What was the situation?
- What were the unsafe habits that contributed to this accident?
- What was the unsafe action?
- What was the accident?
- What was the result?

ACTIVITY

As a class, discuss the answers to the questions. Individually, bring in a newspaper clipping about a recreational accident. In small groups, identify the situation, the unsafe habits and actions, the accident itself, and the result. Write a paragraph describing how the accident chain could have been broken. Post your clippings and paragraphs on the bulletin board.

Water Safety

Swimming, boating, and other water sports are great summer activities. However, drowning is the second leading cause of injury-related death. The four major causes of drowning are failure to wear a life jacket, alcohol use, lack of swimming skill, and hypothermia. Follow these safety precautions for water-related activities.

SWIMMING

▶ Learn how to swim. Know your abilities, and always swim with a buddy.

▶ Swim only in designated areas where a lifeguard is present.

▶ If you get a muscle cramp, relax, float, and press and squeeze the muscle until it relaxes.

DIVING

▶ Learn the proper diving technique. Always check water depth before diving. The American Red Cross recommends a minimum depth of nine feet.

▶ Never dive in unfamiliar areas or into dark or shallow water. Make sure the area is clear of swimmers and floating objects.

BOATING AND PERSONAL WATERCRAFT

▶ Learn how to handle a boat or personal watercraft (PWC) correctly, and know the laws governing their use.

▶ Always wear approved personal flotation devices on boats and PWC.

▶ At the first indication of bad weather, return to shore.

▶ Never ride in a boat or PWC with an operator who has been using alcohol or other drugs.

Figure 27.4 shows survival techniques you can use if you fall into deep water.

Always wear a Coast Guard-approved personal flotation device when boating or using a personal watercraft.

FIGURE 27.4

DROWNING PREVENTION

If you fall into cold water while boating, assume one of these positions. They can help you stay afloat and reduce the risk of hypothermia until help arrives.

A. Lessen heat loss by drawing your knees up to your chest and keeping your upper arms close to the sides of your body. You lose a lot of heat through your head, so try to keep it out of the water.

B. If you are with one or more people, huddle close together in a circle to preserve body heat. A child or smaller person who loses heat faster should be placed in the center of the circle.

Lake, River, and Ocean Safety

Swimming in lakes, rivers, or the ocean presents added safety concerns. Keep these precautions in mind:

▶ **Swim in supervised areas only.** Select an area that is clean and well maintained.

▶ **Enter feet first.** Hidden objects, unexpected drop-offs, and aquatic life may be lurking beneath the surface.

▶ **Watch for marine warnings.** Check to see whether the warning flag is up, or ask the lifeguard whether the water is safe for swimming. If you are at the ocean, check the tides and surf conditions before entering the water. Don't enter the water in an area marked "No Swimming."

▶ **Be aware of surroundings.** Be sure rafts and docks are in good condition. Stay away from piers, pilings, and diving platforms when in the water. Never swim under a raft or dock.

▶ **Plan ahead.** Always make sure that you have enough energy to swim back to shore. If you are pulled offshore by rapid currents or undertows, swim gradually out of the current by swimming across it, often parallel to the shore.

 Always stay within designated swimming areas that are supervised by a lifeguard.

Lesson 2 *Review*

Reviewing Facts and Vocabulary

1. Why is it risky to drink from lakes, rivers, or streams?
2. Analyze and identify three strategies for preventing accidental injuries while camping or hiking.
3. Define the term *hypothermia*.

Thinking Critically

4. **Synthesizing.** You and your family are taking a boat out on the lake for the afternoon. What supplies and safety equipment should you bring with you?
5. **Analyzing.** You and your friend Jake are skiing. He suggests that you try the advanced slope, even though both of you are beginners. What negative consequences are associated with taking this risk?

Applying Health Skills

Practicing Healthful Behaviors. Choose a sport that you would like to learn, and make a list of the proper equipment and safety precautions associated with that sport. Review your list before you participate. Be sure to incorporate all safety precautions, wear the proper clothing, and use safety equipment.

WORD PROCESSING Use word processing to make your list of proper equipment and safety precautions for your chosen sport. Find help in using word-processing software at health.glencoe.com.

Safety on the Road

VOCABULARY

vehicular safety
graduated driver's license
road rage
defensive driver

YOU'LL LEARN TO

- Analyze strategies for preventing accidental injuries while driving or riding in a car or operating another type of vehicle.

- Associate risk-taking while driving a car or operating another type of vehicle with consequences such as unintentional injury.

QUICK START Make a list of strategies for preventing an unintentional injury while operating a vehicle. Include all of the safety measures that you think apply.

According to the CDC, motor vehicle crashes are the leading cause of death among teens—more than 5,700 teens died in 2001. The fatality rate for teen drivers is about four times higher than the rate for drivers from 25 to 65 years old. The number of teen drivers involved in fatal car crashes is decreasing. However, the percentages are still staggering:

▶ 14 percent of *all* drivers involved in fatal crashes were between the ages of 15 and 20.

▶ 21 percent of these drivers were drinking and driving.

▶ 80 percent of these drivers were not wearing safety belts.

Automobile Safety

When teens are entrusted with driving a car, they have a responsibility to themselves, their families, their passengers, and the people in other vehicles. That responsibility is to behave in a manner that reduces the risk of injury and death. Behaving responsibly means practicing **vehicular safety**—*obeying the rules of the road, as well as practicing common sense and good judgment.* Obeying the rules means driving within the speed limit, yielding the right-of-way when indicated, and observing local traffic regulations.

Automobile safety begins even before you start the car—buckle up!

To exercise common sense and good judgment as a driver:

▶ **Pay attention to your vehicle.** Before you start the car, adjust the mirrors and seat to positions that are best for you. Buckle your safety belt. Adjust other items such as the radio, heater, or air conditioner before the car starts moving.

▶ **Pay attention to other drivers.** A popular TV public service announcement sponsored by the National Safety Council advised drivers to "watch out for the other guy." This advice is still sound. At night or when inclement weather reduces visibility, turn on your headlights so that other drivers can see you. In general, drive as though the other driver is going to act irresponsibly. If you do this, you will always be prepared for the unexpected.

▶ **Pay attention to road conditions.** This includes reducing your speed when the road is icy or wet, when a lane narrows, or when there is construction or congestion.

▶ **Pay attention to your physical state.** Don't drive when you are sleepy. If you are tired, do something to refresh yourself, such as rolling down the window or turning on the radio. If you are extremely tired, pull over at the nearest rest stop and call home.

▶ **Pay attention to your emotional state.** If you are angry or feeling other strong emotions, don't drive. Your mental state can affect your judgment and reaction time as much as your physical state can.

Teen Driving Safety

The National Center for Statistics and Analysis reports that 8,155 drivers between 15 and 20 years old were killed in automobile accidents in the year 2000. According to the CDC, teen drivers are more likely than older drivers to speed, run red lights, make illegal turns, ride with an intoxicated driver, and drive after using alcohol or drugs. Teens are also more likely than older drivers to underestimate the dangers in hazardous situations, and they have less experience adjusting to these situations. In an effort to reduce the number of teen deaths in car crashes, some states have adopted a graduated driver's licensing program. A **graduated driver's license** is *a licensing program that gradually increases a new driver's driving privileges over time as experience and skill are gained.* This system allows a new driver to improve his or her driving skills while under the supervision of an older driver. Over time, a teen driver gains more skill, and the driving restrictions are lifted.

Being supervised by an experienced driver can help a teen improve his or her driving skills. *What are three of the common-sense rules of vehicular safety?*

Exploring Issues

Should All States Adopt Graduated Licensing for Teen Drivers?

Some states have adopted a system of graduated driver licensing (GDL) for teens. This system is based on the idea that a teen with a new driver's license needs time and guidance to gain driving experience and skills in reduced-risk settings. More than half of all states have GDL laws. Should the remaining states also adopt GDL laws for new drivers? Here are two points of view.

Viewpoint 1: Ryan D., age 17

Studies have shown that states with GDL laws have experienced reductions in crashes and traffic violations. I think all states should adopt these laws. When you're behind the wheel, you're responsible for yourself and others.

Viewpoint 2: Shandra L., age 16

I see Ryan's point, but I'm not sure all states need to adopt this system. I think the privilege of driving should be based on skill, not on age, especially in states that don't have high crash rates involving teens.

ACTIVITIES

1. Are graduated licensing laws a good idea for all states?
2. Do you think these laws make a difference or would make a difference in your state in terms of fewer lives lost and reduced number of traffic violations? Explain.

Being a Responsible Driver

As you learn to drive and make decisions behind the wheel, be considerate. Other drivers are trying to anticipate your next move, just as you are trying to anticipate theirs. Follow these safety tips:

▶ Always signal when you are about to make a turn or change lanes. Turn the signal off after the maneuver is complete.

▶ Follow all traffic signals and signs, including speed limits.

▶ Don't tailgate. Following too closely can cause an accident. Other drivers may view tailgating as a hostile act.

▶ Let other drivers merge safely into traffic. Cutting them off or not allowing them to merge is unsafe for you and others.

Always:

▶ Assume other drivers' mistakes are not meant to annoy you personally.

▶ Be polite, even if the other driver is not.

▶ Avoid conflict if possible.

Never:

▶ Block the right-hand turn lane.

▶ Use high-beams unnecessarily.

▶ Exchange hostile gestures or words with other drivers.

▼ **When caught in a traffic slowdown, allow other drivers to merge. Such actions diminish the risks of road rage.** *Identify three other actions that could help diffuse road rage.*

ROAD RAGE

Sometimes people who are otherwise emotionally stable become enraged in certain driving situations. **Road rage** is *a practice of endangering drivers by using a vehicle as a weapon.* It can be triggered by a variety of acts, including disputes over a parking space, obscene gestures, loud music, overuse of the horn, and slow driving. A driver consumed with road rage may run red lights, tailgate, or pass on a shoulder. Some enraged drivers have been known to use guns or other weapons. If you see someone who is truly a danger on the road, keep your distance. Get the vehicle's license plate number, and report it promptly to the police.

Other Preventive Measures

Safety belts save lives. Yet according to the CDC's statistics on teen driving, 1 in 5 high school students report that they rarely or never wear safety belts when riding with someone else. Drivers and passengers who fail to use safety belts are more likely to be thrown from the vehicle in a crash. Make sure everyone in the car is buckled up, and take these precautions:

▶ Never engage in high-risk driving behavior such as speeding, drag racing, or daredevil stunts.

▶ Alcohol and other drugs impair judgment, coordination, and reaction time. *Never* use these substances and drive—the consequences could be fatal.

▶ Don't let distractions such as eating or adjusting the radio or CD player take your attention away from the road. Don't use cell phones while driving.

▶ Realize that you have no control over what other drivers are doing, so for the sake of your safety, drive defensively. A **defensive driver** is *a driver who is aware of potential hazards and reacts to avoid them.* A defensive driver acquires driving skills and knowledge to stay safe on the road.

Safety on Wheels

It is important to use proper safety equipment and common sense when bicycling; skateboarding; riding a scooter; or operating a motorcycle, off-road vehicle, or moped. Almost half of the motorcycle drivers who were killed in the year 2000 were not wearing helmets. Many of these drivers could have survived if they had been wearing helmets.

BICYCLE SAFETY

Bicycles are a main form of transportation in many nations around the world. Their popularity in the United States has grown dramatically in recent years because cycling is a great way to stay fit. For safe cycling:

▶ Always wear a safety-approved, hard-shell helmet that fits properly.

▶ Ride with traffic. Always yield the right-of-way—you will not win against a car or truck.

▶ Watch for cars pulling into traffic and for car doors that swing open suddenly in your path.

▶ Obey the same rules as drivers, such as signaling before you turn and stopping for red lights and stop signs.

▶ Learn to use the hand signals for making turns and stopping.

▶ Except when signaling, keep both hands on the handlebars.

▶ Make sure your bike has a bright headlight and a red rear light and reflector for night riding.

▶ Wear reflective, or at least light-colored, clothing when riding at dawn, dusk, after dark, or in the rain.

SKATING SAFETY

Skateboarding and in-line skating can be a lot of fun. Follow these tips to help keep these activities safe:

▶ Wear protective equipment—wrist guards, elbow and knee pads, and a safety-approved, hard-shell helmet.

▶ Watch for pedestrians and keep your speed under control.

▶ If you begin to fall, curl up into a ball and roll, staying loose.

▶ Do not hold anything in your hand, such as a portable radio. Doing so will not allow you to fall properly.

By behaving safely and using proper safety equipment, you can avoid injury while riding a scooter, skateboarding, or in-line skating.

When riding ATVs in unfamiliar areas, be alert for wires, fences, and downed trees that can cause serious accidents.

MOTORCYCLES AND ALL-TERRAIN VEHICLES

Motorcycles and mopeds are subject to the same traffic laws as cars. All-terrain vehicles (ATVs) are driven off-road. A driver's license is not required to operate an ATV, but operators still need to use common sense and know the rules of the road. Cyclists and ATV operators can also reduce the likelihood of injury by following these safety tips.

▶ Be aware of potential hazards, such as a car door opening or the presence of pedestrians.

▶ Wear a helmet and proper clothing, including eye protection.

▶ Be cautious in wet weather when tire traction is poor.

▶ Do not carry an additional rider unless you have a second seat and an additional set of safety equipment, including a helmet.

▶ Do not grab onto objects or other vehicles while moving.

▶ Do not use ATVs on paved roads or streets. Ride four-wheeled ATVs only; they are less likely to flip than three-wheeled ones.

▶ Lesson 3 Review

Reviewing Facts and Vocabulary

1. Define the term *vehicular safety*.

2. Analyze and identify three strategies for preventing accidental injuries while driving a car.

3. What is a *defensive driver*?

Thinking Critically

4. **Evaluating.** What does the saying "it's better to be alive than right" mean when it comes to vehicular safety?

5. **Synthesizing.** Drinking and driving can have serious consequences. List three negative consequences associated with this risk behavior.

Applying Health Skills

Advocacy. Choose a type of vehicle you learned about in this lesson. Think of ways to teach teens about the safety rules and equipment that a person must use to operate that vehicle safely. With classmates, create a video, public service announcement, or comic book that encourages teens to stay safe by following the tips in your presentation.

TECHNOLOGY *OPTION*

WEB SITES Use your video, public service announcement, or comic book as part of a Web page demonstrating the safety tips for your chosen vehicle. See **health.glencoe.com** for help in planning and building your own Web site.

Weather Emergencies and Natural Disasters

VOCABULARY

severe weather
emergency
  survival kit
hurricane
flash flood
tornado
blizzard
earthquake

YOU'LL LEARN TO

- Analyze strategies for preventing accidental injuries during severe weather and natural disasters.

- Explain how technology has impacted the health status of communities by increasing the survival rate during a severe weather event.

- Demonstrate the ability to communicate safety procedures that should be followed during a severe weather event or natural disaster.

QUICK START   Identify a natural disaster that is common in your region of the country, and make a list of safety precautions that you should follow during such an emergency.

The sky turns dark, and an ominous funnel appears on the horizon. You're driving home when a sudden thunderstorm strikes, and visibility is drastically reduced. These situations can occur without warning. However, careful planning and preparation can help you survive weather emergencies and natural disasters.

Severe Weather

Familiarize yourself with the types of severe weather that occur in your area. **Severe weather** refers to *harsh or dangerous weather conditions*. Some types of severe weather, such as tornadoes, hurricanes, and blizzards, usually occur in certain regions and at certain times of the year. When severe weather threatens, the National Weather Service (NWS) uses the media to issue watches and warnings. A *watch* means that the weather conditions are right for a specific weather event to occur. A *warning* means that severe weather has been sighted and is heading toward your area.

Severe weather warnings are broadcast on television and radio stations.

Emergency Survival Preparation

Discuss with your family where to go during an emergency, where to meet if family members get separated, and whom to contact if help is needed. Prepare an **emergency survival kit**—*a group of items that can be used for a short time until an emergency situation has stabilized.* Here are some supplies to collect before disaster strikes:

▶ **Water and food.** Plan on 1 gallon of water per person per day. Store canned and ready-to-eat foods, and a can opener.

▶ **Phone, radio, lighting, and blankets.** A charged cell phone is helpful when phone service is disrupted. Keep a battery-operated radio, flashlights, and extra batteries for each on hand. Blankets can be used for both warmth and shelter.

▶ **Other supplies.** Items such as medications and money may need to be added to your kit at the last minute.

Health Skills Activity

Goal Setting: Preparing an Emergency Survival Kit

Dean and his sister Tara are watching the news about a recent flood in a nearby town.

"I'm glad that's not us!" exclaims Tara. "I'd hate to have our house full of mud. It would ruin my CDs."

"That would be the least of our worries," Dean says. "It wouldn't be safe to drink water from the tap. We wouldn't have food, lights, or a place to sleep."

Tara replies, "I hadn't thought about that. I don't even know Mom's work number without looking it up. Do you?" Tara asks.

"We aren't very prepared, are we? I think we need to put together a survival kit for emergencies," Dean says.

What Would You Do?
Apply the five goal-setting steps to Dean and Tara's situation.

1. Identify a specific goal and write it down.
2. List the steps you will take to reach your goal.
3. Identify potential problems and ways to get help and support from others.
4. Set up checkpoints to evaluate your progress.
5. Reward yourself when you have achieved your goal.

Hurricanes

A **hurricane** is *a powerful storm that originates at sea, characterized by winds of at least 74 miles per hour, heavy rains, flooding, and sometimes tornadoes.* Hurricanes strike mainly on the eastern and southern coasts of the United States and usually occur from June through November, with the peak months being August and September. The NWS tracks hurricanes and issues warnings when they are approaching. If a hurricane watch is issued, secure your property. Bring in items from outside that may blow away in strong winds, such as lawn furniture, children's toys, bicycles, and trash cans. Board up windows and doors, or tape any glass if you are unable to cover it. If a hurricane warning is issued, seek shelter. Evacuate if the NWS instructs you to do so. The farther inland you go, the safer you will be.

 Floods are one type of natural disaster. *Why do you need to drink bottled water in the event of a flood?*

Floods

Floods occur throughout the United States and can happen at any time of year. Flooding is often the result of severe rains that accompany hurricanes. If a flood is likely to occur, move valuables and furniture to a safe location or to higher ground. Listen to radio bulletins while you watch for rising water, and be prepared to evacuate. Before leaving, turn off the utilities in your home. Never walk, swim, ride a bike, or drive a car through flood waters. Both drowning and electrocution are risks in flooded areas. Drink only bottled water because floods can pollute the water supply. Learn under what conditions to abandon your home and when it is safer to stay put until help arrives.

FLASH FLOODS

A **flash flood** is *a flood with great volume and of short duration that is usually caused by heavy rainfall.* If you are in an area that is under a flash-flood warning, leave low-lying areas immediately. Do not attempt to drive through floodwaters or to cross police barricades. Stay away from streams, creeks, storm drains, and irrigation ditches, all of which become treacherous during flash floods.

Severe Thunderstorms

Thunderstorms can occur anywhere in the United States. Most thunderstorms include heavy rains, strong winds, lightning, and sometimes hail. Storm clouds and darkening skies indicate that a

Can lightning strike twice in the same place?

Yes! The saying, "Lightning never strikes the same place twice" is a myth. Tall buildings are often hit repeatedly in successive storms. Even the same bolt of lightning can strike the same place multiple times. The flickering effect you sometimes see in a lightning bolt is actually multiple strokes of lightning following the same path.

If a tornado warning is issued, seek shelter immediately. *Where is the best place in your community to seek shelter if a tornado warning is issued?*

HEALTH
Online

For information from the American Red Cross on how to prepare for and stay safe during natural disasters, go to **health.glencoe.com**.

thunderstorm is approaching. If you are on the water, go to shore. If you are outdoors, get inside. If you can't get inside, take shelter to avoid being struck by lightning. However, stay away from tall structures and trees, because lightning is attracted to tall objects. As a safety precaution, do not use computers, telephones, or televisions during a severe thunderstorm.

Tornadoes

Tornadoes have occurred in every state and can occur at any time of year. The peak months for tornadoes are March through August. A **tornado** is *a whirling, funnel-shaped windstorm that drops from the sky to the ground and produces a narrow path of destruction on land.* Tornadoes are often associated with severe thunderstorms. The winds of a tornado can reach speeds of up to 200 miles per hour, destroying everything in their path. If a tornado approaches, take these precautions:

▶ If you are outside or in a car, seek shelter inside a sturdy building, not a tent or mobile home. If you cannot get to a shelter, lie down in a ditch or low-lying area. Cover yourself with bulky clothing or a blanket. Protect your head with your hands.

▶ If you are indoors, stay away from windows. A storm cellar, basement, or crawl space is the safest place to be. If such an area is not available, go to an interior room, such as a bathroom, hallway, or closet. Cover yourself and protect your head with a mattress or blanket. As a last resort, get under a piece of heavy furniture and hold onto it.

Winter Storms

A severe winter storm called a **blizzard**, *a snowstorm with winds of at least 35 miles per hour,* is common in the northern areas of the United States. To protect yourself during blizzards or other winter storms, follow these steps:

▶ **Stay inside.** The safest place to be during a blizzard is indoors.

▶ **Wear protective clothing.** If you must go outside, prepare for the extremely cold temperatures and the blowing snow. Put on several layers of loose-fitting, lightweight clothing. Choose an outer layer that is wind- and water-resistant. Use a scarf to protect your mouth and neck. Wear a hat, mittens or gloves to protect your hands and fingers. Wear insulated, water-resistant boots to keep your feet warm and dry.

▶ **Avoid getting lost.** Use landmarks to find your way, or stay where you are until help arrives.

Earthquakes

An **earthquake** is *a violent shaking movement of the earth's surface.* Earthquakes can occur in all parts of the United States, but they are most common west of the Rocky Mountains. California alone averages almost 5,000 weak but detectable quakes each year. Most casualties during earthquakes are caused by falling objects or collapsing structures. If you live in an area prone to earthquakes, make sure bookcases and other tall or heavy furniture are bolted to the wall. Follow these safety procedures in the event of an earthquake:

▶ If you are inside a building, stand or crouch in a strongly supported doorway, brace yourself in an inside corner of the building, or get under a piece of sturdy furniture. Cover your head with your arms or a pillow.

▶ If you are outdoors when the earthquake hits, stay away from buildings, trees, and power lines.

▶ Use caution after the tremors have stopped. Stay out of damaged buildings. Be aware that utilities such as electrical or gas lines may be damaged and hazardous. Be prepared for aftershocks—smaller quakes that occur after the main earthquake.

The hazards of an earthquake continue after the shaking has stopped. *Identify measures established in your community to prepare for disasters.*

▶ Lesson 4 *Review*

Reviewing Facts and Vocabulary

1. Define *severe weather*, and list three examples.
2. What is an *emergency survival kit*?
3. How does a hurricane differ from a tornado?

Thinking Critically

4. **Analyzing.** Imagine that a tornado is approaching your home. What strategies can help prevent accidental injuries during this severe weather event?

5. **Evaluating.** Explain how technology and the media have impacted the health status of communities by improving the chances of surviving a severe weather event. What suggestions might you make to further improve their ability to reach a wide range of the population?

Applying Health Skills

Accessing Information. Use online or print resources to obtain a recommended list of items that should be included in an earthquake emergency kit. Write a PSA detailing the items in the kit. Post the information on a public display board.

WEB SITES Post the list of items to be included in an earthquake emergency kit on a Web site. List safety procedures to be followed in the event of an earthquake. See **health.glencoe.com** for help in planning and building your own Web site.

Middle School Safe Behaviors Project

People of different ages respond to different types of media. For instance, recent studies show that, as children become teens, they start to listen to more music whereas younger children spend more time watching television and playing video games. In this activity, you will plan an instructional program on injury prevention and safe behaviors for middle-school students using media that would appeal to their age group.

	Type of Media	Description
Lesson 1: Safety at Home and at Work	Skit	Students will learn what they need to know about fire safety by watching a skit in which a family develops a fire-safety and escape plan for their household.
Lesson 2: Recreation and Water Safety		
Lesson 3: Safety on the Road		
Lesson 4: Weather Emergencies and Natural Disasters		

ACTIVITY

For each lesson, develop a lesson plan that uses a specific form of media to instruct middle-school students on a particular topic. Consider forms such as video games, comic books, skits, print materials, and Web activities. Complete a chart like the one shown above.

EXPRESS YOUR VIEWS

With a partner, select one of your lesson plans and complete the project that you proposed. Pool your projects as a class, and ask permission to present your safety instructional program to a group of middle-school students.

CROSS-CURRICULUM CONNECTIONS

Conduct an Interview. A good way to gather accurate information is to interview knowledgeable people. As a class, brainstorm a list of experts on injury prevention, weather emergencies, and natural disasters, such as health care professionals, driver education teachers, and meteorologists. Your teacher will divide the class into teams and assign each team an expert to interview. Report your findings to the class.

Write a Report. Firefighters, including volunteer firefighters, not only put out fires, they also teach the community how to prevent them. Research the development of the volunteer fire department in American history. Write a brief report that discusses how the demands on volunteer fire departments have changed throughout the years, as well as how fire departments teach fire safety.

Calculate the Magnitude. Earthquakes are measured using the Richter Scale, which was developed in 1935 by Charles Richter at the California Institute of Technology. It is a logarithmic scale, which means that each number represents a power of 10. Therefore a magnitude 4.3 quake can also be written as $10^{4.3}$. How many times more powerful is a magnitude 3 earthquake than a magnitude 1 earthquake?

Research a Topic. Certain activities, such as typing on a computer keyboard, require that specific muscles and tendons perform repetitive motions. This can lead to carpal tunnel syndrome, a condition characterized by varying degrees of numbness, pain, and tingling in the hands and forearms. Research carpal tunnel syndrome and write a report on your findings.

CAREER Corner

Paramedic

Are you interested in helping other people in emergency situations? Paramedics are trained to give immediate and skilled care to people in all types of medical emergencies. These emergencies range from car crashes, heart attacks, and drownings to helping with childbirth. Lives depend upon the quick and competent care of paramedics as they provide assistance to and transport sick or injured people.

Would you like to study to be a paramedic? To enter this profession, you'll need emergency medical training. Find out more about this and other health careers by clicking on Career Corner at **health.glencoe.com**.

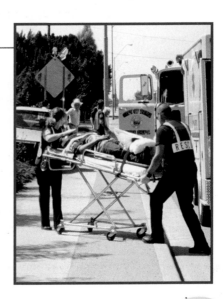

► EXPLORING HEALTH TERMS *Answer the following questions on a sheet of paper.*

Lesson 1 *Match each definition with the correct term.*

unintentional injury	Occupational Safety
smoke alarm	and Health
fire extinguisher	Administration
accident chain	(OSHA)

1. A sequence of events that leads to an unintentional injury.

2. A portable device that puts out small fires by ejecting fire-extinguishing chemicals.

3. An injury resulting from an unexpected event, or accident.

4. The agency in the federal government that is responsible for promoting safe and healthful conditions in the workplace.

Lesson 2 *Identify each statement as True or False. If false, replace the underlined term with the correct term.*

hypothermia   heat exhaustion

5. An overheating of the body that results in cold, clammy skin and symptoms of shock is known as hypothermia.

6. Heat exhaustion is a condition in which body temperature becomes dangerously low.

Lesson 3 *Match each definition with the correct term.*

vehicular safety	defensive driver
graduated driver's license	road rage

7. A driver who is aware of potential hazards and reacts to avoid them.

8. A practice of endangering drivers by using a vehicle as a weapon.

9. A licensing program that gradually increases a new driver's driving privileges over time as experience and skill are gained.

Lesson 4 *Replace the underlined words with the correct term.*

severe weather	hurricane	tornado
emergency survival kit	flash flood	blizzard
earthquake		

10. A flash flood is a violent shaking movement of the earth's surface.

11. A hurricane is a flood with great volume and of short duration that is caused by heavy rainfall.

12. A tornado is a snowstorm with winds of at least 35 miles per hour.

► RECALLING THE FACTS *Use complete sentences to answer the following questions.*

Lesson 1

1. Explain why the pattern of events that can lead to an unintentional injury is known as the "accident chain."

2. Why should every home be equipped with smoke alarms and a fire extinguisher?

3. Why is mixing household chemicals an unsafe procedure?

Lesson 2

4. Why should everyone learn to swim?

5. What can you do to protect yourself from heat exhaustion?

Lesson 3

6. Why are some states adopting a graduated driver's license program?

7. Why is it important to be aware of your emotional state when driving?

8. What are two safety behaviors that can keep you safe on a skateboard?

9. What precautions should you take if a hurricane watch is issued for your area?

10. Where is the safest place to be during a blizzard?

11. Where do earthquakes occur most often in the United States?

➤ THINKING CRITICALLY

1. **Applying.** Alicia spends a lot of time working on the computer. Lately, her neck and back have begun to ache, and her eyes often feel tired. What advice would you give her? *(LESSON 1)*

2. **Evaluating.** Josie lives on a lake and is a good swimmer. On Monday she got home before her parents and decided that she wanted to go for a quick swim. Why is this risky? *(LESSON 2)*

3. **Summarizing.** Though a driver's license is not required to operate an ATV, all ATV operators should use common sense and have a knowledge of road rules. Write a paragraph summarizing safety rules that all ATV operators should know. *(LESSON 3)*

4. **Analyzing.** Experts suggest that homeowners bolt heavy household items such as bookcases to the wall in earthquake-prone areas. How might this procedure prevent accidental injuries? *(LESSON 4)*

➤ HEALTH SKILLS APPLICATION

1. **Advocacy.** Write a letter that stresses the importance of on-the-job training for teen workers in your community. Research your local and state laws and include them in your letter. Submit your letter to your school or local newspaper for publication. *(LESSON 1)*

2. **Refusal Skills.** Mary is excited to be invited out on a boat for a day of water skiing and swimming. However, when she arrives at the boat, Mary learns that the driver of the boat has been drinking alcohol. What should Mary do? *(LESSON 2)*

3. **Decision Making.** Imagine that you attended a party that lasted longer than you had planned. Because your license is graduated, you are not allowed to drive your car at this time of night. Use the decision-making steps to determine what to do. *(LESSON 3)*

4. **Practicing Healthful Behaviors.** Create an informative poster on how to stay safe during severe weather events. Make your poster available to other teens in your school. *(LESSON 4)*

BEYOND the Classroom

Parent Involvement

Accessing Information. Learning to swim can save your life. Research recreation and water-safety programs in your community. With your parents, find out how your family can become involved in these educational programs. If programs do not already exist in your community, find out how you can bring them to your community.

School and Community

American Red Cross. The American Red Cross helps communities during and immediately after a weather emergency or natural disaster. It also offers first-aid, recreation, and water-safety education classes. Contact the agency and find out what volunteer positions are available. Share your findings with the rest of the class.

First Aid and Emergencies

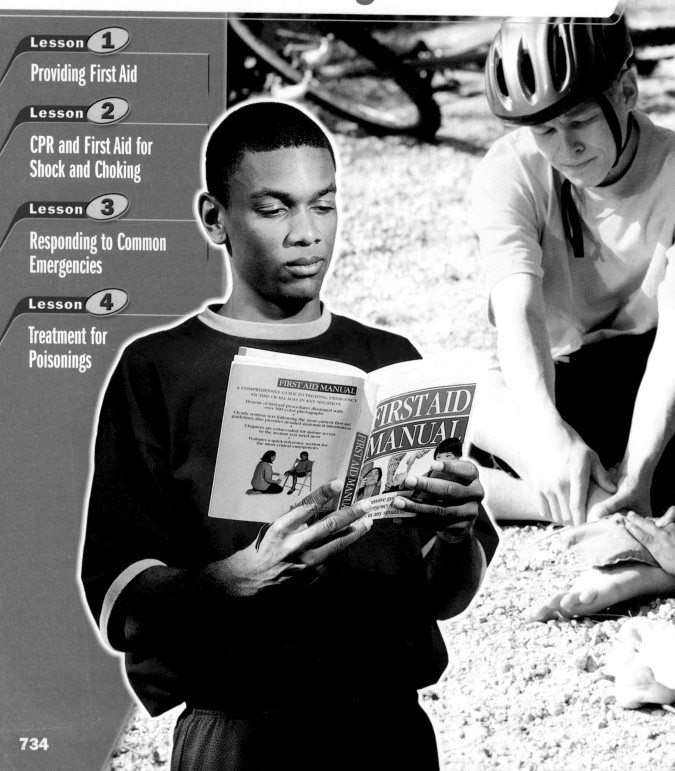

FIRST AID MANUAL

A COMPREHENSIVE GUIDE TO TREATING EMERGENCY VICTIMS OF ALL AGES IN ANY SITUATION

Dozens of first-aid procedures illustrated with over 500 color photographs

Clearly written text following the most current first-aid guidelines also provides detailed anatomical information

Chapters are color-coded for instant access to the section you need most

Features a quick-reference section for the most critical emergencies

FIRST AID MANUAL

What's Your Health Status?

Read each statement below and respond by writing *yes* or *no* for each item.

1. I have the contact information for my family's health care providers.

2. I keep a list of emergency numbers near a telephone in my home.

3. I can help someone who has swallowed a poison.

4. I take small bites of food when eating and chew each bite thoroughly before swallowing.

5. I know what actions to take to help someone who is choking.

6. I know all of the medications that members of my family take.

7. I am trained and certified to administer CPR.

8. I know what steps to take to stop heavy bleeding.

9. I am able to tell the difference between minor and serious burns and can treat first- and second-degree burns.

10. I know how to help with common emergencies such as nosebleed, fainting, foreign objects in the eye, and insect bites.

HEALTH Online

For instant feedback on your health status, go to Chapter 28 Health Inventory at **health.glencoe.com**.

Quick *Write*

Using Visuals. Your response to a medical emergency can be critical to the recovery of an injured person. In what specific ways do you think providing the correct first-aid techniques will help the recovery of this injured person?

Providing First Aid

VOCABULARY
first aid
universal precautions

YOU'LL LEARN TO

• Relate the nation's goals and objectives for improving individual, family, and community health to learning and using appropriate first-aid procedures.

• Understand the importance of learning first aid.

• Analyze strategies for responding to accidental injuries.

QUICK START Write a paragraph explaining the importance of learning first-aid procedures.

▼ Universal precautions protect both the caregiver and the victim from coming into contact with blood and other body fluids that may contain pathogens.

Imagine that you are taking care of your neighbor's son when he suddenly falls off his bike and cuts his knee. Suppose that you are in the school lunchroom and your best friend begins to choke. Do you know what to do in either of these situations? Your response to an accident or an emergency can minimize injury and might even save a life.

First Aid

First aid is *the immediate, temporary care given to an ill or injured person until professional medical care can be provided.* First aid is administered in the seconds and minutes following an emergency situation in which someone becomes ill or injured. Learning first-aid procedures is an important step in meeting the nation's health goals in *Healthy People 2010.* Using the proper first-aid procedures can reduce the number of people who sustain further injury or die in the absence of early and effective treatment.

Universal Precautions

Some infectious agents, such as the HIV and hepatitis B viruses, can be transmitted through contact with blood and other body fluids. Because of this risk, it is important that you use universal precautions when you administer first aid. **Universal precautions** are *actions taken to prevent the spread of disease by treating all blood and other body fluids as if they contained pathogens.* Universal precautions include wearing protective gloves when there is a possibility of touching blood or other body fluids, using a mouthpiece or other protective ventilation devices for breathing emergencies, and washing your hands before and after providing first aid.

Responding to an Emergency

Recognizing an emergency is the first step in responding to it. Common indicators of an emergency include unusual sights, sounds, odors, and behaviors. If you find yourself at the scene of an emergency, remain calm and follow the steps in **Figure 28.1,** which were developed by the American Red Cross.

FIGURE 28.1

CHECK, CALL, CARE

These are the first steps to take in an emergency situation.

1. **Check the scene and the victim.**
   Look around to be sure that the scene is safe. Be alert for dangers such as spilled chemicals, traffic, fire, escaping steam, downed electrical lines, and smoke. Determine the number of victims. If no immediate danger is evident, do not move the victim. Move the victim only if his or her life is threatened.

2. **Call for help.**
   Call the local emergency number or 911. Answer all of the dispatcher's questions. Do not hang up until the dispatcher does. If possible, have someone else make the call so that you can stay with the victim. If you are the one calling for help, finish the call as quickly as possible, and return to the victim.

3. **Provide care for the victim.**
   If possible, get the victim's permission before giving first aid. Always address life-threatening emergencies first. Take care of anyone who is unconscious; who is not breathing or is having trouble breathing; who shows no signs of circulation, such as moving or coughing; or who is bleeding severely. If you aren't sure that the victim is conscious, tap him or her on the shoulder and ask, "Are you okay?"

Types of Injuries

Not all injuries are emergencies. Splinters and scrapes, for example, are relatively minor injuries, and the first-aid treatment for them is usually quick and simple. Other injuries are severe enough to endanger life or cause serious physical damage.

Open Wounds

Open wounds are one type of injury. Treatment depends on the severity and type of wound:

Knives and other sharp objects can cause lacerations. When using any sharp tool, pay attention to what you are doing. *What other steps can you take to reduce the risk of lacerations?*

▶ **Abrasion.** If the skin is scraped against a hard surface, tiny blood vessels in the outer layers of the skin break, resulting in an abrasion. Because of the way the injury occurs, dirt and bacteria can easily enter the site. Therefore, it's especially important to clean the wound to prevent infection and speed healing.

▶ **Laceration.** A laceration is a cut caused by a sharp object, such as a knife or broken glass, slicing through the layers of skin. This type of laceration usually has smooth edges. A hard blow from a blunt instrument or the skin being torn may cause lacerations with jagged edges. All lacerations are accompanied by bleeding. Deep lacerations can result in heavy bleeding, as well as damage to nerves, large blood vessels, and other soft tissues. Infection may also occur.

▶ **Puncture.** A puncture wound is a small but deep hole caused by a pin, nail, fang, or other object that pierces the skin. Puncture wounds do not usually cause heavy external bleeding, but they may cause internal bleeding if the penetrating object damages major blood vessels or internal organs. Puncture wounds carry a high risk of infection, including tetanus.

▶ **Avulsion.** An avulsion results when tissue is partially or completely separated from the body. A partially avulsed piece of skin may remain attached, but it hangs like a flap. Heavy bleeding is common. Sometimes a body part, such as a finger, may be severed. With today's medical technology, severed body parts can sometimes be reattached surgically. Pack the severed part in ice or ice water, if possible, to preserve the tissue. Immediately call for professional medical assistance.

Health Skills Activity

How to Handle a Puncture Wound

Jamie, 16, is looking after Jason, her 7-year-old neighbor, for the afternoon. They are in the backyard playing with toy cars and trucks. After a while, Jason gets up and walks over to the tool shed.

"Jason," Jamie calls, "you're not supposed to go over there. Come back here and pull out my car with your tow truck. I'm stuck in the mud."

Jason starts to walk back, and suddenly starts screaming and holding his foot.

"Oh, my gosh!" Jamie cries. She looks at Jason's foot.

Jason has stepped on a nail, which has punctured his foot. Jamie notes that the wound looks deep but doesn't appear to be bleeding heavily.

What should Jamie do?

What Would You Do?
Describe in detail how you would apply these first-aid steps to Jamie's situation.
1. Protect yourself from infections spread by contact with blood.
2. Control any bleeding.
3. Clean the wound.
4. Protect the wound.
5. Get medical attention if necessary.

First Aid for Bleeding

To stop blood flow from an open wound, first put on clean protective gloves, if possible. Wash a minor wound with mild soap and running water to remove dirt and debris. Do not attempt to clean a severe injury such as an avulsion. Always wash your hands before and after providing care, even if you wear gloves.

To control bleeding:

▶ Cover the wound with sterile gauze or a clean cloth and press firmly.

▶ If possible, elevate the wound above the level of the heart.

▶ Cover the gauze or cloth dressing with a sterile bandage.

▶ If necessary, cover the dressing with a pressure bandage and/or use pressure point bleeding control (see next page).

▶ Call for help or have someone else do so.

Applying pressure to a wound will often stop the flow of blood. *What precautions should you take before assisting someone with an open wound?*

A pressure bandage may be used to maintain continuous pressure on a wound. *Identify a situation that would require the use of a pressure bandage.*

How to Apply a Pressure Bandage

Roller bandages can be used to maintain continuous pressure on a wound and control bleeding. A bandage applied snugly to the injured area will hold the dressing in place and facilitate blood clotting. To use a roller bandage:

▶ Place a dressing over the wound.

▶ Secure the roller bandage over the dressing.

▶ Using overlapping turns, cover the dressing completely, as shown in the diagram at the left.

▶ Secure the roller bandage in place by splitting its end into two strips. Tie the split bandage ends tightly over the wound.

▶ Make sure that the bandage is not so tight that it cuts off circulation. It should be just tight enough to maintain pressure on the wound.

Pressure Point Bleeding Control

If elevating the wound and applying a pressure bandage do not stop the bleeding, pressure point bleeding control must be used. This procedure involves pressing the main artery against a bone to stop blood supply to the injured area. Because this technique stops normal blood circulation, it should be used only when absolutely necessary. The diagram at the left shows the location of the points at which pressure should be applied when using this technique.

A person who requires pressure point bleeding control is seriously injured and possibly in shock. Professional medical assistance is necessary and should be consulted before this procedure is applied.

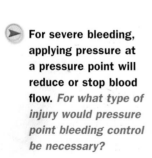

For severe bleeding, applying pressure at a pressure point will reduce or stop blood flow. *For what type of injury would pressure point bleeding control be necessary?*

Burns

Heat, radiation from the sun, certain chemicals, and electricity can all burn the skin and soft tissues of the body. Burns caused by heat are the most common. Those caused by chemicals or electricity require special first-aid procedures—for information on treating these types of burns, contact the American Red Cross.

Burns are classified according to depth: first-degree burns are superficial, and second- and third-degree burns are deep. Minor burns can be treated at home. Severe burns, however, require professional medical care. **Figure 28.2** shows the three classifications of burns and the treatment for each.

FIGURE 28.2

TYPES OF BURNS AND TREATMENT

The severity of the burn determines the type of burn and treatment.

First-degree burn	Second-degree burn	Third-degree burn
In a **first-degree burn,** only the outer layer of skin is burned and turns red. Cool the burn with cold running water or by immersing it in cold water (not ice) for 10 minutes. A clean, cold, wet towel will help reduce pain. Pat the area dry, and cover it with a sterile bandage.	A **second-degree burn** is one in which the top several layers of skin are damaged. The skin will have blisters and appear blotchy. Cool the burn with cold water (not ice), and elevate the burned area. Wrap the area loosely with a sterile, dry dressing. Do not pop blisters or peel loose skin. Seek professional medical attention.	A **third-degree burn** is a serious burn in which deeper layers of skin and possibly fat, muscle, nerves, and bone are damaged. Call for professional medical help immediately. Cool the burn with large amounts of cold water (not ice). Cover the area with a dry sterile dressing or clean cloth.

▶ Lesson 1 Review

Reviewing Facts and Vocabulary

1. Define *first aid.*
2. Relate the nation's health goals and objectives to individual, family, and community health: Explain why knowing first-aid procedures can help achieve the goals of *Healthy People 2010.*
3. Why is it necessary to use universal precautions when giving first aid to a person who is bleeding?

Thinking Critically

4. **Synthesizing.** Analyze and develop a strategy for responding to a minor laceration.
5. **Analyzing.** Describe a strategy for responding to a second-degree burn.

Applying Health Skills

Communication Skills. What would you say to a teen who isn't sure why he or she should learn first aid? Write a dialogue in which you use effective communication skills to explain to the teen the importance of knowing first aid.

TECHNOLOGY O P T I O N

WORD PROCESSING   Use word-processing software to write your dialogue. See **health.glencoe.com** for tips on using word-processing software.

CPR and First Aid for Shock and Choking

VOCABULARY

**chain of survival
defibrillator
cardiopulmonary
   resuscitation (CPR)
shock**

YOU'LL LEARN TO

• Identify the appropriate steps for responding to life-threatening emergencies.

• Analyze strategies for responding to an emergency situation requiring CPR.

• Analyze strategies for responding to a shock or choking victim.

QUICK START   Write a paragraph describing what you know about CPR.

(A) The increased availability of AEDs has lead to improved survival rates for heart-attack victims.

I n an emergency, you need to act quickly—the first few minutes after a medical crisis are usually the most critical. The key is knowing what to do, remaining calm, and making a decision to act.

Life-Threatening Emergencies

I f the victim in an emergency is unresponsive, you must begin immediately the **chain of survival**, *a sequence of actions that maximize the victim's chances of survival.* If the victim is an adult, you can begin the first two links in the chain: call 911 and begin CPR. The next two links, early defibrillation and transfer to advanced care, are usually the responsibility of the emergency medical personnel when they arrive. A **defibrillator** is *a device that delivers an electric shock to the heart to restore its normal rhythm.* An automated external defibrillator (AED) is a handheld device that almost anyone can be trained to use. AEDs have not been approved for use on children who are younger than eight years old or who weigh under 55 pounds.

CPR

A person whose breathing and heartbeat have stopped may need CPR. **Cardiopulmonary resuscitation (CPR)** is *a life-saving first-aid procedure that combines rescue breaths with chest compressions, supplying oxygen to the body until normal body functions can resume.* You must be properly trained by a professional and certified before administering CPR.

CPR for Adults

The steps of CPR are known as the ABCs—airway, breathing, and circulation. If an adult victim is unresponsive, tap him or her and ask in a loud voice, "Are you okay?" If the victim doesn't respond, start the chain of survival. First, call 911 or have someone else do so. Then kneel beside the victim and follow the steps developed by the American Heart Association, which are shown in **Figures 28.3** and **28.4.**

FIGURE 28.3

THE ABCs OF ADULT CPR

A Airway. Look inside the victim's mouth. Remove anything you see blocking the airway. If you don't suspect head or neck injuries, lay the person flat on a firm surface. Gently tilt the head back by lifting the chin with one hand while pushing down on the forehead with the other. If you suspect head or neck injuries, do not move the victim. Open his or her airway by lifting the jaw instead.

B Breathing. Look, listen, and feel for breathing. *Look* for chest movement. *Listen* at the victim's mouth for breathing. *Feel* for exhaled air on your cheek. If the victim is not breathing normally, begin rescue breathing:

1. Keeping the victim's head in the proper position, pinch the nostrils shut.

2. Place your mouth over the victim's mouth, forming a seal. Give 2 slow breaths, each about 2 seconds long. The victim's chest should rise with each breath.

C Circulation. Check for signs of circulation, such as breathing, coughing, or movement. If there are no signs of circulation, a person trained in CPR should begin chest compressions immediately (see **Figure 28.4**). If the victim responds (coughs or moves, for example) but is still not breathing normally, give 1 rescue breath every 5 seconds.

FIGURE 28.4

ADULT CPR CYCLES

1 **Position your hands.** To begin chest compressions, find a spot on the lower half of the victim's breastbone, right between the nipples. Place the heel of one hand on that point, and interlock your fingers with the fingers of the other hand. Don't allow your fingers to rest on the victim's ribs.

2 **Begin chest compressions and rescue breathing.** Lean over the victim so that your shoulders are directly above your arms and hands. Lock your elbows and press straight down quickly and firmly at a rate of about 100 compressions per minute. Allow the chest to spring back between compressions. After every 15 compressions, give 2 rescue breaths. Complete 4 continuous cycles (just over 1 minute) of CPR, then check for signs of circulation. Continue CPR, checking for signs of circulation every few minutes. If the victim begins to respond, stop chest compressions. If the victim coughs or moves but is still not breathing, give 1 rescue breath every 5 seconds until help arrives. If the victim begins breathing normally, turn the victim onto his or her side and wait for professional medical help.

Exploring Issues

Should Schools Require Teens to Take a CPR Course?

Heart attacks are the most common medical emergencies in the United States. Many deaths could be prevented, however, by people performing CPR. As a result, organizations such as the American Heart Association and the American Red Cross have certified thousands of people in CPR. To increase the number of trained rescuers, many people think CPR certification should be a high-school graduation requirement. Others disagree. Here are two points of view.

Viewpoint 1: Michael P., age 15

I don't think that all high-school students should be required to take a CPR course. It should be a personal choice. Health courses need to focus more on risk behaviors that affect young people, such as using tobacco, alcohol, and other drugs. Teens who want CPR training can go to their local chapter of the Red Cross or American Heart Association.

Viewpoint 2: Sydney J., age 15

Every year in the United States, 350,000 people die of sudden heart attacks. Many of these people could be saved if CPR were administered. It makes sense that the more people who are trained in CPR, the fewer people who may die. Many of these courses are taught by teachers who instruct students in the use of AEDs as well as in oxygen administration. Both of these technologies have improved the survival rates of heart attack victims.

ACTIVITIES

1. **Should high schools require teens to take a CPR course? Why or why not?**
2. **CPR training "obligates" people to use their skills when they witness an emergency situation. How well do you think teens could handle this responsibility?**

CPR for Infants and Children

Infants and children in life-threatening emergencies aren't treated in exactly the same way that adults are. For example, you shouldn't use an AED on an infant or a child. Likewise, you can't use the same amount of force in chest compressions. **Figures 28.5** and **28.6** on the next page show how to perform CPR on infants and children. These steps were developed by the American Heart Association. For an infant or child, provide about one minute of CPR *before* calling 911 for help.

FIGURE 28.5

THE ABCs OF INFANT AND CHILD CPR

A Airway. Look inside the victim's mouth. Remove anything you see blocking the airway. If you don't suspect head or neck injuries, lay the victim flat on a firm surface. Gently tilt the head back by lifting the chin with one hand while pushing down on the forehead with the other. If you suspect head or neck injuries, do not move the victim. Instead, open his or her airway by lifting the jaw.

B Breathing. Look, listen, and feel for breathing. *Look* for chest movement. *Listen* at the victim's mouth for breathing. *Feel* for exhaled air on your cheek. If the victim is not breathing, begin rescue breathing:

Keep the victim's head in position. For a child, pinch the nostrils shut and seal your mouth over the victim's mouth. For an infant, seal your mouth over the mouth and nose. Give 2 slow breaths, each about 1 to 1½ seconds long. The chest should rise with each breath.

C Circulation. Check for signs of circulation, such as breathing, coughing, or movement. If there are no signs of circulation, a person trained in CPR should begin chest compressions immediately (see **Figure 28.6**). If the victim responds (coughs or moves, for example) but is still not breathing normally, give 1 rescue breath every 3 seconds for either a child or an infant.

FIGURE 28.6

INFANT AND CHILD CPR CYCLES

1 Position your hands. With one hand, keep the victim's head tilted, unless you suspect head or neck injury. For a child, place the heel of your other hand on the lower half of the breastbone and position your shoulder directly over your straightened arm and hand. For an infant, imagine a line drawn between the nipples. Place two or three fingers of your hand on the lower half of the infant's breastbone, about one finger's width below the imaginary nipple line.

2 Begin chest compressions and rescue breathing. Compress the victim's chest downward approximately ⅓ to ½ the depth of the chest at a rate of *about* 100 times per minute for a child, and *at least* 100 times per minute for an infant. Release pressure completely between compressions. After every 5 compressions, give 1 rescue breath (see **Figure 28.5**). Complete 20 continuous cycles (just over 1 minute) of CPR, and then check for signs of circulation. Continue CPR, checking for signs of circulation every few minutes. If the victim shows signs of circulation, stop chest compressions and continue rescue breathing if necessary (1 rescue breath every 3 seconds).

First Aid for Shock

When something happens to reduce blood flow throughout the body, limiting the amount of oxygen carried to the cells, shock may occur. **Shock** is *a failure of the cardiovascular system to keep an adequate supply of blood circulating to the vital organs of the body.* This life-threatening emergency requires immediate medical attention. Common symptoms of shock include restlessness or irritability; altered consciousness; nausea; pale or ashen appearance; cool, moist skin; and rapid breathing and pulse.

If you suspect a head or spinal injury, don't move the victim. Otherwise, have the victim lie down if he or she has not already done so. This position often minimizes pain and keeps the victim calm. You should also

▶ phone 911 or the local emergency number.

▶ control any external bleeding.

▶ elevate the legs about 12 inches, unless you suspect head or back injury or broken bones involving the legs or hips. If you aren't sure, leave the victim lying flat. This helps the blood return to the heart.

▶ never give the victim anything to eat or drink. Eating or drinking could cause vomiting.

▶ reassure the victim.

Did You Know ?

One cause of shock is losing a large volume of fluid, usually as a result of bleeding. However, shock can result from a significant loss of *any* body fluids. This means that even diarrhea or vomiting, if prolonged and severe, can lead to shock.

First Aid for Choking

Choking occurs when a person's airway becomes blocked by food or a swallowed object. If the obstruction is not removed, the victim can die from lack of oxygen within a few minutes.

To help someone who is choking, you must first recognize the signs. A person may clutch his or her throat with one or both hands, which is the universal sign for choking. The victim may also cough weakly, make high-pitched sounds, or turn blue in the face. If someone appears to be choking but can cough forcefully or speak, do not attempt first aid. A strong cough can expel the object from the airway.

If you suspect that someone is choking, ask, "Are you choking?" and look for the universal choking sign. Then ask, "Can you speak?" If the person cannot speak in reply, the airway is completely blocked and the victim needs immediate first aid.

Be alert for the universal choking sign.

> Use abdominal thrusts on a choking adult, but never on a choking infant. Use back blows alternating with chest thrusts for an infant. *Why do you think different methods are used for adults and infants?*

If the choking victim is an adult or a child, use abdominal thrusts—quick inward and upward pulls to the diaphragm—to force the obstruction out of the airway. To perform this procedure, stand behind the victim and place your arms around him or her. Make a fist with one hand, and grasp it with your other hand. Pull inward and upward just under the rib cage.

If you begin to choke while you are alone, use your own fist and hand to perform the procedure on yourself. You can also try pressing your abdomen forcefully against the back of a chair.

If the choking victim is an infant, hold the baby face down on your forearm. Support the infant's head and neck with your hand and point the head downward so that it is lower than the chest. With the heel of your hand, give the infant five blows between the shoulder blades. If the object is not dislodged, turn the infant over and perform five chest thrusts as described in the CPR section. Alternate the five blows between the shoulders with five chest thrusts until the object is dislodged or the infant begins to breathe or cough. Call 911 if the object is not dislodged within one minute. If the infant loses consciousness, phone 911 and begin CPR if you are trained and certified in the procedure.

Lesson 2 *Review*

Reviewing Facts and Vocabulary

1. Define *cardiopulmonary resuscitation*.
2. Why should you never give a shock victim anything to eat or drink?
3. What is the universal sign for choking?

Thinking Critically

4. **Evaluating.** Explain why it's important to check the airway before beginning CPR.
5. **Analyzing.** Compare the strategy for responding to a choking adult with the strategy for responding to a choking infant.

Applying Health Skills

Advocacy. Make a video encouraging teens to learn basic first-aid techniques for choking and shock. Make the video available to your class.

TECHNOLOGY OPTION

WORD PROCESSING Use word processing to write the script for your video. See **health.glencoe.com** for help in using word-processing software.

Responding to Common Emergencies

VOCABULARY
fracture
unconsciousness
concussion

YOU'LL LEARN TO

- Analyze strategies for responding to muscle, joint, and bone injuries.
- Analyze strategies for responding to unconsciousness.
- Analyze strategies for responding to animal bites.
- Analyze strategies for responding to nosebleeds and to foreign objects in the eye.

QUICK START Write down three situations that come to mind when you hear the word *emergency.* Next to each situation, describe how you would respond to the emergency.

Suppose that you and a friend are out jogging when your friend falls and sprains an ankle. How can you be sure that the injury is a sprain and not a fracture? Would you know what to do in either case? As with major emergencies, knowing the proper response when dealing with common emergencies can help prevent further injury or complications.

Muscle, Joint, and Bone Injuries

When too much stress is put on an area of the body, an injury may occur. These injuries vary in severity and can affect the bones, muscles, tendons, or ligaments. Some injuries, such as muscle strain, will usually feel better in a few days. Other injuries, such as a broken bone, may take several weeks to heal and require professional medical treatment for a full recovery to occur.

Bone, muscle, and joint injuries can be serious, but they are usually not life threatening.

Applying ice to a sprain reduces swelling and eases pain. *Why is it a good idea to see a health care professional if you suspect that you have a sprain?*

h⊙t link

R.I.C.E. For more information on R.I.C.E., see Chapter 4, page 102.

Muscle Cramps

A muscle cramp is the sudden and painful tightening of a muscle. Muscle cramps can occur when you are physically active or at rest. Some medications can also cause them. If a muscle cramp occurs:

▶ Stretch out the affected muscle to counteract the cramp.

▶ Massage the cramped muscle firmly.

▶ Apply moist heat to the area.

▶ Get medical help if the cramp persists.

Strains and Sprains

A strain is an injury to a muscle, usually resulting from overuse of the muscle. The symptoms of a strain include pain, swelling, bruising, and loss of movement caused by small tears in the muscle. A sprain is an injury to a ligament. Sprains usually result from a sudden twisting force. Sprains also cause pain and swelling from badly stretched or torn ligaments. Although serious sprains require professional medical attention, minor sprains and strains may be treated with the **R.I.C.E.** procedure:

▶ **R**est—Avoid any movements or activities that cause pain, including any use of the affected muscle or joint. Help the victim find a comfortable position.

▶ **I**ce—Ice helps reduce pain and swelling. Place ice cubes in a plastic bag, and wrap a towel or cloth around the bag. Hold the bag on the affected area for 20 minutes, remove it for 20 minutes, and then reapply it. Repeat this process every 3 waking hours over the course of 72 hours.

▶ **C**ompression—Light pressure from wearing an elastic wrap or bandage can help reduce swelling. The wrap should be firm but not uncomfortable.

▶ **E**levation—Raising the affected limb above the level of the heart helps reduce pain and swelling.

Fractures and Dislocations

Fractures and dislocations are similar. A **fracture** is *a break in the bone.* If a joint is under extreme stress, it may dislocate, or disconnect. First-aid procedures are the same for both fractures and dislocations. If possible, keep the victim still and call 911. If the victim must be moved, keep the fractured area immobilized by securing a splint to the body part with clean lengths of cloth. You can fashion a splint from everyday materials such as rolled newspapers and heavy cardboard. Seek professional medical care immediately.

Unconsciousness

Unconsciousness is *a condition in which a person is not alert and aware of his or her surroundings.* There are different levels of unconsciousness, ranging from drowsiness to coma. An unconscious victim can choke to death because of his or her inability to cough, clear the throat, or react to a blocked airway. The primary goal when providing first aid to an unconscious victim is to prevent choking until professional medical help arrives. If the victim is unconscious, place him or her in the recovery position shown in **Figure 28.7** and seek professional medical help immediately.

Fainting

Fainting occurs when the blood supply to the brain is temporarily inadequate. Loss of consciousness is usually brief. Although fainting doesn't always indicate a medical problem, it might be symptomatic of a serious disorder. Treat fainting as a medical emergency until the symptoms are relieved and the cause is known.

If you feel faint, lie down or sit down and place your head between your knees. If someone else faints, position the person on his or her back with legs elevated 8 to 12 inches above the heart unless you suspect head or neck injury. Do not place a pillow under the person's head. This can block airflow. Loosen any tight clothing. Sponge the person's face with water. Do not splash water on the face; this may cause the person to choke. If the person vomits, quickly roll him or her into the recovery position shown in **Figure 28.7** to prevent choking. If the person fails to revive promptly, seek medical help.

CHARACTER CHECK

Citizenship. If you see someone who has just suffered an injury, don't assume that someone else will stop and help. Everyone else might be making that same assumption. **Be a responsible member of your community. If you see someone who needs medical assistance, do what you can to help, even if all you can do is call 911.**

FIGURE 28.7

THE RECOVERY POSITION

The recovery position is the safest placement for an unconscious person because the airway is protected. Put the person in the recovery position only if no spinal or head injury is suspected.

This position helps an unconscious person breathe and allows fluids such as blood and vomit to drain. Do not move a person if you suspect spinal or head injuries. Movement can worsen these injuries.

Concussion

A **concussion** is *a jarring injury to the brain that affects normal brain function.* Even if there are no external signs of injury, the brain can strike the inside of the skull and be damaged. To avoid causing spinal injury, do not move an unconscious victim if you suspect a head injury or concussion. Check the person's airway, breathing, and circulation, and get professional medical help immediately. If you suspect that a person has a concussion:

▶ Have a conscious victim lie down.

▶ Use first aid for any bleeding.

▶ If the victim is unconscious and you do not suspect head or neck injury, place him or her in the recovery position, as shown in **Figure 28.7** on page 751. Call 911 immediately.

Animal Bites

One of the most serious possible consequences of an animal bite is rabies, a viral disease of the nervous system that eventually causes paralysis and death if left untreated. There is no cure for rabies after symptoms develop. However, if a person is vaccinated promptly after being bitten, he or she can develop immunity before symptoms appear.

When someone is bitten, report the incident to your community health department or animal control department. It's important to determine whether the animal has rabies. If you find the animal, do not try to capture it. Give its description and location to the proper authorities or the police. The animal will be captured for testing and observation.

Animal bites also carry the risk of infection, including tetanus, an often fatal disease. Although tetanus can be treated, the treatment is long, difficult, and often unsuccessful. Tetanus can be prevented, however, by keeping your immunizations up to date. First aid for animal bites includes the following:

▶ Wash the bite area with mild soap and warm water for five minutes to remove saliva and any other foreign matter.

▶ Use direct pressure or pressure point bleeding control to stop any bleeding.

▶ If the wound is swollen, apply ice wrapped in a towel for 10 minutes.

▶ Cover the wound with a clean dressing or bandage.

Never approach a strange dog. Always ask the owner's permission before approaching or touching a dog that you do not know. *What two diseases are associated with animal bites?*

Nosebleeds

Nosebleeds often occur if the nose is struck or if the mucous membranes in the nose dry out from breathing dry air. Seek professional medical attention if nosebleeds occur often.

To treat a nosebleed, keep the person quiet. Walking, talking, and blowing the nose may increase bleeding. Tell the person to breathe through his or her mouth. Have the person sit down and lean forward. Do not tilt the person's head back—doing so may cause the person to choke as blood runs down the back of the throat. Using a protective barrier, press on the bleeding nostril. Maintain pressure for 15 minutes. If the person's nose is still bleeding after 15 minutes, repeat the procedure. If bleeding continues, seek professional medical help.

Applying direct pressure to a nosebleed usually stops the bleeding. *Why might dry air cause a nosebleed?*

Hands-On Health ACTIVITY

First-Aid Stations

In this activity you will set up learning stations for common emergencies and rotate through them.

What You'll Need

- pen or pencil and notebook paper
- poster board and markers
- props (optional)

What You'll Do

1. In small groups, research the following information for the emergency assigned by your teacher:
   - how to recognize it
   - appropriate steps to take in the correct sequence
   - what to do after first aid has been provided
2. Decide on a creative way to present your material at a learning station, such as a poster, a board game, a quiz show, a puzzle, a news story, or demonstrations with props such as bandages.
3. Each group will set up a learning station. One person in each group coordinates the activities at each learning station while all other students rotate through the stations. Group members take turns supervising their station.

Apply and Conclude

Write a script for a skit about a teen or a group of teens who encounter a medical emergency. The script should show one teen experiencing the emergency while the others administer proper first aid.

Object in the Eye

To flush an object out of your own eye, gently pour water from a small clean glass into the eye.

Foreign objects such as dirt, sand, or slivers of wood or metal that enter the eye are irritating and can cause damage. Encourage the victim not to rub the eye, an action that may scratch the cornea, but to blink several times. If blinking does not dislodge the object, try to find it in the eye. First, wash your hands. Gently pull the lower eyelid down while the person looks up. If you don't see anything, hold the upper lid open and examine the eye while the person looks down. If you see the object on the surface of the eye, lightly touch it with a moistened cotton swab or the corner of a clean cloth.

You can also flush the eye with sterile saline solution or tap water. If the person is wearing contact lenses, do not remove the lens before flushing the eye. To flush the eye, tilt the person's head to the side so that the affected eye is lower than the unaffected eye. Gently hold the eye open with one hand. With the other hand, pour a steady stream of cool water into the eye, from the inside corner toward the outside corner. The water should wash over the surface of the eye. Seek professional medical help if the object is not removed.

▶ Lesson 3 Review

Reviewing Facts and Vocabulary

1. What is a *fracture*?
2. What is the primary goal when providing first aid to an unconscious person?
3. What are two common causes of nosebleeds?

Thinking Critically

4. **Analyzing.** While hiking with you, a friend stumbles on a tree root and falls. By the time you get home, her ankle is badly swollen and she can't walk without leaning on you. Analyze and describe the strategy you would use to respond to this accidental injury.

5. **Evaluating.** Why should you seek professional medical care if a sprain or strain doesn't improve or if you suspect that the injury might be a fracture?

Applying Health Skills

Accessing Information. Use online and print resources to find additional information about rabies. Using the information you have obtained, write a newspaper article about giving first aid to someone who has been bitten by an animal, including how to prevent rabies.

WEB SITES Use your newspaper article as part of a Web site you develop on rabies. See **health.glencoe.com** for help in planning and building your Web site.

Treatment for Poisonings

VOCABULARY

poison
venom
poison control center

YOU'LL LEARN TO

• Analyze strategies for responding to poisonings.

• Analyze strategies for responding to bites and stings.

• Analyze strategies for preventing and responding to skin irritation caused by contact with poisonous plants.

QUICK START Accidental poisonings are often associated with toddlers. What are some safety procedures that can help prevent accidental poisoning in a home with young children? Compile a list of at least five tips.

Knowing how to respond to poisoning emergencies is an important part of first aid. A **poison** is *any substance—solid, liquid, or gas—that causes injury, illness, or death when introduced into the body.* Approximately 90 percent of poisonings occur in the home, and more than half of these poisonings involve children under the age of six.

Types of Poisoning

Poisoning results when substances that are not meant to enter the body do so. The substance could be a chemical that is swallowed, a pesticide that is absorbed through the skin, or **venom**, *a poisonous substance secreted by a snake, spider, or other creature,* that is injected into the body through a sting or bite. Even certain plants and foods can be poisonous. Gases or vapors may also be poisonous, such as carbon monoxide from hot water heaters and furnaces, exhaust fumes from automobiles, and fumes from gas- or oil-burning stoves. Your poison control center can tell you the correct procedure to follow in the event of a poisoning. A **poison control center** is *a 24-hour hot line that provides emergency medical advice on treating poisoning victims.*

Many household products become poisons if they are used incorrectly. *Where can you find information about the toxicity of various household products?*

Poison can enter the body in four ways: ingestion, inhalation, absorption, and injection. *What can you do to prevent accidental poisonings?*

First Aid for Poisoning

Proper treatment of poisoning requires professional guidance. The best resource in handling poison emergencies is the local poison control center. Have the phone number of your poison control center posted near your phone.

Time is critical when a poisoning has occurred. Some poisoning situations require quick action to minimize the amount of damage to the victim or to prevent death. First, call 911 for help. Then follow these first-aid tips for poisonings.

▶ **Swallowed poisons** vary in their first-aid treatment because the substances that can be swallowed affect the body differently. Quickly try to determine what was swallowed, and call your poison control center. Follow the instructions given to you. It is important that you call the poison control center first. You may be instructed to give the victim something that dilutes the poison, such as milk or water, or you may be directed to induce vomiting. Do not try to induce vomiting unless you are told to do so. Some poisons can be aspirated into the lungs and cause even more damage; others can burn the esophagus if the victim vomits.

▶ **Inhaled poison** is serious because of the damage that can be done to the lungs and other organs of the respiratory system. Quickly get the person to fresh air. Do not breathe in the fumes. If the victim is not breathing, start rescue breathing.

▶ **Poison on the skin** must be removed as quickly as possible to limit the exposure to the body. Remove contaminated clothing. Rinse skin continuously with water for 15 minutes. Then rinse the skin with mild soap and water. Rinse again with fresh water. If possible, have someone call 911 while you are rinsing the skin.

▶ **Poison in the eye** is absorbed quickly. Immediately start flushing the eye with lukewarm water and continue for 15 minutes. Have the victim blink the eye as much as possible while flooding the eye. Do not force the eye open, and do not rub the eye. Have someone call 911 while you are rinsing the eye.

When you call the poison control center:

▶ Be prepared to give your name, location, and telephone number.

▶ Provide the name of the substance, when it was ingested, and the amount involved. If possible, give the brand name of the product and a list of the ingredients.

▶ Describe the state of the victim, as well as his or her age and weight.

▶ Be prepared to follow instructions and answer any questions.

Real-Life Application

Contacting a Poison Control Center

Poisonous products often display warning labels that provide instructions on what to do if someone swallows, inhales, or has skin or eye contact with the product. For cases of poisoning in which the specific product is known, use this information when you contact the poison control center.

The WORKS Toilet Bowl Cleaner

WARNING: KEEP OUT OF REACH OF CHILDREN
CONTAINS: HYDROXYACETIC ACID ✪

FIRST AID:
If in eyes: Hold eye open and rinse slowly and gently with water for 15–20 minutes.
Remove contact lenses, if present, after the first five minutes, ✪ and then continue rinsing eye.
If on skin or clothing: Remove contaminated clothing. ✪
Rinse skin immediately with plenty of water for 15–20 minutes.
If swallowed: Have person sip a glass of water if he or she is able to swallow.
Do not induce vomiting unless told to do so by a poison control center. ✪
Do not give anything by mouth to an unconscious person. ✪

- Why is it important for a poison control center to know the specific poison?

- Why should you remove contact lenses if a chemical has entered the eye?

- Why must contaminated clothing be removed at once?

- What is a poison control center? Where is the one nearest you?

- Why is it dangerous to give an unconscious person something to drink?

ACTIVITY

With a partner, role-play a scenario that involves contacting a poison control center when a child has ingested the product shown above. Write your dialogue, and then practice asking and giving information clearly and calmly. One of you will be the caller; the other will be a health professional at the poison control center. The latter will ask for the caller's name and telephone number, as well as questions about

- the child's condition, age, and weight.

- the suspected poison and what instructions/warnings/ingredients appear on the label.

- the time the poisoning may have occurred.

- what first aid the caller may have already provided.

Conclude the role-play with what you think the health professional might tell the caller to do. Then switch roles and repeat the role-play.

FIGURE 28.8

FIRST AID FOR SNAKEBITE

Use the following steps to administer first aid to a snakebite victim:

- Get the victim to a hospital. This is the most important step. Keep the victim calm and in a reclining position, if possible. The more the victim moves, the greater the risk that venom will circulate throughout the body.

- Keep the bitten area at or below the level of the heart. If the bitten area is on a limb, immobilize that limb.

- Call 911, or have someone else do so. Follow any instructions that are given.

- Do not apply ice or heat. Applying heat will diffuse the venom more rapidly. Applying ice will cause tissue damage. Also, do not give the victim aspirin or other drugs. Some substances can interact dangerously with the venom or thin the blood, causing the venom to spread more rapidly into tissues.

- Maintain breathing and prevent aggravation of the wound. If you are the victim of a snakebite and are alone, walk slowly and rest periodically to help minimize blood circulation.

First Aid for Poisonous Bites and Stings

Insect and animal stings and bites are among the most common sources of injected poisonings. A poisonous bite or sting can come from several sources, including insects, spiders, ticks, scorpions, snakes, marine life, and other animals.

Snakebite

There are about 20 species of venomous snakes in the United States. Most are rattlesnakes, copperheads, coral snakes, and water moccasins (also called cottonmouths). Usually, the bite of a venomous snake is not fatal; however, a bite can cause severe pain, loss of function, and, in rare situations, loss of a limb. The first-aid procedures for snakebite are found in **Figure 28.8.**

Insect Bites and Stings

Some insects, such as the bee, hornet, yellow jacket, wasp, and fire ant, cause painful stings that can produce a strong allergic reaction. For people who are highly allergic to the venom of these insects even one sting can cause a life-threatening condition. These people need immediate medical attention if they are stung. However, for most people, insect bites are uncomfortable but not life threatening. Follow these first-aid procedures for insect bites and stings:

- Move to a safe area to avoid further harm. Try to remove the stinger by scraping it off with a firm, sharp-edged object such as a credit card or fingernail.

- Wash the area with mild soap and water to help prevent infection. To reduce pain and swelling, apply a cold compress. Apply hydrocortisone cream, calamine lotion, or a baking soda paste to the area several times a day until the pain is gone.

- If the victim was bitten by a venomous spider or scorpion and begins to have trouble breathing or shows other signs of a severe reaction, call 911 immediately.

These are common poisonous plants.

Poison Oak

Poison Ivy

Poison Sumac

First Aid for Poisonous Plants

About 85 percent of Americans will develop an allergic skin reaction if exposed to poison ivy, poison oak, or poison sumac. Symptoms include blistering, swelling, burning, and itching at the point of contact, and the person may develop fever.

The first defense against poisonous plants is to recognize and avoid them. If you come into contact with a poisonous plant, remove contaminated clothing. Flush affected areas with water, and then wash thoroughly with soap and water. Certain over-the-counter preparations can be used to wash the affected areas. If a rash develops, use calamine lotion to relieve the itching. For severe discomfort or pain, seek medical attention.

 Lesson 4 *Review*

Reviewing Facts and Vocabulary

1. Define the terms *poison* and *venom*.
2. What information should you have ready when you call a poison control center?
3. Analyze and describe the strategy for responding to insect bites and stings.

Thinking Critically

4. **Analyzing.** Analyze and describe a strategy for preventing an accidental poisoning in your kitchen.
5. **Synthesizing.** Develop a list of items needed to administer first aid to a bee-sting victim who is not allergic to bee venom.

Applying Health Skills

Practicing Healthful Behaviors. Prepare a pamphlet that shows the first-aid procedures for responding to poisonings. Include each type of poisoning mentioned in this lesson. Make your pamphlet available to other students in your school.

PRESENTATION SOFTWARE Use the material from your pamphlet and computer software to create a presentation. See **health.glencoe.com** for information on how to create a presentation.

Emergency and Rescue Workers in the Media

Firefighters, police officers, paramedics, and other emergency and rescue workers are receiving increased media attention for their acts of heroism and bravery. In this activity, you will analyze print media coverage of emergency and rescue workers.

- What kind of story is it? For example, is it a news article about an emergency situation? Is it a human interest piece about the good deeds of the emergency or rescue worker?
- What is the general tone of the article?
- How does the headline help tell the story?
- Where does the story appear in the newspaper or magazine? How does the article's placement help determine what type of story it is?
- Does the story refer to the rescue worker by name, or does it mention only that a rescue worker was on the scene? If a person's name is mentioned, explain why.
- Does a photograph accompany the story? What effect does it have on the story?
- Does the story show the rescue worker in a positive light? If so, identify the specific passages in which his or her deeds are shown positively.
- In what other ways does the story bring recognition to the work of rescue professionals?

ACTIVITY

Search through newspapers or magazines for stories about rescue and emergency workers. Choose an article and analyze it by answering the questions in the chart above. Write your analysis in the form of a report, and share it with the class.

EXPRESS YOUR VIEWS

Prepare a list of ten interview questions for the emergency or rescue worker featured in the article that you analyzed. Questions might focus on background, training, and coping with high-stress situations.

CROSS-CURRICULUM CONNECTIONS

Write a Dialogue. When a medical emergency occurs, it takes a team to deal with the crisis. Imagine that your job is to calm the injured person. Write a paragraph describing what you would say to reassure the victim. Use descriptive words in your dialogue, and keep in mind that your audience is someone who is scared.

Work in Teams. Developments such as 911 and CPR have improved the chances of survival in the event of an emergency. Organizations such as the American Red Cross have also made contributions to the field of emergency care. Your teacher will divide your class into teams and assign each team a research topic on the subject of emergency care. Present your findings to the class.

Determine the Amount. In the year 2000, there were 172,000 people employed as emergency medical technicians (EMTs) or paramedics in the United States. Of those, 40 percent were employed by private ambulance services, 30 percent were employed by government agencies, and 20 percent were employed by hospitals. How many of the 172,000 EMTs and paramedics were employed by private ambulance services? How many were employed by government agencies?

Research a Topic. In 1628, William Harvey demonstrated that a system of arteries and veins circulated blood throughout the body. Research to learn more about Harvey's findings as well as the theories that his work eventually displaced. Discuss these ideas in light of current concepts of health and first aid.

 CAREER Corner

Emergency Physician

Can you make fast and accurate decisions? As an emergency physician, you often have to make quick diagnoses under extreme conditions. You also need to be able to communicate.

To become an emergency physician, you need a four-year college degree and a medical degree. After finishing medical school, you'll need one year of internship and two to three years of residency. Find out more about this and other health careers by clicking on Career Corner at **health.glencoe.com**.

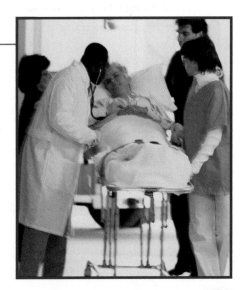

Chapter 28 *Review*

► EXPLORING HEALTH TERMS *Answer the following questions on a sheet of paper.*

Lesson 1 *Match each definition with the correct term.*

universal precautions   first aid

1. The immediate, temporary care given to an ill or injured person until professional medical care can be provided.
2. Actions taken to prevent the spread of disease by treating all blood and other body fluids as though they contained pathogens.

Lesson 2 *Match each definition with the correct term.*

defibrillator   shock
chain of survival
cardiopulmonary resuscitation

3. A failure of the cardiovascular system to keep an adequate supply of blood circulating to the vital organs of the body.
4. A device that delivers an electric shock to the heart to restore its normal rhythm.
5. A sequence of events that maximize the victim's chances of survival.

Lesson 3 *Fill in the blanks with the correct term.*

concussion   unconsciousness
fracture

A blow to the head can cause a (__6__), which is a jarring injury to the brain, without actually causing (__7__). If the blow is hard enough, it can cause a skull (__8__).

Lesson 4 *Fill in the blanks with the correct term.*

venom   poison
poison control center

A (__9__) provides emergency medical advice on treating poisoning victims. Snake (__10__) is a (__11__) when it is introduced into the human body.

► RECALLING THE FACTS *Use complete sentences to answer the following questions.*

Lesson 1

1. What are two universal precautions that a person should follow when giving first aid to another person?
2. What are the first three things you should do when you recognize an emergency situation?
3. What are the four types of open wounds?

Lesson 2

4. What is the chain of survival for adults?
5. What are the ABCs of CPR?
6. What are the symptoms of shock?

Lesson 3

7. What is the first-aid procedure for a person who has a muscle cramp?
8. What is the first-aid procedure for a person who has fainted?
9. Why is the recovery position the safest position for a person who is unconscious?

Lesson 4

10. What is the first-aid procedure for a person who has inhaled poison?
11. What is the first-aid procedure for poison in the eye?
12. Why is it important to wash a poisonous bite or sting with mild soap and water?

➤ THINKING CRITICALLY

1. **Applying.** While you are jogging through town with some friends, you see that a car has just struck someone on a bicycle. Analyze and describe a strategy for responding to this type of accidental injury. *(LESSON 1)*

2. **Synthesizing.** Why can quick abdominal thrusts dislodge an obstruction in the airway? *(LESSON 2)*

3. **Analyzing.** Explain why you should not try to capture an animal that has bitten someone. *(LESSON 3)*

4. **Evaluating.** Which of the first-aid techniques covered in the chapter would be especially important for a camper or hiker to know? Explain your choices. *(LESSON 4)*

➤ HEALTH SKILLS APPLICATION

1. **Advocacy.** Prepare a talk that encourages younger students in your community to learn first aid. Compile lists of local emergency telephone numbers for distribution. *(LESSON 1)*

2. **Analyzing Influences.** Evaluate the effect of technology on first aid. For example, what techniques and capabilities are available today that were not available 50 years ago? *(LESSON 2)*

3. **Accessing Information.** Research to learn whether your state has a high incidence of rabies and what measures are taken to keep the disease under control. *(LESSON 3)*

4. **Practicing Healthful Behaviors.** Find out which poisonous plants are in your area, how they can be recognized, and what to do in case of exposure to them. Use what you have learned to create a teaching tool, such as a poster or a comic book, for elementary school children. *(LESSON 4)*

BEYOND the Classroom

Parent Involvement

Accessing Information. Learn more about where members of your community can become certified in CPR. With your parents, find out how your family can become involved in promoting CPR certification for everyone. If classes are not available in your community, find out how you can arrange for someone to provide classes in your community.

School and Community

CPR Certification. Train to become certified in CPR. Then research to find out how you can volunteer to help teach others the lifesaving techniques of CPR.

Environmental Health

Recycling Center

How Do You Rate?

Read each statement below and respond by writing *yes, no,* or *sometimes* for each item. Write *yes* only for items that you practice regularly.

1. I conserve water in my home.
2. I turn out lights when leaving a room.
3. I don't litter.
4. I buy products in refillable containers when possible.
5. I avoid buying disposable products when reusable alternatives are available.
6. I use fans instead of turning on the air conditioning whenever possible.
7. I reuse paper and plastic bags that are brought home from the store.
8. I buy recycled paper products when I have the choice.
9. I actively participate in a recycling program in my community.
10. I put on a second layer of clothing rather than turning up the heat if I feel cold at home.

HEALTH Online

For instant feedback on your health status, go to Chapter 29 Health Inventory at **health.glencoe.com**.

Quick *Write*

Using Visuals. Taking care of the environment is everyone's responsibility. In what specific ways do you and your family actively take part in protecting the environment?

Air Quality

VOCABULARY

air pollution
smog
Air Quality Index (AQI)
asbestos
radon
noise pollution
decibel

YOU'LL LEARN TO

- Relate the nation's environmental health goals and objectives to individual, family, and community health.

- Identify sources of air pollution and strategies for reducing it.

- Develop strategies to evaluate information relating to critical environmental health issues.

QUICK START Breathing is something you do without thinking. Write a paragraph explaining how you think breathing polluted air could negatively affect your health.

Air quality affects all living organisms, including humans. *Why is it important to alert the public when air pollution levels are extremely high?*

Modern technology has improved the lives of many people in the world. However, the pollution of air, land, and water that may result from technological advances can harm the environment and therefore people's health.

Air Pollution

Air pollution is a serious problem in this nation. It is linked to an estimated 50,000 to 120,000 premature deaths each year. The U.S. health care costs associated with outdoor air pollution range from $40 to $50 billion per year. For this reason, one goal of *Healthy People 2010* is to reduce the proportion of persons exposed to air that does not meet the U.S. Environmental Protection Agency's (EPA) health-based standards for ozone, a major component of air pollution.

Air pollution is *the contamination of the earth's atmosphere by substances that pose a health threat to living things.* The EPA monitors air quality and sets U.S. air quality standards. The agency has identified five major air pollutants whose levels need to be regulated in order to have cleaner air nationwide. These pollutants are described in **Figure 29.1**.

FIGURE 29.1

FIVE COMMON AIR POLLUTANTS

The EPA has set national air quality standards for these pollutants.

Air Pollutant	Sources	Primary Health Concerns
Ozone (O_3) is a gas composed of three oxygen atoms. Ground-level ozone is a major component of smog, *a yellow-brown haze that forms when sunlight reacts with air pollution.*	O_3 forms from a chemical reaction between nitrogen oxide compounds and volatile organic compounds (VOCs). Motor vehicle exhaust, industrial emissions, gasoline vapors, and chemical solvents are the primary sources of nitrogen oxides and VOCs.	O_3 can irritate and inflame lung airways. It is linked to aggravated asthma, reduced lung capacity, and increased susceptibility to respiratory illnesses such as pneumonia and bronchitis.
Particulate Matter (PM) is a general term for particles such as dust, dirt, soot, smoke, mold, and liquid droplets that are found in the air.	PM may be emitted directly into the air from sources such as motor vehicle exhaust and factories. PM may also form in the air through chemical reactions between gases.	PM is linked to aggravated asthma, chronic bronchitis, decreased lung function, and premature death.
Carbon Monoxide (CO) is a colorless, odorless gas that contains carbon and oxygen. It is formed when carbon in fuel is not burned completely.	Outdoor sources of CO include motor vehicle exhaust and industrial processes. Indoor sources include gas stoves, cigarette smoke, and unvented gas and kerosene space heaters.	CO is poisonous. It prevents the body from receiving the oxygen it needs. It affects people with heart disease and can harm the central nervous system. Large quantities are fatal.
Sulfur Dioxide (SO_2) is a gas made up of sulfur and oxygen. It dissolves in water to form an acid, and it reacts with other gases in the air to form sulfates and other harmful particles.	SO_2 is formed when fuel that contains sulfur (such as coal and oil) is burned, when gasoline is extracted from oil, and when metals are extracted from their ores.	SO_2 contributes to respiratory illnesses and aggravates existing heart and lung diseases.
Nitrogen Oxides (NO_X) is a general term for a group of highly reactive gases that contain varying amounts of nitrogen and oxygen.	These substances form when fuel is burned at high temperatures. Primary sources include motor vehicles and electric utilities.	Nitrogen oxides help form ground-level ozone. They form particles that cause or trigger serious respiratory problems.

Reducing Air Pollution

The Clean Air Act of 1990 regulates the five pollutants described in Figure 29.1. Even with such laws in place, air quality can vary. The **Air Quality Index (AQI)**, developed by the EPA, is *an index for reporting daily air quality.* Shown in **Figure 29.2,** the AQI informs the public about local air quality and whether air pollution levels pose health risks.

You and your family can take the following actions to help reduce air pollution.

▶ **Reduce car use.** Walk or bicycle, take public transportation, or carpool to your destination.

▶ **Conserve energy.** Turn off lights when not in use. Set the air conditioner at a higher temperature. Put on extra layers of clothing instead of turning up the heat.

▶ **Use air-friendly machinery.** Small motors such as those found on mowers, chain saws, and leaf blowers emit pollutants. Use manual machinery when possible.

FIGURE 29.2

AIR QUALITY INDEX (AQI)

The AQI alerts people to possible health concerns of breathing polluted air.

Range	Air Quality	Color Code
0 to 50	**Good:** There is little or no health risk.	Green
51 to 100	**Moderate:** Some pollutants may pose a health concern for a small number of individuals.	Yellow
101 to 150	**Unhealthy for Sensitive Groups:** Unless a person has specific health concerns, pollution levels in this range are not likely to cause health problems.	Orange
151 to 200	**Unhealthy:** All individuals may experience some minor negative effects.	Red
201 to 300	**Very Unhealthy:** More serious effects may be felt by all individuals.	Purple
301 to 500	**Hazardous:** Entire population is at risk.	Maroon

Indoor Air Pollution

Most people spend about 90 percent of their time indoors. EPA studies indicate that indoor levels of certain pollutants may be 2 to 5 times—and on occasion more than 100 times—higher than outdoor levels. Sources of indoor air pollution include building and furnishing materials such as carpeting and furniture made of certain pressed woods. Another source is old insulation containing **asbestos** (as-BES-tuhs), *a fibrous mineral that has fireproof properties*. When materials containing asbestos deteriorate, tiny fibers of the mineral are released into the air. Household cleaning products and other chemicals also contribute to indoor air pollution. Another major source is the particles and gases that form as a result of combustion. Stoves, furnaces, fireplaces, heaters, and tobacco smoke can all contaminate indoor air. Inadequate ventilation increases the problem. Energy-efficient homes may have so little air exchange that pollutants build up to dangerous levels.

Health Concerns of Indoor Air Pollution

The effects of indoor air pollution depend on the contaminant and the length of exposure. Immediate health concerns include irritation of the eyes, nose, and throat; headaches; dizziness; and fatigue. Long-term exposure to some pollutants can cause asthma. Exposure to lead, especially in children, can damage the kidneys, liver, brain, and nerves. Asbestos has been linked to lung cancer, especially in people who smoke. High levels of carbon monoxide can cause death.

The EPA estimates that **radon**, *an odorless, radioactive gas,* causes at least 14,000 lung cancer deaths per year. Radon is produced during the natural breakdown of the element uranium in soil, rocks, and water. It can seep into a house through cracks in the foundation. Home testing is the only way to assess exposure to radon. Homes with high levels of radon require increased indoor-outdoor air exchange. Some may need structural work to reduce radon levels.

Managing Indoor Air Pollution

To manage indoor air pollution, you must first identify the contaminants. Often, removing or replacing an object or appliance and providing sufficient indoor-outdoor air exchange will solve the problem. Make sure that hot water heaters and furnaces are properly vented and operating efficiently to avoid a buildup of carbon monoxide. Many families have installed carbon monoxide detectors to warn of a toxic buildup. Similar detectors are available for radon. Homeowners who discover the presence of asbestos or lead should seek professional help in removing these contaminants.

What is sick building syndrome?

The term *sick building syndrome* (SBS) refers to a situation in which the occupants of a building experience health problems that seem to be linked to the atmosphere within the building. Symptoms of SBS include headache; itchy and irritated eyes, throat, or nose; dizziness and nausea; fatigue; inability to concentrate; and a sensitivity to odors. SBS sufferers often report relief soon after leaving the building.

For more information on ways to minimize indoor air pollution, click on Web Links at health.glencoe.com.

Real-Life Application

Indoor Air Pollution and Asthma: What You Can Do

The incidence of asthma in people of all ages is increasing. Indoor air pollution has been identified as a major contributor to this increase. Study the graph, answer the questions on the right, and then complete the activity.

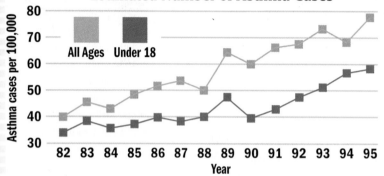

Estimated Number of Asthma Cases

All Ages   Under 18

Asthma cases per 100,000

Year: 82 83 84 85 86 87 88 89 90 91 92 93 94 95

Source: National Center for Health Statistics, National Health Survey, 1982–1995

ACTIVITY

Work with a small group. Use reliable library and online sources to investigate additional measures that can improve indoor air quality. Cite your sources, and provide an explanation of why each source is reliable.

What can be done to reduce the levels of such triggers as dust and pet dander in the home?

In the 1960s children and teens were outside at least three hours each day. Today, they are outside less than two hours each day. How might these facts relate to the increase in asthma?

Today's homes allow less air to circulate. How might this contribute to the increase in asthma? What can be done to increase ventilation?

Tobacco smoke is one of the leading contributors to asthma attacks. How can exposure to tobacco smoke be limited or prevented?

Noise Pollution

Traffic, loud music, and power tools such as mowers and construction equipment are all sources of noise pollution. **Noise pollution** is *harmful and unwanted sound of sufficient intensity to damage hearing.* Hearing impairment caused by noise rarely leads to total deafness; however, the hearing loss is permanent, and hearing aids often do not compensate for the damage.

A **decibel** is *a unit used to express the relative intensity of loudness of sound.* Normal conversation is about 65 decibels. Exposure to noise levels of 85 decibels and above can result in temporary hearing loss, often accompanied by ringing in the ears. Normal hearing will usually return, but continued exposure can lead to permanent hearing loss. **Figure 29.3** shows the decibel levels of various sounds.

FIGURE 29.3

DECIBEL LEVELS OF COMMON SOUNDS

Weakest sound heard by the average ear

Constant exposure at 85 decibels or greater may cause hearing loss.

Tractor, motorcycle, snowmobile

Ambulance siren, amplified music

Rocket launch

Normal conversation

Hair dryer, power lawn mower

Chain saw

Jet engine at takeoff

| 0 | 65 | 85 | 90 | 100 | 110 | 120 | 140 | 180 |

Reducing Noise Pollution

There are several ways to reduce noise pollution in your environment. Be sure to keep the volume down on stereos, radios, and television sets. Avoid unnecessary use of the car horn. When possible, use manual tools instead of power tools.

Lesson 1 Review

Reviewing Facts and Vocabulary

1. Define *air pollution* and *noise pollution*.
2. Describe the EPA's role in monitoring air quality.
3. List two actions you can take to help reduce noise pollution.

Thinking Critically

4. **Evaluation.** Relate the nation's environmental health goals and objectives in *Healthy People 2010* to the health of individuals, families, and communities.
5. **Analyzing.** Imagine that the media has reported an AQI of 175. Paul, who has asthma, can't decide whether he wants to go in-line skating outdoors or play basketball in the air-conditioned gym. Determine which choice is healthier for Paul and explain your decision.

Applying Health Skills

Accessing Information. Think of a specific critical health issue related to air pollution. Find information on this topic, and develop strategies to evaluate the source of your information. Make a list of these strategies.

TECHNOLOGY OPTION

WORD PROCESSING   Use word processing to produce your list of strategies. See health.glencoe.com for help in using word-processing software.

Protecting Land and Water

VOCABULARY
biodegradable
landfill
hazardous waste
deforestation
urban sprawl
wastewater

YOU'LL LEARN TO

• Identify sources of land and water pollution.

• Assess the impact of population on community and world health.

• Analyze the influence of laws on health-related environmental issues.

• Examine strategies for reducing land and water pollution.

QUICK START Write a brief public service announcement encouraging people to help keep lakes, rivers, and streams free of pollution.

Most wastes are disposed of in landfills and covered with soil to prevent the spread of disease by insects and rodents.

The wastes generated by human activity can pollute both land and water. However, there are many actions people can take to reduce pollution and help preserve land and water resources.

Waste Disposal

Many wastes are **biodegradable**, or *able to be broken down by microorganisms in the environment*. However, when biodegradable materials are discarded in quantities too large for nature to handle, or when materials are not biodegradable, other waste disposal solutions must be found.

Solid Waste

Much solid waste ends up in landfills. A **landfill** is *an area that has been safeguarded to prevent disposed wastes from contaminating groundwater*. Landfills must be located away from certain areas to protect groundwater (water that collects under the earth's surface) and must be lined with special materials to prevent leakage. Landfill operators must follow practices that reduce odor and control disease-carrying insects and rodents.

FIGURE 29.4

HAZARDOUS WASTES

Source/Activity That Generates Waste	Type of Waste Produced
Arts and crafts (e.g., painting, building models)	Solvents, paints, adhesives
Dry cleaning	Solvents
Construction	Oils, solvents, paints
Vehicle maintenance	Solvents, paints, ignitable wastes, used oil and batteries
Yardwork and gardening	Pesticides, herbicides, solvents
Household tasks	Solvents, oils, cleaning materials, paints, paint thinner

Hazardous Waste

A **hazardous waste** is *a substance that is explosive, corrosive, highly reactive, or toxic to humans or other life forms.* Industrial processes generate some hazardous wastes. Others are generated by common activities, including those described in **Figure 29.4.** Household products such as batteries are also considered hazardous wastes. Many of these wastes are banned from landfills and must be disposed of at special collection sites so that they don't contaminate the environment.

Nuclear wastes, a collection of radioactive materials that pose serious hazards to humans and other life forms, are a type of hazardous waste. Exposure to radiation can increase the risk of cancer. It can also alter a person's sex cells, causing genetic abnormalities to be passed on to offspring. Because of the long decay rates of some radioactive materials, these materials must be isolated in secure facilities for thousands of years.

Expansion and Development

Throughout history population growth has been accelerating. It took half a million years for humankind to reach a population size of 1 billion, but the next billion people were born in a span of only 80 years, and close to 1½ billion more have been born since 1975. In certain U.S. and world regions where population growth is rapid, there is a low quality of life and much human suffering. Rapid population growth also leads to swift deterioration of the land and to a severe drain on resources such as water.

Urban development can also have a dramatic impact on the land. As new cities are built, room for them must be cleared. This clearing has been at the expense of wilderness areas and rain forests.

Disappearing Forests

Developing nations in Central America, Africa, and Southeast Asia are rapidly expanding in agriculture and industry. These nations have been clearing tropical forests on a massive scale for fuel and to make way for farms and ranch land. This **deforestation**, or *destruction of forests,* has upset the fragile balance of nature.

Aside from providing a home to countless plant and animal species, the world's great forests play a vital part in controlling soil erosion, flooding, and sediment buildup in rivers, lakes, and reservoirs. Deforestation interferes with these processes. It can also change regional patterns of rainfall as a result of altered rates of evaporation, transpiration (vapor exhaled from the surface of green plants), and run-off. Without trees, precipitation declines and the region grows hotter and drier. Ultimately, desertlike conditions prevail where there were once rich, tropical grasslands.

Using public transportation instead of driving reduces pollution and helps conserve resources. *How might an efficient public transportation system improve community health?*

Urban Sprawl

The spreading of city development (houses, shopping centers, businesses, and schools) onto undeveloped land is called **urban sprawl**. As the land surrounding cities becomes developed, environmental problems can occur. Runoff from parking lots and fertilized lawns may contaminate the drinking water supply. Air quality worsens as increased automobile and lawnmower usage adds more engine exhaust to the air.

To help address the problem of urban sprawl, city planners are rethinking the way suburbs are organized to help reduce consumption of natural resources and decrease the amount of pollution. In planned communities, schools and businesses are located within walking distance of homes, and sidewalks are required. Walking the short distances from home to work, school, or shopping provides physical activity for pedestrians, saves resources, and reduces pollution. The inclusion of efficient public transportation in these communities helps reduce the number of people driving to work. Consequently, fewer vehicles are on the highways, reducing both the level of pollution and the number of injuries and deaths caused by traffic accidents.

Water Supplies and Pollution

The EPA requires water suppliers to monitor and test water before sending it through municipal or community water systems. If the water is contaminated, the supplier must shut down the system and fix the problem. No agencies monitor the quality of water coming from private wells, however. Water treatment and purity depend on actions taken by those who use the well.

All drinking water is susceptible to pollution. Because the water can come from large sources such as rivers, lakes, or aquifers (water-bearing layers of rock, sand, or gravel) that underlie several counties or states, the pollution source can be far away from where the water is used.

Polluted Runoff

About 40 percent of the nation's rivers, lakes, and coastal waters are not safe for swimming or other types of water recreation. Water pollution is sometimes caused by illegal dumping of industrial chemical wastes, but a greater contamination problem is created by pollution that comes from many sources throughout the environment. Most surface water contamination is caused by polluted runoff—rainwater or snowmelt that runs over the land, picking up such contaminants as pesticides, fertilizers, and wastes. Polluted runoff can also contaminate groundwater, the primary source of drinking water for millions of people in the United States.

Wastewater

Wastewater, *used water that comes from homes, communities, farms, and businesses,* is another source of water pollution. Along with sewage, wastewater includes water that is generated and discharged from industries, feedlots, and many other sources. Wastewater contains harmful substances such as human or animal wastes, metals, and pathogens. Some wastewater must be treated by cooling in order to prevent thermal pollution. Thermal pollution occurs when the temperature of discharged water is higher than the temperature of a body of water in the environment. Because this hot water can disrupt aquatic ecosystems, it must be cooled before it enters the environment. The EPA regulates the treatment and discharge of wastewater under the Clean Water Act. Treated water that is released back into the environment must be safe for humans and other living organisms.

Other Sources of Water Pollution

Other sources of water pollution include:

▶ **Sediment.** Sediment from land erosion can destroy aquatic ecosystems and clog lakes, stream channels, and harbors.

▶ **Oil.** Some oil contamination comes from the cleaning of oil tankers and the release of oil from offshore drilling rigs. Problems can also occur when people dump used motor oil or household chemicals down household and storm drains.

Polluted runoff is a major source of water pollution in the United States.

Reducing the Risks

You and your family can take steps to help keep our land and water clean.

▶ Recycle materials whenever possible to reduce the amount of waste going to landfills. You'll learn more about reducing solid wastes in Lesson 3.

▶ Dispose of all materials properly. Don't put oil paints, paint solvents, or batteries into the trash. Don't pour household chemicals or motor oil down the drain or onto the ground. Instead, take these and other hazardous materials to the appropriate collection sites.

▶ Follow directions when using chemicals such as cleaning products, fertilizers, and pesticides, and don't overuse them.

▶ Reduce water usage. Repair leaky faucets. Follow the recommendations for landscape watering that apply to your area. Reducing water usage decreases the amount of water that must be treated.

▶ Lesson 2 *Review*

Reviewing Facts and Vocabulary

1. What is a *landfill*?
2. Assess the impact of population on community and world health.
3. How can polluted runoff contaminate water supplies?

Thinking Critically

4. **Applying.** Analyze how laws like the Clean Water Act positively influence health and prevent disease.
5. **Analyzing.** You have probably heard the saying, "Water, water everywhere, but not a drop to drink." Explain this statement in terms of available drinking water.

Applying Health Skills

Advocacy. Create a comic book about a superhero named Captain Cleanup and his or her adventures cleaning up land and water pollution. The comic book should be targeted to elementary school students and contain a strong message about what young people can do to reduce land and water pollution.

WEB SITES Use your comic book as part of a Web page you develop on reducing pollution. See **health.glencoe.com** for help in planning and building your own Web site.

Advocating for a Healthy Environment

VOCABULARY
conservation
precycling
recycling

YOU'LL LEARN TO

* Identify strategies for conserving resources, precycling, and recycling.

* Develop strategies for protecting the environment.

* Describe a variety of community and world environmental protection programs.

QUICK START   Make a list of the environmental benefits of participating in a recycling program.

Many of today's environmental problems result from the lifestyle and consumer choices we make. In this lesson you'll learn about what you can do to protect the health of the environment.

Conserving Resources

Most natural resources don't exist in an endless supply. The coal, natural gas, and petroleum we use for fuel took millions of years to form. It takes about 20 years for a tree to become large enough to cut for use as paper. These examples illustrate the need to conserve our natural resources. **Conservation** is *the protection and preservation of the environment by managing natural resources to prevent abuse, destruction, and neglect.* The actions that you and your family take at home have an impact on the environment. Some actions you can take to conserve natural resources are featured on the next page.

Planting trees helps replenish this natural resource. *How do trees benefit the environment?*

Heating and Cooling

▶ Seal leaks around doors, windows, and electrical sockets to prevent heated or cooled air from escaping. Keep doors and windows shut and close fireplace vents when the fireplace is not in use to keep cooled or heated air inside the home.

▶ During heating season, wear an extra layer of clothing instead of turning up the thermostat. Keep the thermostat at about 68°F. For further conservation, turn the thermostat down at bedtime.

▶ Keep the thermostat at about 78°F during air-conditioning season. Use a fan to keep air circulating— this will make the area feel cooler.

Water Conservation

▶ Wash clothes in warm or cold, not hot, water. Accumulate a full load before washing laundry or running the dishwasher.

▶ Fix leaky faucets, and never let water run unnecessarily. Turning off the water while brushing your teeth or shaving can save 4.5 gallons of water per minute.

▶ If you have a large-capacity toilet tank, fill plastic bottles with water, seal them, and place them in the tank. The bottles will keep the tank from filling completely, which will save up to a gallon of water per flush.

Lighting and Appliances

▶ Replace traditional lightbulbs with compact fluorescent bulbs, which use less energy and last longer.

▶ Switch off lights when you leave a room.

▶ Turn off televisions, radios, computers, and other appliances when they are not in use.

▶ Use a microwave or toaster oven instead of a conventional oven when cooking a small amount of food.

▶ Don't preheat a conventional oven for longer than necessary. Avoid opening the oven door unnecessarily while the appliance is in use.

Precycling and Recycling

The easiest, most cost-efficient way of conserving natural resources is reducing the quantity of waste. Precycling and recycling are two ways of accomplishing this goal.

Precycling

Precycling—*reducing waste before it is generated*—means purchasing and using products wisely. How can you precycle? Reduce your use of products that are used once and then discarded. For example, try using cloth napkins instead of paper ones. Purchase products in bulk or in the largest package appropriate for your use to reduce excess packaging. Buying products such as laundry detergent or fruit juice as concentrates also reduces packaging. Choose products designed to be recycled. For example, look for the code on plastic packages. Those that carry a 1, 2, or 3 are most easily recycled.

Precycling also involves reusing materials. Reusing paper or plastic shopping bags or carrying your own cloth bags is a form of precycling. So is donating unneeded household goods or clothing to charities instead of discarding them.

▼ **Carrying your own cloth bags instead of using paper or plastic ones is one way to precycle.**
What is another example of precycling?

Recycling

Recycling is *the processing of waste materials so that they can be used again.* Recycling has several benefits:

▶ **Recycling conserves resources.** Both energy and raw materials are conserved by recycling. For example, making a can from recycled aluminum takes only 10 percent of the energy needed to make a new can from raw materials.

▶ **Recycling reduces reliance on landfills.** Landfill space is limited, and it cannot keep up with increasing demands. Because of this, it is important to reduce the amount of waste that gets deposited in landfills.

▶ **Recycling protects environmental health.** Recycling utilizes materials that might otherwise harm the environment if disposed of in landfills. Thus, recycling efforts lead to a cleaner and more healthful environment.

Hands-On Health ACTIVITY

One Planet—Your Role

In this activity you will create a chart that demonstrates the need to conserve resources.

What You'll Need

- pen or pencil and notebook paper
- poster board or construction paper
- markers

What You'll Do

1. Divide a sheet of paper into three columns. Label the columns "Items I Throw Away Every Week," "Ways of Precycling or Recycling," and "Why It Matters."

2. List at least five items in the first column, and complete the other two columns for those items.

3. Work in a small group. Combine the best ideas and create a poster-sized chart, similar to the one on your sheet of paper, that includes several ways to precycle or recycle commonly used items. Use persuasive language, and illustrate your group's chart.

4. Present the chart to the class. Then display it in the classroom or in a school hallway.

Apply and Conclude

Find statistics on how precycling and recycling help reduce waste and pollution. Be sure to relate the data to the actions described in your poster.

Manufacturers put codes on plastic containers to give consumers information on how to recycle.

TIPS FOR RECYCLING AND REDUCING WASTE

More than 80 percent of household waste can be recycled. The following are some guidelines for specific recyclable materials.

▶ **Aluminum.** Rinse cans and other aluminum items such as pie pans and frozen food trays. Crush them to save space.

▶ **Cardboard.** Flatten cardboard boxes and tie them together.

▶ **Glass.** Rinse all glass containers. Recycle metal lids separately.

▶ **Plastics.** Look for the code on the container. Most recyclers take those marked with a 1, 2, or 3.

▶ **Newspaper.** Stack newspapers and tie the bundles with string or rope, or place the papers in paper shopping bags for easy handling.

▶ **Glossy Paper.** Contact services that help you remove your name from mailing lists. Find out whether a local retirement or community center can use discarded magazines. What you can't eliminate or redistribute, recycle.

Protecting the Environment

Here are some practical suggestions for becoming involved in protecting the environment:

▶ **Become an informed consumer.** Evaluate products with regard to their impact on natural resources. Give feedback to companies on ways they can help protect the environment.

▶ **Contact organizations that promote the conservation of resources and educate people on environmental issues.** Ask for ideas on how to conserve natural resources. Consider joining an environmental organization. Most of these organizations can give you information on current environmental issues. They can also suggest ways to promote the health of the environment.

▶ **Take action against local polluters.** The environmental problems in your community directly affect your health. Targeting local polluters is an effective way of protecting your health and that of your family and neighbors. Join with others to inform elected officials of your concerns.

 Lesson 3 *Review*

Reviewing Facts and Vocabulary

1. Define the term *conservation*.
2. What is the difference between *precycling* and *recycling*?
3. List three environmental benefits of recycling.

Thinking Critically

4. **Analyzing.** How does conserving resources protect the health of the environment?
5. **Applying.** Develop strategies to conserve natural resources in your home. List three strategies not included in this lesson that your family can undertake to conserve resources.

Applying Health Skills

Accessing Information. Research and describe a variety of environmental protection programs, both in your community and in countries throughout the world. Create a chart to display the information that you obtain. Include the name of the community or country, the name of the program, and a brief description of the program's mission.

SPREADSHEETS Use a spreadsheet to organize your information and create your chart. See **health.glencoe.com** for tips on how to create and use a spreadsheet.

Environmental Health in the News

In this activity, you will answer the following questions in order to compare and contrast how articles from two different print media cover the same environmental health issue.

Questions to Answer

1. What aspect of the environmental health issue does each article address?

2. How does each article convey the subject matter to the reader?

3. How does each article link the environmental issue to specific health problems?

4. Does each article include comments from environmental health experts, scientists, physicians, and/or politicians?

5. Can you detect any bias in either article?

6. Do the articles provide relevant information about how the issue affects a specific community?

7. Do the articles provide a regional or global perspective on the issue?

8. In your opinion, which source provides better coverage of the issue? Why?

ACTIVITY

Think of a specific environmental health issue. Then, locate articles in two different types of print media that pertain to this topic. You can choose from your local newspaper; a major city newspaper, such as the *New York Times* or the *Washington Post;* or a national news magazine, such as *Time* or *Newsweek*. Write an analysis of how these two different sources cover the same topic. Use the answers to the questions above to guide your analysis.

EXPRESS YOUR VIEWS

Healthy People 2010 has a number of goals that relate to environmental health issues that affect all Americans. Review these goals, and write a position paper that suggests how the media sources you analyzed have played or can play a role in helping reach the goals.

CROSS-CURRICULUM CONNECTIONS

Compose a Haiku. Think about something in the natural environment that inspires you, such as a bird in flight, a shooting star, or the soothing sounds of a stream. Compose a haiku, a Japanese form of poetry that often focuses on nature, on the subject you've chosen. Use vivid language to describe a certain aspect of your subject, such as its shape, size, or color.

Conduct Team Research. The health of humans is undeniably linked to the health of the environment. Over the past 40 years, the environmental movement has worked to clean up the earth. Work with a team to research a specific environmental organization, such as the Sierra Club or the U.S. Fish & Wildlife Service. Report to the class on the history of the organization and its purpose and goals.

Compute the Cost. The health-related costs of outdoor air pollution range from $40 to $50 billion per year. Suppose that in a certain year, the health costs of air pollution were $45 billion. Given a U.S. population of 281.4 million people, how much does health care related to air pollution cost each person in this particular year?

Write a Report. Some people may think that air pollution is solely the result of human activity. However, there have always been natural sources of air pollution, such as dust storms. Use reliable online and print resources to find information on various natural sources of air pollution. Summarize your findings in a brief report.

Environmental Engineering Technician

Would you like to improve the quality of the environment? If so, you might enjoy a career as an environmental engineering technician.

Environmental engineering technicians work closely with environmental engineers and scientists in developing methods and devices used in the prevention, control, or correction of environmental hazards.

To become an environmental engineering technician, you will need a two-year associate's degree or extensive on-the-job training. Find out more about this and other health careers by clicking on Career Corner at **health.glencoe.com**.

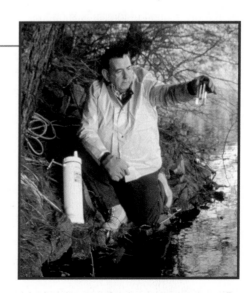

Chapter 29 *Review*

> **EXPLORING HEALTH TERMS** *Answer the following questions on a sheet of paper.*

Lesson 1 *Match each definition with the correct term.*

air pollution   noise pollution
asbestos   radon
decibel   smog
Air Quality Index (AQI)

1. A yellow-brown haze that forms when sunlight reacts with air pollution.
2. An index for reporting daily air quality.
3. A fibrous mineral that has fireproof properties.
4. An odorless, radioactive gas that can cause cancer.
5. A unit used to express the relative intensity of loudness of sound.

Lesson 2 *Fill in the blanks with the correct term.*

landfill   biodegradable
deforestation   urban sprawl
hazardous waste   wastewater

6. _____ wastes can be broken down by microorganisms in the environment.
7. A substance that is explosive, corrosive, highly reactive, or toxic to humans or other life forms is known as _____ .
8. The destruction of forests is known as _____ .
9. The spreading of city development onto undeveloped land is called _____ .
10. _____ is used water that comes from homes, communities, farms, and businesses.

Lesson 3 *Replace the underlined words with the correct term.*

precycling   conservation
recycling

11. <u>Recycling</u> is the protection and preservation of the environment by managing natural resources.
12. <u>Conservation</u> involves making decisions about products *before* you purchase them in order to reduce waste.
13. The processing of materials so that they can be used again in some form is <u>precycling</u>.

> **RECALLING THE FACTS** *Use complete sentences to answer the following questions.*

Lesson 1

1. Name five common air pollutants.
2. List two strategies for managing indoor air pollution.
3. Temporary hearing loss may occur when a person is exposed to noise levels at or above what decibel level?

Lesson 2

4. If many wastes are biodegradable, why are landfills necessary?
5. What is nuclear waste?
6. List three sources of water pollution and two ways of reducing this type of pollution.

Lesson 3

7. Name three ways to conserve natural resources.
8. List three precycling strategies.
9. What are three practical ways to become involved in protecting the environment?

➤ THINKING CRITICALLY

1. **Evaluating.** Explain how keeping your automobile engine in good condition can reduce air pollution. *(LESSON 1)*

2. **Analyzing.** Before the development of modern landfills, trash was discarded in pits or open dumps. Explain how today's landfills are an improvement over this waste-disposal strategy. *(LESSON 2)*

3. **Applying.** List three grocery store items that create excessive waste. Suggest an alternative for each item. *(LESSON 3)*

➤ HEALTH SKILLS APPLICATION

1. **Accessing Information.** Choose one of the five air pollutants tracked by the EPA. Research whether that pollutant is present in the air in your community. Write a brief report summarizing your findings. *(LESSON 1)*

2. **Advocacy.** Polluted runoff may occur as a result of heavy rains that pick up fertilizers and pesticides from lawns. Write a public service announcement encouraging people to carefully follow application instructions for these products. *(LESSON 2)*

3. **Goal Setting.** Talk with your family about ways to conserve natural resources. Then use the goal-setting steps to choose and work toward a family conservation goal. As part of the goal-setting process, have each family member sign a pledge to do his or her part to conserve resources. *(LESSON 3)*

BEYOND the Classroom

Parent Involvement

Accessing Information. Find out what materials are recycled in your community. Work with a parent or other adult family member to interview managers of several recycling centers or hazardous waste collection sites. Put together an informative pamphlet that describes local waste management and recycling services. Make your pamphlet available to other families in your neighborhood.

School and Community

Volunteering Opportunities. Locate a recycling center or charitable organization in your community that collects donated items for resale. Contact the agency to find out what volunteer positions are available. Share what you have learned with your classmates.

Appendix Table of Contents

		HEALTH SKILLS	NATIONAL HEALTH EDUCATION STANDARDS
		Comprehending Concepts	Students will comprehend concepts related to health promotion and disease prevention.
ACCESSING INFORMATION		Accessing Information	Students will demonstrate the ability to access valid health information and health-promoting products and services.
PRACTICING HEALTHFUL BEHAVIORS	STRESS MANAGEMENT	Practicing Healthful Behaviors Stress Management	Students will demonstrate the ability to practice health-enhancing behaviors and reduce health risks.
ANALYZING INFLUENCES		Analyzing Influences	Students will analyze the influence of culture, media, technology, and other factors on health.
COMMUNICATION SKILLS / CONFLICT RESOLUTION / REFUSAL SKILLS		Communication Skills Conflict Resolution Refusal Skills	Students will demonstrate the ability to use interpersonal communication skills to enhance health.
DECISION MAKING / GOAL SETTING		Decision Making Goal Setting	Students will demonstrate the ability to use goal-setting and decision-making skills to enhance health.
ADVOCACY		Advocacy	Students will demonstrate the ability to advocate for personal, family, and community health.

Healthy People 2010

Healthy People 2010 is a set of 28 health objectives established for the nation to achieve over the first decade of the new century. The objectives, listed on these pages, were created after the Surgeon General's Report in 2000 identified specific National Health Promotion and Disease Prevention goals. The chapters and lessons in *Glencoe Health* provide strategies for addressing many of the objectives of *Healthy People 2010.*

1. **Access to Quality Health Services** Improve access to comprehensive, high-quality health care services.

2. **Arthritis, Osteoporosis, and Chronic Back Conditions** Prevent illness and disability related to arthritis and other rheumatic conditions, osteoporosis, and chronic back conditions.

3. **Cancer** Reduce the number of new cancer cases as well as the illness, disability, and death caused by cancer.

4. **Chronic Kidney Disease** Reduce new cases of chronic kidney disease and its complications, disability, death, and economic costs.

5. **Diabetes** Through prevention programs, reduce the disease and economic burden of diabetes, and improve the quality of life for all persons who have or are at risk for diabetes.

6. **Disability and Secondary Conditions** Promote the health of people with disabilities, prevent secondary conditions, and eliminate disparities between people with and without disabilities in the U.S. population.

7. **Educational and Community-Based Programs** Increase the quality, availability, and effectiveness of educational and community-based programs designed to prevent disease and improve health and quality of life.

8. **Environmental Health** Promote health for all through a healthy environment.

9. **Family Planning** Includes preventing unintended pregnancy.

10. **Food Safety** Reduce foodborne illnesses.

11. **Health Communication** Use communication strategically to improve health.

12. **Heart Disease and Stroke** Improve cardiovascular health and quality of life through the prevention, detection, and treatment of risk factors; early identification and treatment of heart attacks and strokes; and prevention of recurrent cardiovascular events.

13. **HIV** Prevent human immunodeficiency virus (HIV) infection and its related illness and death.

14. Immunization and Infectious Diseases Prevent disease, disability, and death from infectious diseases, including vaccine-preventable diseases.

15. Injury and Violence Prevention Reduce injuries, disabilities, and deaths due to unintentional injuries and violence.

16. Maternal, Infant, and Child Health Improve the health and well-being of women, infants, children, and families.

17. Medical Product Safety Ensure the safe and effective use of medical products.

18. Mental Health and Mental Disorders Improve mental health and ensure access to appropriate, quality mental health services.

19. Nutrition and Overweight Promote health and reduce chronic disease associated with diet and weight.

20. Occupational Safety and Health Promote the health and safety of people at work through prevention and early intervention.

21. Oral Health Prevent and control oral and craniofacial diseases, conditions, and injuries, and improve access to related services.

22. Physical Activity and Fitness Improve health, fitness, and quality of life through daily physical activity.

23. Public Health Infrastructure Ensure that Federal, Tribal, State, and local health agencies have the infrastructure to provide essential public health services effectively.

24. Respiratory Diseases Promote respiratory health through better prevention, detection, treatment, and education efforts.

25. Sexually Transmitted Diseases Promote responsible sexual behaviors, strengthen community capacity, and increase access to quality services to prevent sexually transmitted diseases (STDs) and their complications.

26. Substance Abuse Reduce substance abuse to protect the health, safety, and quality of life for all, especially children.

27. Tobacco Reduce illness, disability, and death related to tobacco use and exposure to secondhand smoke.

28. Vision and Hearing Improve the visual and hearing health of the Nation through prevention, early detection, treatment, and rehabilitation.

40 Developmental Assets

Search Institute has identified the following building blocks of healthy development that help young people grow up healthy, caring, and responsible.

External Assets

Support

1. **Family support**—Family life provides high levels of love and support.
2. **Positive Family Communication**—Young person and her or his parent(s) communicate positively, and young person is willing to seek advice and counsel from parents.
3. **Other Adult Relationships**—Young person receives support from three or more nonparent adults.
4. **Caring Neighborhood**—Young person experiences caring neighbors.
5. **Caring School Climate**—School provides a caring, encouraging environment.
6. **Parent Involvement in Schooling**—Parent(s) are actively involved in helping young person succeed in school.

Empowerment

7. **Community Values Youth**—Young person perceives that adults in the community value youth.
8. **Youth as Resources**—Young people are given useful roles in the community.
9. **Service to Others**—Young person serves in the community one hour or more per week.
10. **Safety**—Young person feels safe at home, school, and in the neighborhood.

Boundaries and Expectations

11. **Family Boundaries**—Family has clear rules and consequences and monitors the young person's whereabouts.
12. **School Boundaries**—School provides clear rules and consequences.
13. **Neighborhood Boundaries**—Neighbors take responsibility for monitoring young people's behavior.
14. **Adult Role Models**—Parent(s) and other adults model positive, responsible behavior.
15. **Positive Peer Influence**—Young person's best friends model responsible behavior.
16. **High Expectations**—Both parent(s) and teachers encourage the young person to do well.

Constructive Use of Time

17. **Creative Activities**—Young person spends three or more hours per week in lessons or practice in music, theater, or other arts.
18. **Youth Programs**—Young person spends three or more hours per week in sports, clubs, or organizations at school and/or in the community.
19. **Religious Community**—Young person spends one or more hours per week in activities in a religious institution.
20. **Time at Home**—Young person is out with friends "with nothing special to do" two or fewer nights per week.

Internal Assets

Commitment to Learning

21. **Achievement Motivation**—Young person is motivated to do well in school.
22. **School Engagement**—Young person is actively engaged in learning.
23. **Homework**—Young person reports doing at least one hour of homework every school day.
24. **Bonding to School**—Young person cares about her or his school.
25. **Reading for Pleasure**—Young person reads for pleasure three or more hours per week.

Positive Values

26. **Caring**—Young person places high value on helping other people.
27. **Equality and Social Justice**—Young person places high value on promoting equality and reducing hunger and poverty.
28. **Integrity**—Young person acts on convictions and stands up for her or his beliefs.
29. **Honesty**—Young person "tells the truth even when it is not easy."
30. **Responsibility**—Young person accepts and takes personal responsibility.
31. **Restraint**—Young person believes it is important not to be sexually active or to use alcohol or other drugs.

Social Competencies

32. **Planning and Decision Making**—Young person knows how to plan ahead and make choices.
33. **Interpersonal Competence**—Young person has empathy, sensitivity, and friendship skills.
34. **Cultural Competence**—Young person has knowledge of and comfort with people of different cultural/racial/ethnic backgrounds.
35. **Resistance Skills**—Young person can resist negative peer pressure and dangerous situations.
36. **Peaceful Conflict Resolution**—Young person seeks to resolve conflict nonviolently.

Positive Identity

37. **Personal Power**—Young person feels he or she has control over the "things that happen to me."
38. **Self-Esteem**—Young person reports having a high self-esteem.
39. **Sense of Purpose**—Young person reports that "my life has a purpose."
40. **Positive View of Personal Future**—Young person is optimistic about her or his personal future.

PHYSICAL ACTIVITY AND FITNESS GUIDELINES

The Surgeon General's Report on Physical Activity and Health, along with the President's Council on Physical Fitness and Sports, identified fitness as a major public health concern. The Physical Fitness Objectives from *Healthy People 2010* for children and adolescents appear below.

Physical Activity in Children and Adolescents

- Increase the proportion of adolescents who engage in moderate physical activity for at least 30 minutes on 5 or more of the previous 7 days.

- Increase the proportion of adolescents who engage in vigorous physical activity that promotes cardiorespiratory fitness 3 or more days per week for 20 or more minutes per occasion.

- Increase the proportion of the nation's public and private schools that require daily physical education for all students.

- Increase the proportion of adolescents who participate in daily school physical education.

- Increase the proportion of adolescents who spend at least 50 percent of school physical education class time being physically active.

- Increase the proportion of adolescents who view television 2 or fewer hours on a school day.

PHYSICAL FITNESS GUIDELINES

Regular physical activity performed on a daily basis reduces the risk of developing illness or disease. Moderate physical activity can be achieved in a variety of ways, and the Centers for Disease Control and Prevention have developed this list of examples showing moderate amounts of activity that can contribute to an individual's health.

Physical Activities Arranged by Energy Level and Time

- Washing and waxing a car for 45–60 minutes
- Washing windows or floors for 45–60 minutes
- Playing volleyball for 45 minutes
- Playing touch football for 30–45 minutes
- Gardening for 30–45 minutes
- Wheeling self in wheelchair for 30–40 minutes
- Walking 1 $\frac{3}{4}$ miles in 35 minutes (20 min/mile)
- Basketball (shooting baskets) for 30 minutes
- Bicycling 5 miles in 30 minutes
- Dancing fast (social) for 30 minutes
- Pushing a stroller 1 $\frac{1}{2}$ miles in 30 minutes

- Raking leaves for 30 minutes
- Walking 2 miles in 30 minutes (15 min/mile)
- Water aerobics for 30 minutes
- Swimming laps for 20 minutes
- Wheelchair basketball for 20 minutes
- Basketball (playing a game) for 15–20 minutes
- Bicycling 4 miles in 15 minutes
- Jumping rope for 15 minutes
- Running 1 $\frac{1}{2}$ miles in 15 minutes (10 min/mile)
- Shoveling snow for 15 minutes
- Stair walking for 15 minutes

Source: CDC, Physical Activity and Health, A Report of the Surgeon General

A

Absorption The passage of digested food from the digestive tract into the cardiovascular system (Ch. 17, 442)

Abstinence A deliberate decision to avoid harmful behaviors, including sexual activity before marriage and the use of tobacco, alcohol, and other drugs (Ch. 1, 20; Ch. 12, 318; Ch. 25, 649)

Abuse Physical, mental/emotional, or sexual mistreatment of one person by another (Ch. 13, 348)

Accident chain A sequence of events that leads to an unintentional injury (Ch. 27, 706)

Acquired immune deficiency syndrome (AIDS) A disease in which the immune system of the patient is weakened (Ch. 25, 658)

Action plan A multistep strategy to identify and achieve your goals (Ch. 2, 36)

Active immunity Immunity your body develops to protect you from disease (Ch. 24, 631)

Active listening Paying close attention to what someone is saying and communicating (Ch. 10, 256)

Addiction A physiological or psychological dependence on a drug (Ch. 23, 595)

Addictive drug A substance that causes physiological or psychological dependence (Ch. 21, 540)

Additive interaction Medicines working together in a positive way (Ch. 23, 589)

Adolescence The period from childhood to adulthood (Ch. 20, 514)

Adoption The legal process of taking a child of other parents as one's own. (Ch. 20, 527)

Adrenal glands Glands that help the body recover from stress and respond to emergencies (Ch. 18, 466)

Advertising A written or spoken media message designed to interest consumers in purchasing a product or service (Ch. 3, 49)

Advocacy Taking action to influence others to address a health-related concern or to support a health-related belief (Ch. 2, 32)

Aerobic exercise Any activity that uses large muscle groups, is rhythmic in nature, and can be maintained continuously for at least 10 minutes three times a day or for 20 to 30 minutes at one time (Ch. 4, 83)

Affection A feeling of fondness for someone (Ch. 12, 313)

Affirmation Positive feedback that helps others feel appreciated and supported (Ch. 11, 278)

Aggressive Overly forceful, pushy, hostile, or otherwise attacking in their approach (Ch. 12, 312)

Air pollution The contamination of the earth's atmosphere by substances that pose a health threat to living things (Ch. 29, 766)

Air Quality Index (AQI) An index for reporting daily air quality (Ch. 29, 768)

Alcohol abuse The excessive use of alcohol (Ch. 22, 565)

Alcohol poisoning A severe and potentially fatal physical reaction to an alcohol overdose (Ch. 22, 571)

Alcoholic An addict who is dependent on alcohol (Ch. 22, 576)

Alcoholism A disease in which a person has a physical or psychological dependence on drinks that contain alcohol (Ch. 22, 576)

Alienation Feeling isolated and separated from everyone else (Ch. 9, 230)

Allergy A specific reaction of the immune system to a foreign and frequently harmless substance (Ch. 26, 688)

Americans with Disabilities Act A law prohibiting discrimination against people with physical or mental disabilities in the workplace, transportation, public accommodations, and telecommunications (Ch. 26, 699)

Amniocentesis A procedure in which a syringe is inserted through a pregnant female's abdominal wall into the amniotic fluid surrounding the developing fetus (Ch. 19, 501)

Amniotic sac A thin, fluid-filled membrane that surrounds and protects the developing embryo (Ch. 19, 487)

Anabolic-androgenic steroids Synthetic substances similar to the male hormone testosterone (Ch. 4, 94; Ch. 23, 601)

Anaerobic exercise Intense short bursts of activity in which the muscles work so hard that they produce energy without using oxygen (Ch. 4, 84)

Analgesics Pain relievers (Ch. 23, 588)

Anemia A condition in which the ability of the blood to carry oxygen is reduced (Ch. 16, 426)

Angina pectoris Chest pain that results when the heart doesn't get enough oxygen (Ch. 26, 677)

Anorexia nervosa A disorder in which the irrational fear of becoming obese results in severe weight loss from self-imposed starvation (Ch. 6, 154)

Antagonistic interaction Occurs when the effect of one medicine is canceled or reduced when taken with another medicine (Ch. 23, 589)

Antibody A protein that acts against a specific antigen (Ch. 24, 631)

Antigen A substance that is capable of triggering an immune response (Ch. 24, 630)

Anxiety The condition of feeling uneasy or worried about what may happen (Ch. 8, 210)

Anxiety disorder A condition in which real or imagined fears are difficult to control (Ch. 9, 225)

Appendicitis Inflammation of the appendix (Ch. 17, 450)

Appendicular skeleton The 126 bones of the upper and lower limbs, shoulders, and hips (Ch. 15, 387)

Appetite A desire, rather than a need, to eat (Ch. 5, 111)

Arrhythmia Irregular heartbeats (Ch. 26, 677)

Arteries Blood vessels that carry blood away from the heart (Ch. 16, 419)

Arthritis A group of more than 100 different diseases that cause pain and loss of movement in the joints (Ch. 26, 693)

Asbestos A fibrous mineral that has fireproof properties, once widely used as an insulator. (Ch. 29, 769)

Assailant A person who commits a violent act against another (Ch. 13, 341)

Assault An unlawful attack on a person with the intent to harm or kill (Ch. 13, 344)

Assertive Standing up for your rights and beliefs in firm but positive ways (Ch. 12, 310; Ch. 13, 332)

Asthma An inflammatory condition in which the trachea, bronchi, and bronchioles become narrowed, causing difficulty in breathing (Ch. 16, 434; Ch. 26, 690)

Asymptomatic stage A period of time during which a person infected with HIV has no symptoms (Ch. 25, 662)

Atherosclerosis The process in which plaques accumulate on artery walls (Ch. 26, 675)

Auditory ossicles Three small bones linked together that connect the eardrum to the inner ear (Ch. 14, 377)

Autoimmune disease A condition in which the immune system mistakenly attacks itself, targeting the cells, tissues, and organs of a person's own body (Ch. 26, 691)

Autonomy The confidence that a person can control his or her own body, impulses, and environment (Ch. 19, 505)

Axial skeleton The 80 bones of the skull, spine, ribs, vertebrae, and sternum, or breastbone (Ch. 15, 387)

B

Bacteria Single-celled microorganisms (Ch. 24, 623)

Behavior therapy A treatment process that focuses on changing unwanted behaviors through rewards and reinforcements (Ch. 9, 237)

Benign Noncancerous (Ch. 26, 681)

Bile A yellow-green, bitter fluid important in the breakdown and absorption of fats (Ch. 17, 445)

Binge drinking Drinking five or more alcoholic drinks at one sitting (Ch. 22, 571)

Binge eating disorder A disorder characterized by compulsive overeating (Ch. 6, 155)

Biodegradable Able to be broken down by microorganisms in the environment (Ch. 29, 772)

Biomedical therapy The use of certain medications to treat or reduce the symptoms of a mental disorder (Ch. 9, 237)

Biopsy The removal of a small piece of tissue for examination (Ch. 26, 686)

Birthing center A facility in which females with low-risk pregnancies can deliver their babies in a homelike setting (Ch. 19, 492)

Bladder A hollow muscular organ that acts as a reservoir for urine (Ch. 17, 455)

Blizzard A snowstorm with winds of at least 35 miles per hour (Ch. 27, 728)

Blood alcohol concentration (BAC) The amount of alcohol in a person's blood expressed as a percentage (Ch. 22, 570)

Blood pressure A measure of the amount of force that the blood places on the walls of blood vessels, particularly large arteries, as it is pumped through the body (Ch. 16, 424)

Body composition The ratio of body fat to lean body tissue, including muscle, bone, water, and connective tissue such as ligaments, cartilage, and tendons (Ch. 4, 81)

Body image The way you see your body (Ch. 6, 144)

Body language Nonverbal communication through gestures, facial expressions, behaviors, and posture (Ch. 10, 258; Ch. 13, 332)

Body mass index (BMI) A ratio that allows you to assess your body size in relation to your height and weight (Ch. 6, 145)

Brain stem A three-inch-long stalk of nerve cells and fibers that connects the spinal cord to the rest of the brain (Ch. 15, 403)

Bronchi The airways that connect the trachea and the lungs (Ch. 16, 431)

Bronchitis An inflammation of the bronchi caused by infection or exposure to irritants such as tobacco smoke or air pollution (Ch. 16, 433)

Bulimia nervosa A disorder in which some form of purging or clearing of the digestive tract follows cycles of overeating (Ch. 6, 154)

Bullying The act of seeking power or attention through the psychological, emotional, or physical abuse of another person (Ch. 13, 336)

C

Calories Units of heat that measure the energy used by the body and the energy that foods supply to the body (Ch. 5, 110)

Cancer Uncontrollable growth of abnormal cells (Ch. 26, 681)

Capillaries Small vessels that carry blood between arterioles and small vessels called venules (Ch. 16, 419)

Carbohydrates The starches and sugars present in foods (Ch. 5, 114)

Carbon monoxide A colorless, odorless, and poisonous gas (Ch. 21, 541)

Carcinogen A cancer-causing substance (Ch. 21, 541; Ch. 26, 682)

Cardiac muscle A type of striated muscle that forms the wall of the heart (Ch. 15, 395)

Cardiopulmonary resuscitation (CPR) A life-saving first-aid procedure that combines rescue breaths with chest compressions, supplying oxygen to the body until normal body functions can resume (Ch. 28, 743)

Cardiorespiratory endurance The ability of the heart, lungs, and blood vessels to use and send fuel and oxygen to the body's tissues during long periods of moderate-to-vigorous activity (Ch. 4, 80)

Cardiovascular disease (CVD) A disease that affects the heart or blood vessels (Ch. 26, 674)

Cartilage A strong, flexible connective tissue (Ch. 15, 387)

Cerebellum The second largest part of the brain (Ch. 15, 403)

Cerebral palsy A group of nonprogressive neurological disorders that are the result of damage to the brain before, during, or just after birth or in early childhood (Ch. 15, 409)

Cerebrum The largest and most complex part of the brain (Ch. 15, 402)

Cervix The opening to the uterus (Ch. 18, 476)

Chain of survival A sequence of actions that maximize the victim's chances of survival (Ch. 28, 742)

Character Those distinctive qualities that describe how a person thinks, feels, and behaves (Ch. 2, 37)

Child abuse Domestic abuse directed at a child (Ch. 11, 288)

Chlamydia A bacterial infection that affects the reproductive organs of both males and females (Ch. 25, 654)

Chorionic villi sampling (CVS) A procedure in which a small piece of membrane is removed from the chorion, a layer of tissue that develops into the placenta (Ch. 19, 501)

Choroid A thin structure that lines the inside of the sclera (Ch. 14, 372)

Chromosomes Threadlike structures found within the nucleus of a cell that carry the codes for inherited traits (Ch. 19, 499)

Chronic stress Stress associated with long-term problems that are beyond a person's control (Ch. 8, 204)

Chyme A creamy, fluid mixture of food and gastric juices (Ch. 17, 444)

Citizenship The way you conduct yourself as a member of the community (Ch. 10, 249)

Clique A small circle of friends, usually with similar backgrounds or tastes, who exclude people viewed as outsiders (Ch. 12, 304)

Club drugs Drugs associated with concerts, dance clubs, and all-night parties called raves. (Ch. 23, 606)

Cluster suicides A series of suicides occurring within a short period of time and involving several people in the same school or community (Ch. 9, 233)

Cognition The ability to reason and think out abstract solutions (Ch. 20, 516)

Cognitive therapy A treatment method designed to identify and correct distorted thinking patterns that can lead to feelings and behaviors that may be troublesome, self-defeating, or self-destructive (Ch. 9, 237)

Commitment A promise or a pledge (Ch. 20, 524)

Communicable disease A disease that is spread from one living thing to another or through the environment (Ch. 24, 622)

Communication The ways in which you send messages to and receive messages from others (Ch. 10, 250)

Comparison shopping A method of judging the benefits of different products by comparing several factors, such as quality, features, and cost (Ch. 3, 50)

Compromise A problem-solving method that involves each participant's giving up something to reach a solution that satisfies everyone (Ch. 10, 251)

Concussion A jarring injury to the brain that affects normal brain function (Ch. 28, 752)

Conduct disorder A pattern of behavior in which the rights of others or basic social rules are violated (Ch. 9, 228)

Confidentiality Respecting the privacy of another and keeping details secret (Ch. 10, 267)

Conflict Any disagreement, struggle, or fight (Ch. 10, 262)

Conflict resolution The process of ending a conflict through cooperation and problem solving (Ch. 2, 30; Ch. 10, 264)

Congenital A condition that is present at birth (Ch. 16, 425)

Conservation The protection and preservation of the environment by managing natural resources to prevent abuse, destruction, and neglect (Ch. 29, 777)

Constructive criticism Nonhostile comments that point out problems and encourage improvement (Ch. 7, 183; Ch. 10, 260)

Consumer advocate People or groups whose sole purpose is to take on regional, national, and even international consumer issues (Ch. 3, 63)

Cool-down An activity that prepares the muscles to return to a resting state (Ch. 4, 91)

Cooperation Working together for the good of all (Ch. 10, 250)

Coping Dealing successfully with difficult changes in your life (Ch. 9, 239)

Cornea A transparent tissue that bends and focuses light before it enters the lens (Ch. 14, 372)

Crisis center A facility that handles emergencies and provides referrals to an individual needing help (Ch. 11, 291)

Cross-contamination The spreading of bacteria or other pathogens from one food to another (Ch. 5, 136)

Culture The collective beliefs, customs, and behaviors of a group (Ch. 1, 14)

Cumulative risks Related risks that increase in effect with each added risk (Ch. 1, 19)

Curfew A set time at which you must be home at night (Ch. 12, 317)

Custody A legal decision about who has the right to make decisions affecting the children in a family and who has the responsibility of physically caring for them (Ch. 11, 281)

Cycle of violence Pattern of repeating violent or abusive behaviors from one generation to the next (Ch. 11, 289)

Cystitis An inflammation of the bladder (Ch. 17, 456)

D

Dandruff A condition that can occur if the scalp becomes too dry and dead skin cells are shed as sticky, white flakes (Ch. 14, 365)

Date rape When one person in a dating relationship forces the other person to participate in sexual intercourse (Ch. 13, 350)

Decibel A unit used to express the relative intensity of loudness of sound (Ch. 29, 770)

Decision-making skills Steps that enable you to make a healthful decision (Ch. 2, 33)

Defense mechanisms Mental processes that protect individuals from strong or stressful emotions and situations (Ch. 7, 189)

Defensive driver A driver who is aware of potential hazards and reacts to avoid them (Ch. 27, 722)

Defibrillator A device that delivers an electric shock to the heart to restore its normal rhythm (Ch. 28, 742)

Deforestation Destruction of forests (Ch. 29, 774)

Depressants Drugs that tend to slow the central nervous system (Ch. 22, 563; Ch. 23, 606)

Depression A prolonged feeling of helplessness, hopelessness, and sadness (Ch. 8, 211)

Dermis The thicker layer of the skin beneath the epidermis that is made up of connective tissue and contains blood vessels and nerves (Ch. 14, 360)

Designer drugs Synthetic substances meant to imitate the effects of hallucinogens and other dangerous drugs (Ch. 23, 610)

Detoxification A process in which the body adjusts to functioning without alcohol (Ch. 22, 578)

Developmental assets Building blocks of development that help young people grow up as healthy, caring, and responsible individuals (Ch. 7, 179)

Developmental task An event that needs to happen in order for a person to continue growing toward becoming a healthy, mature adult (Ch. 19, 504)

Diabetes A chronic disease that affects the way body cells convert food into energy (Ch. 26, 691)

Diaphragm The muscle that separates the chest from the abdominal cavity (Ch. 16, 429)

Dietary Guidelines for Americans A set of recommendations for healthful eating and active living (Ch. 5, 122)

Dietary supplement A nonfood form of one or more nutrients (Ch. 6, 161)

Digestion The mechanical and chemical breakdown of foods for use by the body's cells (Ch. 17, 442)

Disability Any physical or mental impairment that limits normal activities, including seeing, hearing, walking, or speaking (Ch. 26, 695)

Divorce A legal end to a marriage contract (Ch. 11, 281)

DNA (deoxyribonucleic acid) The chemical unit that makes up chromosomes (Ch. 19, 499)

Domestic violence Any act of violence involving family members (Ch. 11, 286)

Drug watches Organized community efforts by neighborhood residents to patrol, monitor, report, and otherwise try to stop drug deals and drug abuse (Ch. 23, 612)

Drug-free school zone An area within 1,000 feet of a school and designated by signs, within which people caught selling drugs receive especially severe penalties (Ch. 23, 612)

Drugs Substances other than food that change the structure or function of the body or mind (Ch. 23, 586)

E

Earthquake A violent shaking movement of the earth's surface (Ch. 27, 729)

Eating disorder An extreme, harmful eating behavior that can cause serious illness or even death (Ch. 6, 153)

EIA A test that screens for the presence of HIV antibodies in the blood (Ch. 25, p. 663)

Electrolytes Minerals that help maintain the body's fluid balance (Ch. 6, 158)

Elimination The expulsion of undigested food or body wastes (Ch. 17, 442)

Embryo The developing child from the time of implantation until about the eighth week of development (Ch. 19, 486)

Emergency survival kit A group of items that can be used for a short time until an emergency situation has stabilized (Ch. 27, 726)

Emerging infection A communicable disease whose incidence in humans has increased within the past two decades or threatens to increase in the near future (Ch. 24, 640)

Emotional abuse A pattern of behavior that attacks the emotional development and sense of worth of an individual (Ch. 11, 287)

Emotional intimacy Ability to experience a caring, loving relationship with another person with whom you can share your innermost feelings (Ch. 20, 523)

Emotional maturity State at which the mental and emotional capabilities of an individual are fully developed (Ch. 20, 520)

Emotions Signals that tell your mind and body how to react (Ch. 7, 184)

Empathy The ability to imagine and understand how someone else feels (Ch. 7, 186)

Emphysema A disease that progressively destroys the walls of the alveoli (Ch. 16, 435)

Empty-nest syndrome Feelings of sadness or loneliness that accompany children's leaving home and entering adulthood (Ch. 20, 531)

Endocrine glands Ductless—or tubeless—organs or group of cells that secrete hormones directly into the bloodstream (Ch. 18, 464)

Environment The sum of your surroundings (Ch.1, 13)

Environmental tobacco smoke (ETS) Air that has been contaminated by tobacco smoke (Ch. 21, 551)

Epidemics Occurrences of diseases in which many people in the same place at the same time are affected (Ch. 25, 648)

Epidemiology The scientific study of patterns of disease in a population (Ch. 3, 65)

Epidermis The outer, thinner layer of the skin that is composed of living and dead cells (Ch. 14, 360)

Epilepsy A disorder of the nervous system that is characterized by recurrent seizures—sudden episodes of uncontrolled electrical activity in the brain (Ch. 15, 409)

Ethanol The type of alcohol in alcoholic beverages (Ch. 22, 562)

Euphoria A feeling of intense well-being or elation (Ch. 23, 605)

Exercise Purposeful physical activity that is planned, structured, and repetitive and that improves or maintains personal fitness (Ch. 4, 81)

Extended family Your immediate family and other relatives such as grandparents, aunts, uncles, and cousins (Ch. 11, 277)

Extensor The muscle that opens a joint (Ch. 15, 395)

External auditory canal A passageway about one inch long that leads to the remaining portion of the outer ear, the eardrum (Ch. 14, 376)

F

Fad diets Weight-loss plans that are popular for only a short time (Ch. 6, 151)

Fallopian tubes A pair of tubes with fingerlike projections that draw in the ovum (Ch. 18, 475)

Family The basic unit of society (Ch. 11, 274)

Family counseling Therapy to restore healthy relationships in a family (Ch. 11, 294)

Fermentation The chemical action of yeast on sugars (Ch. 22, 562)

Fertilization Union of a male sperm cell and a female egg cell (Ch. 19, 486)

Fetal alcohol syndrome (FAS) A group of alcohol-related birth defects that includes both physical and mental problems (Ch. 19, 494; Ch. 22, 576)

Fetus Developing embryo in the uterus (Ch. 19, 486)

Fiber An indigestible complex carbohydrate (Ch. 5, 115)

Fire extinguisher A portable device that puts out small fires by ejecting fire-extinguishing chemicals (Ch. 27, 708)

First aid The immediate, temporary care given to an ill or injured person until professional medical care can be provided (Ch. 28, 736)

F.I.T.T. Frequency, intensity, time/duration, and type of activity (Ch. 4, 90)

Flash flood A flood with great volume and of short duration that is usually caused by heavy rainfall (Ch. 27, 727)

Flexibility The ability to move a body part through a full range of motion (Ch. 4, 81)

Flexor The muscle that closes a joint (Ch. 15, 395)

Food additives Substances intentionally added to food to produce a desired effect (Ch. 5, 131)

Food allergy A condition in which the body's immune system reacts to substances in some foods (Ch. 5, 133)

Food Guide Pyramid A guide for making healthful daily food choices (Ch. 5, 123)

Food intolerance A negative reaction to a food or part of food caused by a metabolic problem, such as the inability to digest parts of certain foods or food components (Ch. 5, 134)

Foodborne illness Food poisoning (Ch. 5, 134)

Foster care A temporary arrangement in which a child is placed under the guidance and supervision of a family or an adult who is not related to the child by birth (Ch. 11, 292)

Fracture A break in the bone (Ch. 28, 750)

Fraud Deliberate deceit or trickery (Ch. 3, 61)

Friendship A significant relationship between two people that is based on caring, trust, and consideration (Ch. 10, 249; Ch. 12, 303)

Frostbite A condition that results when body tissues become frozen (Ch. 4, 100)

G

Gametes Reproductive cells (Ch. 20, 515)

Gang A group of people who associate with one another to take part in criminal activity (Ch. 13, 337)

Gastric juices Secretions from the stomach lining that contain hydrochloric acid and pepsin, an enzyme that digests protein (Ch. 17, 444)

Gene therapy The process of inserting normal genes into human cells to correct genetic disorders (Ch. 19, 503)

Genes The basic units of heredity (Ch. 19, 499)

Genetic disorder A disorder caused partly or completely by a defect in genes (Ch. 19, 500)

Genital herpes An STD caused by the herpes simplex virus (HSV) (Ch. 25, 654)

Goal Something you aim for that takes planning and work (Ch. 2, 34)

Gonads The ovaries and testes (Ch. 18, 466)

Gonorrhea A bacterial STD that usually affects mucous membranes (Ch. 25, 655)

Graduated driver's license A licensing program that gradually increases a new driver's driving privileges over time as experience and skill are gained (Ch. 27, 720)

Grief The sorrow caused by the loss of a loved one (Ch. 11, 282)

Grief response An individual's total response to a major loss (Ch. 9, 239)

Group therapy Treating a group of people who have similar problems and who meet regularly with a trained counselor (Ch. 9, 237)

H

Hair follicle A structure that surrounds the root of a hair (Ch. 14, 365)

Hallucinogens Drugs that alter moods, thoughts, and sense perceptions including vision, hearing, smell, and touch (Ch. 23, 609)

Harassment Persistently annoying others (Ch. 12, 308)

Hazardous waste A substance that is explosive, corrosive, highly reactive, or toxic to humans or other life forms (Ch. 29, 773)

Health The combination of physical, mental/emotional, and social well being (Ch. 1, 4)

Health care system All the medical care available to a nation's people, the way they receive care, and the method of payment (Ch. 3, 54)

Health consumer Anyone who purchases or uses health products or services (Ch. 3, 48)

Health education The providing of accurate health information to help people make healthy choices (Ch. 1, 7)

Health fraud Sale of worthless products or services claimed to prevent diseases or cure other health problems (Ch. 3, 61)

Health insurance A plan in which private companies or government programs pay for part or all of a person's medical costs (Ch. 3, 57)

Health literacy A person's capacity to learn about and understand basic health information and services and use these resources to promote his or her health and wellness (Ch. 1, 8)

Health screening A search or check for diseases or disorders that an individual would otherwise not have knowledge of or seek help for (Ch. 4, 95)

Health skills Specific tools and strategies that help you maintain, protect, and improve all aspects of your health (Ch. 2, 28)

Healthy People 2010 A nationwide health promotion and disease prevention plan designed to serve as a guide for improving the health of all people in the United States (Ch. 1, 7)

Heartburn A burning sensation in the center of the chest that may rise from the bottom, or tip, of the breastbone up to the throat (Ch. 17, 448)

Heat cramps Muscle spasms that result from a loss of large amounts of salt and water through perspiration (Ch. 4, 99)

Heat exhaustion An overheating of the body that results in cold, clammy skin and symptoms of shock (Ch. 27, 715)

Heatstroke A condition in which the body loses the ability to rid itself of excessive heat through perspiration (Ch. 4, 99)

Hemodialysis A technique in which an artificial kidney machine removes waste products from the blood (Ch. 17, 457)

Hemoglobin The oxygen-carrying protein in blood (Ch. 16, 418)

Herbal supplement A chemical substance from plants that may be sold as a dietary supplement (Ch. 6, 161)

Heredity All the traits that are biologically passed from parents to their children (Ch. 1, 12; Ch. 19, 498)

Hernia When an organ or tissue protrudes through an area of weak muscle (Ch. 15, 398)

Hiatal hernia A condition in which part of the stomach pushes through an opening in the diaphragm (Ch. 17, 448)

Hierarchy of needs A ranked list of those needs essential to human growth and development, presented in ascending order starting with basic needs and building toward the need for reaching your highest potential (Ch. 7, 172)

Histamines Chemicals that can stimulate mucus and fluid production in an area (Ch. 26, 689)

Hodgkin's disease A type of cancer that affects the lymph tissue (Ch. 16, 427)

Homicide The willful killing of one human being by another (Ch. 13, 344)

Hormones Chemical substances that are produced in glands and help regulate many of your body's functions (Ch. 7, 185; Ch. 18, 464; Ch. 20, 514)

Hostility The intentional use of unfriendly or offensive behavior (Ch. 7, 187)

Human immunodeficiency virus (HIV) A virus that attacks the immune system (Ch. 25, 658)

Human papillomavirus (HPV) A virus that can cause genital warts or asymptomatic infection (Ch. 25, 652)

Hunger A natural physical drive that protects you from starvation (Ch. 5, 111)

Hurricane A powerful storm that originates at sea, characterized by winds of at least 74 miles per hour, heavy rains, flooding, and sometimes tornadoes (Ch. 27, 727)

Hydration Taking in fluids so that the body functions properly (Ch. 4, 94)

Hypertension High blood pressure (Ch. 26, 675)

Hypothermia A condition in which body temperature becomes dangerously low (Ch. 4, 101; Ch. 27, 715)

I

Illegal drugs Chemical substances that people of any age may not lawfully manufacture, possess, buy, or sell (Ch. 23, 592)

Illicit drug use The use or sale of any substance that is illegal or otherwise not permitted (Ch. 23, 592)

"I" message A statement in which a person describes how he or she feels by using the pronoun "I" (Ch.10, 256)

Immune system A network of cells, tissues, organs, and chemicals that fights pathogens (Ch. 24, 627)

Immunity The state of being protected against a particular disease (Ch. 24, 630)

Implantation The attachment of the zygote to the uterine wall (Ch. 19, 486)

Indigestion A feeling of discomfort in the upper abdomen (Ch. 17, 448)

Infatuation Exaggerated feelings of passion for another person (Ch. 12, 313)

Infection A condition that occurs when pathogens enter the body, multiply, and damage body cells (Ch. 24, 622)

Infertility The inability to conceive a child (Ch. 18, 478)

Inflammatory response A reaction to tissue damage caused by injury or infection (Ch. 24, 628)

Inhalants Substances whose fumes are sniffed and inhaled to achieve a mind-altering effect (Ch. 23, 600)

Integrity A firm adherence to a moral code (Ch. 20, 532)

Interpersonal communication The exchange of thoughts, feelings, and beliefs between two or more people (Ch. 2, 28)

Interpersonal conflict Disagreement between groups of any size, from two people to entire nations (Ch. 10, 262)

Intoxication The state in which the body is poisoned by alcohol or another substance and the person's physical and mental control is significantly reduced (Ch. 22, 563)

J

Jaundice A yellowing of the skin and eyes (Ch. 24, 638)

L

Labor The final stage of pregnancy in which the uterus contracts and pushes the baby out of the mother's body (Ch. 19, 490)

Labyrinth The inner ear (Ch. 14, 377)

Lacrimal gland The gland that secretes tears into ducts that empty into the eye (Ch. 14, 371)

Landfill An area that has been safeguarded to prevent disposed wastes from contaminating groundwater (Ch. 29, 772)

Larynx Voice box (Ch. 16, 431)

Leukemia A form of cancer in which any one of the different types of white blood cells is produced excessively and abnormally (Ch. 16, 426)

Leukoplakia Thickened, white, leathery-looking spots on the inside of the mouth that can develop into oral cancer (Ch. 21, 542)

Ligament A band of fibrous, slightly elastic connective tissue that attaches bone to bone (Ch. 15, 389)

Lipid A fatty substance that does not dissolve in water (Ch. 5, 117)

Long-term goal A goal that you plan to reach over an extended period of time (Ch. 2, 35)

Lymph The clear fluid that fills the spaces around body cells (Ch. 16, 421)

Lymphocytes Specialized white blood cells that provide the body with immunity (Ch. 16, 421; Ch. 24, 630)

M

Mainstream smoke The smoke exhaled from the lungs of a smoker (Ch. 21, 551)

Malignant Cancerous (Ch. 26, 681)

Malpractice Failure by a health professional to meet accepted standards (Ch. 3, 61)

Manipulation An indirect, dishonest way to control or influence others (Ch. 12, 308)

Marijuana Plant whose leaves, buds, and flowers are usually smoked for their intoxicating effects (Ch. 23, 598)

Marital adjustment How well a person adjusts to marriage and to his or her spouse (Ch. 20, 525)

Mastication The process of chewing (Ch. 17, 443)

Media The various methods of communicating information (Ch. 1, 15; Ch. 3, 49)

Mediation A process in which specially trained people help others resolve their conflicts peacefully (Ch. 10, 267)

Mediator A person who helps others resolve issues to the satisfaction of both parties (Ch. 11, 294)

Medical history Complete and comprehensive information about your immunizations and any health problems you have had to date (Ch. 3, 58)

Medicines Drugs that are used to treat or prevent diseases or other conditions (Ch. 23, 586)

Megadose Very large amount of a dietary supplement (Ch. 6, 161)

Melanin A pigment that gives the skin, hair, and iris of the eyes their color (Ch. 14, 361)

Melanoma The most serious form of skin cancer (Ch. 14, 364)

Menopause The end of the reproductive years for a female (Ch. 18, 476)

Menstruation Shedding of the uterine lining (Ch. 18, 476)

Mental disorder An illness of the mind that can affect the thoughts, feelings, and behaviors of a person, preventing him or her from leading a happy, healthful, and productive life (Ch. 9, 224)

Mental retardation The below-average intellectual ability present from birth or early childhood and associated with difficulties in learning and social adaptation (Ch. 26, 697)

Mental/emotional health The ability to accept yourself and others, adapt to and manage emotions, and deal with the demands and challenges you meet in life (Ch. 7, 170)

Metabolism The process by which the body breaks down substances and gets energy from food (Ch. 4, 78; Ch. 22, 569)

Metastasis Spread of cancer from the point where it originated to other parts of the body (Ch. 26, 681)

Minerals Substances that the body cannot manufacture but that are needed for forming healthy bones and teeth and for regulating many vital body processes (Ch. 5, 120)

Miscarriage The spontaneous expulsion of a fetus that occurs before the twentieth week of a pregnancy (Ch. 19, 496)

Modeling Observing and learning from the behaviors of those around you (Ch. 7, 175)

Mood disorder An illness, often with an organic cause, that involves mood extremes that interfere with everyday living (Ch. 9, 226)

Mourning The act of showing sorrow or grief (Ch. 9, 240)

Muscle cramp A spasm or sudden tightening of a muscle (Ch. 4, 102)

Muscle tone The natural tension in the fibers of a muscle (Ch. 15, 396)

Muscular endurance The ability of the muscles to perform physical tasks over a period of time without becoming fatigued (Ch. 4, 80)

Muscular strength The amount of force a muscle can exert (Ch. 4, 80)

N

Narcotics Specific drugs derived from the opium plant that are obtainable only by prescription and are used to relieve pain (Ch. 23, 608)

Neglect Failure to provide for a child's physical or emotional needs (Ch. 11, 288)

Negotiation The use of communication and often compromise to settle a disagreement (Ch. 10, 266)

Nephrons The functional units of the kidneys (Ch. 17, 454)

Neurons Nerve cells (Ch. 15, 400)

Nicotine The addictive drug found in tobacco leaves (Ch. 21, 541)

Nicotine substitute A product that delivers small amounts of nicotine into the user's system while he or she is trying to give up the tobacco habit (Ch. 21, 549)

Nicotine withdrawal The process that occurs in the body when nicotine, an addictive drug, is no longer used (Ch. 21, 548)

Noise pollution Harmful and unwanted sound of sufficient intensity to damage hearing (Ch. 29, 770)

Noncommunicable disease A disease that is not transmitted by another person, a vector, or from the environment (Ch. 26, 674)

Nutrient-dense foods Foods that are high in nutrients as compared with their calorie content (Ch. 6, 148)

Nutrients Substances in food that your body needs to grow, to repair itself, and to supply you with energy (Ch. 5, 110)

Nutrition The process by which the body takes in and uses food (Ch. 5, 110)

O

Obesity Having an excess amount of body fat (Ch. 6, 146)

Occupational Safety and Health Administration (OSHA) The agency in the federal government that is responsible for promoting safe and healthful conditions in the workplace (Ch. 27, 713)

Online shopping Using the Internet to buy products and services (Ch. 3, 52)

Opportunistic infection An infection that occurs in an individual who does not have a healthy immune system (Ch. 25, 659)

Ossification The process by which bone is formed, renewed, and repaired (Ch. 15, 387)

Osteoarthritis A disease of the joints in which cartilage breaks down (Ch. 26, 693)

Osteoporosis A condition in which there is the progressive loss of bone tissue (Ch., 4, 78; Ch. 15, 391)

Ova Female reproductive cells (Ch. 18, 474)

Ovaries The female sex glands that store the ova and produce female sex hormones (Ch. 18, 474)

Overdose A strong, sometimes fatal reaction to taking a large amount of a drug (Ch. 23, 594)

Overexertion Overworking the body (Ch. 4, 99)

Overload Working the body harder than it is normally worked (Ch. 4, 90)

Over-the-counter (OTC) medicines Medicines that you can buy without a prescription (Ch. 23, 590)

Overweight A condition in which a person is heavier than the standard weight range for his or her height (Ch. 6, 146)

Ovulation The process of releasing a mature ovum into the fallopian tube each month (Ch. 18, 474)

P

Pancreas Gland that serves two systems—the digestive and the endocrine systems (Ch. 18, 465)

Pandemic A global outbreak of infectious disease (Ch. 25, p. 665)

Paranoia Irrational suspiciousness or distrust of others (Ch. 23, 600)

Parathyroid glands Glands that produce a hormone that regulates the body's calcium and phosphorus balance (Ch. 18, 465)

Passive A tendency to give up, give in, or back down without standing up for rights and needs (Ch. 12, 312)

Passive immunity Temporary immunity received from another person or from antibodies (Ch. 24, 631)

Pasteurization The process of treating a substance with heat to destroy or slow the growth of pathogens (Ch. 5, 135)

Pathogen An organism that causes disease (Ch. 24, 622)

Peer mediation A process in which trained students help other students find fair ways to resolve conflict and settle their differences (Ch. 13, 339)

Peer mediators Students trained to help other students find fair resolutions to conflicts and disagreements (Ch. 10, 267)

Peer pressure The influence that people your age may have on you (Ch. 12, 307)

Peers People of similar age who share similar interests (Ch. 1, 13; Ch. 12, 302)

Penis A tube-shaped organ that extends from the trunk of the body just above the testes (Ch. 18, 469)

Peptic ulcer A sore in the lining of the digestive tract (Ch. 17, 451)

Perception The act of becoming aware through the senses (Ch. 8, 198)

Periodontal disease An inflammation of the periodontal structures (Ch. 14, 370)

Periodontium The area immediately around the teeth (Ch. 14, 367)

Peristalsis A series of involuntary muscle contractions that move food through the digestive tract (Ch. 17, 443)

Personal identity Your sense of yourself as a unique individual (Ch. 7, 178)

Personality A complex set of characteristics that makes you unique (Ch. 7, 175)

Phagocyte A white blood cell that attacks invading pathogens (Ch. 24, 629)

Pharynx Throat (Ch. 16, 431)

Physical abuse The intentional infliction of bodily harm or injury on another person (Ch. 11, 287; Ch. 13, 349)

Physical activity Any form of movement that causes your body to use energy (Ch. 4, 74)

Physical fitness The ability to carry out daily tasks easily and have enough reserve energy to respond to unexpected demands (Ch. 4, 74)

Physical maturity State at which the physical body and all its organs are fully developed (Ch. 20, 520)

Physiological dependence A condition in which the user has a chemical need for a drug (Ch. 23, 595)

Pituitary gland Regulates and controls the activities of all other endocrine glands (Ch. 18, 465)

Placenta A thick, blood-rich tissue that lines the walls of the uterus during pregnancy and nourishes the embryo (Ch. 19, 487)

Plaque A sticky, colorless film that acts on sugar to form acids that destroy tooth enamel and irritate gums (Ch. 14, 368)

Plasma The fluid in which other parts of the blood are suspended (Ch. 16, 418)

Platelets Cells that prevent the body's loss of blood (Ch. 16, 420)

Platonic friendship A friendship with a member of the opposite gender in which there is affection, but the two people are not considered a couple (Ch. 12, 303)

Pleurisy An inflammation of the lining of the lungs and chest cavity (Ch. 16, 433)

Pneumonia An inflammation of the lungs commonly caused by a bacterial or viral infection (Ch. 16, 433; Ch. 24, 636)

Poison Any substance—solid, liquid, or gas—that causes injury, illness, or death when introduced into the body (Ch. 28, 755)

Poison control center A 24-hour hot line that provides emergency medical advice on treating poisoning victims (Ch. 28, 755)

Post-traumatic stress disorder A condition that may develop after a person's exposure to a terrifying event that threatened or caused physical harm (Ch. 9, 226)

Precycling Reducing waste before it is generated (Ch. 29, 779)

Prejudice An unfair opinion or judgment of a particular group of people (Ch. 10, 260; Ch. 13, 342)

Prenatal care Steps that a pregnant female can take to provide for her own health and for the health of her baby (Ch. 19, 492)

Prescription medicine Medicines that cannot be used without the written approval of a licensed physician (Ch. 23, 590)

Prevention Practicing health and safety habits to remain free of disease and injury (Ch. 1, 6)

Preventive care Actions that prevent the onset of disease or injury (Ch. 3, 55)

Primary care physician Medical doctor who provides physical checkups and general care (Ch. 3, 54)

Priorities Those goals, tasks, and activities that you judge to be more important than others (Ch. 12, 319)

Profound deafness A hearing loss so severe that a person affected cannot benefit from mechanical amplification, such as a hearing aid (Ch. 26, 696)

Progression The gradual increase in overload necessary to achieve higher levels of fitness (Ch. 4, 90)

Protective factors Conditions that shield individuals from the negative consequences of exposure to risk (Ch. 8, 216)

Proteins Nutrients that help build and maintain body cells and tissues (Ch. 5, 116)

Psychoactive drugs Chemicals that affect the central nervous system and alter activity in the brain (Ch. 23, 603)

Psychological dependence Condition in which a person believes that a drug is needed in order to feel good or to function normally (Ch. 23, 595)

Psychosomatic response A physical reaction that results from stress rather than from an injury or illness (Ch. 8, 202)

Psychotherapy An ongoing dialogue between a patient and a mental health professional (Ch. 9, 237)

Puberty The time when a person begins to develop certain traits of adults of his or her own gender (Ch. 20, 514)

Public health A community-wide effort to monitor and promote the welfare of the population (Ch. 3, 64)

Pulp The tissue that contains the blood vessels and nerves of a tooth (Ch. 14, 368)

R

Radon An odorless, radioactive gas (Ch. 29, 769)

Random violence Violence committed for no particular reason (Ch. 13, 344)

Rape Any form of sexual intercourse that takes place against a person's will (Ch. 13, 346)

Recovery The process of learning to live an alcohol-free life (Ch. 22, 578)

Recycling The processing of waste materials so that they can be used again in some form (Ch. 29, 779)

Reflex A spontaneous response of the body to a stimulus (Ch. 15, 404)

Refusal skills Communication strategies that can help you say no when you are urged to take part in behaviors that are unsafe, unhealthful, or that go against your values (Ch. 2, 30; Ch. 12, 310)

Rehydration Restoring lost body fluids (Ch. 6, 158)

Relationship A bond or connection you have with other people (Ch. 10, 248)

Relaxation response A state of calm that can be reached if one or more relaxation techniques are practiced regularly (Ch. 8, 209)

Remission A period of time when symptoms disappear (Ch. 26, 687)

Repetitive motion injury Damage to tissues caused by prolonged, repeated movements (Ch. 15, 393)

Reproductive system The system of organs involved in producing offspring (Ch. 18, 468)

Resiliency The ability to adapt effectively and recover from disappointment, difficulty, or crisis (Ch. 8, 214; Ch. 11, 285)

Respiration The exchange of gases between the body and the environment (Ch. 16, 428)

Resting heart rate The number of times your heart beats in one minute when you are not active (Ch. 4, 92)

Retina The light-sensitive membrane on which images are cast by the cornea (Ch. 14, 372)

Rheumatoid arthritis A disease characterized by the debilitating destruction of the joints due to inflammation (Ch. 26, 694)

Risk behaviors Actions that can potentially threaten your health or the health of others (Ch. 1, 17)

Road rage A practice of endangering drivers by using a vehicle as a weapon (Ch. 27, 722)

Role A part you play in a relationship (Ch. 10, 250)

Role model Someone whose success or behavior serves as an example for others (Ch. 2, 40)

S

Sclera The white part of the eye (Ch. 14, 372)

Scoliosis An abnormal lateral, or side-to-side, curvature of the spine (Ch. 15, 391; Ch. 19, 507)

Scrotum An external skin sac that extends outside the body and contains the testes (Ch. 18, 469)

Sebaceous glands Structures within the skin that produce an oily secretion called sebum (Ch. 14, 361)

Sedentary lifestyle A way of life that involves little physical activity (Ch. 4, 77)

Self-actualization The striving to become the best you can be (Ch. 7, 174)

Self-control A person's ability to use responsibility to override emotions (Ch. 12, 319)

Self-defense Any strategy for protecting oneself from harm (Ch. 13, 332)

Self-directed Able to make correct decisions about behavior when adults are not present to enforce rules (Ch. 20, 528)

Semen A thick fluid containing sperm and other secretions from the male reproductive system (Ch. 18, 469)

Separation A decision between married individuals to live apart from each other (Ch. 11, 281)

Severe weather Harsh or dangerous weather conditions (Ch. 27, 725)

Sex characteristics The traits related to a person's gender (Ch. 20, 515)

Sexual abuse Any sexual contact that is forced upon a person against his or her will (Ch. 11, 287)

Sexual assault Any intentional sexual attack against another person (Ch. 13, 346)

Sexual harassment Uninvited and unwelcome sexual conduct directed at another person (Ch. 13, 336)

Sexual violence Any form of unwelcome sexual conduct directed at an individual, including sexual harassment, sexual assault, and rape (Ch. 13, 345)

Sexually transmitted diseases (STDs) Infectious diseases spread from person to person through sexual contact (Ch. 12, 318; Ch. 25, 648)

Sexually transmitted infections (STIs) Infectious diseases spread from person to person through sexual contact (Ch. 25, 648)

Shock A failure of the cardiovascular system to keep an adequate supply of blood circulating to the vital organs of the body (Ch. 28, 747)

Short-term goal A goal that you can reach in a short length of time (Ch. 2, 35)

Sibling A brother or sister (Ch. 11, 278)

Side effects Reactions to medicine other than the one intended (Ch. 23, 589)

Sidestream smoke The smoke from the burning end of a cigarette, pipe, or cigar (Ch. 21, 551)

Sinusitis Inflammation of the tissues that line the sinuses (Ch. 16, 435)

Skeletal muscles Muscles that are attached to bone and cause body movements (Ch. 15, 395)

Smog A yellow-brown haze that forms when sunlight reacts with air pollution (Ch. 29, 767)

Smoke alarm An alarm that is triggered by the presence of smoke (Ch. 27, 708)

Smokeless tobacco Tobacco that is sniffed through the nose, held in the mouth, or chewed (Ch. 21, 542)

Smooth muscles Muscles that act on the lining of passageways and internal organs (Ch. 15, 395)

Sobriety Living without alcohol (Ch. 22, 578)

Specialist Medical doctor trained to handle particular kinds of patients or medical conditions (Ch. 3, 54)

Specificity Particular exercises and activities that improve particular areas of health-related fitness (Ch. 4, 90)

Sperm Male reproductive cells (Ch. 18, 468)

Spousal abuse Domestic violence directed at a spouse (Ch. 11, 287)

Sprain An injury to the ligament surrounding a joint (Ch. 4, 102)

Stalking The repeated following, harassment, or threatening of an individual to frighten or cause him or her harm (Ch. 13, 349)

Stereotype An exaggerated and oversimplified belief about an entire group of people, such as an ethnic or religious group, or a gender (Ch. 12, 305)

Sterility The inability to reproduce (Ch. 18, 472)

Stillbirth A dead fetus expelled from the body after the twentieth week of pregnancy (Ch. 19, 496)

Stimulant A drug that increases the action of the central nervous system, the heart, and other organs (Ch. 21, 541; Ch. 23, 605)

Strain A condition resulting from damaging a muscle or tendon (Ch. 4, 102)

Stress The reaction of the body and mind to everyday challenges and demands (Ch. 8, 198)

Stress management Ways to deal with or overcome the negative effects of stress (Ch. 2, 31)

Stress-management skills Skills that help an individual handle stress in a healthful, effective way (Ch. 8, 208)

Stressor Anything that causes stress (Ch. 8, 199)

Stroke A condition where an arterial blockage interrupts the flow of blood to the brain (Ch. 26, 678)

Substance abuse Any unnecessary or improper use of chemical substances for nonmedical purposes (Ch. 23, 592)

Suicide The act of intentionally taking one's own life (Ch. 9, 230)

Suppression Holding back or restraining (Ch. 7, 189)

Sweat glands Structures within the dermis that secrete perspiration through ducts to pores on the skin's surface (Ch. 14, 361)

Symptomatic stage The stage in which a person infected with HIV has symptoms as a result of a severe drop in immune cells (Ch. 25, 663)

Synergistic effect Interaction of two or more medicines that results in a greater effect than when the medicines are taken alone (Ch. 23, 589)

Syphilis An STD that attacks many parts of the body and is caused by a small bacterium called a spirochete (Ch. 25, 655)

—————————— **T** ——————————

Tar A thick, sticky, dark fluid produced when tobacco burns (Ch. 21, 541)

Tartar The hard, crustlike substance formed when plaque hardens (Ch. 14, 370)

Tendon A fibrous cord that attaches muscle to the bone (Ch. 15, 389)

Tendonitis The inflammation of a tendon (Ch. 15, 398)

Testes Two small glands that produce sperm (Ch. 19, 469)

Testosterone Male sex hormone (Ch. 18, 469)

Thyroid gland Produces hormones that regulate metabolism, body heat, and bone growth (Ch. 18, 465)

Tinnitus A condition in which a ringing, buzzing, whistling, roaring, hissing, or other sound is heard in the ear in the absence of external sound (Ch. 14, 379)

Tolerance The ability to accept others' differences and allow them to be who they are without expressing disapproval (Ch. 10, 260)

Tolerance A condition in which the body becomes used to the effects of a medicine. (Ch. 23, 589)

Tornado A whirling, funnel-shaped windstorm that drops from the sky to the ground and produces a narrow path of destruction on land (Ch. 27, 728)

Toxin A substance that kills cells or interferes with their functions (Ch. 24, 623)

Trachea Windpipe (Ch. 16, 431)

Training program A program of formalized physical preparation for involvement in a sport or another physical activity (Ch. 4, 93)

Transitions Critical changes that occur at all stages of life (Ch. 20, 529)

Trichomoniasis An STD caused by a microscopic protozoan that results in infections of the vagina, urethra, and bladder (Ch. 25, 655)

Tuberculosis A contagious bacterial infection that usually affects the lungs (Ch. 16, 435)

Tumor An abnormal mass of tissue that has no natural role in the body (Ch. 26, 681)

U

Umbilical cord A ropelike structure that connects the embryo and the mother's placenta (Ch. 19, 487)

Unconditional love Love without limitation or qualification (Ch. 20, 528)

Unconsciousness A condition in which a person is not alert and aware of his or her surroundings (Ch. 28, 751)

Underweight A condition in which a person is less than the standard weight range for his or her height (Ch. 6, 147)

Unintentional injury An injury resulting from an unexpected event, or accident (Ch. 27, 706)

Universal precautions Actions taken to prevent the spread of disease by treating all blood and other body fluids as if they contained pathogens (Ch. 28, 737)

Urban sprawl The spreading of city development (houses, shopping centers, businesses, and schools) onto undeveloped land (Ch. 29, 774)

Ureters Tubes that connect the kidneys to the bladder (Ch. 17, 454)

Urethra The tube that leads from the bladder to the outside of the body (Ch. 17, 455)

Urethritis The inflammation of the urethra (Ch. 17, 456)

Urine Liquid waste material (Ch. 17, 453)

Uterus A hollow, muscular, pear-shaped organ inside a female's body (Ch. 18, 474)

V

Vaccine A preparation of dead or weakened pathogens that are introduced into the body to stimulate an immune response (Ch. 23, 587; Ch. 24, 631)

Vagina A muscular, elastic passageway that extends from the uterus to the outside of the body (Ch. 18, 475)

Values The ideas, beliefs, and attitudes about what is important that help guide the way you live (Ch. 2, 34)

Vector An organism, such as a tick, that carries and transmits pathogens to humans or other animals (Ch. 24, 625)

Vegan Vegetarians who eat only foods of plant origin (Ch. 6, 160)

Vegetarian A person who eats mostly or only foods that come from plant sources (Ch. 6, 159)

Vehicular safety Obeying the rules of the road, as well as exercising common sense and good judgment (Ch. 27, 719)

Veins Blood vessels that return blood to the heart (Ch. 16, 419)

Venom A poisonous substance secreted by a snake, spider, or other creature (Ch. 28, 755)

Verbal abuse Using words to mistreat or injure another person (Ch. 13, 349)

Violence Threatened or actual use of physical force or power to harm another person or to damage property (Ch. 13, 335)

Virus A form of genetic material that invades living cells to reproduce (Ch. 24, 623)

Vitamins Compounds that help regulate many vital body processes, including the digestion, absorption, and metabolism of other nutrients (Ch. 5, 119)

W

Warm-up An activity that prepares the muscles for work (Ch. 4, 90)

Warranty A company's or a store's written agreement to repair a product or refund your money should the product not function properly (Ch. 3, 50)

Wastewater Used water that comes from homes, communities, farms, and businesses (Ch. 29, 775)

Weight cycling The repeated pattern of loss and regain of body weight (Ch. 6, 152)

Wellness An overall state of well-being, or total health (Ch. 1, 5)

Western blot (WB) The most common confirmation test for HIV in the United States (Ch. 25, 664)

Withdrawal A condition that occurs when a person stops using a medicine on which he or she has a chemical dependency (Ch 23. 589)

Workout The part of an exercise program when the activity is performed at its highest peak (Ch. 4, 90)

Absorption/absorción Proceso mediante el cual la comida digerida pasa desde el aparato digestivo al sistema cardiovascular.

Abstinence/abstinencia Una decisión deliberada de evitar una conducta considerada arriesgada o dañina como la actividad sexual prematrimonial, el consumo de tabaco, alcohol, y otras drogas.

Abuse/abuso El maltrato físico, mental/emocional o sexual de una persona por otra.

Accident chain/cadena de accidentes Una serie de sucesos que generan una herida sin intención.

Acquired immune deficiency syndrome (AIDS)/síndrome de inmunodeficiencia adquirida (SIDA) Enfermedad en la cual el sistema inmunológico del paciente se encuentra debilitado.

Action plan/plan de acción Una estrategia que ayuda a identificar y lograr metas.

Active immunity/inmunidad activa La inmunidad que desarrolla el cuerpo para protegerse de enfermedades.

Active listening/audición activa Escuchar atentamente lo que alguien dice o comunica.

Addiction/adicción La dependencia psicológica o fisiológica a las drogas.

Addictive drug/droga adictiva Una substancia que causa la dependencia psicológica o fisiológica.

Additive interaction/interacción aditiva Medicinas que trabajan en conjunto de una manera positiva.

Adolescence/adolescencia La etapa entre la infancia y la edad adulta.

Adoption/adopción Proceso legal para tener como hijo un niño de otros padres.

Adrenal glands/glándulas suprarrenales Glándulas que ayudan al cuerpo a recuperarse del estrés y a actuar ante emergencias.

Advertising/publicidad Un mensaje, oral o escrito, diseñado para incentivar a los consumidores a comprar un producto o servicio.

Advocacy/apoya Apoyar o defender acciones que tienen como objetivo influenciar a otras personas para que respalden asuntos o creencias relacionadas con la salud.

Aerobic exercise/ejercicio aeróbico Cualquier actividad física que sea rítmica, que implique el uso de grupos de músculos grandes y que pueda ser mantenida por al menos 10 minutos tres veces al día o por 20 a 30 minutos en una acción continua.

Affection/afecto El sentimiento de cariño por otra persona.

Affirmation/afirmación Una reacción positiva que ayuda a que otras personas se sientan apreciadas y respaldadas.

Aggressive/agresivo Excesivamente fuerte, insistente, hostil, o de predisposición belicosa.

Air pollution/contaminación atmosférica La contaminación de la atmósfera de la tierra por sustancias que presentan peligro a la salud de los seres vivos.

Air Quality Index (AQI)/índice de calidad del aire Un indicador para informar sobre la calidad del aire diario.

Alcohol abuse/abuso de alcohol Uso excesivo de alcohol.

Alcohol poisoning/envenenamiento alcohólico Una reacción física severa y algunas veces fatal a una sobredosis de alcohol.

Alcoholic/alcohólico Una persona que es adicta al alcohol.

Alcoholism/alcoholismo Enfermedad en que la persona es adicta física o psicológicamente a bebidas alcohólicas.

Alienation/alienación Sentirse solo y separado de todo el mundo.

Allergy/alergia Una reacción específica del sistema inmunológico a una substancia extraña que es usualmente inofensiva.

Americans with Disabilities Act/Ley para Americanos Incapacidados Una ley que prohíbe la discriminación de personas discapacitadas por parte de los lugares de trabajo, transporte, lugares públicos y telecomunicaciones.

Amniocentesis/amniocentesis Un procedimiento en la cual se inserta una jeringa a través de la pared abdominal de una mujer embarazada hasta llegar al líquido amniótico alrededor del embrión en desarrollo.

Amniotic sac/saco amniótico Una membrana delgada llena de líquido que envuelve y protege al embrión.

Anabolic-androgenic steroids/esteroides anabolizantes-androgénicos Substancias sintéticas semejantes a la testosterona, la hormona masculina.

Anaerobic exercise/ejercicio anaeróbico Períodos cortos de actividad física intensiva en la cual los músculos trabajan tan fuerte que producen energía sin usar oxígeno.

Analgesics/analgésicos Medicamentos que alivian el dolor.

Anemia/anemia Condición en la cual la habilidad de la sangre de transportar oxígeno disminuye.

Angina pectoris/angina de pecho Un dolor en el pecho que es causado porque el corazón no está recibiendo suficiente oxígeno.

Anorexia nervosa/anorexia nerviosa Un desorden de alimentación en el cual el miedo irracional a convertirse obeso/a resulta en la pérdida extrema de peso por una dieta de hambre autoimpuesta.

Antagonistic interaction/interacción antagónica Situación en la cual el efecto de un medicamento se elimina o reduce por tomar otro medicamento.

Antibody/anticuerpo Una proteína que ataca antígenos específicos.

Antigen/antígeno Una substancia que es capaz de liberar un agente inmune.

Anxiety/ansiedad La condición de sentirse abrumado o preocupado acerca de lo que que pasará.

Anxiety disorder/trastorno de ansiedad Una condición en la cual el miedo, ya sea real o imaginado, es difícil de controlar.

Appendicitis/apendicitis La inflamación del apéndice.

Appendicular skeleton/esqueleto apendicular Los 126 huesos de las extremidades superiores e inferiores, los hombros, y las caderas.

Appetite/apetito El deseo, mas que la necesidad, de comer.

Arrhythmia/arritmia Palpitaciones irregulares del corazón.

Arteries/arterias Vasos sanguíneos que llevan la sangre desde el corazón a otras partes del cuerpo humano.

Arthritis/artritis Un grupo de mas de 100 condiciones que causan dolor y la pérdida de movimiento en las articulaciones.

Asbestos/asbesto Una fibra mineral que tiene propiedades contra combustión y que fue comúnmente usada como aislante.

Assailant/agresor Una persona que comete un acto violento contra otra persona.

Assault/asalto Un ataque ilegal contra una persona con la intención de hacerle daño o matarla.

Assertive/firme Sostener de manera positiva los derechos y creencias propios.

Asthma/asma Una condición inflamatoria en que la traquea, los bronquios y los bronquiolos se estrechan provocando dificultad para respirar.

Asymptomatic stage/Etapa sin síntomas Un período de tiempo durante el cuál una persona infectada por el VIH no tiene síntomas.

Atherosclerosis/artereosclerosis El proceso en el cual depósitos se acumulan en las paredes de las arterias.

Auditory ossicles/huesecillos auditorios Tres pequeños huesos que se encuentran unidos y conectan el tímpano con el oído.

Autoimmune disease/enfermedad autoinmunológica Una condición en la cuál el sistema inmune se ataca a sí mismo por error, afectando a las células, los tejidos, y los órganos del cuerpo de la misma persona.

Autonomy/autonomía La capacidad que una persona tiene para controlar su propio cuerpo, impulsos y medio ambiente.

Axial skeleton/esqueleto axial Los 80 huesos del cráneo, la columna vertebral, el esternón.

B

Bacteria/bacteria Microorganismos compuestos de una sola célula.

Behavior therapy/terapia de comportamiento Un terapia cuyo objetivo es cambiar conductas indeseadas a través de recompensas y refuerzos.

Benign/benigno No canceroso.

Bile/bilis Un líquido amargo de color amarillo-verde que es importante para la descomposición y absorción de las grasas.

Binge drinking/borrachera El consumo de cinco o más bebidas alcohólicas en un corto plazo.

Binge eating disorder/trastorno de la alimentación excesiva Un desorden de alimentación caracterizado por comer demasiado y de manera compulsiva.

Biodegradable/biodegradable Algo que se descompone por los microorganismos del medio ambiente.

Biomedical therapy/terapia biomédica El uso de ciertos medicamentos para tratar o reducir los síntomas de un desorden mental.

Biopsy/biopsia La extirpación diagnóstica de una pequeña muestra de tejido.

Birthing center/centro de partos Un lugar en el cual mujeres con un embarazo de bajo riesgo pueden dar a luz en un ambiente hogareño.

Bladder/vejiga Un órgano muscular hueco que actúa como recipiente para la orina.

Blizzard/ventisca Una tormenta de nieve con vientos que superan las 35 millas por hora.

Blood alcohol concentration (BAC)/concentración de alcohol en la sangre La cantidad de alcohol contenida en la sangre expresada como un porcentaje.

Blood pressure/tensión arterial Una medida de la presión que la sangre genera en las paredes de los vasos sanguíneos, especialmente en las arterias grandes, cuando la sangre es impulsada por el cuerpo.

Body composition/composición del cuerpo La proporción entre tejido graso y tejido magro incluyendo los músculos, los huesos, el agua, y los tejidos conjuntivos tales como ligamentos, cartílagos y tendones.

Body image/imagen corpora La forma en que uno se ve a su propio cuerpo.

Body language/lenguaje del cuerpo Comunicación no-verbal a través de gestos, expresiones faciales, comportamientos y postura.

Body mass index (BMI)/índice de masa corporal Una medida que permite la evaluación del tamaño de un cuerpo en relación con su peso y estatura.

Brain stem/vástago del cerebro Un ramificación de neuronas y fibras de tres pulgadas de largo que conecta la médula espinal al resto del cerebro.

Bronchi/bronquios Los pasajes que conectan la traquea con los pulmones.

Bronchitis/bronquitis Una inflamación de los bronquios causada por la infección o exposición a irritantes como el humo de tabaco o contaminación ambiental.

Bulimia nervosa/bulimia nerviosa Un trastorno de episodios de comer con exceso seguidos de alguna forma de auto-purgación o limpieza del aparato digestivo.

Bullying/intimidación Buscar poder o atraer atención por abuso psicológico, emocional o físico de otra persona.

C

Calories/calorías Unidades de calor que miden la energía que usa el cuerpo y la energía que la comida proporciona al cuerpo.

Cancer/cáncer El crecimiento incontrolable de células anormales.

Capillaries/capilares Vasos muy pequeños que transportan la sangre entre las arteriolas y las vénulas.

Carbohydrate/carbohidrato Las féculas y azúcares contenidos en los alimentos.

Carbon monoxide/monóxido de carbono Un gas sin color, inodoro, y venenoso.

Carcinogen/cancerígeno Un substancia que produce cáncer.

Cardiac muscle/músculo cardiaco Un tipo de músculo estriado que forma las paredes del corazón.

Cardiopulmonary resuscitation (CPR)/resucitación cardiopulmonar Un procedimiento de primeros auxilios que combina la respiración artificial con presiones en el pecho, proveyendo oxígeno hasta que las funciones vitales puedan resumir.

Cardiorespiratory endurance/resistencia cardio-respiratoria La habilidad que tienen el corazón, los pulmones y los vasos sanguíneos de utilizar y enviar energía y oxígeno a los tejidos del cuerpo durante largos períodos de tiempo con actividad moderada hasta enérgica.

Cardiovascular disease (CVD)/enfermedad cardio-vascular Una enfermedad que afecta el corazón o los vasos sanguíneos.

Cartilage/cartílago Tejido conjuntivo que es fuerte y flexible.

Cerebellum/cerebelo La segunda parte más grande del cerebro.

Cerebral palsy/parálisis cerebral Un grupo de desordenes neurológicos no progresivos y que son el resultado de daños al cerebro antes, durante, o justo después del nacimiento o durante la niñez temprana.

Cerebrum/cerebro La parte más grande y compleja del cerebro.

Cervix/cuello del útero La entrada del útero.

Chain of survival/cadena de supervivencia Una secuencia de acciones que tiene como objetivo maximizar las posibilidades de supervivencia de una víctima.

Character/carácter Las características distintivas que describen como una persona piensa, siente y actúa.

Child abuse/maltrato infantil Abuso doméstico dirigido hacia los niños.

Chlamydia/clamidia Una infección bacteriana que afecta los órganos reproductores de los hombres y mujeres.

Chorionic villi sampling (CVS)/biopsia de vellosidades coriónicas Un procedimiento mediante el cual se remueve una pequeña muestra de membrana de una capa de tejido que se desarrolla en la placenta llamada corión.

Choroid/coroides Una estructura delgada que cubre la parte interna de la esclerótica.

Chromosomes/cromosomas Estructuras parecidas a hilos encontradas dentro del núcleo de una célula y que cargan los códigos para rasgos heredados.

Chronic stress/estrés crónico El estrés relacionado con problemas de largo plazo y fuera del control de una persona.

Chyme/chyme Una mezcla cremosa y líquida de alimento y jugos gástricos.

Citizenship/ciudadanía La manera de comportarse como miembro de la comunidad.

Clique/pandilla Un grupo pequeño de amigos generalmente con gustos y experiencias similares que excluyen a otras personas vistas como ajenas a ellos.

Club drugs/drogas de club Drogas asociadas con conciertos, clubes de baile, y fiestas nocturnas conocidas como "raves".

Cluster suicides/serie de suicidios Una serie de suicidios que ocurren en un período de tiempo corto que involucran a varias personas de un mismo colegio o comunidad.

Cognition/cognición La habilidad de razonar y pensar con soluciones abstractas.

Cognitive therapy/terapia cognoscitiva Una terapia diseñada para identificar y corregir modelos de pensamientos los cuales pueden generar comportamientos que sean problemáticos, contraproducentes, o destructivos para sí mismo.

Commitment/compromiso Una promesa u obligación.

Communicable disease/enfermedad contagiosa Una enfermedad que se puede transmitir de un ser vivo a otro o a través del medio ambiente.

Communication/comunicación Las maneras de enviar los mensajes a otros y de recibir mensajes enviados por otros.

Comparison shopping/compras comparadas Evaluar los beneficios de diferentes productos comparando factores tales como calidad, características y precio.

Compromise/acuerdo Un método para resolver problemas en que cada participante debe sacrificar algo con el fin de solucionar el problema.

Concussion/conmoción cerebral Una situación que es el resultado de un golpe en el cerebro y que afecta su normal funcionamiento.

Conduct disorder/desorden de conducta Un patrón de comportamiento en el cual los derechos de otros o las reglas sociales básicas son violados.

Confidentiality/confidencialidad Respetar la vida privada de otros y guardar detalles secretos.

Conflict/conflicto Cualquier desacuerdo, pelea o enojo.

Conflict resolution/resolución de conflicto Proceso de resolver un desacuerdo a través de la cooperación y solución de problemas.

Congenital/congénito Una condición que se presenta al nacimiento.

Conservation/conservación La protección y preservación del medio ambiente a través de la prevención de abusos, destrucción e incorrecto uso de los recursos naturales.

Constructive criticism/crítica constructiva Comentarios no hostiles acerca del problema que tienen como objetivo mejorar un comportamiento o situación.

Consumer advocate/defensor del consumidor Gente o grupos cuyo único propósito es confrontar los problemas regionales, nacionales, y hasta internacionales del consumidor.

Cool-down/enfriamiento Una actividad que prepara los músculos para volver a un estado de relajación.

Cooperation/cooperación Trabajar juntos para el beneficio de todos.

Coping/hacer frente a Ocuparse exitosamente de los cambios difíciles de la vida.

Cornea/córnea Un tejido transparente que refracta y enfoca la luz antes de pasar al cristalino.

Crisis center/centro para crisis Un plante que maneja emergencias y envía a un individuo que necesita ayuda a especialistas.

Cross-contamination/traspasar la contaminación La dispersión de bacteria u otros microbios patogénicos de una comida a otra.

Culture/cultura Las creencias, costumbres y comportamiento colectivos de un grupo de personas.

Cumulative risks/riesgos acumulados Riesgos relacionados que aumentan en efecto con cada riesgo más.

Curfew/toque de queda Un período de tiempo de restricción en casa nocturno.

Custody/custodia Una decisión legal acerca de quién tiene el derecho de tomar las decisiones que afectarán a un niño, y quién tiene la responsabilidad de hacerse cargo de él.

Cycle of violence/ciclo de violencia Patrón de comportamiento violento o abusivo repetido de una generación a la próxima.

Cystitis/cistitis La inflamación de la vejiga.

D

Dandruff/caspa Una condición que puede resultar si el cuero cabelludo se seca y las células muertas de la piel se desprenden como partículas blancas pegajosas.

Date rape/violación Cuando una persona que se encuentra en una cita obliga a la otra a participar en una actividad sexual.

Decibel/decibelios Una medida que se usa para expresar la intensidad relativa del volumen del sonido.

Decision-making skills/habilidades para tomar decisiones Los pasos necesarios para tomar una correcta decisión.

Defense mechanisms/mecanismos de defensa Procesos mentales que protegen a individuos de emociones y situaciones fuertes o estresantes.

Defensive driver/manejo defensivo Un conductor consciente de peligros posibles que reacciona para evitarlos.

Defibrillator/máquina de defibrilación Un aparato que proporciona choques eléctricos al corazón para restaurar su ritmo normal.

Deforestation/desforestación Destrucción de los bosques.

Depressants/sedantes Sustancias que tienden a disminuir la función del sistema nervioso central.

Depression/depresión Un sentimiento prolongado de soledad, desesperación y tristeza.

Dermis/dermis La capa más gruesa de la piel que se encuentra debajo de la epidermis que está compuesta de tejidos conectivos y contiene vasos sanguíneos y nervios.

Designer drugs/droga de diseño Sustancias sintéticas que tratan de imitar los efectos de los alucinógenos y otras drogas peligrosas.

Detoxification/desintoxicación Un proceso mediante el cual el cuerpo se ajusta para funcionar sin alcohol.

Developmental assets/recursos para el desarrollo Componentes básicos del desarrollo que ayudan a que los jóvenes crecen saludables, afectuosos, y responsables.

Developmental task/tareas requeridas para el desarrollo Sucesos necesarios para que una persona continúe creciendo y se convierta en un adulto saludable y maduro.

Diabetes/diabetes Una enfermedad crónica que afecta el modo en que las células del cuerpo conviertan los alimentos en energía.

Diaphragm/diafragma El músculo que separa los pulmones de la cavidad abdominal.

Dietary Guidelines for Americans/Pautas alimenticias para los estadounidenses Una serie de recomendaciones para la alimentación saludable y la vida activa de los estadounidenses.

Dietary supplement/suplemento alimenticio Uno o más alimentos nutritivos que no son comida.

Digestion/digestión La descomposición mecánica y química de la comida para uso por las células corporales.

Disability/incapacidad Cualquier impedimento físico o mental que limita el desarrollo de actividades normales inclusive ver, oír, caminar o hablar.

Divorce/divorcio Un fin legal de un contrato de matrimonio.

DNA (deoxyribonucleic acid)/ADN (acido desoxirribonucleico La unidad química que compone los cromosomas.

Domestic violence/violencia doméstica Cualquier acto de violencia que incluya a los miembros de una familia.

Drug watches/vigilantes de la droga Un grupo de personas de un vecindario organizadas para espiar, seguir, denunciar o directamente frenar el abuso y venta de drogas.

Drug-free school zone/zona de escuela libre de drogas Un área que comprende 1,000 pies alrededor de una escuela y se encuentra señalizada, en la cual las personas que son atrapadas vendiendo drogas son severamente penalizadas o castigadas, más que lo usual.

Drugs/drogas Sustancias, excepto alimentos, que cambian la estructura o funcionamiento del cuerpo o mente de las personas.

--- **E** ---

Earthquake/terremoto Un temblor que mueve fuertemente la superficie de la tierra.

Eating disorder/desorden alimenticio Un comportamiento que se caracteriza por comer en forma extrema y dañina causando que la persona se pueda enfermar o morir.

EIA/ensayo inmunoenzimático de enzimas Un análisis que estudia la presencia de VIH en la sangre.

Electrolytes/electrolitos Minerales que ayudan a mantener el equilibrio de los fluidos del cuerpo.

Elimination/eliminación La expulsión de comida no digerida o desechos del cuerpo.

Embryo/embrión El estado de desarrollo de un organismo que va desde la implantación hasta las ocho semanas de desarrollo.

Emergency survival kit/botiquín de primeros auxilios Un grupo de artículos que pueden ser utilizados por un corto plazo hasta que la situación de emergencia se haya estabilizado.

Emerging infection/infección emergente Una enfermedad infecciosa cuya incidencia en humanos ha aumentado durante las últimas dos décadas o que amenaza con incrementar en el futuro cercano.

Emotional abuse/abuso emocional Un comportamiento que ataca el desarrollo emocional y la estima de un individuo.

Emotional intimacy/intimidad emocional La habilidad de experimentar una relación de amor y cuidado con otra persona con la cual también se pueden compartir los sentimientos más íntimos.

Emotional maturity/madurez emocional Un estado en el cual las capacidades mentales y emocionales de una persona se encuentran totalmente desarrolladas.

Emotions/emociones Señales que le comunican a la mente y el cuerpo como actuar.

Empathy/empatía La habilidad para imaginar y entender como otra persona siente.

Emphysema/enfisema Una enfermedad que destruye progresivamente las paredes de los alveolos.

Empty-nest syndrome/síndrome del nido vacío Sentimiento de tristeza y soledad que ocurre cuando los hijos, quienes ya se convirtieron en adultos, se van de la casa de sus padres.

Endocrine glands/glándulas endocrinas Órganos o grupos de células sin conductos o tubos que secretan directamente en el flujo sanguíneo.

Environment/medio ambiente Todo lo que nos rodea.

Environmental tobacco smoke (ETS)/ambiente con humo de cigarro Aire que ha sido contaminado por el humo de cigarrillos.

Epidemic/epidemia Una situación en la cual mucha gente contrae una enfermedad al mismo tiempo y en el mismo lugar.

Epidemiology/epidemiología El estudio científico de los patrones de las enfermedades en una población.

Epidermis/epidermis La capa más fina y externa de la piel la cual se encuentra compuesta de células vivas y muertas.

Epilepsy/epilepsia Un desorden del sistema nervioso caracterizado por convulsiones continuas —repentinos episodios de incontrolable actividad eléctrica del cerebro.

Ethanol/etanol El alcohol que se encuentra en las bebidas alcohólicas.

Euphoria/euforia El sentimiento de un intenso bienestar o alegría.

Exercise/ejercicio Actividad física que es planeada, estructurada y repetitiva, y que tiene como objetivo el mantenimiento o el mejoramiento del estado físico de una persona.

Extended family/familia extensa La familia inmediata (padres y hermanos) y otros parientes, como por ejemplo tíos, tías, primos y abuelos.

Extensor/extensor Un músculo que abra una articulación.

External auditory canal/canal auditivo externo Un pasaje de cerca de una pulgada de largo el cual conecta el oído externo con el tímpano.

F

Fad diets/dietas de moda Planes para perder peso que son populares por un corto plazo.

Fallopian tubes/trompas de Falapio Un par de conductos con terminaciones en forma de dedos que ayudan al óvulo en su camino hacia el útero.

Family/familia La unidad básica de una sociedad.

Family counseling/terapia familiar Terapia que ayuda a restaurar las relaciones entre los miembros de una familia.

Fermentation/fermentación La reacción química de la levadura en el azúcar.

Fertilization/fertilización La unión del espermatozoide y el óvulo.

Fetal alcohol syndrome (FAS)/síndrome de alcoholismo fetal Un grupo de defectos de nacimiento causados por el alcohol y que incluyen problemas físicos y mentales.

Fetus/feto El embrión en desarrollo que se encuentra dentro del útero.

Fiber/fibra Un carbohidrato que no es digerible.

Fire extinguisher/extintor de incendios Un aparato portátil que ayuda a apagar incendios a través de la aplicación de químicos extinguidores de fuego.

First aid/primeros auxilios La atención inmediata y temporal que se le proporciona a una persona enferma o herida hasta que una atención medica profesional pueda ser proporcionada.

F.I.T.T./F.I.T.A. Frecuencia, intensidad, tiempo/ duración, y tipo de actividad.

Flash flood/inundación repentina Una inundación de gran volumen y corta duración que es comúnmente causada por fuertes lluvias.

Flexibility/flexibilidad La habilidad de mover una parte del cuerpo fácilmente y en muchas direcciones.

Flexor/músculo flexor Los músculos que cierran las articulaciones.

Food additives/aditivos alimentarios Substancias que son adicionadas a los alimentos en forma intencional para generar un efecto deseado.

Food allergy/alergia a comida Una condición en la cuál el sistema inmunológico del cuerpo reacciona a substancias contenidas en algunos alimentos.

Food Guide Pyramid/pirámide alimenticia Una guía para la elección diaria de alimentos saludables.

Food intolerance/intolerancia a la comida Una reacción negativa a los alimentos (o un elemento particular del alimento) causado por un problema metabólico, como por ejemplo la inhabilidad de digerir ciertos alimentos o algunos de sus componentes.

Foodborne illness/enfermedad alimenticia Intoxicación alimenticia.

Foster care/custodia temporal Un arreglo temporal en el cual un niño es entregado a una familia o adulto no emparentado para que lo guíe y supervise.

Fracture/fractura La rotura de un hueso.

Fraud/fraude Engaño deliberado.

Friendship/amistad Una relación importante entre dos personas que esta basada en solidaridad, confianza y consideración.

Frostbite/congelación Una condición en la cual los tejidos del cuerpo se congelan.

G

Gametes/gametos Células reproductoras.

Gang/banda criminal Un grupo de personas quienes se encuentran vinculados por haber participado en una actividad criminal.

Gastric juices/jugos gástricos La secreciones que provienen del revestimiento del estómago y que contienen ácido clorhídrico y pepsina, una enzima que digiere la proteína.

Gene therapy/terapia genética Un proceso que consiste en introducir genes normales en las células humanas para corregir trastornos genéticos.

Genes/genes Las unidades básicas de la herencia.

Genetic disorder/trastorno genético Un trastorno causado parcial o completamente por defectos en los genes.

Genital herpes/herpes genital Infección de transmisión sexual causada por el virus herpes simple.

Goal/objetivo Algo que una persona desea y para el cual hace planes y trabaja.

Gonads/gónadas Los ovarios y los testículos.

Gonorrhea/gonorrea Una infección bacteriana de transmisión sexual que comúnmente afecta a las membranas mucosas.

Graduated driver's license/licencia de manejar graduada Un programa de licencias que incrementa los privilegios de los conductores nuevos con el tiempo como premio a la experiencia y habilidad.

Grief/aflicción La pena causada por la pérdida de un ser querido.

Grief response/aflicción La respuesta de un individuo a una gran pérdida.

Group therapy/terapia de grupo Tratamiento de un grupo de personas quienes tienen problemas similares.

H

Hair follicle/folículo de pelo Una estructura que rodea la raíz de un pelo.

Hallucinogens/alucinógenos Drogas que alteran el estado de ánimo, el pensamiento, y la percepción, incluso la vista, oído, olfato y tacto.

Harassment/acoso Molestar persistentemente a otra persona.

Hazardous waste/desechos peligrosos Substancia que es explosiva, corrosiva, altamente reactiva, o tóxica para los seres humanos o otras formas de vida.

Health/salud La combinación de bienestar físico, mental/emocional y social.

Health care system/sistema de asistencia médica Toda la asistencia médica disponible para la población de una nación, la forma en que la atención es recibida y la forma en que se paga.

Health consumer/consumidor de servicios de salud Cualquier persona que consume o usa productos o servicios de salud.

Health education/educación de la salud Proveer a las personas con información adecuada de tal manera que puedan tomar decisiones que sean saludables.

Health fraud/engaño sobre la salud La venta de productos o servicios inútiles que supuestamente sirven para prevenir enfermedades o mejorar otros problemas de la salud.

Health insurance/seguro de salud Un plan mediante el cual compañías privadas o el gobierno pagan parte o todos los gastos médicos de una persona.

Health literacy/instrucción sobre la salud La capacidad que tiene una persona para aprender y comprender información básica acerca de la salud y los servicios relacionados, y de usar esos conocimientos para mejorar su propia salud y bienestar.

Health screening/diagnóstico de la salud Estudiar o chequear la salud de una persona con el objetivo de detectar anticipadamente enfermedades u otros problemas de salud.

Health skills/habilidades de la salud Herramientas y estrategias que ayudan a mantener, proteger, y mejorar todos los aspectos de la salud.

Healthy People 2010/Gente saludable 2010 Un plan nacional de salud y prevención de enfermedades que fue diseñado para promover el mejoramiento de la salud de todas las personas en los Estados Unidos.

Heartburn/acidez Una sensación de quemadura en el centro del pecho que puede subir desde la parte inferior del esternón hasta la garganta.

Heat cramps/calambre debido al calor Espasmos musculares que son el resultado de la pérdida de grandes cantidades de sal y agua a través del sudor.

Heat exhaustion/agotamiento debido al calor Un sobrecalentamiento del cuerpo que produce síntomas de un estado de choque y que hace que la piel se ponga helada y húmeda.

Heatstroke/insolación Una condición en la cuál el cuerpo pierde la habilidad para deshacerse del calor excesivo a través del sudor.

Hemodialysis/hemodiálisis Una técnica a través de la cual una máquina de diálisis limpia los desechos de la sangre.

Hemoglobin/hemoglobina La proteína que lleva el oxígeno en la sangre.

Herbal supplement/suplemento herbario Una substancia química de hierbas las cuales se pueden vender como suplemento nutritivo.

Heredity/herencia Todos los rasgos que biológicamente son transferidos de los padres a los hijos.

Hernia/hernia Cuando un órgano o tejido sobresale en un área de músculos débiles.

Hiatal hernia/hernia de hiato Una condición en la cuál una parte del estómago se sale por una abertura en el diafragma.

Hierarchy of needs/pirámides de las necesidades Una graduación de tales necesidades esenciales al crecimiento y desarrollo humano, presentadas en orden ascendiente desde las necesidades más básicas hasta la realización personal.

Histamines/histaminas Substancias químicas que pueden estimular la mucosa y la producción de fluidos en una área del cuerpo.

Hodgkin's disease/enfermedad de Hodgkin Un tipo de cáncer que afecta el tejido linfático.

Homicide/homicidio Cuando una persona mata a otra.

Hormones/hormonas Substancias químicas producidas por las glándulas y que ayudan a regular muchas funciones del cuerpo humano.

Hostility/hostilidad Un comportamiento intencional que es antipático, desagradable u ofensivo.

Human immunodeficiency virus (HIV)/virus de inmunodeficiencia humana (VIH) Un virus que ataca al sistema inmunológico.

Human papillomavirus (HPV)/papovavirus humano (HPV) Un virus que puede causar verrugas genitales o infecciones asintomáticas.

Hunger/hambre La necesidad física y natural de alimentos que nos protege de la inanición.

Hurricane/huracán Una tormenta muy fuerte que se origina en el mar, y que se caracteriza por vientos de al menos 74 millas por hora, fuertes lluvias, inundaciones, y algunas veces tornados.

Hydration/hidratación Tomar los líquidos necesarios para mantener las funciones corporales normales.

Hypertension/hipertensión Presión arterial alta.

Hypothermia/hipotermia Una condición en la cual la temperatura del cuerpo baja demasiado.

— I —

Illegal drugs/drogas ilegales Substancias químicas que ninguna persona, cualquiera sea su edad, puede legalmente producir, poseer, comprar o vender.

Illicit drug use/uso ilegal de drogas El uso o venta de cualquier substancia que es ilegal o no permitida.

"I" message/mensaje "YO" Una declaración en la cual una persona describe como él o ella se siente usando el pronombre "yo."

Immune system/sistema de defensas Una combinación de células, tejidos, órganos, y substancias químicas que combaten agentes patógenos.

Immunity/inmunidad El estado de estar protegido contra una enfermedad en particular.

Implantation/implantación La fijación del zigoto en la pared del útero.

Indigestion/indigestión Un sentimiento de molestia en la parte superior del abdomen.

Infatuation/adoración Los sentimientos de pasión exagerados por otra persona.

Infection/infección Una condición que ocurre cuando agentes patógenos entran al cuerpo, se multiplican y dañan las células.

Infertility/infertilidad La incapacidad de poder concebir un hijo.

Inflammatory response/respuesta inflamatoria Una reacción al daño a los tejidos causada por una lesión o infección.

Inhalants/inhalantes Substancias cuyos gases se aspiran o inhalan para alcanzar un estado alucinante.

Integrity/integridad Una adherencia firme al código moral.

Interpersonal communication/comunicación entre personas El intercambio de pensamientos, sentimientos y creencias entre dos o más personas.

Interpersonal conflict/conflicto entre personas Desacuerdo entre dos o más personas.

Intoxication/Intoxicación Un estado en el cual el cuerpo se encuentra embriagado por alcohol u otra substancia, y el control físico y mental de la persona se encuentra reducido significativamente.

J

Jaundice/ictericia Estado en el cual la piel y los ojos se ponen de color amarillo.

L

Labor/parto El estado final del embarazo en el cual el útero se contrae y empuja el bebé hacia afuera del cuerpo de la madre.

Labyrinth/laberinto Oído interno.

Lacrimal gland/glándula lagrimal La glándula que produce las lágrimas y que las libera por los canales que se vacían en el ojo.

Landfill/terraplenes sanitarios Un área en donde se deposita la basura y que garantiza que no contaminará el medio ambiente.

Larynx/laringe Lugar donde se encuentran las cuerdas vocales.

Leukemia/leucemia Un tipo de cáncer en el cual los glóbulos blancos de la sangre se reproducen excesiva y anormalmente.

Leukoplakia/leucoplaquia Granos con apariencia de piel blanca dura y espesa que se encuentran dentro de la boca y que pueden llegar a producir un cáncer oral.

Ligament/ligamento Un tejido fuerte y elástico que une los huesos.

Lipid/lípido Una substancia grasosa que no se disuelve en el agua.

Long-term goal/objetivo de largo plazo Un objetivo que se planea alcanzar en un periodo largo de tiempo.

Lymph/linfa Un líquido claro que llena los espacios entre las células del cuerpo.

Lymphocytes/linfocitos Células blancas de la sangre que son especialistas en proporcionar la inmunidad al cuerpo humano.

M

Mainstream smoke/humo directo El humo exhalado por los pulmones de un fumador.

Malignant/maligno Canceroso.

Malpractice/mala práctica médica Condición en la que un profesional de la salud no cumple con los estándares aceptados.

Manipulation/manipulación Controlar o influenciar a otros de manera indirecta y desonesta.

Marijuana/marihuana Una planta cuyas hojas, brotes y flores son generalmente fumadas para su efecto embriagador.

Marital adjustment/adaptación matrimonial La manera como una persona se ajusta al matrimonio y a su esposo o esposa.

Mastication/masticación El proceso de masticar.

Media/medios de comunicación Los métodos diferentes usados para comunicar información.

Mediation/mediación Proceso mediante el cual la gente especializada ayuda a resolver conflictos de manera pacífica.

Mediator/mediador Una persona quien ayuda a otros a resolver problemas de manera que las dos partes queden satisfechas.

Medical history/historia médica La información completa acerca de las vacunas y problemas de salud que una persona ha tenido a lo largo de su vida.

Medicines/medicamentos Drogas que son tomadas para terminar o prevenir una enfermedad u otra condición de la salud.

Megadose/megadosis Una cantidad grande de suplemento alimenticio.

Melanin/melanina El pigmento que da el color a la piel, cabello y el iris del ojo.

Melanoma/melanoma El cáncer de la piel más grave de todos.

Menopause/menopausia La época que marca el fin de la vida reproductora de una mujer.

Menstruation/menstruación La eliminación de materia procedente del útero.

Mental disorder/desorden mental Una enfermedad mental que afecta la manera de pensar, el comportamiento y los sentimientos de una persona, y que le impide tener una vida feliz, saludable y productiva.

Mental retardation/retardo mental La habilidad intelectual inferior al promedio que se presenta desde el nacimiento o niñez y que se relaciona con dificultades de aprendizaje y adaptación social.

Mental/emotional health/salud mental/emocional La habilidad de aceptarse a sí mismo y a otras personas, y de adaptarse y hacer frente a las emociones, cambios y nuevas demandas de la vida.

Metabolism/metabolismo Proceso mediante el cual el cuerpo procesa y obtiene energía de los alimentos.

Metastasis/metástasis La extensión del cáncer desde el punto de origen a otras partes del cuerpo.

Minerals/minerales Substancias no producidas por el cuerpo pero que son necesarias para la formación de huesos y dientes saludables, y para regular otros procesos vitales del cuerpo.

Miscarriage/aborto (natural) La expulsión espontánea del feto que ocurre antes de la semana número veinte del embarazo.

Modeling/modelando El proceso de observar y aprender del comportamiento de las personas de alrededor.

Mood disorder/desorden del carácter Una enfermedad, comúnmente de causa orgánica, que se caracteriza por cambios extremos del humor de una persona y que afecta la vida diaria.

Mourning/luto El acto de mostrar pena o dolor.

Muscle cramp/calambre muscular El espasmo o endurecimiento repentino de un músculo.

Muscle tone/tono muscular La tensión natural de los tejidos de los músculos.

Muscular endurance/resistencia muscular La habilidad de los músculos para hacer actividades físicas sin fatigarse.

Muscular strength/fuerza muscular La fuerza que un músculo puede ejercer.

N

Narcotics/narcóticos Drogas específicas que se obtiene de una planta llamada opio, que se usan para aliviar el dolor y que sólo se pueden obtener con receta médica.

Neglect/abandono La no-satisfacción de las necesidades físicas y emocionales de un niño.

Negotiation/negociación El uso de comunicación y compromiso para resolver un desacuerdo.

Nephron/nefrona La unidad de funcionamiento de los riñones.

Neurons/neuronas Células nerviosas.

Nicotine/nicotina Una droga adictiva que se encuentra en las hojas del tabaco.

Nicotine substitute/substituto de nicotina Un producto que libera una pequeña cantidad de nicotina en el cuerpo de una persona que está tratando de dejar de fumar.

Nicotine withdrawal/reacción al retiro de nicotina El proceso que ocurre en el cuerpo cuando la nicotina, una droga adictiva, deja de ser consumida.

Noise pollution/contaminación auditiva Un nivel de ruido no deseado que es lo suficientemente alto para dañar la audición de las personas.

Noncommunicable disease/enfermedad no contagiosa Una enfermedad que no se transmite entre las personas o por un vector, y que tampoco proviene del medio ambiente.

Nutrient-dense foods/alimentos fuertes en elementos nutritivos Alimentos que proporcionan una alta cantidad de elementos nutritivos comparados con las calorías contenidas.

Nutrients/nutrientes Substancias contenidas en los alimentos y que el cuerpo necesita para crecer, mantener un buen estado de salud y generar energía.

Nutrition/nutrición Proceso mediante el cual el cuerpo absorbe y usa los alimentos.

O

Obesity/obesidad El exceso de gordura en el cuerpo.

Occupational Safety and Health Administration (OSHA)/Agencia de Seguridad y Salud Ocupacional Agencia del gobierno federal que es responsable de promover el uso de condiciones de trabajo seguras y saludables.

Online shopping/compras en Internet Comprar bienes o servicios vía Internet.

Opportunistic infection/infección oportunista Una infección que ataca a un individuo con sistema inmunológico debilitado.

Ossification/osificación El proceso mediante el cual el hueso se forma, renueva y repara.

Osteoarthritis/osteoartritis Una enfermedad de las articulaciones en la cual el cartílago se deteriora.

Osteoporosis/osteoporosis Una condición que se caracteriza por la pérdida progresiva de los tejidos de los huesos.

Ova/óvulos Células reproductoras femeninas.

Ovaries/ovarios Las glándulas sexuales femeninas que contienen los óvulos y producen hormonas sexuales.

Overdose/sobredosis Una reacción fuerte, y algunas veces fatal, al consumo de una gran cantidad de drogas.

Overexertion/sobresfuerzo Cuando el cuerpo trabaja demasiado.

Overload/sobrecarga Hacer trabajar el cuerpo más fuerte de lo normal.

Over-the-counter (OTC) medicines/medicamento sin receta Medicamentos que pueden ser comprados sin una receta médica.

Overweight/sobrepeso Una condición en la cual una persona pesa más de lo apropiado para su estatura.

Vector/vector Un organismo, como por ejemplo un insecto, que lleva y transmite agentes patógenos a personas y otros animales.

Vegan/vegetariano estricto Vegetariano quien come exclusivamente alimentos de origen vegetal.

Vegetarian/vegetariano Una persona que come principalmente o solamente alimentos que provienen de las plantas.

Vehicular safety/seguridad vehicular Usar el sentido común, un buen criterio y obedecer las reglas de la carretera.

Veins/venas Vasos sanguíneos que llevan la sangre al corazón.

Venom/veneno Una substancia venenosa secretada por serpientes, arañas u otra criatura viviente.

Verbal abuse/abuso verbal Usar palabras para maltratar o dañar a otras personas.

Violence/violencia Cualquier amenaza o acto físico para dañar o maltratar a una persona o propiedad.

Virus/virus Material genético que invade las células vivas para reproducirse.

Vitamins/vitaminas Substancias que ayudan a regular las funciones vitales del cuerpo inclusive la digestión, la absorción de líquidos y el metabolismo de otros elementos nutritivos.

W

Warm-up/precalentamiento Una actividad que prepara los músculos para el ejercicio.

Warranty/garantía Una promesa escrita, en la cual una empresa o compañía se compromete a reparar un producto o devolver el dinero si éste no funciona bien.

Wastewater/agua de desperdicio Agua sucia que proviene de casas, comunidades, granjas, e industrias.

Weight cycling/ciclo de peso La situación repetida de subir y bajar de peso corporal.

Wellness/bienestar El estado de buena salud.

Western blot (WB)/Western Blot La prueba para confirmar el SIDA mas usada en los Estados Unidos.

Withdrawal/síndrome de abstinencia Es una condición en alguien con farmacodependencia que se presenta al quitársele el medicamento.

Workout/entrenamiento La parte de un programa de actividad física en la que los ejercicios se realizan al más alto nivel.

Note: Page numbers in italic type refer to a picture or feature only.